Making Health Systems Work in Low and Middle Income Countries

"There has been a critical need for a textbook on health systems in developing countries. Siddiqi et al. have filled this void very competently. The text touches all the important topics of this field. Making Health Systems Work in Low and Middle Income Countries *will become a cherished reference for both health systems scholars and practitioners.*"

Julio Frenk, MD, MPH, PhD
President and Professor of Public Health Sciences,
University of Miami

"This textbook presents theoretical concepts and the scientific grounds of interventions for strengthening health systems, fostered by implementation experiences from a wide range of countries. It offers an impressive blend for policy makers, public health practitioners and scholars in various settings, especially low- and middle-income countries, to progressively realize universal health coverage for the benefit of humankind."

Anutin Charnvirakul,
Deputy Prime Minister and Minister of Public Health, Thailand

"This textbook on health systems is a leading resource for public health professionals from low- and middle-income countries. It is an outstanding effort by authors from around the world and will go a long way in bridging the gap between the 'What' and 'How' of achieving universal health coverage and health security as the world confronts the COVID-19 pandemic."

Mamta Murthi, World Bank Vice President for Human Development

"A timely and much needed book that would guide policy and decision makers, and practitioners in low- and middle-income countries in their efforts to reconfigure health systems towards universal health coverage and to enhance health security based on lessons learned over decades from primary health care to current times of the COVID-19 pandemic. The book brings together conceptual clarity on health system thinking along with implementation imperatives in a seamless manner."

Dr. Ahmed Al Mandhari, WHO Regional Director for the Eastern Mediterranean

Making Health Systems Work in Low and Middle Income Countries

Textbook for Public Health Practitioners

Edited by

Sameen Siddiqi
Aga Khan University, Karachi

Awad Mataria
WHO Regional Office for the Eastern Mediterranean, Cairo

Katherine D. Rouleau
University of Toronto, Toronto

Meesha Iqbal
UTHealth School of Public Health, Houston

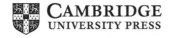

CAMBRIDGE
UNIVERSITY PRESS

University Printing House, Cambridge CB2 8BS, United Kingdom

One Liberty Plaza, 20th Floor, New York, NY 10006, USA

477 Williamstown Road, Port Melbourne, VIC 3207, Australia

314–321, 3rd Floor, Plot 3, Splendor Forum, Jasola District Centre, New Delhi – 110025, India

103 Penang Road, #05–06/07, Visioncrest Commercial, Singapore 238467

Cambridge University Press is part of the University of Cambridge.

It furthers the University's mission by disseminating knowledge in the pursuit of education, learning, and research at the highest international levels of excellence.

www.cambridge.org
Information on this title: www.cambridge.org/9781009211093
DOI: 10.1017/9781009211086

© Cambridge University Press 2023

First published 2023

A catalogue record for this publication is available from the British Library.

ISBN 978-1-009-21109-3 Paperback

....

In Memory of Nehdia Sameen
Nehdia embodied the sort of balance between head
and heart that is critical in any person of excellence.

Contents

Section 2 Transforming Health Systems: Confronting Challenges, Seizing Opportunities

About the Editors

Sameen Siddiqi is Professor and Chair, Department of Community Health Sciences, Aga Khan University, Pakistan. He has previously served as Director, Health System Development WHO Regional Office for the Eastern Mediterranean, where he spearheaded the work on universal health coverage, WHO's Representative to Lebanon and Iran, and worked for the World Bank in Pakistan.

Awad Mataria is the Director of Universal Health Coverage/Health Systems at the WHO Regional Office for the Eastern Mediterranean. He has more than 18 years' experience in health systems strengthening, health economics, and health financing.

Katherine D. Rouleau is a family physician at Unity Health, St. Michael's Hospital in Toronto, Canada, Vice-Chair of the Global Health & Social Accountability program, and Director of the WHO Collaborating Centre on Family Medicine and Primary Care at the Department of Family and Community Medicine, University of Toronto.

Meesha Iqbal is a PhD student at UTHealth School of Public Health, Houston, USA, with interest in health systems governance and strengthening, private sector engagement, and universal health coverage.

Contributors

Abdinasir Abubakar
Manager, Infectious Hazard Prevention and Preparedness, Regional Office for the Eastern Mediterranean, World Health Organization, Cairo, Egypt

Mohammad Abu-Zaineh
Doha Institute for Graduate Studies, Doha, Qatar Aix-Marseille University, CNRS, AMSE, Marseille, France

Francisca Ayodeji Akala
World Bank Practice Manager for the Africa Region, Health, Nutrition and Population Global Practice, Derwood, MD, USA

Shatha Albeik
Public Health Officer, UNRWA, Amman, Jordan

Luke N. Allen
Clinical Research Fellow, London School of Hygiene and Tropical Medicine, London, UK, Family Physician, Hedena Health, Oxford, UK

Olakunle Alonge
Associate Professor, Johns Hopkins Bloomberg School of Public Health, Baltimore, MD, USA

Ala Alwan
WHO Regional Director Emeritus Professor, Global Health, London School of Hygiene and Tropical Medicine, London, UK, Professor, University of Washington, Seattle, WA, USA

Sharon Ametepeh
Health Planner, Ghana Health Service, Accra, Ghana

Noor Ataya
Senior Researcher, Faculty of Health Sciences, American University of Beirut, Beirut, Lebanon

Koku Awoonor-Williams
Director, Policy Planning Monitoring and Evaluation, Ghana Health Service, Accra, Ghana

Eduardo Banzon
Principal Health Specialist, Southeast Asia Regional Department, Asian Development Bank, Manila, Philippines, Honorary Visiting Associate Professor, Saw Swee Hock School of Public Health, National University of Singapore, Singapore

Shannon Barkley
Technical Officer, Primary Health Care, World Health Organization, Geneva, Switzerland

Zulfiqar A. Bhutta
Founding Director, Institute of Global Health and Development, Aga Khan University, Karachi, Pakistan, Robert Harding Inaugural Chair in Global Child Health, Hospital for Sick Children, Toronto, Canada

Lynsey Brown
Research Fellow, Flinders University of South Australia, Adelaide, Australia

Kaara Calma
Lecturer, School of Nursing and Midwifery, Deakin University, Victoria, Australia

Cheryl Cashin
Managing Director, Results for
Development, New York, USA

Somtanuek Chotchoungchatchai
Researcher, International Health Policy
Program, Ministry of Public Health,
Bangkok, Thailand

Dheepa Rajan
Health Systems Adviser, World Health
Organization, Geneva, Switzerland

Daniel Cotlear
Health Financing Advisor, Consultant and
Volunteer, Former Manager of the World
Bank UHC Study Series

Suraya Dalil
Director, WHO Special Programme on
Primary Health Care, Geneva, Switzerland

Jai K. Das
Assistant Professor (Research),
Department of Paediatrics and Child
Health, Aga Khan University, Karachi,
Pakistan, Assistant Director, Institute of
Global Health and Development, Aga Khan
University, Karachi, Pakistan

Delanyo Dovlo
Chair, Faculty of Public Health, Ghana
College of Physicians and Surgeons, Accra,
Ghana

Fadi El-Jardali
Professor and Director K2P Center, Faculty
of Health Sciences, American University of
Beirut, Beirut, Lebanon

Sameh El-Saharty
Lead Health Policy Specialist, World Bank,
Washington, DC, USA

Samer Ellahham
Medical Director of Continuous
Improvement, Director of Accreditation in

the Quality and Safety Institute, and Senior
Cardiovascular Consultant, Heart and
Vascular Institute, Cleveland Clinic, Abu
Dhabi, United Arab Emirates

David B. Evans
Consultant, World Bank Global Solutions
Group Former Director, Health Systems
Governance and Financing, World Health
Organization, Geneva, Switzerland

Hamish Fraser
Associate Professor of Medical Science,
Brown University, Providence, RI, USA

F. Gulin Gedik
Coordinator, Health Workforce, World
Health Organization, Regional Office for
Eastern Mediterranean, Cairo, Egypt

Abdul Ghaffar
Executive Director, Alliance for Health
Policy and Systems Research, World Health
Organization, Geneva, Switzerland

Richard Gregory
Senior Policy Advisor, Global Health Security,
Foreign, Commonwealth and Development
Office (FCDO), London, UK

Ann-Lise Guisset
Hospital Integration Lead, Clinical Services
and Systems Unit, Integrated Health
Services Department, World Health
Organization, Geneva, Switzerland

Rana Hajjeh
Director of Program Management,
Regional Office for the Eastern
Mediterranean, World Health
Organization, Cairo, Egypt

Victoria Haldane
Research Assistant, Dalla Lana School of
Public Health, University of Toronto,
Toronto, Canada, PhD Candidate, Institute
of Health Policy, Management, and

Evaluation, University of Toronto, Toronto, Canada

Samar Hassan
Senior Accreditation Officer, Health Care Accreditation Council, Amman, Jordan

Arian Hatefi
Associate Professor, Department of Epidemiology and Biostatistics, University of California, San Francisco, CA, USA

Christopher H. Herbst
Senior Health Specialist, Health Nutrition and Population, Middle East and North Africa, World Bank, Riyadh, Saudi Arabia

Meesha Iqbal
PhD Student, UTHealth School of Public Health, Houston, TX, USA

Mohamed R. Ismail
Technical Officer, Essential Drugs and Other Medicines, WHO Country Office, Dhaka, Bangladesh

Samer Jabbour
Professor of Public Health Practice, Faculty of Health Sciences, American University of Beirut, Beirut, Lebanon

Dean T. Jamison
Edward A. Clarkson Professor, Emeritus, Institute of Global Health Sciences, University of California, San Francisco, CA, USA

Salma W. Jaouni
Chief Executive Officer, Health Care Accreditation Council, Amman, Jordan

Nirmal Kandel
Unit Head, Evidence and Analytics for Health Security, Department of Health Security Preparedness, WHO Emergency Program, World Health Organization, Geneva, Switzerland

Toby Kasper
Independent Consultant

Edward Kelley
Global Health Lead, ApiJect, Stamford, CT, USA

Christoph Kurowski
Health Financing Global Lead, World Bank, Washington, DC, USA

Aku Kwamie
Alliance for Health Policy and Systems Research, World Health Organization

Arush Lal
MPhil/PhD Candidate, Department of Health Policy, London School of Economics and Political Science, London, UK

John C. Langenbrunner
Former Lead Health Economist/Team Leader, World Bank, Washington, DC, USA

Mondher Letaief
Regional Adviser, World Health Organization, EMRO, Cairo, Egypt, Professor of Public Health, Monastir University, Monastir, Tunisia

Vivian Lin
Executive Associate Dean, Professor of Practice (Public Health), LKS Faculty of Medicine, University of Hong Kong, Hong Kong SAR

Jenny X. Liu
Associate Professor, Institute for Health and Aging, University of California, San Francisco, CA, USA

Beatriz Lobo-Valbuena
Intensive Care Unit, Hospital Universitario del Henares. Coslada (Madrid), Spain

Farihah Malik
PhD Candidate, University College London, London, UK

Aukje K. Mantel-Teeuwisse
Professor of Pharmacy and Global Health, Pharmaceutical Sciences, Utrecht University, Utrecht, the Netherlands

Alejandro Martin-Gorgojo
Dermatologist-Venereologist, STI/ Dermatology Department, Madrid City Council, Madrid, Spain

Jose M. Martin-Moreno
Professor, Department of Preventive Medicine and Public Health and INCLIVA Clinical Hospital, Valencia, Spain, Medical School, University of Valencia, Valencia, Spain

Fadi Martinos
Faculty of Health Sciences, American University of Beirut, Beirut, Lebanon

Awad Mataria
Director, UHC/Health Systems, Regional Office for the Eastern Mediterranean, World Health Organization, Cairo, Egypt

Sumit Mazumdar
Research Fellow, Centre of Health Economics, University of York, York, UK

Zafar Mirza
Professor of Health System & Population Health, School of Universal Health Coverage, Shifa Tameer-e-Millat University, Islamabad, Pakistan, Former State Minister of Health, Pakistan

Ali H. Mokdad
Chief Strategy Officer of Population Health, University of Washington, Seattle, WA, USA, Professor, Health Metrics Sciences, IHME, School of Medicine UW, Seattle, WA, USA

Dominic Montagu
Professor of Epidemiology and Biostatistics, University of California, San Francisco, CA, USA

Nyambura Muriuki
Faculty of Health Sciences, American University of Beirut, Beirut, Lebanon

Carine Naim
Faculty of Health Sciences, American University of Beirut, Beirut, Lebanon

Naima Nasir
Center for Tropical Medicine and Global Health, Nuffield Department of Medicine, University of Oxford, Oxford, UK

Lundi-Anne Omam
PhD Student, University of Cambridge, Cambridge, UK

Walaiporn Patcharanarumol
Director, International Health Policy Program, Ministry of Public Health, Bangkok, Thailand, Director, Global Health Division, Ministry of Public Health, Bangkok, Thailand

Enrico Pavignani
Independent Public Health Consultant

David H. Peters
Professor and Chair, Johns Hopkins Bloomberg School of Public Health, Baltimore, MD, USA

Mario Dal Poz
Professor, Institute of Social Medicine, University of the State of Rio de Janeiro, Rio de Janeiro, Brazil

Nattadhanai Rajatanavin
Research Fellow, International Health Policy Program, Ministry of Public Health, Bangkok, Thailand

Raffaella Ravinetto
Senior Researcher and Policy Advisor, Department of Public Health, Institute of Tropical Medicine, Antwerp, Belgium

Eric de Roodenbeke
International Health Policy and Services Expert

Katherine Rouleau
Vice Chair Global Health and Social
Accountability and Director, WHO
Collaborating Centre on Family Medicine
and Primary Care, Department of Family
and Community Medicine, University of
Toronto, Toronto, Canada

Senjuti Saha
Director and Scientist, Child Health
Research Foundation, Dhaka, Bangladesh

Haniye Sadat Sajadi
Associate Professor of Health Services
Management, University Research and
Development Center, Tehran University of
Medical Sciences, Tehran, Iran

Rehana A. Salam
Assistant Professor (Research), Department
of Paediatrics and Child Health, Aga Khan
University, Karachi, Pakistan

Hiba Sameen
Economic Advisor, Department of Health
and Social Care, London, UK

Malabika Sarker
Professor, BRAC James P Grant School of
Public Health, BRAC University, Dhaka,
Bangladesh

Martin Schmidt
Consultant, Health Financing Global
Solutions Group, World Bank, Geneva,
Switzerland

Akhiro Seita
Director, Health Programme, UNWRA,
Amman, Jordan

Sayed Masoom Shah
Head, Health Policy and Planning,
UNRWA, Amman, Jordan

Kabir Sheikh
Policy Advisor, Alliance for Health Policy
and Systems Research, World Health
Organization, Geneva, Switzerland

Sameen Siddiqi
Professor and Chair, Department
of Community Health Sciences,
Aga Khan University, Karachi, Pakistan

Agnès Soucat
Director, Health Systems Governance and
Financing, World Health Organization,
Geneva, Switzerland

Amirhossein Takian
Professor and Director, Department of
Global Health & Public Policy,
School of Public Health, Tehran University
of Medical Sciences (TUMS), Tehran, Iran.

Ajay Tandon
Lead Economist, Global Practice on Health,
Nutrition, and Population, World Bank,
Washington, DC, USA

Viroj Tangcharoensathien
Senior Advisor, International
Health Policy Program, Ministry
of Public Health, Bangkok, Thailand

Titiporn Tuangratananon
Researcher, International Health Policy
Program, Ministry of Public Health,
Bangkok, Thailand

A. Venkat Raman
Professor, Faculty of Management
Studies, University of Delhi, Delhi, India

Shaheda Viriyathorn
Researcher, International Health Policy
Program, Ministry of Public Health,
Bangkok, Thailand

Michelle Wen
Director, Strategy Planning Management,
Financial Services for the Poor, Bill and
Melinda Gates Foundation, Seattle,
WA, USA

Veronika J. Wirtz
Professor and Director of the World
Health Organization Collaborating Center

in Pharmaceutical Policy, Department of Global Health, Boston University School of Public Health, Boston, MA, USA

Jeremy C. Wyatt
Emeritus Professor of Digital Healthcare, University of Southampton, UK

Kenneth Yakubu
PhD Candidate and Research Assistant, George Institute for Global Health, Sydney, Australia

Shehla Zaidi
Professor, Department of Community Health Sciences, Aga Khan University, Karachi, Pakistan

Mariam Zameer
Senior Manager and Team Lead, Health Systems, Village Reach (Non Profit), Seattle, WA, USA

Preface

It is unimaginable in the twenty-first century to embark on a health reform, structural or programmatic, without considering *health systems* and adopting what is increasingly being recognized as *health systems thinking*. Health systems have come a long way over the last quarter-century and serve as a foundation for such reforms as universal health coverage (UHC), health security, and those associated with the achievement of health-related Sustainable Development Goals. Despite the undisputed role of health systems and a global consensus regarding their importance, many countries, especially the low- and middle-income countries (L&MICs) struggle to "make health systems work" so as to ultimately contribute to improved population health and social and economic development.

Health systems are diverse and complex, and a lot has been published in peer-reviewed articles, journals, and books on their organization, components, interactions, and goals. Although there is a growing consensus among thought leaders as to *what* needs to be done to strengthen health systems in L&MICs, *how* to do so often remains unclear. Recognizing that there is no one-size-fits-all approach to strengthening health systems, this book endeavors to narrow the gaps between *what* and *how*.

The work on the book formally commenced in March 2020, coinciding with the rapid global spread of COVID-19. As much as the pandemic affected our personal and professional lives over the last two years, it also inevitably influenced the contents of this book. As the world strives to adapt to this new phase of COVID-19, the pandemic has allowed us to rethink health systems and their role in health security and multisectorality. Not only is there a chapter in the book devoted to COVID-19 and health systems, but several others include examples illustrating how COVID-19 has impacted and shaped health systems as well as other health-related sectors.

As editors, we are honored and delighted by the diversity and richness of the authorship of this book. There are just about 100 authors altogether who have contributed to the book, coming from 36 countries across 7 regions of the world, stretching from Peru to Australia. Over 40% of the authors are women, with 30% of the chapters led by women authors. More importantly, this book is the result of an outstanding collaboration among authors from the South and the North. We take pride and are indebted to the authors, many of whom are global experts on different aspects of health systems, as well as young emerging thinkers poised to transform our world, for their time and commitment in contributing to different chapters of the book.

While the book is meant for L&MICs, its target readership is by no means restricted to public health practitioners from these countries. Never has health been so obviously a common global stake. This volume is therefore meant for academics at all levels – students, faculty, researchers, and analysts who are working in public health or health systems in L&MICs, as well as those committed to learning and working with L&MICs. Equally, the book is relevant for public health professionals working for civil society organizations, think tanks, and international development agencies. Importantly, we hope that this book would find space on the tabletops of policymakers and health system managers in the Ministries of Health, as well as other related government departments in L&MICs.

Unsurprisingly, the term *low- and middle-income countries* appears hundreds of times throughout the book, from its title page to the last chapter. For this term, and after due deliberation with the contributing authors, we have decided to use the acronym L&MICs. This clarification is important because the acronym LMIC has also been used in the published literature to denote low- and middle-income countries, while most development agencies classify countries by income status into four categories: low-income countries (LICs); lower middle-income countries (LMICs); upper middle-income countries (UMICs); and high-income countries (HICs). Since, this book is aimed at addressing the health system challenges of LICs, LMICs, and UMICs, the acronym of L&MICs has been carefully chosen to include the entire range of low- and middle-income countries, and not just the lower middle-income countries (i.e., LMICs). We hope that L&MICs will become widely accepted and used by all in the future as the standard acronym for low- and middle-income countries.

A bit about the book! It has 37 chapters, organized in two sections. Section 1 is titled "Analyzing Health Systems: Concepts, Components, Performance." It includes 14 chapters and deals with the conceptual, analytical, and foundational aspects of health systems. Its chapters underscore the unquestionable importance of health systems based on primary health care, and the concepts of UHC and health security as central to strengthening health systems. There are individual chapters devoted to each building block or components of the health system, as well as to the role of communities in building health systems. In addition, the last three chapters of the section are devoted to assessing health system performance and making evidence-informed decisions.

Section 2 of the book is titled "Transforming Health Systems: Confronting Challenges, Seizing Opportunities" and comprises 23 chapters. These chapters systematically analyze health system challenges and opportunities and offer evidence-informed solutions for each building block, as well as the health system as a whole within the context of L&MICs. Multiple chapters have been devoted to the topics of UHC, financing health care, and health care delivery in resource-constrained settings. Given their importance, there are dedicated chapters on the role of health systems in reaching health-related Sustainable Development Goals, tackling health determinants, strengthening essential public health functions, and engaging communities. Similarly, there are separate chapters on engaging in health care recovery during emergencies and health system response to the COVID-19 pandemic.

Additionally, the book recognizes that health systems and their reforms are not just a set of technical interventions. Structural health system reforms by their very nature are as political as they are technical, and when externally supported or financed they require a sound understanding of the development partners' and stakeholders' interests, which can sometimes be contentious. These issues have been dealt with in separate chapters on the role of development partners and political economy of health to enhance the understanding of health professionals in L&MICs while dealing with political aspects of health reforms. The book closes with the last chapter is largely based on the experiences of the editorial team on how to "make health systems work" in L&MICs.

The book received generous support and assistance from many quarters during every phase of its development. We are extremely grateful to Anna Whiting, the commissioning editor at Cambridge University Press (CUP), and her entire team for providing the necessary guidance at each step of the publication process. We are also indebted to the five anonymous external reviewers of the book proposal that was first submitted to CUP, which helped shape the final content of the book. Ahsana Nazish and Muneeb Ullah Siddiqui, from the Community Health Sciences Department, Aga Khan University were a great support in reviewing literature and formatting chapters to align it with the publication requirement at submission. Last but not least, as editors we are indebted to our respective institutions, especially the World Health Organization, Regional Office for the Eastern Mediterranean, the St-Michael's Hospital and the University of Toronto, and the Aga Khan University for giving us the independence and flexibility to work on the book over two years.

We believe that this is the first textbook of its kind. It has immensely benefited from the collective wisdom and vast experience of many authors from the North and the South for solving some of the most recalcitrant health system challenges and problems confronting health care providers, managers, and decision-makers in L&MICs. This is the first edition of the book, and we are confident that it will not be the last. We encourage comments and critique from readers to learn from the vast global expertise and to improve the future editions.

This book has been published in softcover and monocolor format, and there is also a digital version available online. The intent has been to keep the price affordable and have as wide a reach as possible, especially for readers in L&MICs as they embark on the journey to reform the health systems in their countries. We hope that you will find in this book the same richness of learning, the momentum for further exploration, and the invitation for ongoing transformation to "make health systems work" that we experienced in pulling it together!

Sameen Siddiqi
Awad Mataria
Katherine D. Rouleau
Meesha Iqbal

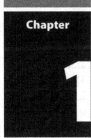

Introduction to Health Systems
Setting the Scene

Sameen Siddiqi, David H. Peters, and Awad Mataria

Key Messages

- Well-performing health systems are critical for pursuing universal health coverage (UHC) and for achieving health and health-related Sustainable Development Goals (SDGs). It is important to understand key concepts such as systems approach, analysis, and thinking before taking a deeper dive into health systems.

- Health systems can be described in broad or restricted terms. The most widely accepted definition of a health system includes all the institutions, actors, and activities whose *primary* purpose is to promote, restore, or maintain health.

- The WHO's health system framework comprising six building blocks and the "Control Knobs" framework with five knobs are the more widely used. Both frameworks have three main goals: improved health status, financial risk protection, and user satisfaction or responsiveness.

- Kielmann's and Roemer's health system models primarily assess health services, although the former defines health systems in broad terms by elaborating the interrelationship between the community, health care delivery, and the external environment.

- No single framework addresses all the aspects of a health system. It is more useful to know the strengths, limitations, purpose, and usefulness of each framework to help achieve a specific objective, such as for analysis, design of reforms, or evaluation of the health system.

1.1 Health Systems from Unfamiliarity to Inevitability

During the 1970s and 1980s, debates within countries and in many international forums indicated a growing dissatisfaction with the state of health and health services. This was accompanied by a broad recognition that the solution needed to include the development of comprehensive *national health systems* [1], a perspective further supported by the *Alma-Ata Declaration on Primary Health Care* as the leading strategy for *Health for All* [2]. While scholarship on strengthening health systems has continued since, questions of what is a health system, what are its boundaries and components, how it should be analyzed, and how to best improve health system performance remain contested and evolving matters. Early work on health systems was influenced by Milton Roemer's descriptive analysis of national health systems [3], while the subsequent reports by WHO in 2000 and 2007 [4, 5] helped solidify a shared understanding of health system functions, goals, and objectives. Given the social and dynamic nature of health systems, new perspectives keep emerging that

1

question the necessity to delineate fixed boundaries of a health system, as every country has a national health system that reflects its history, economic development, and social and political ideologies and decisions [6, 7].

Development partners – international organizations that provide financial, material, or technical assistance to other countries (often labeled "donors"; see Chapter 35) – have often imposed their agendas on low- and middle-income countries (L&MICs) by directing their assistance to prioritized government-run health programs that target specific diseases responsible for major burden in the country. When these efforts are organized, financed, delivered, and monitored around specific types of health conditions (e.g., HIV/AIDS, tuberculosis, malaria, family planning, reproductive health, childhood immunizations, neglected tropical diseases), they are frequently called "vertical" programs. They have typically focused on individual-level interventions, occasionally supplemented by health promotion activities delivered at the population level. Such programs often function in parallel with other programs that can duplicate or fragment efforts if they are not well integrated and coordinated in a health system. While some of these programs have been organized as time-limited campaigns (e.g., smallpox eradication), many are intended as long-term programs, and rely on centralized management and resources to meet their discrete objectives or continued implementation.

Whereas many L&MICs policymakers and development partners are increasingly giving importance to health system strengthening, the success of broader approaches has been mixed. Many governments have not fully appreciated the importance of well-performing health systems as a necessary platform for the successful implementation of public health programs, or to provide a basis for structural reforms. Nonetheless, the crucial importance of health systems has been underscored by recent commitments from most countries to pursue the ambitious target of UHC and for achieving the SDG of Health and Wellbeing (SDG 3) and other health-related SDGs. Yet, societies are increasingly confronted with health, social, and economic crises from disasters due to natural hazards, environmental degradation, pandemics and epidemics, or are constrained by limited access to critical health products that have large social externalities[1] beyond individual use (e.g., COVID-19 vaccines and diagnostics). It is thus apparent that national health systems and international organizations need to be strengthened and reorganized to tackle these neglected *common goods for health* that address population needs [8].

This chapter aims to clarify health system concepts and components, and models and frameworks that are frequently debated in high-level forums and can puzzle public health professionals and organizations working in L&MICs. The purpose is to help develop a systems thinking and approach among these professionals that leads to better-performing health systems and the attainment of UHC and health-related SDGs.

1.2 Health through a Systems Lens

Before taking a deeper dive, it is important to clarify a few fundamental concepts about health systems, recognizing that the terms may take on different meanings in different settings.

---

[1] Social externalities refer to the positive or negative consequences of an economic activity on social capital and on the quality of life of another [9].

A *system* is a set of interconnected parts or components that come together for a given purpose – the word is derived from the Greek term *sunistánai*, meaning "to cause to stand together." A *simple system* will have few parts and stable relationships between the parts, like a rope-and-pulley system to lift heavy objects. A *complicated system* is one that has many parts that interact with each other, may involve subsystems, and typically produces predictable results. Examples include the workings of a mechanical clock or cooking with a recipe. A *complex system* is one with many elements that interact with each other in different and changing ways, typically in a nonlinear fashion, and has multiple subsystems, abilities to adapt, self-organize, or learn, and is not predictable in detail. Because of the central role of adaptation or learning, complex systems are often called *complex adaptive systems*. The Earth's climate is a good example of a complex system, but there are many examples of complex systems in biology (e.g., the human body), ecology (e.g., a coral reef), computer sciences (e.g., artificial intelligence), and social sciences (e.g., cities) and economics (e.g., stock markets).

Since health systems are complex adaptive systems, it is helpful to understand how these systems behave, and their implications for enhancing performance (Figure 1.1). *Feedback loops* are common in health systems and occur when an outcome of a process is fed back into the same system. This can happen in a reinforcing way, such as the vicious cycle between malnutrition and infection, or in a balancing way, such as when there is an equilibrium in a resource-constrained health care system that continues to provide services for a better-off population while failing to reach the poor. *Path dependence* is another characteristic of health systems, where earlier decisions lead to irreversible pathways and different outcomes

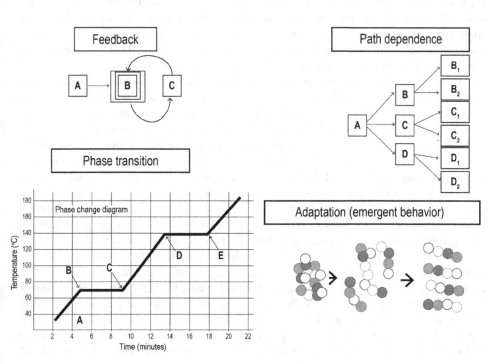

Figure 1.1 Behaviors of complex adaptive systems seen in health systems [10].

based on those initial decisions and choices made along the way. We see this commonly in the different types of technology standards found in different settings, such as why vehicles travel on different sides of the road in different countries. In a health system, it helps explain why complex programs such as health insurance schemes or decentralization of government health services cannot be expected to be simply copied from one place to another and achieve the same results. *Phase transitions* are also a common phenomenon and refer to events that suddenly hit a critical point at which radical changes occur, such as seen in the exponential growth of an epidemic, or in a sudden change in demand for health services. *Adaptation*, or emergent behavior, occurs in a health system with the creation of a new set of behaviors or organization that affects the whole system. This may occur suddenly, such as when community groups organize themselves to respond to a health crisis or when conditions lead to health workers going on strike. They can also happen more deliberately, such as when health teams decide to change how services are implemented through a quality improvement process or how services are provided, perhaps deciding to shift tasks.

Comprehending a system and its interconnected components, while necessary, is by no means sufficient to bring about an improvement in performance. Just as the understanding of systems, and in this context health systems, has evolved, so too have the approaches to examine, analyze, and think about health systems. While not distinctly separate, these approaches build on one another, and are briefly discussed here as systems approach, systems analysis, and systems thinking.

The *systems approach* takes into account the connections and interactions between the components of a system and follows a logical problem-solving method to develop a comprehensive solution to a problem that presents several dimensions. The systems approach follows three general steps: assessment of system vulnerability, implementation of countermeasures, and evaluation of effectiveness [11]. The simplest model of a systems approach is based on input, process, output, and feedback loops, and has been used to analyze systems in different disciplines by *system analysts*. In health, this approach has many uses, such as for assessment of the availability [12] and quality of services (Figure 1.2) [13].

Systems analysis is a problem-solving technique that decomposes or deconstructs a system into its component parts for the purpose of studying how well they work and interact to accomplish their purpose. From a health perspective, systems analysis should be: (1) *broad and inclusive*, considering all characteristics of health system inputs, processes, and performance outcomes; (2) *analytical*, based on how inputs, processes, and outputs interact with each other and with environmental factors to improve performance; (3) *relevant*, considering how reforms to key health system determinants could improve performance; and (4) *evidence-based*, utilizing and sharing information on health system experiences across countries [14]. It should consider politics, history, and institutional arrangements; propose causes of poor health system performance; suggest options and strategies to improve performance; and support implementation and evaluation.

Systems thinking is an analytic process intended to understand how things are connected to each other as part of a whole entity (i.e., a system) [15]. Whenever we talk about how one thing leads to another, or how an event will turn out, we are using a mental model to explain how things fit together. More formally, *systems thinking* involves using explicit rather than implicit models where assumptions are identified, data is used, and the processes can be repeated by others. Note that if the processes are followed in a methodical or orderly fashion, the approach can also be considered *systematic*. There are many different methods,

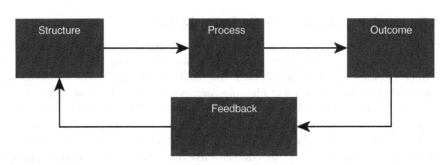

Figure 1.2 Systems approach for analyzing health services.

tools, and approaches that provide different types of insights that are gaining increasing currency in analyzing health systems [15].

Understanding health systems through systems thinking approaches and methods is particularly useful for addressing difficult questions, such as: How does this health program work? What are good entry points to intervene in a health policy and program? How can a health policy or program be scaled up, sustained, or made more effective in reaching marginalized populations? Systems thinking approaches are used to understand the dynamics of disease transmission, or to identify root causes of variations in health behaviors and services. They can also help to address the multisectoral factors that promote the spread of innovation in health, better understand how intended and unintended consequences come about, or facilitate decision-making.

A description of the many quantitative, qualitative, and mixed methods used in systems thinking is beyond the scope of this book, though there are some key systems thinking capabilities that are especially helpful to inform decisions and actions in health systems:

1. mapping actors or stakeholders in a health system (e.g., their interests, capabilities, influence, locations);
2. identifying the types of relationships between actors in a health system (e.g., accountabilities, authorities, financial, organizational, and social connections);
3. engaging with key actors in processes to identify and make a change (e.g., those involved in governance, organization, financing, delivery, and benefit of health policy and programs, with particular attention to ensure there is a "voice" for marginalized and vulnerable groups);
4. identifying and formulating questions that address critical problems;
5. using data and analysis to inform decisions around key questions;
6. focusing on achieving key health results, but looking for unintended consequences of actions that need to be addressed; and

7. learning from and encouraging adaptations that lead to improved performance of health systems.

Ultimately, a systems thinking approach places more attention on local context, incentives, and institutions, anticipates and addresses unintended consequences, and uses approaches to develop and implement policies and programs that engage key actors through the use of data for ongoing problem-solving and adaptation.

1.3 Health System and Its Boundaries

Health systems are not only complex and changing, but are also open systems in that they interact with their external environments and other social systems (e.g., through interactions with people, information, materials, etc.). This makes it challenging to define the boundaries of a health system. Any boundary of a health system is arbitrary and may be contested. The exact boundaries may depend on how stakeholders in a health system view their limits of interaction. This is because a population's health is not only affected by a package of promotive, preventive, curative, rehabilitative, and palliative health care services (typical parts of a health care system), but also by structural and social determinants like education and work opportunities, security, discrimination, clean water, adequate nutrition and housing, or income levels. Yet, as described below, these critical social and structural determinants of health (see Chapter 31) are often considered as outside the boundaries of the health system, even though they interact with it and impact its outcomes. One way this interaction occurs is by having components that fall within a health system, such as nutrition supplementation programs or health education programs that are primarily intended to improve people's health.

Health systems can be described broadly to include the structural and social determinants of health as integral to the system that "produces" good health. One simple health system model illustrates the interrelationship between *environmental ecology, community, and the health care delivery system* interposed between the two (Figure 1.3) [16]. The three components are highly interdependent. The *environmental ecology* – the sociocultural, demographic, economic, and political surroundings – largely determine the health problems and needs of the community, and exert a major influence on the nature, volume, and quality of health services. The *community* largely determines the sociocultural and political milieu and exerts considerable influence on the physical environment. The extent to which the community is involved with health-related matters influences health problems and needs. The range and quality of *health care delivery* thus are determined to a large extent by the environmental ecology and community.

Health systems can be defined more restrictively as a *combination of resources, organization, financing, and management that culminate in the delivery of health services to the population* [17]. This definition is framed around service delivery, which itself may be defined differently in different settings. Such systems frequently focus on individual clinical care and neglect population services (like health regulation, health promotion, or disease surveillance). This definition of a health system does not include all the factors that influence health outside health services, with the argument that if it did, the scope of health systems would be hopelessly broad since virtually all aspects of nature, society, and human relations influence health.

The *World Health Report 2000* defines a health system to include all the *institutions, actors, and activities whose primary purpose is to promote, restore, or maintain health* [4]. A *health activity* is defined as any effort, whether in personal health care, public health

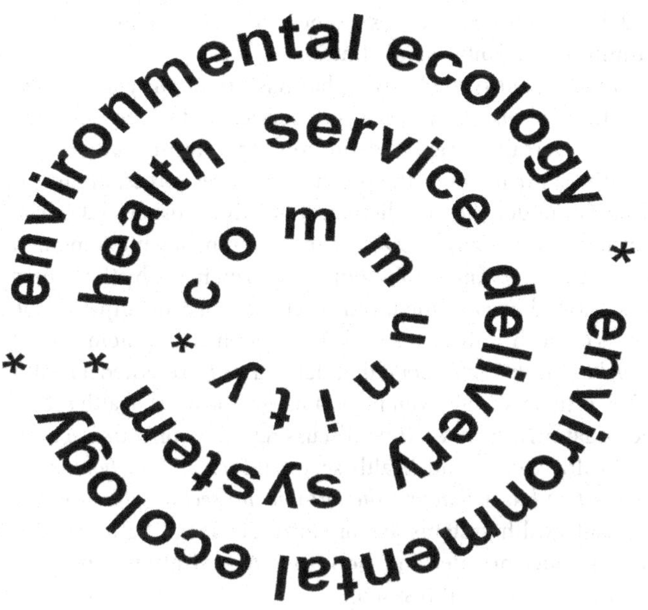

Figure 1.3 Broadly defined health system model [18].

services, or through intersectoral initiatives, whose *primary* purpose is to improve health. The emphasis on the word *primary* is important as it helps define the *boundaries* of the health system. While no one can question the influence of clean water on health, the primary purpose of water supply systems is not to improve health, hence using this definition would not include water supply as part of the health system. On the other hand, the primary purpose of monitoring water quality is better health, and so falls within the boundaries of the health system. Similarly, the primary purpose of women's education is not to improve health, but the primary purpose of health education of women is to improve health. By the same logic, the former would not be considered part of the health system, while the latter would. This distinction is not just theoretical, it has implications for organizing and financing health systems. For example, estimating health expenditures or developing budgets for health organizations depend on what is included in a health system.

This book has chosen to follow the *World Health Report 2000* definition of the health system, while recognizing that health systems are open systems, where structural and social factors interact with the health system and have undeniable importance in affecting people's health.

Whereas *health system* and *health care system* are terms that have been used interchangeably in the literature, a health care system refers to the more limited and specific part of the health system that is concerned with health services and their delivery, financing, organization, and governance. A *health care system* is a formal organizational structure for a defined population whose finance, management, scope, and content are defined by laws and regulations [19]. It may be organized around a set of health facilities providing services to specific populations in a given catchment area, or around an organized network of health care providers or funders of health care. A health care system provides services to people to contribute to their health in defined settings such as homes, educational institutions, workplaces, public places, communities, hospitals, and clinics.

Health system and *health sector* are two related terms that have frequently been used interchangeably. As stated above, the term *health system* is well defined and widely accepted globally [4]; there is, however, no universally accepted definition of the term *health sector*. According to one definition, health sector refers to the policies, laws, resources, organizations, programs, and services that fall under the jurisdiction of health ministries [20]. The term health sector gained prominence during the 1990s as many countries implemented various health sector reforms technically and financially supported principally by the World Bank. Health sector reform was defined as sustained, purposeful change to improve the efficiency, equity, and effectiveness of the health sector [21]. The term health system gained common usage following the *World Health Report 2000* that defined and presented a health system conceptual framework. Nevertheless, and given its past usage, the term health sector continues to be used in specific situations, such as while discussing inter- or multisectoral coordination in health, private health sector, and health sector reforms. *This book shall preferentially use the term health system but will accept the term health sector when used for specific situations.* It recognizes that health systems are organized at local, national, and international levels, and include public, private, and nonprofit organizations and civil society including communities as part of the health system.

1.4 Health System Models and Frameworks

Before plunging into a discussion on health systems, it is important to recognize the theoretical underpinnings of different models and frameworks and the purpose they serve. Theories, models, and frameworks in implementation science have three overarching aims – describing and/or guiding the process of translating research into practice (process models); understanding and/or explaining what influences outcomes (determinant frameworks, classic theories, implementation theories); and evaluating implementation (evaluation frameworks) [22].

A plethora of health system models and frameworks have been proposed that attempt to define, describe, and explain different aspects of health systems [23]. These are arguably helpful in identifying different approaches to health system strengthening, while also creating confusion as to which conceptual model to refer to for designing health system reform interventions. Hence it is important to select models and frameworks according to their proposed aim.

This chapter will discuss four health system frameworks and models: (1) WHO's health system framework; (2) the Control Knobs framework; (3) Kielmann's health system model; and (4) Roemer's health system model. The first two were developed at the beginning of this century, while the last two are from the 1980s and 1990s. Each model or framework was developed for a specific purpose and has its strengths and limitations. Although not discussed here, the Lancet Health Commission on High-Quality Health Systems has also proposed a framework, which is briefly discussed in Chapter 16 [24]. It is more important to be able to comprehend and critique each model than trying to look for the idyllic framework.

From an applied perspective, health system models and frameworks are illustrations of their various components or functions and serve several purposes. In line with Nilsen's proposition, each framework lends itself to *analysis* of the individual components, elements, or subsystems which helps to better understand the extent to which each fulfills its respective *function* within the whole system [22]. Second, frameworks help to assess how the various components *interact* with one another and contribute to achieving the desired objective. Third, they help to *identify* the less well-performing elements and point to remedial measures needed. Finally, frameworks aid in *monitoring* the performance of individual components or the whole system. Indeed, this is an iterative process and the basis for the planning, implementation, monitoring, and evaluation cycle.

1.4.1 The WHO Health System Framework

First presented in the *World Health Report 2000* [4], WHO's health system framework was subsequently modified in 2007 [5]. This framework is widely accepted and used by L&MICs and many have crafted their national health policies and strategies on what has come to be known as the "Building Blocks" framework. The WHO health systems framework has three components – the building blocks and overall goals or outcomes, with intermediary objectives related to service outcomes inserted between the two (Figure 1.4).

Building Blocks. What were previously known as "functions" are now called *"building blocks"* of the health system. The WHO framework has six building blocks: (1) service delivery; (2) health workforce; (3) health information system; (4) medical products, vaccines, and technologies; (5) financing; and (6) leadership and governance. Box 1.1 provides a brief description of each [5].

In this framework, *physical infrastructure* is implicitly considered as part of the building block of service delivery. It is an essential component, especially in low income and conflict settings, where poor physical infrastructure is a critical contributor to dysfunctional health systems. Infrastructure includes the buildings that house health facilities, utilities such as water and electricity, furniture and fixtures, equipment and supplies, transport including ambulances, and backup support for their maintenance and repair.

Overall Goals and Outcomes of the health system as per the framework include improved health, financial risk protection, responsiveness, and efficiency. These are also considered as *intrinsic goals* of the health system as these are valued as an end in themselves.

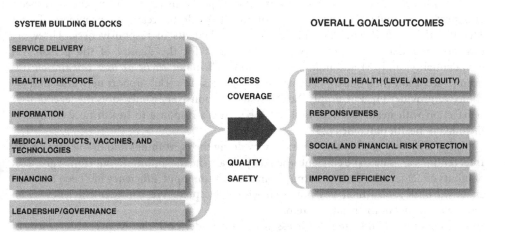

Figure 1.4 The WHO health system framework [5].

> **Box 1.1** The Building Blocks of the Health System [5]
>
> - **Service delivery** refers to delivering effective, safe, quality personal and nonpersonal health interventions to those who need them, when and where needed, with minimum waste of resources.
> - **A health workforce** is one that works in ways that are responsive, fair, and efficient to achieve the best health outcomes possible, and there are sufficient numbers and mix of staff, fairly distributed; they are competent and productive.
> - **A health information system** ensures the production, analysis, dissemination, and use of reliable and timely information on health determinants, health systems performance, and health status.
> - Access to essential **medical products, vaccines, and technologies** of assured quality, safety, efficacy, and cost-effectiveness, and their scientifically sound and efficient use, is crucial for a well-functioning health system.
> - **A health financing** system raises sufficient funds, in ways that these are adequately pooled, and ensures that people are protected from financial catastrophe or impoverishment while using services.
> - **Leadership and governance** involve ensuring strategic policy frameworks exist and are combined with effective oversight, appropriate regulations and incentives, attention to system design, participation, transparency, and accountability.

Health is the defining objective of the health system and can be measured in terms of longevity (life expectancy), mortality (death), morbidity (disease and risk of disease), disability (functionality), fertility (population parameters), or as summary measures of population health, such as health expectancies or health gaps (see Chapter 13).

Financial risk protection is protection against the risk each household faces due to the cost of health care. In a fairly financed system, financial risk is distributed according to the ability to pay rather than to the risk of illness (see Chapter 5). A health system where individuals or households are forced into poverty by paying for needed health care or forced to do without it because of the cost is considered unfair.

Responsiveness refers to how the health system performs relative to nonhealth aspects and meets the population's expectations of how it should be treated by providers of care. The *World Health Report 2000* identifies seven elements of responsiveness. Three are categorized under *respect for persons* – (1) respect for the dignity of the person, (2) confidentiality, and (3) autonomy – while four fall under *client or user orientation*: (4) prompt attention (timeliness), (5) amenities, (6) access to social support networks, and (7) choice of provider [4]. Put simply, health system responsiveness measures the level of user satisfaction with health services and not the system's response to health needs, which is included in health outcomes [25].

Efficiency refers to the value for money by doing the right things and doing them right. Interventions are said to be efficient when they obtain the maximum output from a given set of inputs or achieve the desired output from a minimum input. Efficiency has been included as an *intrinsic goal*, which has not been widely accepted. We consider efficiency as an *instrumental goal* of the health system.

In assessing health systems, it is essential to consider both the overall achievement of stated goals and their distribution across population groups. The latter raises the importance of *equity* as a goal, where equity refers to fairness in the use of limited resources and ensuring equal health outcomes. This particularly applies to the goals of health and responsiveness. By contrast, the goal of financial risk protection is assessed in terms of distribution only. The rationale is that while it is always desirable to achieve more health and more responsiveness, it is not intrinsically valuable to spend an ever-increasing amount of money on the health system. What matters is that available funds should be spent equitably, and the disparity in financial burden should be minimized across groups [26].

Service Outcomes such as access, coverage, quality, and safety are included in the framework as intermediate or instrumental objectives of the health system. The latter is considered as a means and not an end in themselves (Chapter 10). The concept of *equity* is well rooted in access and financial risk protection as it is an intrinsic as well as instrumental goal of the health system. *Intrinsic*, because in egalitarian societies equality is an end and is the value that underpins fair financing; *instrumental* because it underscores the distributional aspects of health services in terms of financial and physical access [26].

Critique. The Building Blocks framework is simple to comprehend and is useful for identifying inputs and key outcomes, and provides a good description of how health system components are functioning. The framework, however, is not strong on assessing how different components relate to one another and lacks the dynamism of informing what sort of interventions are needed to address gaps in the system. It neglects the role of key components like organizations, stakeholders, and processes. This framework also ignores the demand side of the equation or the importance of community engagement. Chapter 11 attempts to present a modified health system framework to address the latter shortcoming.

1.4.2 The "Control Knobs" Framework

Control knobs in this framework have been used metaphorically and derive their name from a system where the managers or operators adjust controls at different steps in the production process to efficiently deliver high-quality products [25]. The control knobs of a health system can be conceived and adjusted in a similar way by the government to enhance performance of the health system.

Before discussing the Control Knobs framework, it is important to understand that this framework was conceived in the 1990s to help countries think through and implement health sector reforms. Four fundamental forces were thought to drive the reform process in countries – rising costs of health care, rising expectations of the citizens who demand more from governments and health systems, limits on the capacity of the governments to pay the costs of health care, and the growing skepticism about conventional approaches to the health sector influenced by the market and diminishing trends toward social solidarity.

The health sector reform process brought together six important elements: (1) the policy cycle and its associated stages; (2) ethical theories underpinning the reform process; (3) systematic political analysis since politics matters at each step of the cycle; (4) a set of core health system performance goals and intermediate performance measures; (5) systematic approaches to health system diagnosis; and (6) a framework of five control knobs that provide options to reformers for influencing health system performance [25].

These five *control knobs* of the health system are thought to reflect the most important factors that determine and can be used deliberately to change health outcomes. These are *financing, payment, organization, regulation, and behavior* (Box 1.2, Figure 1.5). The framework also identifies three *performance goals* similar to the Building Blocks framework, namely health status, financial risk protection, and customer satisfaction.

The health status of the population is the first performance goal and is considered to be politically appropriate, philosophically relevant, and fulfills the test of causal dependence. In deciding which health problems should be given priority, a country may wish to pay special attention to the diseases that are causing the greatest harm.

Financial risk protection is about preventing impoverishment and its associated loss of opportunity as a result of seeking health care. Providing financial risk protection, however, does not allow the population to avoid all costs of health care.

Customer satisfaction is the degree to which citizens are satisfied with services provided by the health sector. This goal allows capturing various features of the health system, apart from its impact on health status.

The framework also proposes three *intermediate performance measures*. These measures are critical links in the chains that connect root causes to the ultimate performance goals. They include efficiency, access, and quality of health services (Chapter 10).

Critique. The Control Knobs framework is robust in helping to think through health system reforms from a policymaker's perspective. The control knobs offer intervention options for reforming the health system, and in this regard the model is dynamic. It does not highlight how different control knobs interact with one another, is primarily supply-driven, and does not emphasize the importance of community engagement. It also assumes that policy interventions have a linear effect while impacting services.

Box 1.2 The Five Control Knobs for Health Sector Reform [25]

- *Financing* refers to all mechanisms for raising money that pays for activities in the health sector. These mechanisms include taxes, insurance premiums, and direct payment by patients. The design of the institutions that collect money (e.g., social insurance funds) is also part of this control knob, along with allocation of resources to different priorities.
- *Payment* refers to the methods for transferring money to health care providers, such as fees, capitation, and budgets. These methods create incentives, which influence how providers behave. Money paid directly by patients is also part of this control knob.
- *Organization* refers to the mechanism to influence the mix of providers in health care markets, their roles and functions, and how the providers operate internally. These mechanisms include measures such as competition, decentralization, and managerial aspects related to providers.
- *Regulation* refers to coercion by the state to alter the behavior of actors in the health systems, including providers, insurance companies, patients, and the population. To be effective, regulation requires sound legislation and enforcement capacity.
- *Behavior* includes efforts to influence how individuals act in relation to health and health care, including both patients and providers. This includes, for example, mass media campaigns on smoking or influencing medical associations to improve physician practices.

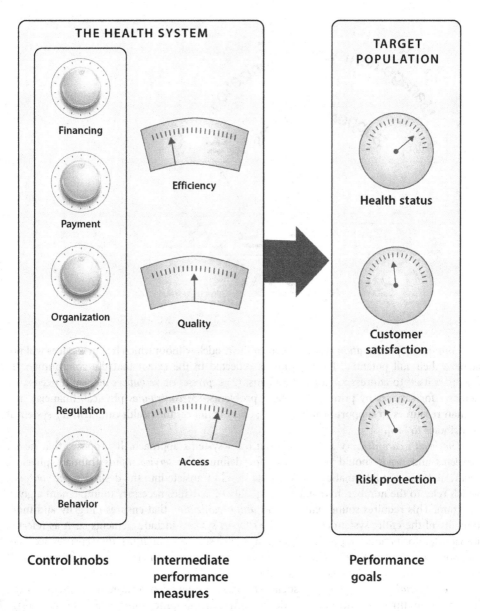

THE HEALTH SYSTEM

Financing

Efficiency

Payment

Organization

Quality

Regulation

Access

Behavior

TARGET
POPULATION

Health status

Customer
satisfaction

Risk protection

| Control knobs | Intermediate performance measures | Performance goals |

Figure 1.5 The five control knobs for health sector reform [25].

1.4.3 Kielmann's Health System Model

Kielmann's health system model was developed in the 1990s primarily to assess the district health system in low-resource settings [27]. Its premise is the *systems approach* that relies on the input, process, output, and feedback loop that lends itself to doing a systems analysis, followed by planning for strengthening the district health system [16]. The model defines health systems in broad terms by elaborating the interrelationship and interdependence between the community, health care delivery system, and external environment (Figure 1.6).

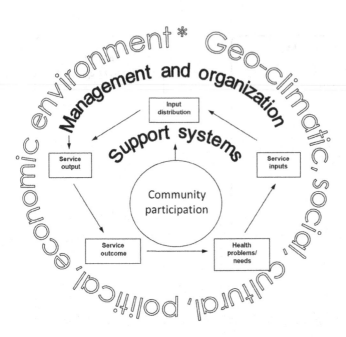

Figure 1.6 Kielmann's health system model.

Community participation is at the heart of the model, without which health services will not achieve their full potential. Participation is reflected in the extent that the community: (1) *organizes* itself to address its health problems; (2) *expresses* or *verbalizes* its health needs and demand for services by prioritizing health problems; (3) *contributes* physical, financial, and human resources to support health services; and (4) *utilizes* the health care delivery system it contributes to [16].

The health care delivery system is based on a systems approach. It proposes that *health problems* and *needs* should be the basis for defining the *service inputs* (human, physical, financial, time, and information). The inputs should translate into the desired *service outputs*, which refer to the number, frequency, and quality of activities necessary to implement a given program. This requires sound *management and organization* that ensures integrity and functionality of the entire system complex. The *support systems* include elements such as referral, transport, information, supply chain, and other subsystems. *Input distribution* ensures access to all population groups. *Service outcomes*, which include both the intermediate (or instrumental) and ultimate (or intrinsic) goals, are directly influenced by the service outputs.

The external environment, the social and environmental determinants, influences the health system through cultural, climatic, economic, geographic, political, and social settings the community lives in. These factors determine the nature of *health problems and needs*, as well as the ways the *community* deals with them. The external environment includes the influence of other sectors – such as education, agriculture, and industry – on health and health services. Such interactions may be mutually beneficial or occasionally detrimental when sectoral activities exert opposing effects.

Critique. Kielmann's model is analytically sound and has an assessment tool that goes with it [18]. The model is comprehensive in that it has three main components – the ecosystem, health care delivery, and the community – and the interactions among these are difficult to miss. The

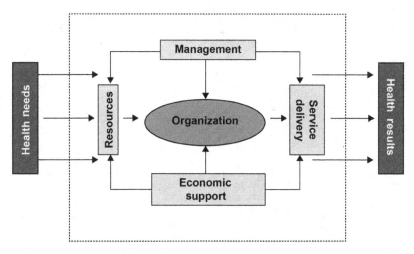

Figure 1.7 Roemer's health system model [3].

model is robust for assessing the delivery of health services especially at the district and subdistrict levels. The model, however, is not suitable for policy analysis or reforms and is rather deficient on issues of governance and financing of the health system.

1.4.4 Roemer's Health System Model

Roemer's health system model, one of the first to be presented, identifies five interconnected activities in a health system [3]. These are: (1) production of resources; (2) organization of programs; (3) economic support mechanisms; (4) management methods; and (5) delivery of services. The health problems and needs feed into the system on one side, and on the other side the health results are produced from the operations of the system. The principal interrelations of these components are shown in Figure 1.7.

The model recognizes that complete mapping of the relation among the five components would require a complex interplay of additional connections. Each component of the health system has numerous subcomponents, many of which can be regarded as subsystems. For example, the component of resources has a subcomponent on human resources, which can be further disaggregated into education of nurses, and the latter can in turn be narrowed down to nursing curriculum and so on. A detailed description of the model can be found elsewhere [3].

Critique. Roemer's model was the first health system model proposed and has historical significance. It follows a systems approach and is fairly descriptive of how health needs get translated into results through five interconnected elements. The model defines the health system rather narrowly without including the external environment and community engagement as essential components.

1.5 Comparative Analysis of the Health System Models and Frameworks

A comparison of characteristics of the health system models and frameworks is presented in Table 1.1. A composite and consensus-based model that includes all the aspects of

Table 1.1 Comparison of health system models

Health system characteristics		WHO health system Building Blocks framework	Control Knobs framework	Kielmann's health system model	Roemer's health system model
Overarching aim [21]	Process models	Yes	No	Yes	Yes
	Determinants frameworks	No	No	Yes	No
	Evaluation framework	Yes	Yes	Yes	Yes
Defining feature		Includes all components whose *primary purpose* is to improve health	*Reform* of the health sector or health policy reform	*Improvement of health services* leading to improved outcomes/results	
Community involvement		No	No	Integral to the model	No
External environmental factors		Not explicitly included		Integral to the model	Not included
Health system goals	Improved health	Yes (aggregate, distributional)	Yes	Yes	Yes
	Financial risk protection	Yes	Yes	No	No
	User satisfaction	Yes (responsiveness)	Yes (customer satisfaction)	Yes (partial through community participation)	No
Follows a systems approach		Partial	Partial	Yes	Yes
Follows a function-based approach		Six building blocks	Five control knobs	Management and organization and support systems	Five interconnected functions
Amenable to policy or systems analysis		Policy and systems analysis		Systems analysis with a focus on services	Systems analysis with a focus on services
Focus of reform		Policy and systems reform, noninterventional	Health policy reforms, with a framework for interventions	Strengthening district health systems	Strengthening health systems

a system has not yet been developed. It is more useful to know the strengths and limitations of each and to use these to achieve a specific objective. For instance, Kielmann's model would serve well if a district-level analysis were desired. Roemer's model would be useful for analyzing a hospital or network of health care institutions. The Control Knobs framework has its strength in health sector reform and for choosing the right mix of structural reform interventions. The WHO Building Blocks framework is best for a comprehensive analysis and for acquiring an overall understanding of the country's health system.

1.6 Conclusion: Thinking Systems, Programs, and Determinants Together

Most health workers in L&MICs are predominantly involved in the implementation of promotive, preventive, curative, rehabilitative, and palliative *programs* to reduce the burden of *problems* associated with reproductive health, communicable diseases, noncommunicable diseases, or injuries. Addressing the underlying *determinants*, especially proximal, is often an integral component of such *programs*. Many health professionals see health from an *illness or program* perspective. This chapter has approached health from a *systems* perspective, which is the aim of this book. Interventions, whether system-led, programmatic, or those targeted at tackling health determinants, are all part of the wider health system and offer the best opportunity for improving health outcomes when addressed together. This is well illustrated through reducing the burden of HIV/AIDS in a population (Figure 1.8). Such an approach advocates for more integrated and universally accessible health systems, building on the principles and a solid foundation of primary health care, which is the subject of the next chapter.

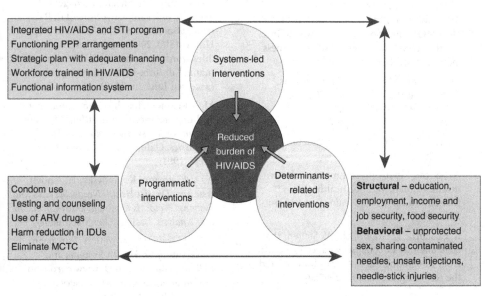

Figure 1.8 Broader systems thinking approach for reducing the burden of HIV/AIDS in a population. ARV, antiretroviral; IDU, intravenous drug users; MCTC, mother-to-child transmission; PPP, public–private partnership; STI, sexually transmitted infections.

References

1. B. M. Kleczkowiski, M. I. Roemer, A. Van der Werff. National health systems and their reorientation towards health for all: guidance for policy-making. 1984. https://apps.who.int/iris/bitstream/handle/10665/41638/WHO_PHP_77.pdf;jsessionid=06AFC07DC9A86CADF27B9D8FC439C712?sequence=1 (accessed June 17, 2021).

2. World Health Organization. Declaration of Alma-Ata International Conference on Primary Health Care, Alma-Ata, USSR, 6–12 September 1978. 1978. www.who.int/docs/default-source/documents/almaata-declaration-en.pdf?sfvrsn=7b3c2167_2 (accessed June 14, 2020).

3. M. I. Roemer. *National Health Systems of the World*. New York, Oxford University Press, 1991.

4. World Health Organization. *The World Health Report 2000: Health Systems – Improving Performance*. Geneva, World Health Organization, 2000. www.who.int/whr/2000/en/whr00_en.pdf?ua=1 (accessed June 14, 2020).

5. World Health Organization. *Everybody Business: Strengthening Health Systems to Improve Health Outcomes: WHO's Framework for Action*. Geneva, World Health Organization, 2007. www.who.int/healthsystems/strategy/everybodys_business.pdf (accessed December, 2020).

6. M. I. Roemer. National health systems throughout the world. *Annu Rev Publ Health* 1993; **14**: 335–353.

7. R. H. Elling. *Cross-National Study of Health Systems*. New Brunswick, Transaction Publishers, 1980.

8. A. Soucat. Financing common goods for health: fundamental for health, the foundation for UHC. *Health Syst Reform* 2019; **5**(4): 263–267.

9. R. Costanza, L. Graumlich, W. Steffen, et al., Sustainability or collapse: what can we learn from integrating the history of humans and the rest of nature? *Ambio* 2007; **36**(7):522–527.

10. L. Paina, D. H. Peters. Understanding pathways for scaling up health services

through the lens of complex adaptive systems. *Health Policy Plan* 2012; **27**(5): 365–373.

11. J. Scott, S. J. Leischow, B. Milstein. Systems thinking and modeling for public health practice. *Am J Public Health* 2014; **96**(3): 403–405.

12. V. A. Navarro. A systems approach to health planning. *Health Serv Res* 1969; **4**(2): 96.

13. A. Donabedian. Evaluating the quality of medical care. *Millbank Mem Fund Q* 1996; **44**(1): 166–203.

14. P. Berman, R. Bitran. The World Bank. Health systems analysis for better health system strengthening. HNP Discussion Paper 65927. 2011. https://openknowledge.worldbank.org/bitstream/handle/10986/13593/659270WP0Healt00Box365730B00PUBLIC0.pdf?sequence=1&isAllowed=y (accessed June 25, 2020).

15. D. H. Peters. The application of systems thinking in health: why use systems thinking? *Health Res Policy Syst* 2014; **12**: 51.

16. A. A. Kielmann, S. Siddiqi, R. K. N. Mwadime. District health planning manual toolkit for district health managers: Ministry of Health Government of Pakistan in collaboration with Multi-donor Support Unit (MSU). 2002. https://msph1blog.files.wordpress.com/2016/10/kielmann-manual-didtrict-health-planning.pdf (accessed June 30, 2020).

17. M. I. Roemer. Health system components and their relationships. *National Health Systems of the World. Volume I, The Countries*. Oxford, Oxford University Press, 1991.

18. A. A. Kielmann, K. Janovsky, H. Annett. *Assessing District Health Needs, Services and Systems: Protocols for Rapid Data Collection and Analysis*. Basingstoke, Macmillan, 1991.

19. World Health Organization, European Observatory on Health Systems and Policies. Glossary. 2009. www.euro.who.int/en/about-us/partners/observatory (accessed July 10, 2020).

20. Public Health Agency of Canada. Canada's response to WHO Commission on Social

Determinants of Health. 2007. www.phac-aspc.gc.ca/sdh-dss/glos-eng.php (accessed December, 2020).

21. P. Berman. Health sector reform: making health development sustainable. *Health Policy* 1995; **32**(1–3): 13–28.

22. P. Nilsen. Making sense of implementation theories, models and frameworks. *Implement Sci* 2015; **10**: 53.

23. G. Shakarishvili, R. Atun, P. Berman, et al. Converging health systems frameworks: towards a concepts-to-actions roadmap for health systems strengthening in low and middle income countries. *Glob Health Govern* 2010; **3**(2).

24. M. E. Kruk, A. D. Gage, C. Arsenault, et al. High-quality health systems in the Sustainable Development Goals era: time for a revolution. *Lancet Glob Health* 2018; **6** (11): e1196–e1252.

25. M. J. Robert, W. Hsiao, P. Berman, et al. *Getting Health Reform Right. A Guide to Improving Performance and Equity.* Oxford, Oxford University Press, 2008.

26. C. J. Murray, J. Frenk. A framework for assessing the performance of health systems. *Bull World Health Organ* 2000; **78** (6): 714–731.

27. A. A. Kielmann, D. Neuvians, W. Kipp, et al. Quality, quantity and utilization of basic health services. In R. Hoda, ed., *Evaluation of the Impact of Health Interventions.* Liege, Derouaux Ordina Editions, 1995.

Chapter

2

Health Systems Based on Primary Health Care

Shannon Barkley, Luke N. Allen, Lynsey Brown, Kaara Calma, Farihah Malik, Lundi-Anne Omam, Suraya Dalil, and Edward Kelley

---

Key Messages

- Primary health care (PHC) is a whole-of-society approach to health that aims to ensure the highest possible level of health and wellbeing and their equitable distribution by focusing on people's needs and preferences (as individuals, families, and communities) as early as possible along the continuum from health promotion and disease prevention to treatment, rehabilitation, and palliative care, and as close as feasible to people's everyday environments.
- The PHC approach comprises three key components:
  1. integrated health services with an emphasis on primary care and essential public health functions;
  2. multisectoral policy and action; and
  3. empowered people and communities.
- Implementation of PHC has been uneven in the decades since its inception, despite strong evidence indicating the effectiveness, equity, and efficiency of the approach.
- There is renewed commitment to PHC to achieve universal health coverage (UHC) and the health-related Sustainable Development Goals (SDGs).

2.1 Introduction

The WHO defines PHC as a

> whole-of-society approach to health that aims to ensure the highest possible level of health and wellbeing and their equitable distribution by focusing on people's needs and preferences (as individuals, families, and communities) as early as possible along the continuum from health promotion and disease prevention to treatment, rehabilitation and palliative care, and as close as feasible to people's everyday environment. [1]

Primary health care acknowledges health as a fundamental human right influenced by biological factors, social and environmental determinants, health services, and public health policies [2]. In 1978 the Declaration of Alma-Ata galvanized the PHC movement, calling on all governments, health care and development workers, and communities to protect and promote the health of all people [3, 4]. Growing health inequities within and between countries were significant drivers for this movement. In the following decades, PHC remained an important foundation for the achievement of equitable improvements in health outcomes globally and at country levels.

> **Box 2.1** Primary Health Care and Primary Care
>
> This chapter differentiates primary health care (an approach) from primary care (a process/platform for service delivery, first-level care) as follows:
>
> **Primary health care** is a whole-of-society approach to health that aims to maximize the level and distribution of health and wellbeing through three components: (1) primary care and essential public health functions as the core of integrated health services; (2) multisectoral policy and action; and (3) empowered people and communities.
>
> **Primary care** is a key process in the health system that supports first-contact, accessible, continued, comprehensive, and coordinated patient-focused care.
>
> This is aligned with WHO definitions.

Research has confirmed that countries with a strong foundation in PHC achieve better health outcomes more effectively, efficiently, and equitably [5, 6]. Additionally, a PHC approach is an essential foundation for risk management and effective response to health emergencies, and for building resilience within health systems [7]. Recognizing the importance of PHC to the achievement of UHC and the health-related SDGs, governments reaffirmed their commitment to PHC in the Declaration of Astana in 2018 [8]. This commitment was further supported by the adoption of the Operational Framework for Primary Health Care at the World Health Assembly in 2020 [9].

2.2 The Evolution of PHC

2.2.1 Before Alma-Ata

The concept of PHC emerged in the 1960s and 1970s and initially drew from the experience of China's "barefoot doctors": village health care workers with an emphasis on rural and preventive care [10]. The period of African decolonization contributed new approaches to health and development which focused on long-term socioeconomic changes rather than specific technical interventions. Criticism of the single disease-focused (vertical) approach to malaria eradication and WHO's evolving consideration of the delivery of so-called basic health services [11] further paved the way to contemporary views of PHC.

In his 1969 book *Health and the Developing World* [12], John Bryant highlighted the shortcomings of hospital-based health care systems in low-income countries, compounded by the lack of attention to preventive services. British historian Thomas McKeown argued that a population's health was less impacted by medical advances than by living standards and nutrition [13]. In 1975, Kenneth Newell's study of medical auxiliaries in low-resource settings demonstrated that interventions limited to the health sector did not result in improved health outcomes [14]. Meanwhile, Carl Taylor, founder of the Johns Hopkins Department of International Health, argued that India provided an instructive model for low- and middle-income countries (L&MICs) [15]. These and other authors contributed to changing the way health was understood [16, 17].

2.2.2 Alma-Ata

Leading up to the landmark 1978 conference, PHC had been identified by the WHO Executive Board as the mechanism of choice to attain the goal of *Health for All*. A background paper highlighted the responsibility of governments to improve their population's health outcomes, while adapting to local economic, political, and social realities, and maintaining a strong focus on community needs, expectations, and participation. In adopting the Declaration of Alma-Ata, governments committed to economic, social, and political actions to attain Health for All by the year 2000 [18]. Health was no longer understood as the mere result of interventions by health workers and health facilities, but also as an outcome of social determinants and social justice (Box 2.2).

2.2.3 The 1980s–2000s

While great strides in health and development were made in the intervening decades, health outcomes fell short of the Declaration's ambitious goal. Some researchers have argued that divergent interpretations of PHC undermined its implementation [19, 20]. Some global actors argued that PHC implementation should focus on narrow (presumably more effective) vertical programs, while others called for more holistic approaches that addressed socioeconomic and political determinants of health [21]. Debates also arose around financing, community

---

Box 2.2 Key Principles of PHC from the Alma-Ata Declaration [3]

- Driven by a country's sociocultural, economic, and political context and its communities
- Based on relevant research and public health experience
- Addresses the community's main health problems
- Includes the following (at a minimum):

  – education concerning prevailing health problems and the methods of preventing and controlling them
  – promotion of food supply and proper nutrition
  – adequate supply of safe water and basic sanitation
  – maternal and child health care, including family planning
  – immunization against major infectious diseases
  – prevention and control of locally endemic diseases
  – appropriate treatment of common diseases/injuries
  – provision of essential drugs

- Requires coordinated efforts across health and related sectors and aspects of national and community development
- Promotes maximum community and individual self-reliance and participation in development and implementation, making the most of available resources and building community capacity
- Sustained by integrated, functional, mutually supportive referral systems enabling comprehensive care provision and prioritization of those most in need
- Relies on health workers (including physicians, nurses, midwives, auxiliaries, community workers, and traditional practitioners) working together and responding to community needs

engagement, equity in service delivery, and the distinction between PHC and primary care. These debates were exacerbated by the global political context of the Cold War, where comprehensive PHC reforms were seen to be closely aligned with communist or socialist ideals. Criticisms of the ambitious goals and comprehensive approach of the Declaration of Alma-Ata culminated at a 1979 Rockefeller Foundation-sponsored conference that promoted a limited PHC approach to address children's health, focusing exclusively on growth monitoring, oral rehydration, breastfeeding, and immunization (GOBI). Female education, family spacing, and food supplementation were later added in recognition of the indissociable link between the health of children and their mothers (GOBI-FFF). This approach, termed *selective primary health care*, was believed to balance impact against achievability [21]. Selective PHC garnered large support from global health donors, lenders, and implementers, particularly from countries with market-based economic systems, further curtailing the support for comprehensive PHC.

In the 1980s and 1990s, the rapid development of health products and technology was accompanied by reduced state intervention, decentralization, and transformation from centrally planned to market-oriented economies. These were associated with emphasis on individual choice and responsibility, and growing expectations about health systems' performance. In addition, the responses to HIV, tuberculosis, and malaria and the creation of disease-specific global health initiatives furthered the debate on vertical vs. horizontal approaches to organization and funding of health systems. Ultimately, the Millennium Development Goals, launched in the year 2000, emphasized vertical health outcomes with minimal consideration of the interplay across sectors.

The *World Health Report 2008: Primary Health Care (Now More Than Ever)* [22] – renewed focus on PHC in the prevailing context of hospital-centrism, commercialization, and fragmentation. The report noted that PHC values of equity, people-centeredness, community participation, and self-determination embraced by the Declaration of Alma-Ata had become widely shared social expectations, despite evidence of persistent challenges in their implementation. The report centered on four reforms to strengthen PHC, aligned with four corresponding social values (Table 2.1). The report was followed by a conceptual pivot toward UHC, embodied in the *World Health Report 2010: Health Systems Financing: The Path to Universal Coverage* [23].

In 2015 the global community adopted the 2030 Agenda for Sustainable Development outlined through 17 SDGs. The concept of UHC, defined as "including financial risk protection, access to quality essential health care services and access to safe, effective, quality and affordable essential medicines and vaccines for all" [24] was included as one of nine health-specific targets, acknowledging its pivotal role in achieving sustainable social, economic, and environmental development.

Table 2.1 The social values that drive PHC and corresponding sets of reforms

Social values	Reforms
Health equity, solidarity, and social inclusion	Universal coverage
People-centered care	Service delivery
Health authorities that can be relied on	Leadership
Communities where health is promoted and protected	Public policy

Despite conceptual and implementation challenges, evidence generated over the decades following Alma-Ata consistently demonstrated that countries and regions embodying the principles of comprehensive PHC (e.g., Brazil, Costa Rica, Cuba, Iran, Kerala (India), Oman, Sri Lanka, and Thailand) saw significant improvements in population health outcomes, with reduced health inequalities at lower cost [25, 26].

2.2.4 Declaration of Astana

In October 2018, all WHO Member States renewed their commitment to PHC by welcoming the Declaration of Astana (Box 2.3). While the Declaration of Alma-Ata was primarily focused on establishing PHC in L&MICs, the political commitments in the Declaration of Astana emphasized the need for PHC in all countries to tackle contemporary challenges to attain UHC and the SDGs [27]. The Declaration called for action to meet the health needs of everyone across the life course through comprehensive preventive, promotive, curative, rehabilitative services and palliative care. It acknowledged the rising significance of noncommunicable diseases, including mental health issues, injuries, and the health impacts of climate change, and the important role of PHC in imparting resilience to health systems.

2.3 Primary Health Care Approach

Primary health care has been repeatedly reinterpreted and redefined since the Declaration of Alma-Ata, leading to fruitful progress in some cases but also confusion, unproductive debates, and unmet needs in others. In some contexts, it is understood as a set of priority health interventions for populations characterized by poverty and marginalization who

---

Box 2.3 The Declaration of Astana: Vision and Commitments

We envision:

Governments and societies that prioritize, promote and protect people's health and well-being, at both population and individual levels, through strong health systems.

Primary care and health services that are high quality, safe, comprehensive, integrated, accessible, available and affordable for everyone and everywhere, provided with compassion, respect and dignity by health professionals who are well-trained, skilled, motivated and committed.

Enabling and health-conducive environments in which individuals and communities are empowered and engaged in maintaining and enhancing their health and well-being.

Partners and stakeholders aligned in providing effective support to national health policies, strategies and plans.

We commit to:

• Make bold political choices for health across all sectors,
• Build sustainable primary health care,
• Empower individuals and communities, and
• Align stakeholder support to national policies, strategies and plans

otherwise have no access to essential health services. In other contexts, PHC refers to the provision of ambulatory or first-contact personal health care services (primary care) [27]. In some languages the terms for PHC and primary care are the same, adding to the confusion. Some understand PHC as intrinsically related to the economic, social, and political aspects of development, rather than narrowly focused on health or health service provision.

These understandings are a simplification of the broader definition from the Declaration of Alma-Ata, and their selective implementation risks missing out on the benefits of a comprehensive PHC approach which comprises three key components (Figure 2.1).

2.3.1 Primary Care and Essential Public Health Functions as the Core of Integrated Services

Integrated, People-Centered Health Services

People-centered services acknowledge that health care design and delivery should engage with and respond to the needs and preferences of people, at both the population and individual levels [28, 29].

Integrated health services target physical, psychological, and social wellbeing and involve collaboration across sites and services, both within and beyond the health sector (including social services, etc.). Integrated health services cross a care continuum spanning health promotion, disease prevention, diagnosis, treatment, management, rehabilitation, and palliative care, delivered at individual or population levels as appropriate.

Approaches to integration may link actors at the same level (horizontal integration). In the context of primary care, for example, this means the integration of general practice and allied health and community services, or the coordination of government agencies, private sector agencies, civil society organizations, and other partners providing health and social services (sectoral integration). Services may also be integrated across different levels (vertical integration), such as connecting primary, secondary, and tertiary providers (see

Figure 2.1 Components of PHC.

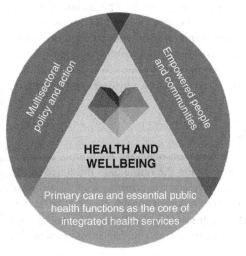

Chapter 27). Additionally, integration may link individual-level services with population-level interventions (see Chapters 24 and 32) [1, 30, 31].

The Role of Primary Care and Essential Public Health Functions

The WHO lists health protection, health promotion, disease prevention, surveillance and response, and disease preparedness as "essential public health functions" [1, 32]. In many health systems, some key population-based functions are delivered by the same primary care teams that are responsible for individual services (e.g., screening and reporting of sexually transmitted diseases, cancer screening, health education, health promotion, and behavior change communication). Efforts to optimally integrate primary care and public health are underway in a number of jurisdictions. Emerging models of care increasingly break down the distinction between family practice and public or population-based health [33].

In PHC-oriented health systems, primary care is the entry point to personal health services for most health problems, delivering accessible, first-contact, continuous, comprehensive, and integrated person-centered care. As an essential component of the health system, primary care also provides services with a family and community orientation, linking public health and personal health. Quality primary care has been linked to increased access to services, better problem recognition and diagnostic accuracy, a reduction in avoidable hospitalization, better health outcomes, attenuation of wealth-based disparities in mortality, and higher life expectancy [34, 35].

In areas with a comprehensive approach to care, combined with well-trained and resourced primary care practitioners including family medicine, primary care can manage the vast majority of health needs without referral, and coordinate secondary and tertiary referrals for the remaining fraction. This involves clear communication between specialists and patients, with family practice teams holding overall responsibility for care coordination.

Primary care services have evolved over time, and in response to the changing disease burden toward more chronic care needs, and have reoriented interventions toward proactive disease prevention, health promotion, chronic disease management, and surveillance and monitoring. Internationally, primary care services are delivered by a diverse range of providers and, increasingly, by multidisciplinary teams. The increased demand for these services has mobilized the expansion of the primary care workforce both in terms of numbers and skill mix. In many countries, primary care teams include physicians (increasingly trained as family physicians), nurse practitioners, practice nurses (registered or diploma-qualified), allied health professionals, community health workers, support workers, and health care assistants [36]. While precise workforce composition will vary across settings, evidence suggests that efforts to optimize comprehensiveness in scope, resilience, and adaptability over time are likely to lead to increased satisfaction by users and providers, and improved outcomes over time.

2.3.2 Multisectoral Policy and Action

Health and wellbeing result primarily from the interaction of social, economic, environmental, and commercial determinants, which are outside the immediate influence of the health sector. As described by the Commission on Social Determinants of Health and reaffirmed in the Rio Declaration on Social Determinants of Health in 2011 [37], it is impossible to achieve Health for All without coordinated and collaborative policy and action across sectors (multisectoral policy and action) to address the determinants of health and the structural underpinnings of social and health inequity that drive toward illness and hinder the attainment of health and wellbeing.

The policy choices and actions taken in other sectors often have significant impacts on health outcomes, even when not their primary intent. For example, policy and actions related to food and agriculture, tobacco control, pollution, and road safety can have a direct impact on health, while policies that enable the education of girls, create safe and equitable workplaces, and provide some degree of social protection can mitigate against social vulnerability and improve health. As important drivers of health and health equity [38], multisectoral policies and actions are essential components of PHC. A PHC approach further recognizes the roles that these other sectors – from finance and industry to education, agriculture, and urban planning – play in contributing to health outcomes.

In order to bring about health-enabling policy changes in other sectors, health ministries must play a robust stewardship role, generating and disseminating evidence on the health impacts of multisectoral determinants and advocating for policies and actions that will protect and promote health from all sectors. This has been demonstrated in areas such as tobacco control and road safety and is increasingly happening in efforts related to air pollution, urban planning, and transport. Notably, efforts to engage other sectors in policy and action to improve health may conflict with vested commercial interests, which can have significant influence over policymakers [8].

In turn, the health sector needs to consider policies and actions to address ways in which it impedes progress in other sectors and on other SDGs, such as the water and air pollution (carbon emission) caused by health facilities. The health sector should be aware of the ways it can impact broader determinants (e.g., climate change, equitable employment opportunities) and take steps to address them.

Key Lessons Learned from Successful Multisectoral Collaboration

Evidence from successful multisectoral action points to key considerations:

- the importance of fully understanding the political ecosystem, especially how history has shaped various stakeholders' interests;
- a common vision and agreed set of objectives with clear leadership roles for each sector and functions to be communicated across sectors;
- ensuring proper oversight and monitoring of implementation processes, aligning monitoring indicators from different sectors, and including shared datasets which better elucidate the contribution of each sector to improving health outcomes; and
- a culture of mutual learning among stakeholders guided by innovation, flexibility, and adaptability.

2.3.3 Empowered People and Communities

The Declaration of Astana highlights the importance of supporting individuals' and communities' participation in policy development and implementation [9]. In the PHC approach, health systems and other sectors contribute to empowerment through enhanced education and dissemination of health information [1]. Health literacy is fundamental to effective self-care and self-efficacy, the communication of health concerns, and the ability to access services; it is also key to prevention and chronic disease management. Health literacy and health empowerment are separate but mutually reinforcing concepts that are required to enable improvements in health-related behaviors and outcomes [39].

Health empowerment is a process that begins with an individual's participation and evolves to *ownership*, where the individual gains control over their own health [40]. Individuals and communities need to be active participants in the creation of health, and this can be achieved through three broad expressions of empowerment and hence participation: as advocates for multisectoral policies and actions for health; as co-developers of health and social services; and as self-carers and caregivers [1].

Advocates for Multisectoral Policies and Actions for Health

By being actively involved in policy development, planning, and implementation, individuals are better able to promote and protect their health, and policies are more likely to respond to their needs and preferences [1]. Advocacy has a vital role in health, as demonstrated in the context of HIV/AIDS, such as in persuading governments to adopt evidence-based approaches, getting new medications approved, decreasing the cost of medications, opposing stigma and discrimination, overturning punitive laws, and mobilizing leadership [41, 42]. For advocacy to be effective, meaningful community engagement in both economic and political arenas is important, and mechanisms that allow input from those particularly disadvantaged by determinants of health are necessary at all levels [1].

Co-developers of Health and Social Services

Beyond active participation on a policy level, the PHC approach promotes the engagement of people in the regulation and delivery of health services in their communities. This empowerment allows services to respond to community needs within the context of social and cultural circumstances of individuals, which consequently improves access to, and effectiveness and responsiveness of services [7, 29]. Furthermore, community engagement improves patient satisfaction and overall health outcomes, and has far-reaching effects on cost-effectiveness [43]. Some countries have demonstrated progressive success through effective community engagement. In Australia, Canada, and Chile, native communities have engaged in the planning and delivery of a range of social and health services that are culturally sensitive, of good quality, and integrated to address disparities in the burden of diseases [1, 5, 44–46]. Community empowerment within the PHC approach transcends consultation and moves toward active involvement of people in decision-making, ensuring diversity through legitimate and meaningful representation and engaging the most disadvantaged parts of the community [1].

Self-Care and Caregiving

The concept of empowerment within the PHC approach acknowledges that individuals experience the impact of their health and are the primary actors in the maintenance of their health on a day-to-day basis – and therefore have a central role in co-creating health, and also share a role in providing informal care to families and peers [1]. Technological advancements have better equipped individuals to manage their health. To date, progressive development of diagnostic tools shows potential to facilitate self-care more effectively. However, consideration is needed to ensure information collected is reliable, and that training is provided to individuals and caregivers to interpret information accurately.

In terms of health literacy, information has increasingly been made available on various platforms, many of which are web-based and easily accessed on mobile phones. However, individuals and communities must be equipped to use and analyze reliable information and technology when needed through the guidance of health experts, and in complex decision-making for themselves or their loved ones [1]. The PHC approach must consider the determinants of health that may affect individuals' ability to make evidence-informed decisions to participate in self-care, including low literacy, poverty, and social exclusion [47].

2.4 The Way Forward

While there has been renewed consensus on the potential of PHC to facilitate the achievement of UHC and other health-related SDGs, implementation of key transformations and reforms is needed. To support this, WHO and UNICEF have developed the *Operational Framework for PHC: Transforming Vision into Action* [9]. The Operational Framework proposes 14 levers (Figure 2.2) needed to translate the global commitments made in the Declaration of Astana into actions and interventions. Such actions and interventions can accelerate progress in strengthening PHC-oriented health systems and ultimately lead to a demonstrable improvement in Health for All without distinction of any kind.

Actions and interventions related to each lever are not intended to be carried out independently: they are intimately interrelated, and impact and enable each other. They need to be an integral part of the national health strategy, prioritized, optimized, and sequenced in ways that guarantee overall results along the three dimensions of UHC. For each lever, a nonexhaustive list of proposed actions and interventions at policy, operational, and implementation levels, and actions and interventions to be carried out by engaged people and communities, are included. It also includes tools and resources to facilitate actions related to each lever.

The Operational Framework is intended to be applicable to a wide range of countries and thus includes a range of actions, not all of which will be appropriate to or should be prioritized in every country. The levers should inform national planning processes and decision-making for PHC implementation. The levers and actions have different significance in countries with different levels of social or economic development, PHC orientation, and health status.

Countries will need to assess, prioritize, optimize, and sequence the levers and their respective actions, while considering specifically how the core strategic levers can facilitate planned actions in the operational levers. This process should occur in the context of an inclusive planning process with community participation that includes the most vulnerable, disadvantaged, and marginalized people. The selection and implementation of specific actions should be informed by a robust evidence base, both local (for example, the social, economic, and environmental situation and trends in the country, disease burden, and strengths and weaknesses of the health system) and global (for example, what has been shown to work/not work in improving PHC), as well as by the values and preferences of diverse stakeholders. In addition, actions should be refined according to progress and as further evidence and experience are generated to advance PHC.

The Operational Framework is further supported by two companion documents: (1) performance measurement and monitoring guidance and (2) a compendium of case studies demonstrating the implementation of levers and related outcomes.

As recognized in the commitments in the Declaration of Astana, the alignment of stakeholders' support to national policies, strategies, and plans under country leadership is

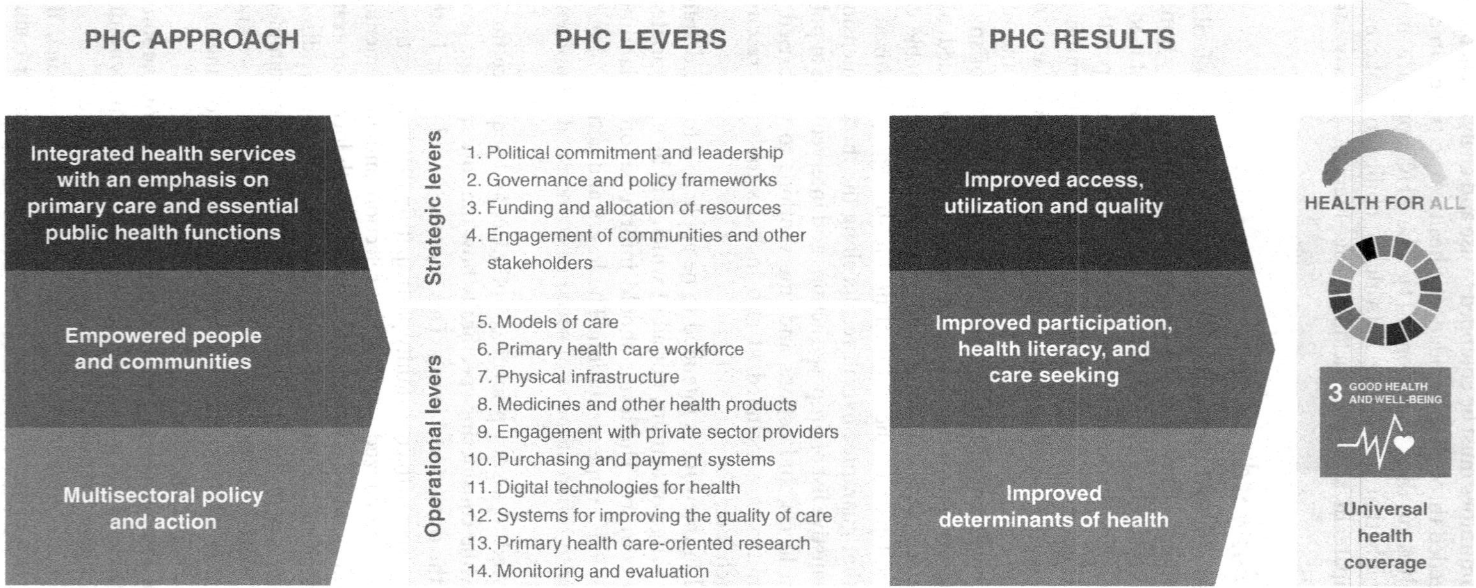

PHC APPROACH

Integrated health services with an emphasis on primary care and essential public health functions

Empowered people and communities

Multisectoral policy and action

PHC LEVERS

Strategic levers
1. Political commitment and leadership
2. Governance and policy frameworks
3. Funding and allocation of resources
4. Engagement of communities and other stakeholders

Operational levers
5. Models of care
6. Primary health care workforce
7. Physical infrastructure
8. Medicines and other health products
9. Engagement with private sector providers
10. Purchasing and payment systems
11. Digital technologies for health
12. Systems for improving the quality of care
13. Primary health care-oriented research
14. Monitoring and evaluation

PHC RESULTS

Improved access, utilization and quality

Improved participation, health literacy, and care seeking

Improved determinants of health

HEALTH FOR ALL

3 GOOD HEALTH AND WELL-BEING

Universal health coverage

Figure 2.2 PHC theory of change.

essential to make sustainable progress on PHC toward UHC. International partners – including organizations in the United Nations system, bilateral and multilateral donors, philanthropies, and partnerships – support PHC in countries in a variety of ways at national, regional, and global levels. This support includes provision of normative guidance, technical assistance, capacity-building, financing, cross-border learning, tool development, and knowledge generation and management. These efforts must be stepped up in order to accelerate progress.

References

1. World Health Organization, United Nations Children's Fund (UNICEF). A vision for primary health care in the 21st century: towards universal health coverage and the Sustainable Development Goals. 2018. https://apps.who.int/iris/handle/10665/328065 (accessed June 18, 2021).

2. D. Guzys. Community and primary health care. In D. Guzys, R. Brown, E. Halcomb, et al., eds., *An Introduction to Community and Primary Health Care*. Victoria, Cambridge University Press, 2017, pp. 3–19.

3. World Health Organization. Declaration of Alma-Ata. 1978. https://cdn.who.int/media/docs/default-source/documents/almaata-declaration-en.pdf?sfvrsn=7b3c2167_2 (accessed June 12, 2021).

4. H. Kluge, E. Kelley, P. N. Theodorakis, et al. Forty years on from Alma Ata: present and future of primary health care research. *Prim Health Care Res Dev* 2018; **19**(5): 421–423.

5. M. E. Kruk, D. Porignon, P. C. Rockers, et al. The contribution of primary care to health and health systems in low- and middle-income countries: a critical review of major primary care initiatives. *Soc Sci Med* 2010; **70**(6): 904–911.

6. B. Starfield, L. Shi, J. Macinko. Contribution of primary care to health systems and health. *Milbank Q* 2005; **83**(3): 457–502.

7. World Health Organization. Primary health care and health emergencies. 2018. www.who.int/docs/default-source/primary-health-care-conference/emergencies.pdf?sfvrsn=687d4d8d_2 (accessed June 11, 2021).

8. World Health Organization, United Nations Children's Fund (UNICEF). Declaration of Astana. 2018. www.who.int/docs/default-source/primary-health/declaration/gcphc-declaration.pdf (accessed June 15, 2021).

9. World Health Organization, United Nations Children's Fund (UNICEF). *Operational Framework for Primary Health Care: Transforming Vision into Action*. Geneva, World Health Organization, 2020. https://apps.who.int/iris/handle/10665/337641 (accessed June 16, 2021).

10. C. Weiyuan. China's village doctors take great strides. *Bull World Health Organ* 2008; **86**(12): 914–915.

11. J. H. Bryant, J. B. Richmond. Alma-Ata and primary health care: an evolving story. In H. K. Heggenhougen, ed., *International Encyclopedia of Public Health*. Boston, MA, Elsevier, 2008, pp. 152–174.

12. J. Bryant. *Health and the Developing World*. New York, Cornell University Press, 1969.

13. T. McKeown. *The Modern Rise of Population*. New York, Academic Press, 1976.

14. K. W. Newell. World Health Organization. Health by the people. 1975. https://apps.who.int/iris/handle/10665/40514 (accessed June 15, 2021).

15. C. E. Taylor, ed. *Doctors for the Villages: Study of Rural Internships in Seven Indian Medical Colleges*. New York, Asia Publishing House, 1976.

16. S. B. Rifkin. Alma Ata after 40 years: primary health care and health for all – from consensus to complexity. *BMJ Glob Health* 2018; **3**(Suppl. 3): e001188.

17. M. Cueto. The origins of primary health care and selective primary health care. *Am J Public Health* 2004; **94**(11): 1864–1874.

18. World Health Assembly. Thirty-second World Health Assembly, Geneva, 7–25 May 1979: resolutions and decisions. 1979. https://apps.who.int/iris/handle/10665/153658 (accessed June 18, 2021).

19. T. Hone, J. Macinko, C. Millett. Revisiting Alma-Ata: what is the role of primary health care in achieving the Sustainable Development Goals? *Lancet* 2018; **392** (10156): 1461–1472.

20. J. Rohde, S. Cousens, M. Chopra, et al. 30 years after Alma-Ata: has primary health care worked in countries? *Lancet* 2008; **372** (9642): 950–961.

21. J. A. Walsh, K. S. Warren. Selective primary health care: an interim strategy for disease control in developing countries. *N Engl J Med* 1979; **301**(18): 967–974.

22. World Health Organization. *The World Health Report 2008: Primary Health Care (Now More Than Ever)*. Geneva, World Health Organization, 2008. https://apps.who.int/iris/handle/10665/43949 (accessed June 18, 2021).

23. World Health Organization. *The World Health Report 2010: Health Systems Financing – the Path to Universal Coverage*. Geneva, World Health Organization, 2010. https://apps.who.int/iris/handle/10665/44371 (accessed June 19, 2021).

24. United Nations Department of Economic and Social Affairs. Goal 3: ensure healthy lives and promote well-being for all at all ages. 2016. https://sdgs.un.org/goals/goal3 (accessed June 18, 2021).

25. World Health Organization. Progressing primary health care: a series of country studies. 2018. www.who.int/publications-detail-redirect/WHO-HIS-SDS-2018.17 (accessed June 18, 2021).

26. A. Edelman, R. Marten, H. Montenegro, et al. Modified scoping review of the enablers and barriers to implementing primary health care in the COVID-19 context. *Health Policy Plan* 2021; **36**(7): 1163–1186.

27. K. T. Jungo, D. Anker, L. Wildisen. Astana declaration: a new pathway for primary health care. *Int J Public Health* 2020; **65**(5): 511–512.

28. P. P. Valentijn, S. M. Schepman, W. Opheij, et al. Understanding integrated care: a comprehensive conceptual framework based on the integrative functions of primary care. *Int J Integr Care* 2013; **13**: e010.

29. L. J. Brown, J. Oliver-Baxter. Six elements of integrated primary healthcare. *Aust Fam Physician* 2016; **45**(3): 149–152.

30. World Health Organization. Integrating health services. Brief, technical series on primary health care. 2018. https://apps.who.int/iris/bitstream/handle/10665/326459/WHO-HIS-SDS-2018.50-eng.pdf (accessed June 18, 2021).

31. World Health Organization. Framework on integrated, people-centred health services: report by the secretariat. 2016. https://apps.who.int/gb/ebwha/pdf_files/WHA69/A69_39-en.pdf (accessed June 13, 2021).

32. L. O. Ngo Bibaa. Primary health care beyond COVID-19: dealing with the pandemic in Cameroon. *BJGP Open* 2020; **4**(4): bjgpopen20X101113.

33. B. Rechel. How to enhance the integration of primary care and public health? Approaches, facilitating factors and policy options. 2020. https://apps.who.int/iris/handle/10665/330491 (accessed June 15, 2021).

34. S. Barkley, B. Starfield, L. Shi, et al. The contribution of primary care to health systems and health. In M. Kidd, I. Heath, A. Howe, eds., *Family Medicine: The Classic Papers*. Boca Raton, FL, CRC Press, 2016, pp. 191–239.

35. World Health Organization. Primary health care: closing the gap between public health and primary care through integration. 2018. www.who.int/publications/i/item/primary-health-care-closing-the-gap-between-public-health-and-primary-care-through-integration (accessed June 18, 2021).

36. T. Freund, C. Everett, P. Griffiths, et al. Skill mix, roles and remuneration in the primary care workforce: who are the healthcare professionals in the primary

care teams across the world? *Int J Nurs Stud* 2015; **52**(3): 727–743.

37. World Health Organization. Rio Political Declaration on Social Determinants of Health. 2011. https://cdn.who.int/media/docs/default-source/documents/social-determinants-of-health/rio_political_declaration.pdf?sfvrsn=6842ca9f_5&download=true (accessed June 18, 2021).

38. S. Salunke, D. K. Lal. Multisectoral approach for promoting public health. *Indian J Public Health* 2017; **61**(3): 163–168.

39. S. C. Lin, I. J. Chen, W. R. Yu, et al. Effect of a community-based participatory health literacy program on health behaviors and health empowerment among community-dwelling older adults: a quasi-experimental study. *Geriatr Nurs* 2019; **40**(5): 494–501.

40. World Health Organization. The Ottawa Charter for Health Promotion. 1986. www.euro.who.int/__data/assets/pdf_file/0004/129532/Ottawa_Charter.pdf (accessed June 18, 2021).

41. UNAIDS. Invest in advocacy: community participation in accountability is key to ending the AIDS epidemic. 2016. www.unaids.org/sites/default/files/media_asset/JC2830_invest_in_advocacy_en.pdf (accessed June 18, 2021).

42. K. Rohrer, D. Rajan, Population consultation on needs and expectations. In G. Schmets, D. Rajan, S. Kadandale, eds., *Strategizing National Health in the 21st Century: A Handbook.* Geneva, World Health Organization, 2016, pp. 35–102.

43. S. Cyril, B. J. Smith, A. Possamai-Inesedy, et al. Exploring the role of community engagement in improving the health of disadvantaged populations: a systematic review. *Glob Health Action* 2015; **8**: 29842.

44. C. Reeve, J. Humphreys, J. Wakerman, et al. Strengthening primary health care: achieving health gains in a remote region of Australia. *Med J Aust* 2015; **202**(9): 483–487.

45. J. Smylie, M. Kirst, K. McShane, et al. Understanding the role of Indigenous community participation in Indigenous prenatal and infant-toddler health promotion programs in Canada: a realist review. *Soc Sci Med* 2016; **150**: 128–143.

46. M. C. Torri. Multicultural social policy and community participation in health: new opportunities and challenges for indigenous people. *Int J Health Plann Manage* 2012; **27**(1): e18–e40.

47. M. V. Williams, D. W. Baker, E. G. Honig, et al. Inadequate literacy is a barrier to asthma knowledge and self-care. *Chest* 1998; **114**(4): 1008–1015.

Universal Health Coverage and Health System Strengthening

Awad Mataria, Sameh El-Saharty, Sumit Mazumdar, Abdinasir Abubakar, Rana Hajjeh, and Sameen Siddiqi

---

Key Messages

- Universal health coverage (UHC) means that all individuals and communities receive good-quality health services without suffering financial hardship. It is described using the three dimensions of service coverage, financial protection, and population coverage.
- UHC is measured by estimating the service coverage index, which tracks progress in 14 tracer indicators, and by the degree of financial protection that estimates the percentage of households that incur catastrophic health expenditures or are impoverished due to direct out-of-pocket payment for health.
- Major challenges to UHC include insufficient investment in health, fragmented and inefficient health systems, lack of private sector engagement, lack of focus on vulnerable groups, and disengaged communities.
- UHC and global health security aim to mitigate potential health and economic threats at individual and collective levels, respectively. Health system strengthening is the policy instrument that brings them together by elevating health and mitigating risk for all.

This chapter examines the evolution in global thinking on UHC and the role of health systems strengthening. It describes the path from primary health care to health systems and UHC. The concept of UHC is elucidated by explaining what it does and does not mean in practice, and by introducing its dimensions, intermediary objectives, and ultimate goals. The chapter also explains how progress toward UHC can be measured and hence monitored as per the Sustainable Development Agenda. It also summarizes the challenges that low- and middle-income countries (L&MICs) face to advance UHC. The chapter concludes by illustrating the interlinkage between UHC and health security based on lessons learned from the COVID-19 pandemic. The chapter does not, however, present the strategies and options for advancing UHC, which are addressed across the whole book especially in Chapters 15–17 and 24.

3.1 Introduction: From Primary Health Care to UHC

The 1978 Declaration of Alma-Ata set out primary health care (PHC) as the approach to achieve Health for All by the year 2000 (see Chapter 2). The Declaration launched a revolutionary movement to reform health systems with significant achievements, which eventually faltered, partly because it was so profoundly misunderstood [1] and partly because its approach was a mixture of idealistic values and operational recommendations on how health services need to be organized and delivered. In 2008, universal coverage was proposed as one of four reforms of PHC renewal [2], and in 2018 was further reiterated as the vehicle to implement the public health and primary care component of PHC under the Astana Declaration [3]. It was, however, the landmark *World Health Report 2010: Health Systems Financing The Path to Universal Coverage*[1] that put UHC on the global health agenda, arguing for a fundamental reorientation of the way health systems are financed to advance UHC [4].

The last decade witnessed increased interest in UHC as a key policy goal – both globally and in L&MICs. This was prompted by the endorsement of the 2030 Agenda for Sustainable Development, for which achieving UHC is one of the overarching health targets (target 3.8) [5]. Accordingly, many national health development plans and development partners' initiatives in several L&MICs adopted UHC as their primary goals, with a focus on strengthening health systems as the engine for its realization and for the achievement of Sustainable Development Goal 3 (SDG 3 – Good Health and Wellbeing) and other health-related targets.

The aspiration of UHC is not new. It goes back to 1883, when the German chancellor Otto von Bismarck put in place the foundation for a national system that insures workers and their families against medical costs [6]. It was also at the heart of the 1942 report by Sir William Beveridge, "Social Insurance and Allied Services" [7], which described the foundation of the modern welfare state in the UK. Concretely, UHC thinking started to take shape following the Second World War as a means to promote health and enhance social cohesion, and was accordingly articulated in the WHO constitution of 1948 [8]. While unarguably a noble goal, UHC still needs to be understood within the boundaries of its definition.

3.2 UHC Definition and Dimensions

3.2.1 UHC Definition

Universal health coverage means that *all* individuals and communities receive the health *services* they need – in *good quality* to be effective – and *without suffering financial hardship* [9]. Accordingly, UHC is commonly described using the three dimensions of service coverage, financial protection, and population coverage, presented in the form of a cube (Figure 3.1). The three dimensions are sometimes labeled as the depth, breadth, and direct costs of coverage. The depth of coverage refers to the extent of services covered by pooled funds, the breadth to the percentage of the population covered, and the direct costs to the financial risk associated with the current coverage arrangement.

Presenting the three UHC dimensions using a cube indicates the policy trade-offs between the three dimensions. Policymakers in all countries have to make the hard choice regarding which dimension to prioritize. In some instances, progress in one dimension might have drawbacks in one or the other two dimensions, provided all other variables remain the same. In addition, the higher the demand for health care, the more important the risk of financial hardship becomes, making the two dimensions of service coverage and financial protection interdependent. Finally, as individual and collective *needs* translate into *wants* and then *demands*, which economists qualify as *unlimited*, the coverage gaps will sustain and might increase, indicating the nonstatic nature of the UHC goal.

---

[1] The WHR 2010 focused on health systems financing and provided reform options for raising sufficient resources, managing them, and removing financial barriers to access needed care.

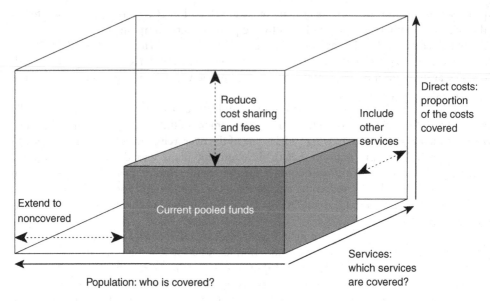

Reduce
cost sharing
and fees

Include
other
services

Direct costs:
proportion
of the costs
covered

Extend to
noncovered

Current pooled funds

Services:
which services
are covered?

Population: who is covered?

Figure 3.1 Three dimensions to consider when moving toward universal coverage [4].

3.2.2 The Three Dimensions of UHC

The *service coverage* dimension is the one that answers the question: *Which services are covered under the UHC goal?* Conceptually, this dimension refers to the ability of individuals and communities to access and use their *needed* health services. The latter includes the full spectrum of health programs and interventions, including promotion, prevention, treatment, rehabilitation, and palliative care [9]. The needs-based definition of UHC implies that individuals and communities should also have a say in what is to be covered. In practice, however, service coverage is reduced to a predefined set of core or essential health programs and interventions, often referred to as the *essential package of health services*, defined based on epidemiological, economic, and social criteria (see Chapter 15). It is worth noting that although this dimension assumes that what is provided is of "good" quality to be effective, some researchers prefer that quality be more emphasized and have called for "embedding quality within UHC"; others propose quality as a "fourth" dimension to the cube shown in Figure 3.1 [10–12].

The *financial protection* dimension answers the question: *What proportion of cost is covered by a prepayment arrangement?* Hence, it addresses what share of costs needs to be paid by individuals directly as they seek their needed health services – that is, paid out-of-pocket (OOP) (see Chapter 5). This dimension emphasizes the importance of prepayment using one of the available options – for instance, through tax-based revenue or health insurance (Chapter 17) to finance a core or an essential set of health services, interventions, and programs (Chapter 15). This dimension is critical because the higher the share of OOP payment in health spending, the higher the risk of financial hardship faced by individuals or households, with the associated economic and social consequences. L&MICs use alternative health financing arrangements to reduce the share of OOP and enhance the goal of financial protection (see Chapters 16 and 18) [13].

The *population coverage* dimension might be the one closest to how policymakers pursue UHC as it is the most politically visible to the public and hence is usually prioritized. It answers the question of *who is covered* and *who is not* by the other two dimensions of *service coverage* and *financial protection*. Assessing this dimension requires distinguishing between those who are *eligible* for coverage and those who are *entitled* to coverage under a certain coverage arrangement, and those who are *actually covered* [14]. While certain population groups might be eligible for coverage by certain prepayment arrangements, given prevailing constitutional rights or legal provisions, it should be noted that being eligible does not necessarily infer an entitlement to financial protection and service coverage; nor does it indicate being able to benefit from effective coverage with quality health services that contribute to improved health outcomes. Hence, moving toward UHC calls for continuously identifying and monitoring which population groups are eligible, entitled, and actually covered under the different prepayment arrangements and via a relevant "model of care" (see Chapter 10).

While describing UHC using its three dimensions is appealing to policymakers, formulating a vision, strategy, and roadmap to advance UHC requires a consideration of UHC's intermediate objectives and final goals. UHC's definition depicts three coverage goals: reducing the gap between utilization and needs, enhancing financial protection and improving quality; and three intermediate instrumental objectives: equity in resource distribution, efficiency, and transparency and accountability [15]. Considering UHC goals and objectives implies that all countries, at their various levels of socioeconomic development, will continually aspire toward UHC.

The above indicates that UHC has more facets than are captured by the "cube" model. It is therefore useful to look at UHC as both a journey and a destination, and as a policy goal that could be materialized only through overarching health system strengthening strategies. Figure 3.2 depicts how, using a health financing perspective, all health system functions

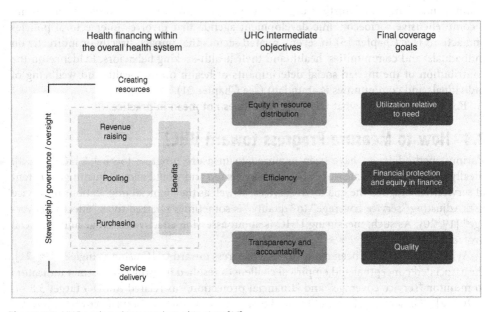

Figure 3.2 UHC goals and intermediate objectives [16].

Box 3.1 UHC: What It Means and What It Does Not Mean [9]

UHC means	UHC does not mean
1. It is a socioeconomic development agenda and hence is everybody's business.	1. It is only about the "cube" model and its three dimensions.
2. Access to predefined entitlements is guaranteed.	2. It provides service coverage and financial protection to the better-off first and the poor later.
3. Health services are covered through certain prepayment arrangements that ensure financial protection.	3. All health services are provided free for all at the point of delivery.
4. It includes individual and population-based services.	4. It is limited to a minimum package of health services.
5. All health system components are needed to ensure progress toward UHC.	5. It is only about health financing and insurance *per se.*
6. It is about progressive expansion of coverage of health services and financial protection.	6. It is about improved health without financial risk protection.
7. It is about social inclusion, equity, and development.	
8. Intersectoral interventions are important for UHC as they impact the health of individuals and populations.	

---

contribute to the progress in the final UHC coverage goals by acting on the three intermediate objectives. The same depiction could be provided for the other health system components. One could further argue that progress toward UHC would even require a comprehensive socioeconomic development agenda that involves intersectoral policies and actions (see Chapter 15) in several related sectors that impact directly or indirectly on individuals' and communities' health and their health-seeking behaviors. Evidence on the contribution of the myriad social determinants of health on the health and wellbeing of individuals and communities is abundant (see Chapter 31).

Box 3.1 summarizes what UHC does and does not mean in practice.

3.3 How to Measure Progress toward UHC?

Various methodologies have been explored to measure progress toward UHC [16–18]. Ideally, a reliable single measure of UHC is preferred and would allow adjusting the extent of services coverage to the quality of services, as well as the financial implications of service use. Adjusting "service coverage" to "quality" is sometimes referred to as "effective coverage" [19, 20]. As such, measuring UHC is about assessing effective coverage and financial protection together.

While attempts have been made to track progress toward UHC using a single index [21], the associated conceptual and empirical challenges resulted in using two distinct indicators to monitor "service coverage" and "financial protection," as related to SDG target 3.8 on UHC [7]. These are SDG indicator 3.8.1, which measures "service coverage" using a composite index, named the Service Coverage Index (SCI); and SDG indicator 3.8.2, which measures the level of financial hardship associated with service use. The two SDG indicators are described here.

3.3.1 Service Coverage Index

The SCI tracks progress in service coverage based on four categories of essential health services (Table 3.1), including: (1) reproductive, maternal, newborn, and child health; (2) infectious diseases; (3) noncommunicable diseases; and (4) service capacity and access. The index is calculated using a geometric mean of 14 tracer indicators and is reported using a unitless scale from 0 to 100. There is no well-defined benchmark, but nearing or reaching 100 on the index can be interpreted as meeting the SDG target. An algorithm is used to convert the SCI values into a percentage and number of people benefiting from service coverage, based on limited survey data and modeling, and is provided in Annex A1.3 of the *UHC Global Monitoring Report 2019* [22].

Although financing was not a focus of the analysis, the GBD 2019 Universal Health Coverage Collaborators estimated that US$1,398 per capita health spending is required as a threshold for achieving a UHC effective coverage score of 80 [17].

3.3.2 Financial Protection

Financial protection (FP) is assessed based on an estimation of the number or percentage of households or individuals who face financial hardship, either by incurring catastrophic health expenditure (CHE) or becoming impoverished due to direct OOP payment on health. CHE is measured using two thresholds: 10% and 25% of total household consumption or income. The lower CHE threshold (10%) obviously results in a larger number of people who face financial hardship due to direct OOP payments. Conversely, impoverishment due to direct OOP payment on health is measured – *mainly* – using two poverty lines: US$3.20 and US$1.90 per person per day in 2011 purchasing power parity (PPP) terms (see Table 3.2).[2]

The *UHC Global Monitoring Report* published in 2019 [22] reported that SCI has increased, globally, from 45 out of 100 in 2000 to 66 out of 100 in 2017, while FP has been going in the opposite direction: the proportion of the population with OOP spending exceeding 10% of their household budget rose from 9.4% to 12.7% between 2000 and 2015, and at the same time the proportion of the population with OOP spending exceeding 25% rose from 1.7% to 2.9%. The gains in service coverage have come at a major cost to individuals and their families. The latest 2021 *UHC Global Monitoring Report* [23] estimated that *globally* almost one billion individuals experienced catastrophic OOP expenditures in 2017, with more than one-quarter of that number spending more than 25% of their budgets (290 million) as OOP payment.

Figure 3.3 plots the incidence of CHE and SCI for most countries [22]. Countries tend to fall into four quadrants: *Quadrant I* countries are those with high SCI and low CHE; *Quadrant II* includes countries with low SCI and low CHE; *Quadrant III* presents countries with high SCI and high CHE; and *Quadrant IV* identifies countries with low SCI and high CHE. As expected, high and upper middle-income countries scored the highest in SCI

---

[2] A method of currency valuation based on the premise that two identical goods in different countries should eventually cost the same. PPP allows economists and investors to determine the exchange rate between currencies for the trade to be on par with the purchasing power of the countries' currencies.

Table 3.1 Calculating the UHC SCI using hypothetical country data

Tracer indicators for UHC SCI		Country example
Reproductive, maternal, newborn, and child health		
1. Family planning	Demand satisfied with modern method among women 15–49 years who are married or in a union (%)	35
2. Pregnancy and delivery care	Antenatal care, four or more visits (ANC4) (%)	65
3. Child immunization	One-year-old children who have received three doses of DTP3 (%)	70
4. Child treatment	Care-seeking behavior for children with suspected pneumonia (%)	60
+RMNCH = (FP • ANC • DTP3 • Pneumonia)$^{1/4}$		**56**
Infectious diseases		
1. Tuberculosis treatment	TB effective treatment coverage (%)	65
2. HIV treatment	People living with HIV receiving antiretroviral therapy (%)	10
3. Malaria prevention	Population at risk sleeping under insecticide-treated bed nets (%)[a]	–
4. Water and sanitation	Households with access to at least basic sanitation (%)	80
Infectious = (ART • TB • WASH • ITN)$^{1/4}$ OR Infectious = (ART • TB • WASH)$^{1/3}$ if low risk of malaria		**36**
Noncommunicable diseases		
1. Prevention of cardiovascular disease	Prevalence of normal blood pressure, regardless of treatment status (%)	80
2. Management of diabetes	Mean fasting plasma glucose (FPG) (mmol/L)	80
3. Cancer detection and treatment	Cervical cancer screening among women aged 30–49 years (%)[b]	–
4. Tobacco control	Adults aged ≥15 years not smoking tobacco in last 30 days (%)	80
NCD = (BP • FPG • Tobacco)$^{1/3}$		**77**
Service capacity and access		
1. Hospital access	Hospital beds per capita (w/ threshold)	39
2. Health worker density	Health professionals per capita (w/ threshold): physicians, psychiatrists, and surgeons	25
3. Access to essential medicines	Proportion of health facilities with WHO-recommended core list of essential medicines available[b]	–
4. Health security	International Health Regulations core capacity index	50
Capacity = (Hospital • HWD • IHR)$^{1/3}$		**35**
UHC SCI = (RMNCH • Infectious • NCD • Capacity)$^{1/4}$		**48**

[a] Malaria low-risk country; [b] Insufficient data currently available.
Adapted from [19]; for precise methods of calculation please refer to Annex 1.2.1 of [19].

Table 3.2 Tracer indicators for measuring FP [22]

Indicator	Explanation of indicator	Thresholds used to measure FP
Incidence of CHE due to OOP health spending (%)	When OOP spending on health care (without reimbursement by a third party) exceeds a household's ability to pay	Catastrophic spending at 10% household total consumption or income Catastrophic spending at 25% household total consumption or income
Incidence of impoverishment due to OOP health spending (%)	When household health care expenses are high enough that its spending on nonmedical budget items such as food, shelter, and clothing are reduced to below the level indicated by the poverty line	Poverty line: at 2011 PPP US$1.90 per day Poverty line: at 2011 PPP US$3.20 per day

(Quadrants I and II). It is worth noting that all low and the majority of lower middle-income countries fall in Quadrants III and IV, indicating low service coverage and a wide spectrum of FP.

The greatest progress in SCI in recent years has been reported in low-income countries – except for countries affected by conflict, which were generally lagging far behind – and has mainly been due to implementation of interventions against infectious diseases. Middle-income countries continue to have the largest population deprived of essential health services, and constitute 75% of the world's population. Table 3.3 presents the evolution in service coverage and FP in selected L&MICs based on the latest available data.

3.3.3 Population Coverage

Policymakers in L&MICs have constantly raised the question of *who is covered* and *who is not covered* as they work to develop policies and strategies to expand service coverage with FP. Accordingly, clustering the population into easily distinguishable categories allows countries to achieve big strides on the path to UHC by identifying and targeting those who remain outside the coverage remit. A common categorization is the one based on the economic activity of individuals – for example, formal sector vs. informal sector workers. The formal sector could be further distinguished into public and private formal sector. The informal sector could also be divided into poor and nonpoor informal sectors. Examples of each subgroup are included in Box 3.2. Using such categorization allows having an overall estimate of the uncovered population at the national level and identifying strategies to target them.

3.4 Challenges to Accelerated Progress toward UHC in L&MICs

As countries progress toward UHC, they face many challenges, starting with the inadequate understanding of what UHC is about [24], including the assumption by some that it would entail that all services would be made available *free* for everyone. This is intimidating for policymakers pursuing UHC. Once these misconceptions are clarified, additional challenges need to be addressed, some of which are considered here.

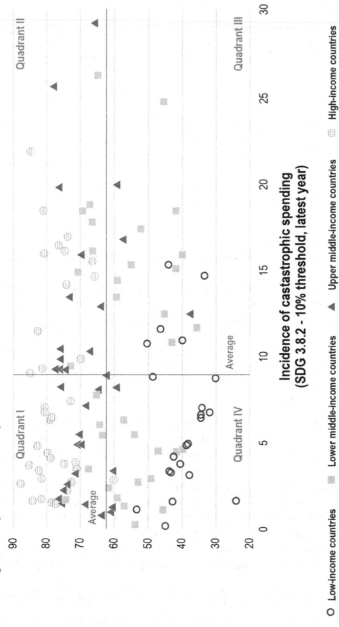

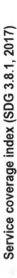

Figure 3.3 UHC status as related to SDG indicators 3.8.1 and 3.8.2 [22].

Table 3.3 Service coverage and FP in selected L&MICs

Country	UHC SCI (out of 100), 2019 (SDG 3.8.1)	Incidence of catastrophic expenditure (%) at 10% of household total consumption or income – most recent available estimate (year) (SDG 3.8.2)	Impoverishment due to OOP health expenditures (US$3.20 per day in 2011 PPP), most recent available estimate (year) [22]
Afghanistan	37	14.6 (2013)*	2.97 (2013)
Bangladesh	51	24.4 (2016)	6.18 (2016)
Brazil	75	11.8 (2017)	2.01 (2008)
Burkina Faso	43	3.1 (2014)	1.04 (2014)
China	≥80	24.0 (2016)	NA
Colombia	78	8.2 (2016)	0.71 (2016)
Cuba	80	NA	NA
Egypt	70	31.1 (2017)	1.07 (2012)
Georgia	65	31.2 (2017)	5.33 (2013)
India	61	17.3 (2017)	4.61 (2011)
Indonesia	59	4.5 (2017)	0.84 (2015)
Iran	77	15.3 (2019)	0.17 (2013)
Kenya	56	5.1 (2015)	1.32 (2015)
Kyrgyzstan	70	3.5 (2016)	1.01 (2016)
Lebanon	72	26.6 (2012)	0.03 (1999)
Pakistan	45	4.5 (2015)*	2.92 (2015)
Qatar	74	NA	NA
South Africa	67	1.0 (2014)	0.61 (2010)

[a] Data from [23], except for the last column, which is from [22].
Reproduced with permission from [22, 23].

3.4.1 Insufficient Investment in Health

While almost 85% of the world population lives in L&MICs [25], the latest global estimates show that in 2019 L&MICs spent only 21% of the US$8.5 trillion spent on health globally (9.8% of global GDP) [26]. In addition, only 21% of what is spent on health in low-income countries comes from government sources (34–38% in middle-income countries) [26]. As a result, the average share of direct OOP spending on health in L&MICs ranges between 34% and 40% in middle-income countries and reaches 44% in low-income countries – compared to around 21% in high-income countries [26].

Box 3.2 UHC from a Population Coverage Perspective

Formal sector	Informal sector
A. Formal public	**A. Informal nonpoor**
1. Public sector employees	1. Self-employed
2. Armed forces	2. Landowners/farmers
3. Parastatal organizations	3. Shopkeepers
B. Formal private	**B. Informal poor**
1. Private enterprises	1. Unemployed
2. Corporations	2. Individuals under the poverty line
3. Nongovernmental organizations (NGOs)	3. Refugees/internally displaced persons (IDPs)
	4. Resident noncitizens

There is no "magic" number to indicate how much should be spent on health as a percentage of GDP or government budget [27]. Nevertheless, countries' experiences show that progress toward UHC requires investing more *public* money for health. Increasing public investment on health depends on two factors: (1) fiscal space and (2) prioritization. While "fiscal space" defines the overall resources available to the government to invest in all sectors, "prioritization" indicates the level of importance given to health in the government budget – for more discussion refer to Chapter 5. An analysis conducted for the countries of the Eastern Mediterranean Region of WHO (EMR) found that the low investment in health is less due to fiscal space constraints and is more a result of the low priority given to health in governments' budgets [28]. General government health expenditure as a percentage of general government expenditure in 2015 in the EMR was around 9% compared to 11% globally [28]. The 2013 Lancet Commission on Global Health 2035 identified many opportunities for increasing public investment in health, mainly from domestic sources [29].

3.4.2 Fragmented, Low-Performing, and Inefficient Health Systems

A major impediment to implementing reforms toward UHC are health systems that are fragmented, low-performing (ineffective), and inefficient. Health systems that lack adequate infrastructure, are under-resourced in terms of workforce capacities and health technologies, are vertically and horizontally fragmented, and that are poorly governed and managed pose a major challenge to UHC. The *World Health Report 2010* [4] identified 10 areas of inefficiency in the health sector impacting its performance in enhancing progress toward UHC (Box 3.3). The list refers to pitfalls in all health system components, including inadequate infrastructure and human resources, poor-quality services, and weak coordination between different programs and service providers, which all result in fragmented and parallel systems. Investment in strengthening health system capacity should precede or at least parallel any reform toward UHC to be successful.

3.4.3 Socioeconomic, Political, and Demographic Factors

Multiple predisposing factors (e.g., age, gender, religion, place of residence, racial or ethnic group, language, disability, and poverty) are known to influence individuals' behaviors and access to health services [30]. Countries with large informal sectors and significant poverty levels, and other vulnerable groups – such as refugees, IDPs, and migrants – are further challenged to ensure effective progress toward UHC.

3.4.4 Incorporating Public Health Programs into Packages of UHC Interventions

Universal health coverage requires developing an essential package of interventions that target the major burden of disease and are cost-effective (Chapters 15). In many countries this requires reconciling with existing priority public health programs, including those for communicable and noncommunicable diseases and maternal and child health, while facilitating integration at all levels. This poses several organizational and management challenges to implementing the UHC agenda. Accordingly, a balance between horizontal and vertical approaches needs to be considered as a basis for health system strengthening as reforms for UHC are rolled out.

3.4.5 Private Sector Engagement

The private sector is a major provider of services in many L&MICs. Yet, in many countries, the private sector operates on objectives that are self-guided and market-oriented, and do not align – and often are not required to align – with the overall goals of the health sector, including the achievement of UHC. Involving the private sector in provision of publicly funded benefit packages for UHC raises key questions of accountability, quality, efficiency, and governance, the answers to which, especially in the context of L&MICs, are at best at a rudimentary stage of development [31]. The delivery of services by the private sector must be understood in a broader sense in the context of the overall health system rather than only private providers in isolation [32]. See Chapters 27 and 28 for more discussion on the role of the private sector in health.

3.4.6 Lack of Focus on Vulnerable Groups

An important challenge is that UHC is much more difficult to achieve than to advocate for. In many instances the poor find themselves in a situation where they can gain little until the final stages of the transition from advocacy to implementation. If UHC is to display a trickle-down pattern of spread marked by increasing the benefits for better-off groups first and only later on benefiting the poor, it may well result in a rise in inequality over an extended period of time, or worse, it may result in a permanent disparity [33].

In order to avoid such an eventuality, Davidson Gwatkins and Alex Ergo proposed what might appropriately be called *progressive universalism* as the adequate approach to advance UHC while continuously ensuring equity [33]. At the center of such an approach lies a determination to ensure that people who are poor gain at least as much as those who are better-off at every step of the way toward UHC, rather than having to wait and catch up as the goal is eventually approached. The Lancet Commission on Global Health 2035: A World Converging within a Generation [29] also proposed an integrative approach to health system strengthening based on the principles of *progressive universalism*. The latter starts by defining the set of entitlements to be guaranteed to everyone, and then builds the systems that ensure their effective delivery (see Chapter 15).

3.4.7 Disengaged Communities

Community engagement describes a complex political process with dynamic negotiation and renegotiation of power and authority between providers and recipients of health care in order to achieve the shared goal of UHC [34]. This requires health systems to shift from an almost exclusively vertical, top-down, and curative paradigm to one that places people at the center of health services [35]. Despite this recognition, the predominant discourse has focused on financing and service provision aspects of UHC, with inadequate attention given to engaging patients, families, and local communities. Though examples of community engagement exist (see Chapters 11 and 29), there is very little guidance on how to implement and embed community engagement as a concerted, integrated, strategic, and sustained component of health systems [34].

3.5 Health System Strengthening, UHC, and Global Health Security: A New Paradigm

COVID-19 unveiled how ill-prepared the world was to face a pandemic of such magnitude and how vulnerable most national health systems are in terms of continuous access to essential health services amid emergencies. UHC and health security have been described as two sides of the same coin [36]. The pandemic signaled the low investment in essential public health functions [37] and other common goods for health in building equitable and resilient health systems that advance UHC and promote health security (see

Chapters 32, 34, and 37) [38–40]. A recent review has stressed the importance of adequate health workforce, effective regulatory policies, equitable and transparent health financing, robust health intelligence, and intersectoral collaboration for achieving UHC and health security [41].

Step 0 in health system recovery from COVID-19 requires adequate investment in essential public health functions and other common goods for health (e.g., policy and coordination, taxes and subsidies, regulation and legislation, information, analysis, and communication, and population services), coupled with rebuilding fit-for-purpose institutions toward UHC and health security [39]. This also calls for integrating health program specificities – such as communicable diseases, noncommunicable diseases, and reproductive, maternal, neonatal, child, and adolescent health – in all endeavors that aim for strengthening health systems.

Both UHC and global health security (GHS) aim to mitigate potential health and economic threats either at the level of the individual (UHC) or the collective (GHS). For UHC, the risk results from individuals' exposure to economic hazard as a result of a health event, while for GHS the risk results from an infectious disease hazard that may result in a large-scale outbreak, threatening a population and/or the economy or political stability [42]. It is argued that health system strengthening can be the policy mechanism which brings GHS and UHC together, elevating health and mitigating the risk for all.

3.6 Conclusion

While UHC contributes to the betterment of individual and population health by improving access to quality health care and ensuring FP, it is also a direct and indirect factor of economic and social development (Figure 3.4) – by enhancing individual productivity and

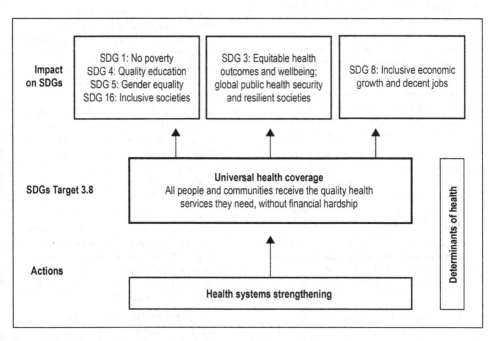

Figure 3.4 UHC and social and economic development [43].

supporting job creation while promoting social equity and solidarity [43]. This makes UHC both a health and socioeconomic development agenda.

Today, UHC is seen by many as the leading health system policy response to the Right to Health principles entrenched in Article 25 of the Universal Declaration of Human Rights [44]. Successful countries' experiences demonstrate that progress toward UHC is first and foremost a political choice and commitment [45].

References

1. World Health Organization. From primary health care to universal coverage: the "affordable dream." 2017. www.who.int/publications/10-year-review/chapter-uhc.pdf?ua=1 (accessed December 14, 2021).

2. World Health Organization. *World Health Report 2008: Primary Health Care (Now More Than Ever)*. Geneva, World Health Organization, 2008. https://reliefweb.int/sites/reliefweb.int/files/resources/98C1FCE13A0C5968C12574E1003F944B-who_oct2008.pdf (accessed December 10, 2021).

3. World Health Organization. Declaration of Astana. 2018. www.who.int/docs/default-source/primary-health/declaration/gcphc-declaration.pdf (accessed December 10, 2021).

4. World Health Organization. *The World Health Report 2010: Health Systems Financing: The Path to Universal Coverage*. Geneva, World Health Organization, 2010. https://apps.who.int/iris/handle/10665/44371 (accessed December 25, 2021).

5. United Nations. Transforming our world: The 2030 Agenda for Sustainable Development. https://sdgs.un.org/2030agenda (accessed December 15, 2021).

6. T. Bärnighausen, R. Sauerborn. One hundred and eighteen years of the German health insurance system: are there any lessons for middle- and low-income countries? *Soc Sci Med* 2002; **54**(10): 1559–1587.

7. W. Beveridge. Social insurance and allied services. 1942. https://apps.who.int/iris/bitstream/handle/10665/57560/scan.pdf?sequence=1&isAllowed=y (accessed July 18, 2021).

8. World Health Organization. Constitution of the World Health Organization. 1948. www.who.int/governance/eb/constitution/en/ (accessed December 10, 2021).

9. World Health Organization. Universal health coverage. 2021. www.who.int/news-room/fact-sheets/detail/universal-health-coverage-(uhc) (accessed December 10, 2021).

10. H. L. Sobel, D. Huntington, M. Temmerman. Quality at the centre of universal health coverage. *Health Policy Plan* 2016; **31**(4): 547–549.

11. National Academies of Sciences, Engineering, and Medicine. *Crossing the Global Quality Chasm: Improving Health Care Worldwide*. Washington, DC: National Academies Press, 2018. www.ncbi.nlm.nih.gov/books/NBK535653/pdf/Bookshelf_NBK535653.pdf (accessed February 3, 2022).

12. P. Barker. Making universal health coverage whole: adding quality as the fourth dimension. 2016. www.ihi.org/communities/blogs/_layouts/15/ihi/community/blog/itemview.aspx?List=7d1126ec-8f63-4a3b-9926-c44ea3036813&ID=340 (accessed February 3, 2022).

13. A. Mataria, S. El-Saharty, M. M. Hamza, et al. Transforming health financing systems in the Arab world toward universal health coverage. 2021. https://link.springer.com/referenceworkentry/10.1007/978-3-030-36811-1_155 (accessed February 3, 2022).

14. WHO Regional Office for the Eastern Mediterranean. Towards universal health coverage: challenges, opportunities and roadmap. 2013. https://applications.emro.who.int/docs/RC_Techn_paper_2013_tech_disc_2_15016_EN.pdf?ua=1 (accessed February 2, 2022).

15. World Health Organization. Developing a national health financing strategy:

a reference guide. 2017. https://apps
.who.int/iris/handle/10665/254757
(accessed December 14, 2021).

16. World Bank. Measuring progress towards
universal health coverage: with an
application to 24 developing countries.
Policy Research Working Paper 7470.
2015. https://openknowledge
.worldbank.org/handle/10986/23432
(accessed July 23, 2021).

17. GBD 2019 Universal Health Coverage
Collaborators. Measuring universal health
coverage based on an index of effective
coverage of health services in 204 countries
and territories, 1990–2019: a systematic
analysis for the Global Burden of Disease
Study 2019. *Lancet* 2020; **396**(10258):
1250–1284.

18. WHO, World Bank. Monitoring progress
towards universal health coverage at
country and global levels: framework,
measures and targets. 2014. http://apps
.who.int/iris/bitstream/handle/10665/
112824/WHO_HIS_HIA_14.1_eng.pdf?
sequence=1 (accessed December 14, 2021).

19. A. Jannati, V. Sadeghi, A. Imani, et al.
Effective coverage as a new approach to
health system performance assessment:
a scoping review. *BMC Health Serv Res*
2018; **18**(1): 886.

20. A. Jha, F. Godlee, K. Abbasi. Delivering on
the promise of universal health coverage.
BMJ 2016; **353**: i2216.

21. A. Wagstaff, S. Neelsen. A comprehensive
assessment of universal health coverage in
111 countries: a retrospective observational
study. *Lancet Glob Health* 2020; **8**(1):
e39–e49.

22. World Health Organization. *Primary
Health Care on the Road to Universal
Health Coverage 2019 Monitoring Report
Conference Edition*. Geneva, World Health
Organization, 2019. www.who.int/docs/
default-source/documents/2019-uhc-
report.pdf (accessed December 13, 2021).

23. World Health Organization, World Bank.
*Tracking Universal Health Coverage: 2021
Global Monitoring Report: Conference Edition*.
Geneva, World Health Organization, 2021.
https://cdn.who.int/media/docs/default-

source/world-health-data-platform/events/
tracking-universal-health-coverage-2021-
global-monitoring-report_uhc-day.pdf?
sfvrsn=fd5c65c6_5&download=true
(accessed January 29, 2022).

24. W. Aftab, F. J. Siddiqui, H. Tasic, et al.
Implementation of health and health-
related sustainable development goals:
progress, challenges and opportunities –
a systematic literature review. *BMJ Glob
Health* 2020; **5**(8): e002273.

25. World Bank. Classifying countries by
income. 2019. https://datatopics
.worldbank.org/world-development-
indicators/stories/the-classification-of-
countries-by-income.html (accessed
December 25, 2021).

26. World Health Organization. Global
expenditure on health: public spending on
the rise? 2021. www.who.int/publications/
i/item/9789240041219 (accessed
December 25, 2021).

27. World Health Organization. Spending
targets for health: no magic number. 2016.
www.who.int/publications/i/item/WHO-
HIS-HGF-HFWorkingPaper-16.1
(accessed December 13, 2021).

28. World Health Organization. Strengthening
health financing systems in the Eastern
Mediterranean Region towards universal
health coverage: health financing atlas
2018. 2019. https://apps.who.int/iris/
handle/10665/311328 (accessed
December 25, 2021).

29. D. T. Jamison, L. H. Summers, G. Alleyne,
et al. Global health 2035: a world
converging within a generation. *Salud
Publica Mex* 2015; **57**(5): 444–467.

30. P. A. Braveman, S. Kumanyika, J. Fielding,
et al. Health disparities and health equity:
the issue is justice. *Am J Public Health* 2011;
101(Suppl. 1): S149–S155.

31. R. Horton, S. Clark. The perils and
possibilities of the private health sector.
Lancet 2016; **388**(10044): 540–541.

32. B. McPake, K. Hanson. Managing the
public–private mix to achieve universal
health coverage. *Lancet* 2016; **388**(10044):
622–630.

33. D. R. Gwatkin, A. Ergo. Universal health coverage: friend or foe of health equity? *Lancet* 2011; **377**(9784): 2160–2161.

34. P. Allotey, D. T. Tan, T. Kirby, et al. Community engagement in support of moving toward universal health coverage. *Health Syst Reform* 2019; **5**(1): 66–77.

35. A. Odugleh-Kolev, J. Parrish-Sprowl. Universal health coverage and community engagement. *Bull World Health Organ* 2018; **96**(9): 660–661.

36. World Health Organization. All roads lead to universal health coverage. 2017. www.who.int/news-room/commentaries/detail/all-roads-lead-to-universal-health-coverage (accessed December 14, 2021).

37. A. Alwan, O. Shideed, S. Siddiqi. Essential public health functions: the experience of the Eastern Mediterranean Region. *East Mediterr Health J* 2016; **22**(9): 694–700.

38. A. Soucat, I. Kickbusch. Global common goods for health: towards a new framework for global financing. *Global Policy* 2020; **11**(5): 628–635.

39. A. Soucat. Financing common goods for health: fundamental for health, the foundation for UHC. *Health Syst Reform* 2019; **5**(4): 263–267.

40. A. Mataria, R. Brennan, A. Rashidian, et al. "Health for All by All" during a pandemic: "Protect Everyone" and "Keep the Promise" of universal health coverage in the Eastern Mediterranean Region. *East Mediterr Health J* 2020; **26**(12): 1436–1439.

41. A. Debie, R. B. Khatri, Y. Assefa. Successes and challenges of health systems governance towards universal health coverage and global health security: a narrative review and synthesis of the literature. *Health Res Policy Sys* 2022; **20**. doi: 10.1186/s12961-022-00858-7.

42. C. Wenham, R. Katz, C. Birungi, et al. Global health security and universal health coverage: from a marriage of convenience to a strategic, effective partnership. *BMJ Glob Health* 2019; **4**(1): e001145.

43. M. P. Kieny, H. Bekedam, D. Dovlo, et al. Strengthening health systems for universal health coverage and sustainable development. *Bull World Health Organ* 2017; **95**(7): 537–539.

44. United Nations. Universal Declaration of Human Rights. www.un.org/en/about-us/universal-declaration-of-human-rights (accessed December 13, 2021).

45. World Health Organization. Universal health coverage: a political choice. 2017. www.who.int/director-general/speeches/detail/universal-health-coverage-a-political-choice (accessed February 8, 2022).

Health System Governance

Concepts, Principles, and Practice

Sameen Siddiqi and Shehla Zaidi

Key Messages

- Health system governance is the aggregation of principles and normative values such as equity, accountability, and transparency within the political system in which a health system functions. There is increasing appreciation of the central role of governance in influencing all elements of the health system.
- Closely related to governance are leadership and management. Good governance, leadership, and management are a precondition for high-performing health systems.
- Several governance principles and elements have been identified; the five key ones are strategic vision, participation, accountability, transparency, and rule of law.
- Governance in practice is seen as a set of organizational and management challenges related to all components of the health system, which managers are frequently unable to see using a health governance lens.
- Multisectoral governance for health involves government and nongovernment agencies in solving multidimensional challenges of differing levels of complexity – those that are win–win, neutral, or with conflicting interests across sectors.
- Ministries of Health need to assume new responsibilities in the twenty-first century for which their four major roles relate to: (1) de jure governance processes; (2) preparation for and response to change in context; (3) relationship management; and (4) values management.

4.1 Introduction and Concepts

The term *governance* was formally recognized as an essential component of the health system as late as the year 2007 [1], and is among the least understood of all its functions. Put simply, it concerns the actions and means adopted by a society to organize itself in the promotion and protection of the health of its population [2]. Transparency International states that health system governance determines the primary objectives of a health system and the direction of policy and legislation needed to achieve these [3]. More recently, *health system governance has been described as an aggregation of principles and normative values such as equity, accountability, and transparency within the political system in which a health system functions* [4]. There is increasing appreciation of the central role of governance and its influence on all aspects of the health system and beyond (Figure 4.1).

The underlying theories, principles, and their practical application lend themselves to a better understanding of health system governance. Before doing so it is essential to explain

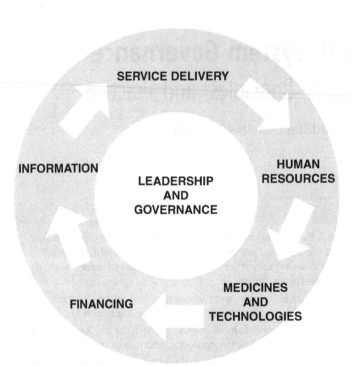

Figure 4.1 Governance and its influence on other health system functions [1].

key terms that are often linked with governance – these are stewardship, leadership, and management. *Stewardship*, mentioned in the *World Health Report 2000* as a function of the health system, and used interchangeably with governance, refers to the function of a government responsible for the welfare of the population, and is concerned about the trust and legitimacy with which its activities are viewed by the citizenry [5]. Although the use of the term stewardship has largely been replaced by governance, Ministries of Health are often recognized as the "steward" of the health system. Closely related to governance are leadership and management. There are multiple definitions of these terms in the literature; Box 4.1 offers just one of many. *While leaders do the "right things," managers do the "things right," and governance provides the "right environment to do things."* Good governance, leadership, and management are preconditions for high-performing health systems.

4.2 Theories Underpinning Governance in Health

The term *governance* was first used by Richard Eells in 1960 [9]. Governance was a less frequently used term in development circles until employed in the World Bank's 1989 report, "From crisis to sustainable growth: sub-Saharan Africa" [10]. *It was defined as the manner in which power is exercised in the management of countries' economic and social resources for development* [11]. Subsequently, Daniel Kaufmann et al. elaborated on how governance in a country is exercised by identifying three areas, with two dimensions for each area (Box 4.2) [12]. It is no surprise that the use of the term governance was much more common in development sectors before it was introduced as a building block of the health system.

Box 4.1 Stewardship, Leadership, and Management

- **Stewardship** refers to a wide range of functions carried out by governments as they seek to achieve national health policy objectives. It comprises six functions: (1) generating intelligence (information and evidence); (2) formulating strategic policy direction; (3) ensuring tools for implementation through incentives and sanctions; (4) building and sustaining partnerships; (5) developing a fit between policy objectives and organizational structures and culture; and (6) ensuring accountability [6].
- **Leadership** is the process of influencing the activities of an organized group toward goal achievement [7]. It is about presenting a vision of what can be achieved, communicating this to others, and evolving strategies for realizing the vision. Leaders motivate people, mobilize resources, and provide the needed support to achieve shared goals.
- **Management** is the art of getting things done through and with people in formally organized groups, and includes the four main functions of planning, organizing, directing, and controlling [8]. Managers have clarity of purpose and tasks, good organizational skills, ability to communicate tasks and expected results, command on administrative and regulatory processes, and good delegation skills.

Box 4.2 Six Dimensions of Governance as Described by the World Bank [12]

1. The process by which governments are selected, monitored, and replaced:

   a. voice and accountability
   b. political stability and absence of violence/terrorism

2. The capacity of the government to effectively formulate and implement sound policies:

   a. government effectiveness
   b. regulatory quality

3. The respect of citizens and the state for the institutions that govern economic and social interactions among them:

   a. rule of law
   b. control of corruption

Several theories relevant to governance have wide applications in economics, political science, public administration, and health. Of these, two that are briefly discussed here are *principal–agent theory* and *public goods theory*.

Principal–agent theory assumes that the goals of principals (e.g., policymakers and managers) and agents (e.g., providers) diverge and that agents are able to maximize their interests at the expense of the principal because of better information (information asymmetry) about what they are doing, while principals seek to increase their oversight over agents without efforts to overcome the information gaps [9]. A health governance lens that focuses on principal–agent relationships among health system actors can provide useful insights into the dynamics of health system performance that can lead to the identification of underlying institutional incentives and problems [13]. In health systems, this concerns a variety of widely disseminated reforms requiring good governance, such as the purchaser–

provider split, managerial autonomy for providers, private sector participation in provision, use of independent regulators and agencies for specialist functions, and outsourcing ancillary functions such as catering and estate management [14].

The **theory of public goods** was postulated by the economist Paul Samuelson in 1954 [15]. It states that public goods are goods that are collectively consumed, and are nonrival and nonexcludable. *Nonexcludable* means that nonpaying consumers cannot be prevented from accessing a good or service and *nonrivalrous* means that the consumption of a good or service by one consumer does not prevent simultaneous consumption by other consumers. This theory is relevant to both health and governance as many health interventions have elements of public goods such as disease surveillance, health promotion, and herd immunity due to vaccination programs. From a governance perspective, such goods or services are not provided efficiently by the market and requires the state to intervene by supplying these directly or by introducing regulatory measures.

A systematic review of the literature to describe the concept of governance and its underpinning theories identified 16 frameworks developed to assess governance in the health system [16]. Of these, only five had been applied and had used the principal–agent theory. The review concluded that a comprehensive assessment of governance would enable policymakers to prioritize solutions for problems identified as well as replicate and scale-up examples of good practice. Drawing on existing frameworks, a recent review has emphasized the need for more theoretically informed empirical research on health system governance in conflict-affected settings [17].

4.3 Relationship between Health and Governance

The relationship of governance to population health was demonstrated by Reidpath and Allotey while examining data on three structural factors for 176 countries: access to improved water, GDP per capita, and governance [18]. The study revealed that healthy populations tend to have better governance, better physical infrastructure, and greater wealth. The relationship is complicated by the fact that these factors are also correlated with each other.

The relevance and influence of governance in health is visible at different levels, from the global to the national and subnational. In addition to health system governance in a country, there are other levels such as global health governance, corporate governance, and clinical governance (Box 4.3). These levels of governance in health are addressed in other chapters (see Chapters 19, 26, 29, and 34), while the rest of this chapter is devoted to the principles and practice of health system governance at the national and subnational levels.

4.4 Health System Governance: Principles

There is a consensus on the importance of governance in health, yet it has been a challenge in terms of defining the key principles, elements, and values, and their remit, that would lend to assessing health system governance distinctly or objectively. There have been several attempts at identifying the key elements, which has helped advance the debate on health system governance. Table 4.1 provides a comparative analysis of the elements of health system governance in selected frameworks [26].

Despite the plethora of governance elements, there is a tacit agreement on the importance of *strategic vision, participation, accountability, transparency,* and *rule of law* being at the heart of good governance in health (Table 4.2). In summary, a well-governed health

> **Box 4.3** Health Governance: Something for All Levels
>
> - **Global health governance** describes the formal and informal institutions, norms, and processes that govern or directly influence global health policies and outcomes [19].
> - **Corporate governance** focuses on how to design organizations that will have appropriate internal controls, strategic development, and shareholder or stakeholder representation in decisions [20].
> - **Clinical governance** is a framework through which organizations are accountable for continually improving the quality of their services and safeguarding high standards of care by creating an environment in which excellence in clinical care will flourish [21].
> - **Participatory governance** is a prerequisite for government responsiveness which aims to increase citizen participation in public policy processes, which in turn increases responsive governance that aims to meet the health needs of citizens and promote and improve access and quality of health services [22]. A related concept of **community health governance** is evolving that entails three local governance mechanisms of horizontal coordination, demand for accountability and self-help as a constant process of learning from the field to strengthen policymaking [23].
> - **People-centered governance** is a framework that contends that understanding of governance is predominantly focused on the role of government, whereas nonstate actors such as the local health market and community, through individual and collective actions, impact on the governance of primary health care [24].
> - **Networked governance** is characterized by dialog and exchange leading to networks and partnerships that provide a motivational force for key public values, rather than relying on rules and use of incentives [25].

system should have clear goals based on the participation of relevant stakeholders, especially those from disadvantaged groups or who may have less power to influence policies, and from which transparent policies are designed and adhered to by promoting accountability and enforcing rule of law [24, 30]. Collectively, all of these contribute to reducing the risk of corruption, which is a fundamental governance problem in many low- and middle-income countries (L&MICs). One governance principle that is essential to health is *ethics*. No health system governance framework can be complete without considering the ethical aspects of health care and research. The commonly accepted principles of health care ethics include respect for autonomy, nonmaleficence, beneficence, and justice.

Most health system governance frameworks focus on the role of governments in governance, and efforts to understand the governance roles of nongovernment health system actors have remained limited. A multilevel governance framework focuses on the governance relations among different health system actors and defines three levels of governance: constitutional governance (e.g., governments), collective governance (e.g., community coalitions), and operational governance (e.g., supply and demand behavior of individuals and providers within the local health market). This has been used as a thinking guide in analyses of primary health care governance in Nigeria [24].

4.5 Health System Governance: Practice

Governance is a practice, dependent on arrangements set at the political or national level, which needs to be operationalized by individuals at lower levels in the health system [16].

Table 4.1 Comparison of governance elements in selected frameworks [26]

Governance element	WHO 2007 [1]	Islam 2007 [27]	Siddiqi et al. 2009 [28]	Lewis and Pettersson 2009 [29]
Accountability	•	•	•	•
Effectiveness/efficiency			•	
Equity			•	
Ethics			•	
Existence of standards		○		•
Incentives	○			•
Information/intelligence	•	•	•	•
Participation/collaboration	•	•	•	
Policy/system design	•	•		
Regulation	•	•		
Responsiveness		•	•	
Rule of law			•	
Transparency	○	○	•	○
Vision/direction	○		•	

Key: • governance element is identified as a discrete element; ○ governance element is mentioned in the context of other elements.

More often these governance elements and principles are seen as management challenges, which health system managers in L&MICs face almost on a daily basis but are unable to see the inefficiencies and inequities in health and health care using a governance lens (Table 4.2). It stands to reason that inappropriate management practices need to be systematically analyzed and understood in the light of governance principles if these are to be addressed by well-meaning health system managers and decision-makers.

It is critically important to be able to recognize gaps in governance as a first step to addressing these challenges. The demonstration of good or bad governance practices in relation to different health system challenges is extensively discussed across the different chapters of this book, while the strategies to address these governance challenges are dealt with in Chapter 19.

Accountability is a critical pillar of governance and can positively impact by ensuring that political leadership acts on behalf of voters, organizational leadership delivers to performance targets and controls opportunities for corruption [31], and citizens' ownership improves the quality of public services [32].

There are two broad approaches to accountability, depending on the pathway through which accountability is streamed. *Top-down accountability* has traditionally been implemented within public sector institutions and typically relies on inculcating a work culture of performance target setting, annual performance review, and improved capacity for evidence

Table 4.2 Core health system governance principles

Explanation	Core areas	Example related to health system challenges
Principle: Strategic vision		
Leaders have a broad and long-term perspective on health and human development, along with a sense of strategic directions for such development. There is also an understanding of the historical, cultural, and social complexities in which that perspective is grounded.	Defined values, instruments of planning, strategic goals and targets, aligned interests	Absence of a long-term health workforce plan that considers labor market dynamics as well as policy levers related to production of various cadres, skill mix, migration, maldistribution, and their regulation.
Principle: Participation and consensus orientation		
All men and women have a voice in decision-making for health, either directly or through legitimate intermediate institutions that represent their interests. Such broad participation is built on freedom of association and speech, as well as capacities to participate constructively.	Deliberative decision-making, coalition building, inclusiveness, community empowerment, and capacity building	District health managers fail to co-produce health plans by engaging other public sectors, private sector, nongovernmental, and community stakeholders, including women, especially to give voice to the marginalized and vulnerable.
Principle: Transparency		
Transparency is built on the free flow of information for all health matters. Processes, institutions, and information should be directly accessible to those concerned with them, and enough information should be provided to understand and monitor health matters.	Conflict of interest, corruption, political nepotism, power abuse, and aggregation and dissemination of data	An inquiry report of potential misappropriation of funds in the health sector is hushed instead of being prepared after a thorough inquiry by an independent team and made available to the public and media.
Principle: Accountability		
Decision-makers in government, the private sector, and civil society organizations involved in health are accountable to the public, as well as to institutional stakeholders. This accountability differs depending on the organization and whether the decision is internal or external to an organization.	Vertical answerability, horizontal answerability, public data and communication, and compliance and liability	Decision-makers are not held accountable for decisions made in the health system that cause wastage of resources due to abuse of power or outright fraud through the use of the public purse for personal gain.

Table 4.2 (cont.)

Explanation	Core areas	Example related to health system challenges
Principle: Rule of law		
Legal frameworks pertaining to health should be fair and enforced impartially, particularly the laws on human rights related to health.	Equality before the law, avoidance of arbitrariness, separation of powers, procedural transparency, and regulatory enforcement	Absent or inadequate legislation, regulatory capacity, and enforcement mechanisms to control the production, marketing, and sales of tobacco and other unhealthy products.

generation. The recent growth in the use of digital technologies offers promising potential for the quick supply of programmatic and expenditure information. *Bottom-up accountability* refers to creating a shared understanding of health care issues and a wider network of commitment to resolve them. It relies on pressure from citizens to improve the local conditions and involves working with civil society organizations that keep communities informed and build demand to affect improvement in local health clinics and services. While promising, citizens have limited leverage over health care providers, and collective action problems can be hard to overcome [33].

Authority and responsibility are two important elements closely related to accountability that need to be briefly explained. As per Henri Fayol [34], *authority* is the right to give orders and the power to exact obedience. Hence, it includes the powers to assign duties to subordinates and make them accept and follow them. Additionally, as per McFarland [35], *responsibility* means the duties and activities assigned to a position or an executive. In other words, it is the obligation of the person to complete the task given. All three – authority, responsibility, and accountability – are interrelated, and each one leads to the initiation of the other two. Hence, before being held accountable an individual or an institution should be given the necessary authority to successfully execute the assigned responsibility.

4.6 Tools for Assessing Health System Governance

Assessing governance has been and continues to be a challenge. The most authentic work on assessing country-level governance has been led by the World Bank [12]. Figure 4.2 shows the trend for the period 2014–2019 in the control of corruption, one of the six dimensions of governance delineated by the World Bank, for four South Asian countries, with Sweden as a comparator. Despite the quantitative nature of assessment, almost all data on governance is perception-based and relies on the views and opinions of different segments of society.

Despite attempts, there have been few if any valid, reliable, and globally acceptable tools developed for assessing health system governance. One such tool assesses health system governance by posing broad and specific questions for different governance principles at three levels – the national level, the health policy formulation level, and the policy implementation level. The logic and sequencing of questions for the governance principle of Strategic Vision is illustrated in Box 4.4 [28]. More recently a new tool for assessing governance of the health policymaking process has been introduced and tested in Lebanon [36].

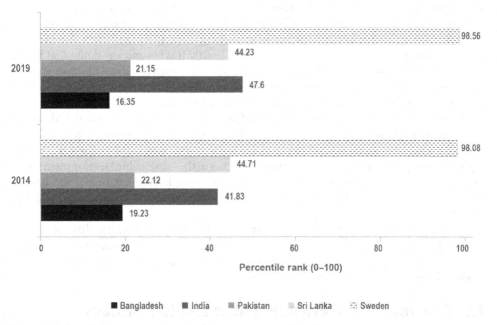

Figure 4.2 Control of corruption in four South Asian countries and Sweden: 2014–2019.

Box 4.4 Analytical Framework for Assessing the Governance Principle of Strategic Vision [28]

One of the **domains** is long-term vision:
The **broad questions** at the different levels are:
- *National level.* What are the broad outlines of economic policy of the government?
- *Health policy formulation level.* Is there a long-term vision (policy) for health?
- *Policy implementation level.* Are implementation mechanisms in line with stated objectives of health policy?

The **specific questions** at the different levels are:
- *National level.* Where does health rank in the overall development framework by resource allocation, and as a percentage of total government expenditure and as a percentage increase in expenditure?
- *Health policy formulation level.* Is there a national health policy/strategic plan available, stating objectives, strategies with a timeframe, and allocated resources?
- *Policy implementation level.* What priority programs are being implemented and how do they correspond to the policy objectives?

4.7 Multisectoral Governance for Health

Multisectoral governance for health is defined as the governance mechanisms where several government agencies and nongovernment actors (including civil society and the private sector) are involved in solving multisectoral and multidimensional health challenges [37].

The importance of multisectoral engagement stems from the wide range of structural determinants and risk factors that influence health outcomes. Air pollution, lack of water and sanitation, poor housing conditions, food insecurity, and unhealthy foods and lifestyles are all well known to adversely impact population health. It is beyond any doubt that health policymakers and managers will need to acquire newer competencies and discover governance arrangements that allow them to work in a multisectoral environment, beyond the provision of health care, if rapid gains in health are to be made.

The need for multisectoral engagement had been recognized even prior to the Alma-Ata Declaration on Primary Health Care in the 1970s, then called intersectoral coordination, and later when the social determinants of health were mainstreamed in the early 2000s. Multisectoral governance has gained further impetus in the Sustainable Development Goals (SDGs) era, requiring innovative means of cross-sectoral implementation if the goal of Better Health and Wellbeing (SDG 3) and other health-related SDGs are to be achieved [38–40].

Chapters 19 and 30 will further detail options on effectively governing multisector action for health. Suffice to state that three types of policy issues require multisectoral governance with different levels of complexity – those that are win–win, neutral or no conflict, or with conflicting interests across sectors (Table 4.3).

4.8 Governance and Essential Public Health Functions

Essential public health functions (EPHFs) are an indispensable set of actions, under the primary responsibility of the state, that are fundamental to achieving the goal of public health through collective action [45]. These have been an important means of indirectly assessing health system governance in the past until efforts to adopt a more direct approach to grasp the subject were initiated following the *World Health Report 2000* [46].

Table 4.3 Policies requiring multisectoral governance with varying levels of complexity [42]

Level of complexity	Example of multisectoral governance
Win–win	Confronting zoonotic diseases which threaten human security, such as H5N1 outbreaks. Wildlife, animal, agriculture, and public health agencies perceive that their institutional mandates could only be achieved by "working together" to gain mutual benefits [41].
Neutral or no conflict	There are no institutional conflicts for achieving reproductive, maternal, newborn, child, and adolescent health targets of SDGs with actors outside the health sector (gender equity, food and nutrition security, rural development) and civil society organizations [42]. Building a shared vision is essential to facilitate multisectoral action, yet challenges remain during implementation [43].
Conflicting interests	Public sector agencies responsible for trade and economic growth (e.g., food, beverage, and alcohol) are at times in conflict with health goals to combat noncommunicable disease and obesity epidemics. In such cases, successful multisectoral action needs negotiation skills where compromises are sought across actors [44].

Table 4.4 The 11 EPHFs for the region of the Americas proposed in 2002 [45]

No.	Description	No.	Description
EPHF 1	Monitoring evaluation and analysis of the health situation of the population	EPHF 7	Evaluation and promotion of equitable access to necessary health services
EPHF 2	Public health surveillance, research, and control of risks	EPHF 8	Human resource development and training in public health
EPHF 3	Health promotion	EPHF 9	Quality assurance in personal and population-based health services
EPHF 4	Social participation in health	EPHF 10	Research in public health
EPHF 5	Development of policies and institutional capacity for planning and management in public health	EPHF 11	Reducing the impact of emergencies and disasters on health
EPHF 6	Strengthening the institutional capacity for regulation and enforcement in public health		

In the 1990s, WHO carried out an international Delphi study to define the concept and to confirm which functions are likely to be the most essential [47]. In 2002, the Centers for Disease Control and Prevention (CDC), the Latin American Center for Health Research, and the Pan American Health Organization proposed a set of 11 EPHFs for the Region of the Americas (Table 4.4) [45]. Since then, many different regions of WHO have developed their own set of EPHFs [48, 49]. These functions constitute an important component of the responsibilities of the state in health and are part of its steering role (see Chapter 31). Measuring these functions helps assess the performance of the national health authority or the Ministries of Health and indirectly ascertains the quality of health system governance.

4.9 Stewardship Role of a Ministry of Health in the Twenty-First Century

The scope of health has rapidly expanded from delivery of health services to Health in All Policies, a collaborative approach that integrates and articulates health considerations into policymaking across sectors to improve the health of all communities and people [50]. This change has been instrumental in "pushing" and "pulling" Ministries of Health of all countries, especially L&MICs, to assume new roles and responsibilities in the twenty-first century, for which many are not prepared. For many ministries, the expanding frontiers of health and health systems are moving goal posts.

A recent review identifies four major roles of Ministries of Health: (1) de jure governance processes; (2) preparation for and response to changing contexts; (3) relationship management; and (4) values management [51]. Figure 4.3 identifies performance areas under each of these roles and functions for Ministries of Health to keep pace with

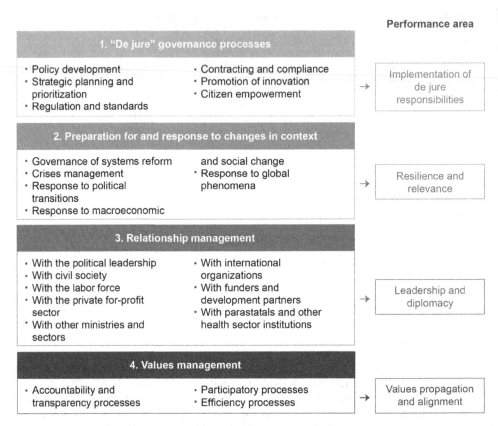

Figure 4.3 Ministry of Health governance roles and performance areas [51].

the vastly changing health system imperatives from the local to the global. While the performance areas are not cast in stone and can be adapted to local requirements, these provide a good listing of the current and future roles of the twenty-first-century Ministries of Health in L&MICs.

4.10 Scope and Influence of Governance on Other Health System Components

As stated earlier, health system governance influences all other components of the health system by virtue of its central role. It permeates all other building blocks and is driven by people and actors in the system [24]. Many health reforms, structural or programmatic, in L&MICs have not achieved their desired objectives due to lack of attention given to the key governance principles of participation, transparency, and accountability during their design and implementation. Good governance is a critical element in any reform intervention, whether it relates to setting up health insurance schemes, public–private partnerships, or implementing hospital autonomy.

China's success in achieving scale-up of rural health insurance schemes has attracted considerable interest in many L&MICs, especially regarding the schemes' designs, coverage, and funding mechanisms. However, health systems governance is critical to enable their development and operation. Strengthening practices in various governance domains could inform the adaptation of these schemes in other L&MICs settings [52]. Similarly, public–private partnerships in health involve a wide range of actors, stakeholders, and types of partnerships, and different types of partnerships may require different governance structures, processes, and practices. The roles of transparency and accountability are critical in the governance of public–private partnerships [53].

Public sector hospitals in Pakistan face major governance challenges, yet they serve as a backbone and are the last resort for seeking health care for poorer segments of society. Improving governance and management of these institutions offers a huge opportunity to enhance efficiency and provide better quality of care. A recent analysis proposes three strategic priorities to reform these hospitals. First, demonstrate consistency and commitment in implementing policies related to hospital governance; second, launch a countrywide program of capacity development of hospital managers; and third, establish a system of e-governance to enhance accountability, transparency, and performance of hospitals [54].

4.11 Conclusion

Health system governance continues to be an uncharted territory that requires concerted efforts to develop consensus on its remit and boundaries, validate assessment tools and indicators to monitor the quality of governance, and most importantly to test and develop interventions that could help improve governance of the health system. The thinking on health system governance has evolved over the last decade due to the several initiatives taken to straighten out its complexities, yet more needs to be done. This chapter has focused on the conceptual aspects of health system governance. Later in the book, Chapter 19 will address the recalcitrant challenges of improving governance in health based on the best current evidence.

References

1. World Health Organization. *Everybody Business: Strengthening Health Systems to Improve Health Outcomes*. Geneva, World Health Organization, 2007. www.who.int/healthsystems/strategy/everybodys_business.pdf (accessed November 11, 2020).

2. R. Dodgson, K. Lee, N. Drager. Global health governance: a conceptual review. 2002. https://apps.who.int/iris/handle/10665/68934 (accessed December 22, 2020).

3. Transparency International Global Health. Health system governance. 2021. https://ti-health.org/health-system-governance (accessed December 26, 2021).

4. D. Balabanova, A. Mills, L. Conteh, et al. Good health at low cost 25 years on: lessons for the future of health systems strengthening. *Lancet* 2013; **381**(9883): 2118–2133.

5. R. B. Saltman, O. Ferroussier-Davis. The concept of stewardship in health policy. *Bull World Health Organ* 2000; **78**(6): 732–739.

6. P. Travis, D. Egger, P. Davies, et al. Towards better stewardship: concepts and critical issues. 2002. www.who.int/healthinfo/paper48.pdf (accessed October 11, 2020).

7. C. F. Rauch Jr., O. Behling. Functionalism: Basis for an alternate approach to the study of leadership. In J. G. Hunt, ed., *Leaders and Managers*. New York, Pergamon, 1984, pp. 45–62.

8. H. Koontz. The management theory jungle. *AMJ* 1961; **4**(3): 174–188.

9. J. W. Pratt, R. J. Zeckhauser. *Principals and Agents: The Structure of Business*. Boston, MA, Harvard Business School Press, 1985.

10. World Bank. From crisis to sustainable growth: sub-Saharan Africa – a long term

perspective study (English). https://documents.worldbank.org/en/publication/documents-reports/documentdetail/498241468742846138/from-crisis-to-sustainable-growth-sub-saharan-africa-a-long-term-perspective-study (accessed June 12, 2020).

11. World Bank. Governance: the World Bank's experience. https://documents.worldbank.org/en/publication/documents-reports/documentdetail/711471468765285964/governance-the-world-banks-experience (accessed June 14, 2020).

12. D. Kaufmann, A. Kraay, M. Mastruzzi. The worldwide governance indicators: methodology and analytical issues. *Hague J. Rule Law* 2011; **3**(2): 220–246.

13. D. W. Brinkerhoff, T. J. Bossert. Health governance: principal–agent linkages and health system strengthening. *Health Policy Plan* 2014; **29**(6): 685–693.

14. S. L. Greer, M. Wismar, J. Figueras. *Strengthening Health System Governance: Better Policies, Stronger Performance.* Milton Keynes, Open University Press, 2016.

15. P. A. Samuelson. The pure theory of public expenditure. *Rev Econ Stat* 1954; **36**(4): 387–389.

16. T. Pyone, H. Smith, N. van den Broek. Frameworks to assess health systems governance: a systematic review. *Health Policy Plan* 2017; **32**(5): 710–722.

17. M. Lokot, I. Bou-Orm, T. Zreik, et al. Health system governance in settings with conflict-affected populations: a systematic review. *Health Policy Plann* 2022; **37**(5): 655–674.

18. D. D. Reidpath, P. Allotey. Structure, (governance) and health: an unsolicited response. *BMC Int Health Hum Rights* 2006; **6**(1): 1–7.

19. K. Lee, A. Kamradt-Scott. The multiple meanings of global health governance: a call for conceptual clarity. *Global Health* 2014; **10**(1): 1–10.

20. N. Woods. Good governance in international organizations. In A. J. Lyon, K. Stiles, A. Edgar, et al., eds., *Global Governance: A Review of Multilateralism and International Organizations.* Leiden, Brill Nijhoff, 1999.

21. R. McSherry, P. Pearce. *Clinical Governance: A Guide to Implementation for Healthcare Professionals.* Chichester, Wiley, 2011.

22. A. I. Marshall, K. Kantamaturapoj, K. Kiewnin, et al. Participatory and responsive governance in universal health coverage: an analysis of legislative provisions in Thailand. *BMJ Glob Health* 2021; **6**(2): e004117.

23. S. Madon, S. Krishna. Theorizing community health governance for strengthening primary healthcare in LMICs. *Health Policy Plann,* 2022; **37**(6): 706–716.

24. S. Abimbola, J. Negin, S. Jan, et al. Towards people-centred health systems: a multi-level framework for analysing primary health care governance in low- and middle-income countries. *Health Policy Plan* 2014; **29**(Suppl. 2): ii29–ii39.

25. G. Stoker. Public value management: a new narrative for networked governance. *Am Rev Public Adm* 2006; **36**(1): 41–57.

26. I. Mikkelsen-Lopez, K. Wyss, D. de Savigny. An approach to addressing governance from a health system framework perspective. *BMC Int Health Hum Rights* 2011; **11**(1): 13.

27. USAID. *The Health System Assessment Approach: A How-to Manual, Version 2.0.* Washington, DC, USAID, 2012. www.hfgproject.org/wp-content/uploads/2015/02/HSAA_Manual_Version_2_Sept_20121.pdf (accessed December 11, 2020).

28. S. Siddiqi, T. I. Masud, S. Nishtar, et al. Framework for assessing governance of the health system in developing countries: gateway to good governance. *Health Policy* 2009; **90**(1): 13–25.

29. M. Lewis, G. Pettersson. *Governance in Health Care Delivery: Raising Performance.* Washington, DC, World Bank, 2009.

30. S. Siddiqi, S. Jabbour. Health system governance. In S. Jabbour, R. Yamout, R. Giacaman, et al., eds., *Public Health in the Arab World.* Cambridge, Cambridge University Press, 2012.

31. L. Wenar. Accountability in international development aid. *Ethics Int Aff* 2006; **20**(1): 1–23.

32. D. Freire, M. Galdino, U. Mignozzetti. Bottom-up accountability and public service provision: evidence from a field experiment in Brazil. *RAP* 2020; 7(2): 2053168020914444.

33. M. Björkman, J. Svensson. Power to the people: evidence from a randomized field experiment on community-based monitoring in Uganda. *Q J Econ* 2009; 124 (2): 735–769.

34. C. P. Uzuegbu, C. O. Nnadozie. Henry Fayol's 14 Principles of Management: implications for libraries and information centres. *JISTaP* 2015; 3(2): 58–72.

35. D. E. McFarland. *Management Principles and Practices*, 4th ed. New York, Macmillan, 1974.

36. R. Hamra, S. Siddiqi, E. Carmel, et al. Assessing the governance of the health policy-making process using a new governance tool: the case of Lebanon. *Health Res Policy Syst* 2020; 18(1): 1–6.

37. C. Kanchanachitra, V. Tangcharoensathien, W. Patcharanarumol, et al. Multisectoral governance for health: challenges in implementing a total ban on chrysotile asbestos in Thailand. *BMJ Glob Health* 2018; 3(Suppl. 4): e000383.

38. S. Siddiqi, W. Aftab, F. J. Siddiqui, et al. Global strategies and local implementation of health and health-related SDGs: lessons from consultation in countries across five regions. *BMJ Glob Health* 2020; 5(9): e002859.

39. W. Aftab, F. J. Siddiqui, H. Tasic, et al. Implementation of health and health-related sustainable development goals: progress, challenges and opportunities – a systematic literature review. *BMJ Glob Health* 2020; 5(8): e002273.

40. Z. A. Bhutta, S. Siddiqi, W. Aftab, et al. What will it take to implement health and health-related sustainable development goals? *BMJ Glob Health* 2020; 5(9): e002963.

41. N. Marano, P. Arguin, M. Pappaioanou, et al. Role of multisector partnerships in controlling emerging zoonotic diseases. *Emerg Infect Dis* 2005; 11(12): 1813.

42. K. Rasanathan, N. Damji, T. Atsbeha, et al. Ensuring multisectoral action on the determinants of reproductive, maternal, newborn, child, and adolescent health in the post-2015 era. *BMJ* 2015; 351: h4213.

43. S. Zaidi, Z. Bhutta, S. S. Hussain, K. Rasanathan. Multisector governance for nutrition and early childhood development: overlapping agendas and differing progress in Pakistan. *BMJ Glob Health*. 2018; 10(3): e000678.

44. A. Ruckert, A. Schram, R. Labonté, et al. Policy coherence, health and the sustainable development goals: a health impact assessment of the Trans-Pacific Partnership. *Crit Public Health* 2017; 27(1): 86–96.

45. Centers for Disease Control and Prevention, Centro Latino Americano de Investigaciones en Sistemas de Salud, Pan American Health Organization, World Health Organization. Performance measurement of essential public health functions. 2000. www.paho.org/hq/dmdocu ments/2010/EPHF_Guidelines_Applying_ Instrument_Performance_Measurement .pdf (accessed December 11, 2020).

46. World Health Organization. *The World Health Report 2000: Health Systems – Improving Performance*. Geneva, World Health Organization, 2000. www.who.int/w hr/2000/en (accessed November 14, 2020).

47. D. W. Bettcher, S. A. Sapirie, E. H. Goon. Essential public health functions: results of the international Delphi study. 1998. https:// apps.who.int/iris/handle/10665/55726 (accessed December 11, 2020).

48. A. Alwan, P. Puska, S. Siddiqi. Essential public health functions for countries of the Eastern Mediterranean Region: what are they and what benefits do they offer. *East Mediterr Health J* 2015; 21(12): 859–860.

49. World Health Organization, Regional Office for Europe. Review of public health capacities and services in the European Region. 2012. www.euro.who.int/__data/ assets/pdf_file/0010/172729/Review-of- public-health-capacities-and-services-in- the-European-Region.pdf (accessed December 11, 2020).

50. Centers for Disease Control and Prevention. Health in all policies. 2016. www.cdc.gov/policy/hiap/index.html (accessed December 24, 2021).

51. V. Sriram, K. Sheikh, A. Soucat. Addressing governance challenges and capacities in ministries of health. 2020. https://hsgovcollab.org/system/files/2020-05/FINAL-WEB-3442-OMS-HSGF-WHO-WorkingPaper.pdf (accessed November 13, 2020).

52. B. Yuan, W. Jian, L. He, et al. The role of health system governance in strengthening the rural health insurance system in China. *Int J Equity Health* 2017; **16**(1): 1–20.

53. R. M. Taylor, J. Alper. *Exploring Partnership Governance in Global Health.* Washington, DC, National Academies Press, 2018.

54. S. Siddiqi, M. Iqbal, W. Aftab. Review of the governance of public sector hospitals in Pakistan: lessons for the future. *WHHS* 2019; **55**(3): 7.

Financing Health Care
Revenue Raising, Pooling, and Purchasing

David B. Evans, Awad Mataria, Christoph Kurowski, and Martin Schmidt

---

Key Messages

- Raising resources to fund progress toward universal health coverage (UHC) is the first necessary, but not sufficient, component of health financing.
- Health financing also requires the development of strategies that pool resources together to share the financial risks of ill-health across populations, and decisions about purchasing either the inputs to provide the health services needed by the population or the services themselves.
- Revenues can come from many sources, but progress toward UHC requires predominant reliance on obligatory prepaid funds – that is, contributions that are made before someone becomes ill, so that they can draw on them in the event of illness. Obligatory prepayment can come from government taxes and charges and mandatory social health insurance contributions.
- Direct out-of-pocket payments (OOPs) that households make for health services discourage their use, reducing both coverage and continuation of treatment. Millions of people who use services also suffer severe financial hardship because of OOPs. Obligatory prepaid funds, therefore, need to be pooled to allow people to seek care, to continue treatment, and to be protected from financial hardship associated with OOPs.
- Purchasing involves decisions about what services to guarantee universally, and how they should be paid for.
- Any decision about the appropriate mix of health services inevitably requires concomitant consideration of what levels of service quality and financial protection are desired, given the available funds.
- Purchasing frameworks, involving choices on the combination of payment methods and payment rates, are critical for giving the incentives for greater efficiency and equity in the use of the available funds.
- The shock of the COVID-19 pandemic has highlighted that health financing policy needs to have two additional capacities to complement day-to-day activities in the three core health financing functions of revenue generation, purchasing, and pooling. The first is the capacity to adjust to shocks that suddenly increase the need for health spending and/or reduce the capacity to raise revenues, called health financing resilience. The second is the capacity to adjust to emerging threats, or opportunities, that effect health costs or revenues more slowly and more predictably. This is called health financing sustainability. Both resilience and sustainability are critical to the search for high-performance health financing on the road to UHC.

5.1 Introduction

The COVID-19 pandemic starkly illustrated how unexpected shocks can suddenly increase the need for countries to spend on health. At the same time, the global recession of 2020 reduced the capacity of virtually all countries to raise the revenues to finance the health response and maintain progress toward UHC [1–3]. Health financing is, however, more than simply mobilizing and collecting necessary resources for health. This chapter focuses on defining health financing and all its components [4–8].

5.2 What Is Health Financing?

Health financing includes three interrelated functions of raising funds for health, pooling them to spread the financial risks of paying for health services, and then using the available funds to purchase or provide the health services that people need [4].

It is widely accepted that the ultimate objective of health financing is to move countries closer to UHC, where all people can use the health services they need (promotive, preventive, curative, rehabilitative, and palliative), of sufficient quality to be effective, while also ensuring that the use of these services does not expose the user to financial hardship [4–7].

While the performance of the three health financing functions are important determinants of how close a country gets to UHC, they are not the only ones. Social and economic factors such as income levels and poverty rates are also critical, as are other factors such as training and motivating the necessary health workers (see Chapter 3) [5]. However, insufficient funds result in inadequate or low-quality health services. Where people have to pay most of the costs OOP, the poor (and often other segments of the population) will not obtain needed services or will suffer severe financial consequences in using them. And where service provision is inefficient and inequitable, the poor cannot obtain quality services and the pace of the journey toward UHC slows.

It has recently become clear that health financing also requires the capacity to systematically assess and respond to threats to health spending and revenue generation that might set back progress toward UHC [6]. Shocks are sudden and unpredictable events that require more health spending, or which reduce revenues, such as the COVID-19 pandemic. Other factors that impact health spending might emerge more slowly, and be more predictable, such as the aging of the population or the rate of formalization of the labor force. The capacity to deal with the first is called *health financing resilience*, and with the second *health financing sustainability*.

Hence, high-performance health financing for UHC can be defined as funding levels that are adequate, sustainable, and resilient; pooling that is sufficient to spread the financial risks of ill-health; and spending that is both efficient and equitable to assure the desired levels of health service coverage, quality, and financial protection for all people [6].

The following sections discuss the three core health financing functions that are critical to ensuring a high-performance health financing system.

5.3 Revenue Generation

Revenue generation, or revenue raising, is the process of mobilizing the funds required to purchase or provide the health services people need. The resulting funds must also cover the activities that make the system work, such as governance, pandemic preparedness and response, and monitoring and evaluation.

The capacity to raise revenues depends critically on the level of a country's national income. For example, in 2019, the most recent year for which health spending data is available, low-income countries (LICs) spent, on average, US$39 per capita, compared to US$119 in lower middle-income countries (LMICs), US$472 in upper middle-income (UMICs), and US$3,191 in high-income countries (HICs) [9, 10].

Sources of revenue can be *obligatory* or *voluntary*. The first source of obligatory revenue comes from taxes and other types of charges levied by governments, both national and subnational. Some of these revenues are then allocated to health. In some countries there is a second source, social health insurance (SHI) contributions – traditionally raised from mandatory wage-based deductions (see Chapter 17).

The largest component of voluntary contributions comes from OOP health payments made by households for the services they receive, supplemented by voluntary health insurance contributions and contributions from the private or nongovernment sector – for example, funding provided by faith-based organizations to run health facilities. Funding from external sources (largely development assistance for health [DAH]) supplements domestic sources in some countries.

The relative importance of these sources varies across country income groups (Figure 5.1). Obligatory sources of finance get increasingly more important, on average, as country incomes grow, while the relative contribution of OOPs declines. External funding is limited largely to the two lower-income groups. Voluntary health insurance and other voluntary contributions are a relatively unimportant source everywhere.

The heavy reliance on OOPs seen in LICs deters many people from using needed health services, reduces adherence to treatment regimens, and can result in financial hardship and impoverishment for those who seek care [5, 12, 13]. Accordingly, health financing policy in

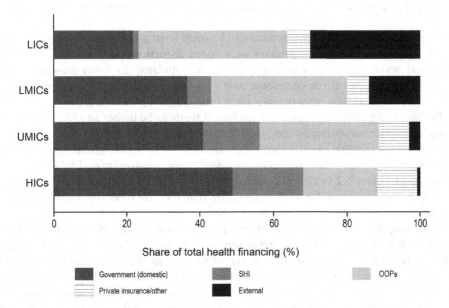

Figure 5.1 Share of total health financing by source by country income group, 2019. Data from [9]; income classifications from [11].

most low- and middle-income countries (L&MICs) aims to reduce reliance on OOPs rather than seeing them as an option for raising additional funds for health.

Revenue generation can only be achieved by increasing the share of general government funds and compulsory social contributions dedicated to health. These contributions are then pooled (see the next section). Because people first pay (through taxes and other contributions) and then draw on the funds if, and only if, they get sick, the contributions are termed *prepayment*. Prepayment with subsequent pooling allows people to use needed health services and protects them from the severe financial consequences of paying OOP [5, 12, 13].

There are three determinants of a government's ability to spend on health from general funds. The first is how much revenue is raised through taxation of different types, charges, other sources of revenue such as royalties from natural resources, and by borrowing. The second is the share of these revenues that it can spend (as opposed to repaying public debt or reducing the budget deficit). The third is the share of overall revenues allocated to health. *Fiscal space*, which refers to the funds available to spend, is determined by the first two. The amount available to spend on health, sometimes loosely called fiscal space for health, is determined by all three.

Economic growth increases government revenues. It accounted for over 60% of the increase in government health spending observed in MICs from 2000 to 2015, and 37% in LICs [14]. The converse is also true: government revenues fall during an economic recession, limiting their capacities to spend [2, 3].

Increasing the share of government revenues in GDP can add spending capacity to economic growth. The proven options to do this include increasing the range or rates of taxes and charges, ensuring that more individuals and firms contribute to a given tax or charge (expanding the tax base), and increasing the efficiency of revenue collection, including the reduction of corruption [6, 13, 15, 16]. Introducing or increasing *pro-health taxes* on products that damage health, like cigarettes, alcohol, or CO_2 emissions, is one example [17, 18].

Social health insurance contributions can be considered a tax, given that contributions are generally raised through mandatory wage-based deductions [19]. Although SHI raises substantial revenues in HICs and is growing in popularity in lower-income settings, Figure 5.1 showed that it can contribute only a small proportion to revenues in LICs and LMICs because of the low rates of labor force formalization [9, 13, 16, 20].

The share of government spending on health tends to be higher in HICs and UMICs than in lower-income settings, where it has remained stubbornly modest (Figure 5.2). There is, however, considerable variation across countries in each income group, with a number allocating relatively low shares to health compared to the group averages [9, 16, 17]. This is illustrated in Figure 5.2, which also highlights two LICs (Liberia and Mali) with shares trending below the mean for LICs, suggesting that there is room for them to increase funding for health by increasing the share.

Increasing the share of government spending on health is partly a political exercise: competition between sectors for increasing budget shares is intense. It is also partly technical because Ministries of Health are often seen as inefficient. Improving public financial management practices in health, for example, allows the allocated funds to be used rapidly rather than remain unspent, improves accountability and transparency, and allows a Ministry of Health to demonstrate the results achieved with their health spending [6].

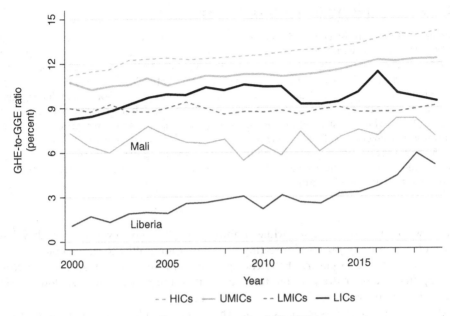

Figure 5.2 The share of health in overall government spending 2008–2010, by country income group and with selected LICs. Data from [9].

Earmarking has been widely used to channel resources to health. The objective of earmarking is to increase health funding in a way that protects it from the political debates associated with the budget negotiations [21, 22]. SHI is an example of this type of *hard earmarking*, with the funds protected for health.

Linking a new source of revenue, or an increase in tax, to the intention to spend more on health is also politically more acceptable to the population than simply increasing taxes. Governments, therefore, sometimes signal their intention to spend more on health through earmarking a revenue source that will go through the budget process – despite the knowledge that the eventual increase in health spending might be smaller than the increase in revenue, something called *soft earmarking*.

In short, the preferred way of increasing revenues for health and to progress toward UHC is to increase obligatory prepaid revenues in the manner described above. In lower-income settings this can be supplemented by increases in DAH. The impact of COVID-19 on revenue generation for health is described briefly in Box 5.1.

5.4 Pooling

Pooling prepaid contributions allows people to use a set of health services without having to pay the full cost from their own pockets when they need them [5, 7, 24]. Beneficiaries can use the set of health services covered by the pooled funds if they get sick, usually with zero or low OOPs to protect them from the financial hardship involved in paying directly for care.

For pooling to work in this way, a pool has to be large enough so that a few people incurring high health care costs do not threaten its financial viability. In any given year, the

Box 5.1 The Impact of COVID-19 on Revenue Generation

Before COVID-19, most LICs, and many LMICs, were off-track to achieve the health-specific SDG (SDG 3). Even with maximum efforts to increase the share of government revenues in GDP, and to allocate a higher proportion to health, they would have been unable to guarantee universal coverage for a set of health services consistent with SDG 3 by 2030 [5, 23].

This shortcoming will be worse for many countries over the next few years following the COVID-19 pandemic. Government revenues per capita fell in all but a handful of countries in 2020 [2, 3]. While most countries are expected to return to economic growth in 2021, government revenues will rise slowly from the 2020 nadir. Of particular concern is a group of 52 countries expected to see overall government spending per capita remain below the 2019 pre-COVID-19 levels from 2021 to 2026, making it difficult for them to spend more on health in the foreseeable future.

sick draw on the pooled funds while healthy people do not, even though they have contributed financially, effectively creating a subsidy from healthy to sick people.

Most countries also ensure that richer people contribute more than poorer people, knowing that the poor draw on the funds more than the rich due to their lower health status. This creates subsidies from rich to poor people.

The final type of cross-subsidy is found where some people are required to contribute less than others, most commonly because they retire from the workforce or are unemployed. They pay less income tax or lower health insurance premiums than employed people. They are also more likely to draw on the pooled funds for their health care because they are older, creating subsidies from people in formal sector employment to those who are not.

Different financing modalities, however, facilitate pooling to different degrees (Table 5.1).

General government revenues are used to provide or purchase health services on behalf of the entire population. This facilitates all of the cross-subsidies described earlier, although the extent of financial risk protection depends on how much is raised compared to health needs.

Obligatory SHI contributions are typically paid into pools held and managed separately from general government revenues. The beneficiaries are the contributors – traditionally only formal sector workers and sometimes their families, so the pools are smaller than under general government revenues. More recently, some governments have expanded the concept of SHI, requiring nonformal workers to purchase insurance if they can afford it, while covering the poor from government revenues.

People who purchase *voluntary health insurance*, including micro-insurance and community-based health insurance, contribute to separate pools to those generated from obligatory contributions. They are smaller than the mandatory pools, covering only the people who have contributed. Various types of voluntary health insurance have developed in LICs, partly because public services are either unavailable or are perceived to be of poor quality [25–28]. Voluntary health insurance has been shown to increase access to health services and improve financial protection for the people who contribute. The very poor, who are most at risk of ill-health, have not, however, been able to afford it, so voluntary mechanisms alone have not been able to ensure universality [5, 6, 26–28]. For example, community health insurance has been promoted in a number of West African countries for

Table 5.1 The degree of pooling possible with different financing modalities

Financing modality	Source of revenue	Voluntary/mandatory	Level of risk pooling	Remarks
General government revenue	Taxes, charges, natural resources, royalties, etc.	Mandatory/automatic	High	Covers formal and informal sector, poor and rich
SHI (formal sector)	Wage-based deductions levied on employees, sometimes employers	Mandatory	Low to medium in lower-income settings depending on the relative size of the formal sector	
SHI (formal and informal sector)	Wage-based deductions, other contributions for those who can pay; government revenues for those who cannot	Mandatory	Can be high where contributions are obligatory and the government covers the contributions of people who cannot pay or from whom it is difficult to collect contributions	Can cover formal and informal sector, poor and rich
Private health insurance	Contributions	Voluntary	Low – covers only people who pay	The poor cannot afford to join
Community health insurance	Contributions	Voluntary	Relatively low – generally small pools	The poor cannot afford to join
Donor financing	Bilateral and multilateral aid come from government revenue in donor countries; foundation contributions come from the wealth of private individuals or companies	Voluntary	On-budget aid helps spread risks	
Medical savings account	Typically, deductions from wages in the formal sector	Mandatory	Very low – spreads risk over the individual's life cycle; sometimes can be used to subsidize family members	
OOPs	Fees; under insurance these include copayments, deductibles, coinsurance	Voluntary in the sense that people can choose not to seek care	Zero	

many years, but population coverage remains low, as does the contribution of this form of insurance to overall revenues [29].

Moreover, if people can opt out of mandatory contributions (taxes or SHI), low-risk people and those who can afford OOP payments will not contribute, leaving the pool to cover only high-risk and poor people: this has been called *adverse selection* [30]. An important lesson, therefore, is that progress toward UHC requires pooling from mandatory contributions. This does not mean there is no room for voluntary insurance, but the predominant form of pooling needs to come from obligatory contributions.

Medical savings accounts are forms of obligatory saving, with deductions from an individual's salary. The individual, and sometimes close family members, can draw on the funds in case of illness. Essentially this spreads the individual's financial risk of ill-health over time, so the degree of pooling is very low.

Historically, most countries have developed multiple pooling arrangements. This can result in *fragmentation*, where the cross-subsidization described earlier occurs only within each pool rather than in the population as a whole. As a result, the contributions of beneficiaries, the range of services offered to them, their quality, and any requirements to make OOPs on top of their prepaid contributions (see Box 5.2) differ, resulting in inequalities and inequities across pools in the coverage with quality health services and with financial protection. Fragmentation also results in inefficiency: multiple administrations increase administration costs while the bargaining capacity of the individual pools to negotiate lower prices with providers is reduced [28, 31].

Merging pools to increase their size and reduce fragmentation has proved politically difficult in many countries, so the government have found ways to reduce the effects of fragmentation. They include *risk equalization mechanisms* that transfer funds from pools that cover low-risk people to those that cover higher-risk people, legislating that the benefits of different pools need to be the same, or increasing government subsidies to the pools that cover poorer people [7].

Out-of-pocket payments do not provide the benefits of pooling. There is no cross-subsidization so that people who cannot afford to use services simply do not seek them. Many of those who seek care suffer severe financial hardship due to the OOPs they make, sometimes forcing people to go into debt and sell assets and pushing some into poverty [32–35]. User fees are the most common form of OOPs, but payments made in the presence of some pooling arrangements (see Box 5.2) are also OOP payments. The different indicators available for tracking progress in reducing financial hardship linked to OOPs are described in Chapter 3.

Box 5.2 Forms of OOPs Sometimes Coexist with Mandatory Pooling

Copayments for services funded by the government are the OOPs which patients must make at the time they receive the services. In health insurance, **copays** are usually a fixed amount an insured person must pay for particular services, such as medicines.

A **deductible** is the amount that must be paid OOP before the health insurance starts to cover the cost.

Some types of insurance require patients to cover a proportion of the costs of particular health services OOP, which is called **coinsurance**.

5.5 Purchasing

Purchasing involves the allocation of funds to obtain health services and ensure financial protection on the behalf of individuals, groups, or populations [4, 8, 36]. Progress toward UHC requires a mix of personal health services, including health promotion, disease prevention, treatment, rehabilitation, and palliation. It also requires a range of complementary activities, including population-based services such as health promotion, and a range of public health and governance functions: for example, pandemic preparedness, health workforce development, setting and enforcement of standards, health information systems and the associated monitoring and evaluation, and health research [37].

One form of purchasing involves buying the inputs needed to produce the desired health services: national health services invest in buildings and equipment, hire health workers, and purchase medicines and other inputs to provide health services. Another form involves buying health services from providers – some health insurance funds do this. Beneficiaries can seek care for a specified range of services, often from a mix of public and private providers, and the fund uses the pooled revenue from beneficiary contributions to pay the providers.[1]

Revenue generation and pooling together provide the funds that allow purchasing for UHC to take place. This sets the boundaries of what can be achieved. The purchasing function, however, determines *what* services are available, to whom, where, at what quality, and whether any OOPs will be required [4, 8]. This function, therefore, determines the coverage with needed services and with financial protection that can be obtained from the available pooled funds. The purchasing function can also give incentives for improved efficiency and equity of health spending, allowing more rapid progress toward UHC for any level of resource availability.

When purchasing uses information on aspects of provider performance, the health needs of the people, and details of service or input costs and expenditures to further health system goals, it is called *strategic purchasing* (see Chapter 18).

Two interrelated decisions are required for purchasing, whether it is strategic or more passive (i.e., nonstrategic): what to purchase and how to purchase. These are broken down into components and discussed below.

5.5.1 What to Purchase?

Who are the beneficiaries? When governments purchase the inputs to provide health services, the entire population is generally eligible to use them, although sometimes eligibility is restricted to citizens. On the other hand, the beneficiaries of health insurance schemes are usually the people who contribute financially or whose contributions are covered by the government.

What health services are guaranteed to beneficiaries and at what level of financial protection? Some form of prioritization is inevitable in making these decisions, even in the richest countries. In LICs and LMICs, however, any guaranteed set of health services will necessarily be smaller than in UMICs and HICs. Progress toward UHC requires progressively increasing the guaranteed benefits over time, something called progressive universalism (see Chapters 3 and 15).

---

[1] Pools are frequently supplemented from general government revenues, and sometimes from DAH.

Selecting which services to guarantee cannot be done in isolation from decisions about the quality and the desired level of financial protection. For example, a government with a given budget would need to choose between providing a set of services free of charge or a larger set with some user-charges.

Decisions then must be made about the mix (sometimes called a basket or package) of services to be guaranteed. Some national health services and insurance schemes do not define a clear and explicit set of services: people can only access what is available at the health facility they attend. Other countries and health insurance schemes explicitly define what services are guaranteed, giving people a better sense of their entitlement. However, a comprehensive, guaranteed set of services is often announced for political reasons without having the adequate resources to finance them all at the desired level of quality. This results in implicit rationing, or poor service readiness, where people obtain only some of the guaranteed services – an example is the frequent stock-outs of medicines in many LICs [37].

Methods of selecting the service mix range from political or bureaucratic decisions, to more formal procedures including health technology assessment (HTA), based heavily on a cost-effectiveness analysis of the possible ways of using the available resources. HTA is more common in higher-income economies, where it has been limited to incremental decisions – whether a proposed new technology is seen as a cost-effective addition to the existing set [4, 6, 38]. Rarely has it been used to derive the entire guaranteed package, although the various iterations of the Disease Control Priorities Project [39] sought to provide information that could be useful to this process in a range of different settings (see Chapter 15).

5.5.2 How to Purchase?

Who will be "contracted" to provide services? Contracting is the formalization of a relationship between actors [4, 40, 41]. Where purchasers buy the inputs to "make" health services, contracting (in the form of employment contracts) specifies the responsibilities of both employees and their employers (see Chapter 28).

Where purchasers buy health services as outputs (instead of service inputs) from service providers on behalf of their beneficiaries, they must negotiate with providers to agree on their mutual obligations. These obligations cover the terms and conditions of payment, which may also specify performance objectives, indicators, targets, data disclosure, and reporting requirements. They can also describe dispute resolution mechanisms [40].

Some countries require health insurance schemes to contract with all empaneled providers, while others allow selective contracting. In the former, the availability of services is determined by where the service providers are located. In the second case, the purchaser can influence not only where services are available, but also the range of services. They are also in a stronger position to negotiate prices and quality [4].

Provider Payment Frameworks

Payment frameworks consist of *payment methods* and *payment rates*, which together determine the size of the financial transfer from the purchaser to the provider(s). They also create financial incentives for different types of behavior by service providers. The challenge in strategic purchasing is to ensure that payment frameworks create the type of provider incentives that are consistent with the goal of moving more rapidly toward UHC.

The main component of a provider payment method is called the *base* or *primary method*. Table 5.2 describes the range of primary provider payment methods that can be observed across health systems, along with the *payment units* associated with each.

Only line-item budgets pay for inputs. The remainder pay for various types of outputs. Four of the output-based payment methods cover activities such as a care episode (global budgets, case-based payment, per diems, fee-for-service), and in two, people form the payment unit (capitation and global capitation).

The extent to which payments for different health services are aggregated across diseases and over time – called *bundling* – varies substantially. On the one hand, the two forms of capitation involve payment bundled for a range of health services over a period of time. On the other hand, fee-for-service pays for each individual service delivered at a particular point in time.

Each combination of payment method with payment unit offers different types of incentives for provider behavior. Some are considered in more detail later in Chapter 18. Focusing here on the examples of capitation and fee-for-service used above, capitation offers incentives for providers to optimize the mix of service outputs (e.g., prevention vs. treatment) and inputs (e.g., generic vs. branded medicines) assuming they can keep any revenues that remain at the end of the period. They also have an incentive to reduce the number of visits per patient, although it is sometimes argued that they have an incentive to under-service as well.

Table 5.2 Provider payment methods and the associated payment unit

Payment method	Payment unit	Examples
Line-item budget	Service inputs (e.g., salaries, medicines)	Predominant form of provider payment methods for public primary health care (PHC) providers in L&MICs.
Capitation	Person	Mostly used to pay for PHC, in some UMICs (e.g., Thailand) and many HICs blended with other provider payment methods.
Global capitation	Population	Became popular in the United States to pay for integrated care starting in the 1990s and again under the Affordable Care Act.
Global budgets	Services or service inputs	Typically used for hospitals – e.g., in China – where payment amount is fixed for a particular population and year, regardless of the services provided.
Case-based payment	Care episode	Typically used for hospitals in HICs, for example, diagnosis-related groups.
Per diems	Day	Typically used for hospitals, especially for some diseases and conditions that are not suitable for case-based payments, in particular mental diseases.
Fee-for-service	Services	Common as part of a blended payment framework for PHC and often for hospitals in LMICs.

Adapted from [4].

Fee-for-service offers incentives for overservicing in terms of the number of visits and investigations and procedures per patient. It does nothing to encourage optimization of the mix of service outputs. On the other hand, fee-for-service is the only payment method that does not deter providers from treating potentially high-cost patients. All the other payment methods, including both forms of capitation, incentivize providers to reject these patients if they can – a phenomenon referred to as "cherry-picking."

The final distinction to make between the primary payment methods is that some are *retrospective* and others are *prospective*. The activity-based payment methods of fee-for-service, per diem, and case-based payment are examples of the former: they reimburse providers ex-post (or retrospectively) for services that have already been delivered. Providers do not risk losing money in this relationship but are reimbursed for the services provided. On the other hand, line-item budgets, global budgets, and the two forms of capitation provide a fixed sum of money ex-ante (i.e., prospectively) for the providers to carry out the agreed services. The providers risk losing money if they have to provide services that exceed the payment received.

Payment rates are the amount the purchaser transfers to a provider for each payment unit. The process of setting payment rates – i.e., the *pricing* – is sometimes fixed administratively (e.g., governments specify prices), but more commonly is developed by negotiation. Pricing agreements with providers for purchasing service outputs, as opposed to those related to the purchase of inputs, usually also define whether the providers can levy additional OOP charges on patients beyond the payments made by the purchaser. Frequently, this type of price negotiation takes place in the context of known expenditure ceilings that the purchaser faces.

Purchasing can, therefore, be a relatively straightforward process, as in the case of line-item budgets used by many Ministries of Health. It can also, however, be extremely complex when purchasers seek to influence provider behavior using mixes of payment methods. Chapter 18 explores this further.

Demand-side financing. Rather than purchasing inputs or services on the supply side, an alternative is to provide funding to individuals or households to allow them to use the available health services, called *demand-side financing*. The most common forms are *cash transfers* and *vouchers*.

Cash transfers are sometimes provided *unconditionally* in the hope they will reduce the financial barriers (e.g., transport costs, OOPs) to accessing needed health services. More commonly in health, they are *conditional* on the recipient taking certain actions, such as obtaining childhood immunizations or seeking regular antenatal care [42, 43]. Vouchers work like money: they can be exchanged with a service provider in return for the specified health services – most frequently associated with maternal and child care [42, 43].

There is increasing evidence that demand-side financing increases coverage with selected health interventions, and in some cases improves health outcomes [42–44]. When combined with supply-side improvements they provide added benefits in terms of increased coverage [42]. On the other hand, despite decades of support, there is little evidence about their relative cost-effectiveness compared to supply-side interventions [42, 43]. Moreover, because they have been funded mainly through DAH, the question of how they can be incorporated into domestic health financing processes without displacing supply-side purchasing is yet to be resolved.

5.6 Health Financing Sustainability and Resilience

Emerging threats and shocks require health financing policymakers not only to develop the core functions of revenue generation, pooling, and purchasing described earlier, but also to have the capacity to undertake a health financing *resilience* and *sustainability* analysis [6, 45].

Health financing sustainability is the capacity to attain and maintain levels of health spending necessary to achieve the desired levels of health service coverage and financial protection in the medium term, taking into account possible sources of revenues in both the public and private sectors. The sustainability assessment considers how much is needed compared to what is available (*sufficiency*), what types of improvements in efficiency are possible, and the impact of emerging threats on the need to spend on health and the capacity to raise revenue.

Health financing resilience is the ability to absorb and respond to the less predictable shocks in both spending and revenue generation, such as pandemics. The onset of these shocks is sudden and difficult to predict. The ability to react rapidly and at scale – most importantly, the ability to immediately access contingency and emergency funding (with rules on its use in place as well as the capacity to deploy and use them effectively) – facilitates resilience to shocks that require increases in health spending. This is an emerging challenge for the development of high-performance health financing.

5.7 Conclusions

This chapter has described the core elements of high-performance health financing for UHC. Each of the three health financing functions must perform its role: revenue generation must obtain the desired prepaid and pooled resources; pooling must allow access to needed health services while spreading the financial risks of seeking care across the population; and purchasing must warrant that spending is efficient and equitable in ensuring that people obtain the services they need, of good quality, and with financial protection.

In addition, health financing decision-makers need to regularly reassess progress and risks, and make adjustments to emerging challenges that might affect health financing sufficiency and sustainability, as well as be prepared for possible shocks that might affect health financing resilience.

This, of course, requires considerable capacity and good governance in health financing, strongly associated with good governance in the health system as a whole. These questions are discussed in other chapters.

References

1. International Monetary Fund. Fault lines widen in the global recovery. 2021. www.imf.org/en/Publications/WEO/Issues/2021/07/27/world-economic-outlook-update-july-2021 (accessed December 29, 2021).

2. C. Kurowski, D. B. Evans, A. Tandon, et al. From double shock to double recovery: implications and options for health financing in the time of COVID-19. 2021. https://open knowledge.worldbank.org/handle/10986/35298 (accessed December 29, 2021).

3. C. Kurowski, D. B. Evans, A. Tandon, et al. From double shock to double recovery: implications and options for health financing in the time of COVID-19. Technical update – widening rifts. 2021. https://openknowledge.worldbank.org/bitstream/handle/10986/35298/From_Double_Shock_to_Double_Recovery%20

Revision%2020210916.pdf?sequence=7 (accessed December 29, 2021).

4. C. Kurowski, D. B. Evans, A. Irwin. et al. Scaling what works: convergence on health financing policies for universal health coverage in low- and middle-income countries (forthcoming).

5. World Health Organization. *The World Health Report 2010: Health Systems Financing – the Path to Universal Coverage.* Geneva, World Health Organization, 2010. https://apps.who.int/iris/handle/10665/44371 (accessed December 29, 2021).

6. World Bank. High-performance financing for universal health coverage: driving sustainable, inclusive growth in the 21st century. 2021. www.worldbank.org/en/topic/universalhealthcoverage/publication/high-performance-health-financing-for-universal-health-coverage-driving-sustainable-inclusive-growth-in-the-21st-century (accessed December 29, 2021).

7. World Health Organization. Financing for universal health coverage: dos and don'ts. 2019. https://p4h.world/en/news/financing-universal-health-coverage-dos-and-donts (accessed December 29, 2021).

8. P. Gottret, G. Schieber, H. R. Waters. Good practices in health financing: lessons from reforms in low and middle-income countries. 2008. https://openknowledge.worldbank.org/handle/10986/6442 (accessed December 29, 2021).

9. World Health Organization. Global health expenditure database. 2021. https://apps.who.int/nha/database (accessed November 29, 2021).

10. World Health Organization. Global expenditure on health: public spending on the rise? 2021. https://apps.who.int/iris/bitstream/handle/10665/350560/9789240041219-eng.pdf (accessed December 29, 2021).

11. N. Hamadeh, C. Van Rompaey, E. Metreau. New World Bank country classifications by income level: 2021–2022. 2021. https://datahelpdesk.worldbank.org/knowledgebase/articles/906519-world-bank-country-and-lending-groups (accessed December 29, 2021).

12. P. Saksena, J. Hsu, D. B. Evans. Financial risk protection and universal health coverage: evidence and measurement challenges. *PLoS Med* 2014; **11**(9): e1001701.

13. World Bank. First universal health coverage financing forum: raising funds for health. Background paper. 2016. https://thedocs.worldbank.org/en/doc/5d7befa83cbafe469a1f9a5d591eb443-0140062021/related/Background-Paper-First-Annual-UHC-Financing-Forum-DRM.pdf (accessed December 29, 2021).

14. A. Tandon, J. Cain, C. Kurowski, et al. Intertemporal dynamics of public financing for universal health coverage: accounting for fiscal space across countries. 2018. https://openknowledge.worldbank.org/handle/10986/31211 (accessed December 29, 2021).

15. A. Baum, A. Hodge, A. Mineshima, et al. Can they do it all? Fiscal space in low-income countries. IMF Working Paper. 2015. www.imf.org/en/Publications/WP/Issues/2017/05/05/Can-They-Do-It-All-Fiscal-Space-in-Low-Income-Countries-44889 (accessed December 29, 2021).

16. H. Barroy, S. Sparkes, E. Dale, et al. Can low- and middle-income countries increase domestic fiscal space for health: a mixed-methods approach to assess possible sources of expansion. *Health Syst Reform* 2018; **4**(3): 214–226.

17. Task Force on Fiscal Policy for Health. Health taxes to save lives: employing effective excise taxes on tobacco, alcohol, and sugary beverages. 2019. www.bloomberg.org/public-health/building-public-health-coalitions/task-force-on-fiscal-policy-for-health (accessed December 29, 2021).

18. World Health Organization. Health taxes: a primer for WHO staff. 2018. https://apps.who.int/iris/bitstream/handle/10665/275715/WHO-HGF-EAE-HealthTaxes-2018-Primer-eng.pdf?sequence=1&isAllowed=y/ (accessed December 29, 2021).

19. International Monetary Fund. Government financial statistics manual. 2001. www.imf.org/external/pubs/ft/gfs/manual/ (accessed December 29, 2021).

20. A. S. Yazbeck, W. D. Savedoff, W. C. Hsiao, et al. The case against labor-tax-financed social health insurance for low- and low-middle-income countries. *Health Aff (Millwood)* 2020; **39**(5): 892–897.

21. C. Cashin, S. Sparks D. Bloom. Earmarking for health: from theory to practice. Health Financing Working Paper 5. 2017. https://apps.who.int/iris/bitstream/handle/10665/255004/9789241512206-eng.pdf (accessed December 29, 2021).

22. C. Ozer, D. Bloom, A. M. Valle, et al. Health earmarks and health taxes: what do we know? 2020. https://openknowledge.worldbank.org/handle/10986/34947 (accessed December 29, 2021).

23. R. M. C. Kaboré, E. Solberg, M. Gates, et al. Financing the SDGs: mobilising and using domestic resources for health and human capital. *Lancet* 2018; **392**(10158): 1605–1607.

24. P. C. Smith, S. N. Witter. Risk pooling in health care financing: the implications for health system performance. Health, Nutrition and Population Discussion Paper. 2004. https://openknowledge.worldbank.org/handle/10986/13651 (accessed December 29, 2021).

25. E. Spaan, J. Mathijssen, N. Tromp, et al. The impact of health insurance in Africa and Asia: a systematic review. *Bull World Health Organ* 2012; **90**(9): 685–692.

26. I. Mathauer, P. Saksena, J. Kutzin. Pooling arrangements in health financing systems: a proposed classification. *Int J Equity Health* 2019; **18**(1): 198.

27. I. Mathauer, B. Mathivet, J. Kutzin. Community based health insurance: how can it contribute to progress towards UHC? Health Financing Policy Brief 3. 2017. www.who.int/publications/i/item/WHO-HIS-HGF-PolicyBrief-17.3 (accessed December 29, 2021).

28. I. Mathauer, J. Kutzin. Voluntary health insurance: its potentials and limits in moving towards UHC. 2017. www.who.int/publications/i/item/WHO-HIS-HGF-Health-Financing-Policy-Brief-18.5 (accessed December 29, 2021).

29. J. Kutzin. Why does public finance matter for UHC? 2016. www.who.int/health_financing/events/JosephKutzin-why-does-public-finance-matter-for-uhc.pdf (accessed December 29, 2021).

30. M. Geruso, T. J. Layton. Selection in health insurance markets and its policy remedies. *J Econ Perspect* 2017; **31**(4): 23–50.

31. S. Thomson, P. Jeurissen. Single vs multiple competing purchasing agencies: analysis of options for the health system in Cyprus. 2017. www.euro.who.int/__data/assets/pdf_file/0011/339662/WHO_005-Cyprus-SCREEN.pdf (accessed December 29, 2021).

32. A. Wagstaff, G. Flores, J. Hsu, et al. Progress on catastrophic health spending in 133 countries: a retrospective observational study. *Lancet Glob Health* 2018; **6**(2): e169–e179.

33. P. Saksena, J. Hsu, D. B. Evans. Financial risk protection and universal health coverage: evidence and measurement challenges. *PLoS Med* 2014; **11**(9): e1001701.

34. O. Smith, S. N. Nguyen. Getting better: improving health system outcomes in Europe and Central Asia. 2013. https://openknowledge.worldbank.org/handle/10986/13832 (accessed December 29, 2021).

35. World Health Organization. *Tracking Universal Health Coverage: 2021 Global Monitoring Report*. Geneva, World Health Organization, 2021. www.who.int/publications/i/item/9789240040618 (accessed December 29, 2021).

36. I. Mathauer, E. Dale, M. Jowett, et al. Purchasing health services for universal health coverage: how to make it more strategic? 2019. https://apps.who.int/iris/handle/10665/311387 (accessed December 29, 2021).

37. A. Fitzpatrick. The impact of public health sector stockouts on private sector prices and access to healthcare: evidence from the anti-malarial drug market. *J Health Econ* 2021; **81**: 102544.

38. World Bank. Second annual UHC financing forum greater efficiency for better

health and financial protection. 2017. https://thedocs.worldbank.org/en/doc/5d7befa83cbafe469a1f9a5d591eb443-0140062021/related/Background-Paper-Second-Annual-UHC-Financing-Forum-FORUM.pdf (accessed December 29, 2021).

39. Disease Control Priorities. Home page. 2018. http://dcp-3.org (accessed December 29, 2021).

40. J. Perrot. Different approaches to contracting in health systems. *Bull World Health Organ* 2006; **84**(11): 859–866.

41. S. Vong, J. Raven, D. Newlands. Internal contracting of health services in Cambodia: drivers for change and lessons learned after a decade of external contracting. *BMC Health Serv Res* 2018; **18**(1): 375.

42. T. Ensor, S. Tiwari. Demand-side financing in health in low-resource settings. In P. Revill, M. Suhrcke, R. Moreno-Serra, et al., eds., *Global Health Economics: Shaping Health Policy in Low- and Middle-Income Countries*. Singapore, World Scientific Publishing, 2020, pp. 217–237.

43. A. Glassman, D. Duran, L. Fleisher, et al. Impact of conditional cash transfers on maternal and newborn health. *J Health Popul Nutr* 2013; **31**(4 Suppl. 2): 48–66.

44. B. M. Hunter, S. Harrison, A. Portela, et al. The effects of cash transfers and vouchers on the use and quality of maternity care services: a systematic review. *PLoS One* 2017; **12**(3): e0173068.

45. S. Kwon, E. Kim. Sustainable health financing for COVID-19 preparedness and response in Asia and the Pacific. 2022. https://ideas.repec.org/a/bla/asiapr/v17y2022i1p140-156.html (accessed February 4, 2022).

Health Workforce in Low and Middle Income Countries
Concepts and Dynamics Unpacked

Christopher H. Herbst, Jenny X. Liu, and Francisca Ayodeji Akala

---

Key Messages

- Health workers are critical agents in a health system, and thus essential to the achievement of health-related Sustainable Development Goals (SDGs).
- Challenges related to their availability, distribution, and performance need to be understood and addressed.
- Evidence-based policy measures are required in the education sector and labor markets to have a sufficiently available, evenly distributed, and well-performing health workforce. Proper planning is also required to address issues related to the behaviors of health workers and institutions, and the factors that drive their behaviors.
- The behavior of the health workforce varies by country, cadre, and context, and therefore requires targeted and tailored solutions.
- Close collaboration between health, education, and finance is critical, given the multisectoral dimensions of the health workforce.

6.1 Background

A well-performing health workforce is critical for the success of any health system. In the broader sense, health workers are the clinical and nonclinical cadres working within and outside the health sector (e.g., technology, government administration) whose job is to protect and improve the health of their communities [1]. A higher density of health workers vis-à-vis the population has been shown to be associated with improved service coverage and health outcomes [2, 3]. However, improving service coverage is dependent on more than just the availability of health workers. The distribution and performance of health workers is equally important to service delivery and coverage goals. Ultimately, what is needed is a health workforce that can effectively respond to the shifting health priorities of the population, given evolving disease burden and epidemiology, and deploy technological resources rationally and cost-effectively. This requires taking into account education and health labor market dynamics, and ultimately matching the supply and skills of health workers to population needs, now and in the future [4].

The importance of the health workforce to the larger global development agenda is reflected in the SDG targets (Box 6.1). SDG 3, which aims to *ensure healthy lives and promote wellbeing for all at all ages*, calls for substantially improving the training, recruitment, and retention of health workers in low- and middle-income countries (L&MICs). This target aligns with the global recognition that countries across all income groups are

> **Box 6.1** 2030 SDGs and Targets for the Health Workforce
>
> **SDG 3. Ensure healthy lives and promote wellbeing for all at all ages.**
> *Target 3.8. Achieve universal health coverage*
> By 2030: *"Achieve universal health coverage, including financial risk protection, access to quality essential health care services and access to safe, effective, quality and affordable essential medicines and vaccines for all."*
> *Indicator 3.8.1* – Coverage of essential health services
> *Target 3.C. Increase health financing and support health workforce in developing countries*
> By 2030, *"Substantially increase health financing and the recruitment, development, training and retention of the health workforce in developing countries, especially in least developed countries and small island developing states."*
> *Indicator 3.C.1* – Health worker density and distribution

facing similar issues in delivering an evidence-based response to the challenges related to the availability, distribution, and performance of their health workforce [5]. Such challenges are especially severe among the least developed countries and small island states, which simultaneously bear the highest burden of disease and face the most barriers to mobilizing adequate resources.

A good understanding of the factors determining health workforce adequacy is critical to inform policy. This chapter provides an overview of some of the theories and evidence related to health workforce planning to better understand common workforce challenges prevalent in L&MICs. The adequacy or gap in the size and composition of the workforce is determined by the degree of alignment between the health needs of the population and the workforce supply. The latter is determined by the difference between the training of new workers and those exiting the workforce. More recently, policymakers have also emphasized labor market demand as a key determinant of the health workforce as it largely determines the fiscal capacity of a given health system to employ the desired workforce. A holistic consideration of these factors taken together, and how they may change in the future, can enable a more systematic, deliberate, and informed approach to evidence-based health workforce policymaking. While it is not feasible to address every aspect of health workforce availability, distribution, and performance comprehensively, more detailed information is available elsewhere in the literature [5, 6].

This chapter highlights some key considerations in identifying the desired health workforce, including critical workforce challenges and the factors that influence them. The chapter begins with a brief overview of some of the conceptual underpinnings for a deeper understanding of the workforce issues, followed by an overview of some of the specific L&MICs challenges and determinants related to workforce availability, distribution, and performance. A few theories and frameworks, which can be used to diagnose existing challenges in a more systematic fashion, are highlighted.

6.2 Conceptual Overview

This section presents a few conceptual underpinnings that explain health workforce availability, distribution, and performance, which can be used to assess and identify policy solutions for the health workforce challenges in L&MICs.

6.2.1 Health Workers as Agents of the Public Sector

Classical theory holds that health workers are where they are because of central-level planning efforts [7]. In this perspective, health workers are government agents with limited choice, who are assigned to a specific position or workplace as determined by the planning efforts of the ministries and agencies that employ them. Centralized regulations and policies are closely aligned with planning efforts [5, 6]. This early conception of workforce planning reflects contexts in which most health workers were employed as civil servants in the predominant public sector. Government actions in terms of planning, recruitment, and renumeration would thus be the decisive factors in determining where health workers would ultimately be placed. Such focus on central health workforce planning, however, neglects other important factors that influence human resource adequacy and capacity, such as the role of the private sector marketplace for health care, labor market dynamics and behavior, and the preferences of health workers that ultimately determine the availability, distribution, and performance of the health workforce [4, 5, 8].

6.2.2 Health Workers as Dynamic Agents within Markets

Today, it is widely accepted that the health workforce needs to be analyzed and understood in the larger context of education and health labor markets [4–6]. The 2006 *World Health Report* [1] was critical in expanding the workforce narrative by including the influence of markets in shaping the availability, distribution, and performance of the health workforce. Many L&MICs were experiencing a proliferation of their private sectors for both health professionals' education and health service delivery, and increasing numbers of health workers in L&MICs were migrating for education and work opportunities abroad. Health workers were no longer considered stagnant agents of the public sector who could simply be deployed, managed, and controlled. Instead, health workers were increasingly seen as agents functioning within dynamic global, national, and subnational labor markets, with choices regarding where they wished to work – whether at home or abroad, in the public or the private sector, at the primary or hospital level, and in remote or urban areas.

The critical importance of the behavior of both health workers and institutions in determining the availability, distribution, and performance is illustrated in Figure 6.1. In contexts with limited government intervention, health workers and the institutions that employ them determine their own decisions. That is to say, the health worker needs to be willing to work or study at the institution, while the institution in turn needs to recruit these workers. Furthermore, to maximize their performance, health workers must be willing to invest effort, be present, and be productive. Health workers' willingness to maximize performance is further reinforced by the willingness of employers to motivate health workers by supporting them, providing necessary equipment and supplies, and by holding workers accountable for their actions.

Neoclassical wage theory suggests that decisions taken by individual workers and institutions – the economic actors within a labor market are driven largely by the capacity of the institutions, the probability of finding employment, and the preferences of individuals [9, 10]. In this sense, it has been argued that a health worker will prefer or accept a particular job if the benefits of doing so outweigh the opportunity cost or the potential gain from an alternative option [11]. The same could be said for the employing institutions and their decisions to accept or recruit a particular health worker in a given labor market or labor submarket (e.g., within a geographic area, specific cadre, or type of position).

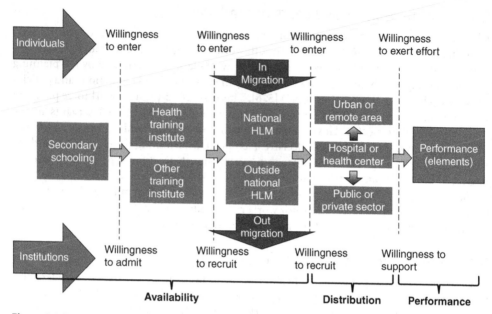

Figure 6.1 Decision-making of individuals and institutions influence health workers' labor market (HLM) outcomes.

Labor market economic theory draws on the above understanding and suggests that uptake of a particular job in that market, whether for example rural or urban, private or public, national or international, is determined by two forces – labor market *supply* and labor market *demand* [5, 6, 12]. Health worker labor market *supply* is defined as the willingness and ability of health workers to take on a particular job. Health worker labor market *demand* reflects the willingness and capacity of *employers* to recruit health workers, which in turn is influenced by the preferences of individual consumers for the amount and types of health services they demand. The worker here refers to anyone who wishes to offer their services for compensation while the employer refers to any entity or organization that needs an individual to do a specific job (regardless of sector). Labor market demand and supply are influenced to a great extent by the wage or level of compensation offered to the health worker.

Theoretically, a well-functioning labor market assumes that workers can freely move to where their services or skills are demanded and in response to the wages or compensation offered. This follows from standard assumptions of perfect competition in the labor market in which there are numerous employers and workers, all of whom are well informed of their choices. Wages are assumed to be fully responsive to a worker's productivity (e.g., the quantity and quality of services provided), which may go up or down. It is further assumed that employers can hire and dismiss workers, and that workers can freely decide to take on or leave a job if a better employer or job is found. Different health workers with different social and economic characteristics (e.g., gender, age, rural background, training experience) have been shown to respond differently to different levels of compensation.

6.2.3 The Imperfection of Health Labor Markets

While it is desirable for a health worker labor market to be in equilibrium, meaning that willingness to work is matched by the willingness to employ, most labor markets are in disequilibrium – in aggregate and/or in submarkets. A situation where there is more labor market supply than demand can result in health workers being unemployed. This kind of situation is more common in urban locations or at the hospital level in many L&MICs, where there is limited absorptive capacity to employ the required health workers [6]. Health workers may thus have part-time work arrangements, be employed outside the labor market of choice (for example in the private sector), or leave the health sector altogether. Conversely, a situation where there is more demand than there is supply can result in a shortage, leaving available resources idle. In such a situation, there are more funded job vacancies than health workers willing or available to fill these vacancies at the wage level offered – this is particularly common in rural areas and in primary care. When the level of resources an employer is willing and able to offer matches the supply of the workers, the market is said to be in equilibrium. Achieving equilibrium prevents waste of financial and human resources, and maximizes efficiency from an economic perspective; however, equilibrium in the health labor market is seldom found.

Figure 6.2 illustrates the unemployment (surplus) as well as the shortage situation. Notwithstanding that there can be several determinants of employment, we focus on compensation or wages in this example to illustrate potential market dynamics. In this figure, the horizontal axis represents the number of workers and the vertical axis the level of compensation. The downward sloping curve (from left to right) indicates that the number of workers that employers demand tends to be lower at higher compensation levels. The upward sloping supply curve indicates that more workers are willing to provide their labor at increasingly higher levels of compensation. The *unemployment situation (surplus)* is often associated with a relatively higher level of compensation, referred to as *CompU*. This means that there are more individuals willing to supply their services (where the vertical dotted line hits the horizontal axis) than there

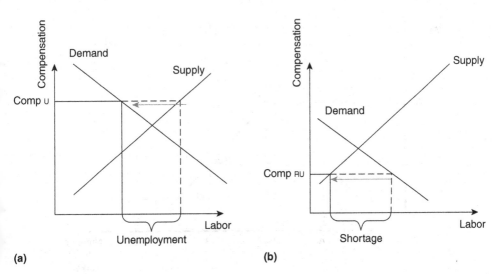

(a)   **(b)**

Figure 6.2 Labor markets in disequilibrium resulting in (a) unemployment (surplus) and (b) shortage. Adapted from [12].

are positions the employers are willing to pay for (where the vertical solid line hits the horizontal axis). This gap is then the number of workers who are not able to be employed, yielding a *surplus* of workers. Conversely, *a worker shortage* is often associated with lower levels of compensation, referred to as *CompRU*, for which the number of workers willing to supply their labor (where the solid vertical line hits the horizontal axis) is relatively few compared to the number of workers that employers want to hire (where the dotted vertical line hits the horizontal axis). Because more workers are demanded than there are available to be employed, a shortage results in this market.

6.2.4 Planning for Needs Is Important

While one priority of policymakers is to help shape the labor market in a way that moves supply and demand toward equilibrium, the ultimate goal is to develop a workforce that meets population needs. In an unemployment situation, a key policy intervention could be to increase the overall absorptive capacity to employ more health workers, for example. Alternatively, in a shortage situation, an intervention could be to introduce incentives – monetary (e.g., bonuses, housing allowances) or nonmonetary (e.g., mentorship, recognition and prestige, career acceleration) – that motivate workers to take a job in the health sector. Even as the market can be moved toward equilibrium, thereby minimizing resource inefficiency and waste, the number of health workers that correspond to a labor market in equilibrium might not meet the service delivery and epidemiological needs of the health system. The need for health workers is not dependent on compensation or the available pool of workers. Rather, it is mainly determined by what health services can be delivered and how to address the health issues prioritized by policymakers.

In Figure 6.3, a labor market in a shortage situation is depicted alongside a vertical line (C) depicting the level of health workers needed for the population. Continuing with our example of the influences of wages on the labor market dynamics, in this particular situation compensation levels are relatively low (W_L), and the number of workers demanded (B) exceeds the

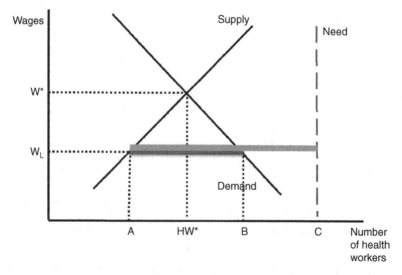

Figure 6.3 Health worker need vis-à-vis market demand and supply. Adapted from [13].

number supplied (A), yielding a *demand-based shortage* ($B - A$). Only A workers can be hired, which is less than the number of workers HW^* that would be otherwise hired if wage compensation levels were optimal (W^*) and equilibrium was achieved. In addition, the level of health workers needed (C) exceeds the number supplied (A), yielding a *need-based shortage* ($C - A$). The existence of both types of shortages indicates that, on the one hand, there is a lack of financial resources to increase compensation that would attract more workers. On the other hand, even if compensation were set at the market optimum (W^*), the number of workers employed is insufficient to meet the needs. Consequently, workforce policies are required not only to shape market dynamics to attract more workers given current wage–quantity trade-offs, but also to increasingly shift both demand and supply curves outward (to the right in this scenario) to maximize available resources and meet health needs.

6.2.5 Needs-Based Estimates Are Highly Context-Dependent

For country-level health workforce planning purposes, needs estimates should be adapted to country-specific contexts. Common global benchmarks of health worker densities to meet health needs have been estimated at 2.28 [1] and 4.5 [4] health workers (physicians, nurses, and midwives) per 1,000 population. These benchmarks are useful for understanding global and regional workforce adequacy. However, neither were developed for detailed country-level workforce planning purposes. Tailored approaches to modeling and calculating needs should be done separately for country-level workforce planning. The organization of health systems, labor market dynamics, population demographics, and disease burdens are all factors that critically determine how health services are delivered, to which people, and for what conditions, and can vary widely.

6.2.6 Workforce Performance as a Multidimensional Concept

Finally, workforce planners need to consider health workforce performance, including productivity and quality. According to health worker labor market economic theory, performance can manifest in multiple ways. One performance dimension involves increasing productivity, which effectively increases workforce supply at any given level of wage (i.e., delivering more services per worker), and would shift the labor supply curve outward to the right in Figure 6.3. Another dimension of performance involves the quality of services, which may or may not affect the quantity of services (for example, more time spent per patient reduces total patients served but may improve diagnostic and treatment accuracy). Quality can be measured in a variety of ways, as described in Chapter 26. Given the performance trade-offs with a focus on quantity or quality, any performance monitoring and accounting system should be carefully crafted to strike an appropriate balance, aligned with overarching health system goals and worker motivations.

Several frameworks have been developed to understand the structural and behavioral underpinnings of health worker performance. A simple framework by Leonard et al. is depicted in Figure 6.4 [14]. This framework considers workforce performance to be a function of health workers' *capacity* and *effort*, which are in turn influenced by workers' education, their educational environment and experience, the workplace environment and related policies, and motivational elements. This framework also highlights the importance of decision-making and behavior of health workers and employers.

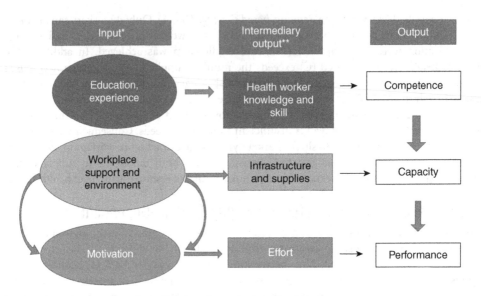

Figure 6.4 Performance unpacked: a function of capacity and effort [14].

6.3 Workforce Availability

The availability of health workers is highly variable among countries, and in L&MICs the number of trained health workers available is often far below the recommended global thresholds of 2.3–4.5 per 1,000 population [1, 4]. Figure 6.5 depicts this wide variation across a selected number of countries for doctors, nurses, and midwives. The lowest densities are generally found in lower income countries, and the highest in upper income countries. For example, whereas Senegal (a low income country) has a density of 0.3 doctors, nurses, and midwives per 1,000 population, France (a high-income country) has 13.7 per 1,000 population. Generally, research has shown a strong positive correlation between national income and health expenditure, and health workforce density [15–17].

Recent modeling has shown that the global workforce shortage, particularly in L&MICs, is expected to worsen as demand and need for health services grow with changing disease burdens and the aging of populations. A 2030 projection of the global supply of doctors, nurses, and midwives for 165 countries revealed that, compared to the 4.45 per 1,000 benchmark, L&MICs are likely to experience a substantial shortage of workers, with supplies insufficient to meet the need (Figure 6.6) [19]. This prediction contrasts with the situation in high- and upper middle-income countries, for which the health workforce density currently exceeds the global benchmark as a whole.[1] The health worker density in these countries is expected to increase further by 2030. This global picture, however, masks shortages of cadres of health workers within some countries. Well-trained community health workers, skilled

---

[1] There are some individual countries in high and upper middle-income countries that also have a current shortage of health workers to meet the estimated global need benchmark. However, estimates aggregated by income group show that the problem of health worker shortages in high- and upper middle-income countries is very small compared to the health worker shortages projected for L&MICs.

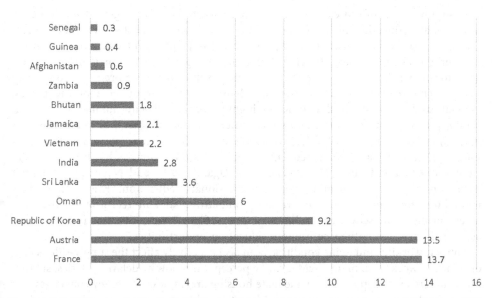

Figure 6.5 Health worker densities in selected low-, middle-, and high-income countries, per 1,000 population [18].

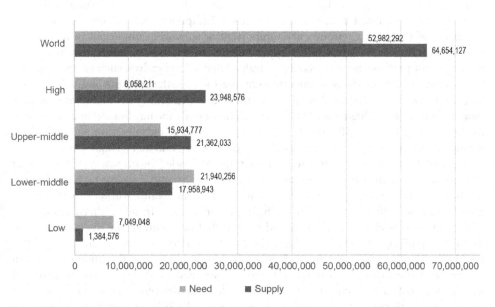

Figure 6.6 The projected health workforce needs-based shortage in 2030, by income group (using the benchmark of 4.45 health workers per 1,000 population). Adapted from [19].

birth attendants, and family practitioners – all critical for the scaling up of preventive and primary care – are often in short supply [4]. A shortage of specialists is also an issue, as is the limited capacity to train specialists in L&MICs. The dearth of faculty able to run specialist and subspecialist programs in many L&MICs precludes the delivery of effective preservice and postgraduate education [20].

A supply deficit of critical workers can be linked to key challenges related to health professionals' education [4]. The inadequate financial, physical, technical, and organizational capacity of education institutions can limit entry and exacerbate drop-out rates among health science students. Public financing for education is often limited, and alternative financing options are often insufficiently explored or considered feasible. The 2012 Sub-Saharan African Medical School Study, one of the biggest regional studies on medical education, highlighted insufficient number of schools, faculty, practical training sites, and study materials, among others, as key bottlenecks for scaling the health workforce [2]. Furthermore, insufficient postgraduate educational opportunities are also a frequent driver for outmigration, as has been shown in countries such as Malawi [21], Poland [22], Uganda [23], and Nepal [24]. In their discussion paper on reforming health professionals' education, Evans et al. [20] highlighted the need for progressive and competitive student recruitment, the need to reform the scale, scope, and value for money of preservice educational institutions, and the need to strengthen continuous education opportunities.

Sub-par working and living conditions can also negatively affect the supply-side behavior of health workers in many L&MICs. The perception of low or delayed salaries, sub-par infrastructure and supplies, and inadequate housing are a few of the many challenges that deter individuals from working in the health sector. Sub-par working and living conditions lead to low levels of recruitment, high turnover, and attrition out of the health care market or health sector altogether. In a study of medical students in six sub-Saharan African countries, 90–95% listed better access to medical equipment and technology and better regulation of the work environment as important or somewhat important in influencing their intention to leave Africa [25]. Supply-side behavior can vary among health workers with different profiles and socioeconomic traits. Higher-level cadres, such as doctors, have been found to be more likely to migrate to markets with better working and living conditions than lower-level cadres [26]. In Nepal, the odds of intending to practice abroad were more than three times higher for those in the highest family income bracket as compared to the lowest [24]. Other traits linked to a larger likelihood of outmigration abroad include having studied abroad [27], having family abroad [28, 29], and being single [30].

Limited fiscal capacity can lead to a shortage of funded positions, and can further exacerbate a health worker shortage. If public or private employers have limited funding to employ workers, it will become difficult for health workers to find a job even if they are willing to work in the health labor market. In our stylized example of a labor market in Figure 6.3, this would be reflected in a shift in the demand curve to the left, resulting in fewer workers being demanded at any given wage. Such a situation is often prevalent in contexts where the public sector dominates the health system, and the private sector remains underdeveloped or disorganized. Similarly, if health care institutions choose to employ workers to deliver services which are not considered a priority but for which consumers are willing to pay, such as cosmetic or selective surgery, workers are effectively diverted away from the delivery of priority health services, creating a shortage of workers to address pressing population needs (e.g., safe deliveries). Ensuring adequate financial capacity to employ and retain health workers within the public and private sectors, and aligning it with population health goals, is critical and too often left out in planning efforts.

6.4 Workforce Distribution

In many L&MICs contexts, much of the higher level and professionally trained workforce tends to be concentrated in urban locations and tertiary care facilities. This is particularly troubling in contexts with large rural and/or poor populations who may simultaneously suffer from higher disease burdens and face the greatest barriers to accessing services. Hence, maldistribution of the health workforce exacerbates existing health inequities. The proportion of the population that lacks access to care due to health worker shortages has been argued to be substantially larger in rural areas than in urban areas (Figure 6.7). A shortage of qualified health workers leaves populations with suboptimal care or without care altogether. Without well-trained formal providers, including allied health professionals and/or community health workers (CHWs) to deliver the full scope of required services, populations typically turn to more accessible untrained and informal service providers, such as street vendors and drug shops, raising questions about the quality of care [31].

Education-related factors influence the supply-side behavior of health workers and contribute to a maldistributed workforce. The financing and location of health training institutions, their recruitment and admissions process, the type of curricula offered, and their training strategies (including rural/urban exposure) influence job location preferences among their graduates. Individuals from, trained in, and trained for rural areas, for instance, have been found to be more likely to work in rural areas in some contexts [33]. A study of medical students in Kenya found that students with rural backgrounds were 2.5 times more likely to practice in rural areas than students with urban origins [27]. In the United States, medical students who felt better prepared in community medicine were found to be more likely to have a preference for rural areas [34]. Selected socioeconomic traits can also influence supply-side preferences for a particular post. Often, lower-level cadres, such as

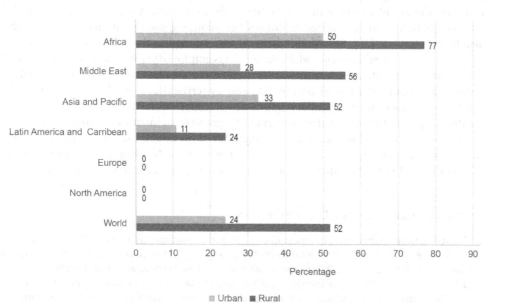

Figure 6.7 Rural/urban populations without access to health care due to health worker shortage (percentages). Adapted from [32].

CHWs or auxiliary cadres and nurses are more likely to work in rural areas than are higher-level cadres, such as physicians or specialists [5]. In Ghana, rural preference of physicians was associated with their parents having lower professional and education status, which suggests that these professionals were similarly from poorer origins [35]. Despite such findings, health professional education often focuses on medical and specialist education, and continues to recruit from and be targeted toward urban elites, and offered in urban areas with little exposure to rural populations or primary care facilities during the course of study [20].

Relatedly, variations in working and living conditions within local health labor markets also contribute to where health workers prefer to work. Rural or remote areas in many L&MICs are often characterized by limited additional income-generating opportunities, inadequate management, challenges related to infrastructure and supplies, and a lack of good housing and schooling for children. Notwithstanding, planners can and should take these factors into account. Discrete choice experiments (Box 6.2), a method for eliciting stated preferences across different choice options, can be used to identify the relative importance of specific job attributes that can increase the likelihood of health workers taking up a particular post. The discrete choice experiment of physicians in Ethiopia, for example, found that a combination of basic housing and equipment can substantially increase the probability of taking up a rural job and offset the need for increasing wages (Figure 6.8) [36]. In Laos, nursing students in rural areas were most willing to give up salary in exchange for permanent job placement alongside housing and transportation provisions [37].

In some contexts, the financing capacity to hire and recruit workers in particular submarkets may be weak and can contribute to an uneven workforce distribution [35]. This can occur in situations where financial and management autonomy in the public sector is low, the private sector is underdeveloped, and health insurance coverage or the population's ability to pay is low. Such a situation is more common in remote areas and can limit the extent to which there is sufficient funding and autonomy to recruit health workers there. Highly centralized health worker financing and recruitment contexts can also be problematic [39]. Situations where salaries are tied to the health worker (that is, salaries follow the health worker wherever he/she is employed) rather than the institutions that employ them (that is, health workers follow the salaries offered) are problematic because the money often flows into urban areas or tertiary-level employment instead of flowing into remote areas or primary care facilities. Policymakers must be cognizant of the positive impacts of decentralizing financing, the granting of institutional autonomy, and the scaling up of health insurance coverage, for achieving a locally adequate health workforce. They should be vigilant for relevant and workable solutions to address labor market demand issues to reduce resource waste and to maximize efficiency and results.

Box 6.2 What Is a Discrete Choice Experiment?

A discrete choice experiment is a quantitative method increasingly used in health care to elicit preferences from participants without directly asking them to state their preferred options. The participants are typically presented with a series of alternative scenarios containing a number of variables or "attributes," each of which may have a number of variations or "levels." Participants are asked to state their preferred choice between two or three competing scenarios, each of which consists of a combination of these attributes/levels [38].

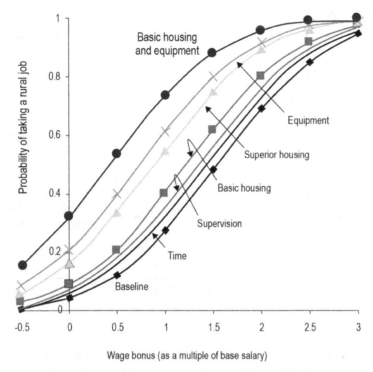

Figure 6.8 Discrete choice experiment to identify incentives needed to shift workers from urban to rural areas [36].

6.5 Workforce Performance

Measuring and identifying the factors that undermine performance are common challenges for health planners. For example, is performance compromised because of lack of skills and competencies, or a lack of equipment and supplies, or because of low motivation, leading to high levels of absenteeism and/or low productivity? These problems require different policy interventions. Identifying the causes of low health worker performance against locally defined performance targets can be effective.

Leonard et al. developed a three-gap performance framework to help identify, measure, and address some of the factors affecting performance [14]. This framework conceptualizes three main performance gaps that can be measured quantitatively (Figure 6.9):

1. the gap between what health workers know (competence) and how they perform (observed performance);
2. the gap between what health workers know (competence) and can actually do (having equipment and supplies); and
3. the gap between what they can do (competence and equipment and supplies) and actually do (the extent to which they apply themselves).

As shown for countries like Tanzania, quantitative data can be collected to measure and address each performance gap using a combination of vignette and direct observation techniques [14]. Attention can then be focused on addressing the biggest gap.

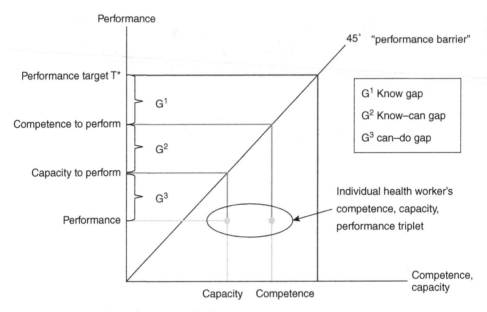

Figure 6.9 Measuring the performance gap [14].

Limited competency resulting from weaknesses in preservice and in-service education in L&MICs are common factors affecting workforce performance. Such weaknesses are related to insufficient financing and inadequate physical, technical, and organizational capacity of preservice institutions (see the discussion above). These translate into key challenges that affect the skills and competencies of health workers, including: the scarcity of skilled teaching faculties, the absence of formalized and accredited residency programs, inadequate continued professional development opportunities, outdated curricula and training strategies, and inadequately supervised practice experience at clinical training sites [20]. Planners do not always consider the importance of a strong regulatory framework for pre- and in-service education, including mechanisms for accreditation, licensing and certification, and renewal [20]. L&MICs often lack the resources to effectively enforce regulations, even if they exist. The private sector for educating health professionals is growing quickly in many L&MICs, and the lack of standards and effective regulatory oversight means that the quality of training is often inadequate, leading to poor-quality health service provision. Planners and policymakers need to work closely with the education sector to address ongoing education- and training-related weaknesses in order to optimize health workers' performance.

Inadequate working environments can be equally detrimental to health workers' performance. While planners and professional associations often turn to education-related solutions to improve workforce performance, other factors may be even more important to address. A quantitative measurement of the "know–can" gap in Tanzania, for instance, revealed that the performance score of health workers did not increase with greater competency scores (Figure 6.10). In addition to lack of motivation and inadequate effort (discussed below), insufficient equipment and supplies are common barriers to optimal performance in L&MICs, even when skills and competencies are appropriate. Without

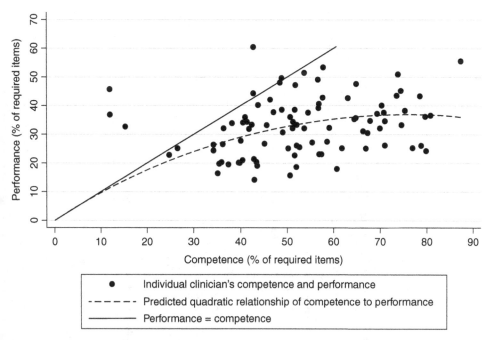

Figure 6.10 Know–can gap: application in Tanzania shows that factors other than education (e.g., competence) affect health worker performance [14].

proper equipment, a well-functioning supply chain, including water, tools, and medicines, health workers are challenged to perform satisfactorily. Sufficient funding and management capacity at national, subnational, and facility levels are key aspects in this regard.

Low levels of productivity and absenteeism can result from perceptions of low or delayed salaries; lack of continuing education opportunities, career advancement, recognition of achievements, or incentives; and limited accountability. Unannounced visits made to health facilities showed absenteeism rates of 35% in Bangladesh, 37% in Uganda, and 40% in India and Peru [40]. Often absenteeism in the public sector is linked to health workers pursuing additional income-generating practices in the private sector. Dual practice or "moonlighting" in the private sector is widespread globally, and particularly prevalent among higher-level cadres such as physicians (see Chapter 27) [41]. While additional income generation is the main motivation, even workers intrinsically motivated toward patient care may become despondent under suboptimal working conditions. Despite perceptions of low salaries, often driven by professional associations, the salaries of health workers in some countries can be relatively high when compared to their productivity levels. Consultations per provider can vary greatly. Overall, adequately designed and tailored accountability and performance management strategies, including ones that contain performance incentives for health workers, are often lacking.

Table 6.1 summarizes the factors that influence health workforce availability, distribution, and performance.

Table 6.1 Summary of factors that influence health workforce availability, distribution, and performance

- **Workforce availability**
  - Availability of health workers globally is highly variable, and in L&MICs is often far below the 2.3–4.5 per 1,000 population global thresholds and country-specific targets.
  - The global workforce shortage in L&MICs is expected to worsen in the future as demand and need for health services grow with changing disease burdens and aging populations.
  - Supply deficit of critical workers can be linked to key challenges related to health professionals' education.
  - Suboptimal working and living conditions negatively affect the supply-side behavior of health workers in many L&MICs.
  - Fiscal shortcomings can lead to a shortage of funded job posts and can further exacerbate a health worker shortage.

- **Workforce distribution**
  - Higher-level and professionally trained workforce in many L&MICs tend to be concentrated in urban locations and tertiary care facilities.
  - Education-related factors influencing supply-side behavior of health workers contribute to a maldistributed workforce.
  - Variations in working and living conditions within local health labor markets contribute to distributional inequities and supply-side behavior among health workers.
  - Limited financing capacity to hire and recruit workers in particular submarkets can contribute to an uneven workforce distribution.

- **Workforce performance**
  - Causes of low health worker performance should be assessed against locally defined performance targets.
  - A three-gap performance framework (related to knowledge, capacity, and actual performance) can identify, measure, and address the factors affecting performance.
  - Weaknesses in preservice and in-service education in L&MICs are common factors affecting workforce performance.
  - Inadequate working environment can be equally detrimental to health workers' performance.

6.6 Conclusion

This chapter provided a brief overview of some of the underlying theories and evidence to better comprehend key health workforce challenges prevalent in L&MICs. Some of the conceptual underpinnings for a deeper understanding of the workforce issues, followed by a synopsis of specific L&MICs challenges and determinants related to workforce availability, distribution, and performance to improve service delivery and coverage goals were discussed. Ultimately the desired health workforce should be able to effectively respond to the shifting health priorities of the population, given evolving disease burden and epidemiology. This requires taking into account education and health labor market dynamics – influencing the behavior of health workers and institutions – and ultimately effectively matching the supply and skills of health workers to population needs, now and in the future.

References

1. World Health Organization. *The World Health Report 2006: Working Together for Health*. Geneva, World Health Organization, 2006. www.who.int/whr/2006/en/ (accessed December 15, 2020).

2. L. Chen, T. Evans, S. Anand, et al. Human resources for health: overcoming the crisis. *Lancet* 2004; **364**(9449): 1984–1990.

3. S. Anand, T. Bärnighausen. Human resources and health outcomes: cross-country econometric study. *Lancet* 2004; **364**(9445): 1603–1609.

4. World Health Organization. *Global Strategy on Human Resources for Health: Workforce 2030*. Geneva, World Health Organization, 2016. www.who.int/hrh/resources/pub_glob strathrh-2030/en/ (accessed December 18, 2020).

5. R. M. Scheffler, C. H. Herbst, C. Lemiere, et al. *Health Labor Market Analyses in Low- and Middle-Income Countries: An Evidence-Based Approach*. Washington, DC, World Bank, 2016.

6. T. A. Ghebreyesus, R. M. Scheffler, A. L. Soucat. Labor market for health workers in Africa: new look at the crisis. 2013. https://openknowledge.worldbank.org/handle/10986/13824 (accessed November 12, 2020).

7. A. Smith, E. Cannan, M. Lerner. *An Inquiry into the Nature and Causes of the Wealth of Nations*. New York, The Modern Library, 1937.

8. B. McPake, A. Maeda, E. C. Araújo, et al. Why do health labour market forces matter? *Bull World Health Organ* 2013; **91**: 841–846.

9. U. Lehmann, M. Dieleman, T. Martineau. Staffing remote rural areas in middle- and low-income countries: a literature review of attraction and retention. *BMC Health Serv Res* 2008; **8**(1): 1–10.

10. A. Marshall. *Principles of Economics*. London, Macmillan, 1890.

11. C. Hongoro, C. Norman, Health workers: building and motivating the workforce. In D. T. Jamison, J. G. Breman, A. R. Measham, et al., eds., *Disease Control Priorities in Developing Countries*, 2nd ed. New York, Oxford University Press, 2006.

12. M. Andalón, G. Fields. A labor market approach to the crisis of health care professionals in Africa. 2011. www.econstor.eu/bitstream/10419/46097/1/662489454.pdf (accessed December 11, 2020).

13. T. Bruckner, J. Liu, R. M. Scheffler. Demand-based and needs-based forecasts for health workers. In R. M. Scheffler, C. H. Herbst, C. Lemiere, et al. eds., *Health Labor Market Analyses in Low- and Middle-Income Countries: An Evidence-Based Approach. Directions in Development*. Washington, DC, World Bank, 2016.

14. K. L. Leonard, M. C. Masatu, C. H. Herbst, et al. The systematic assessment of health worker performance: a framework for analysis and its application in Tanzania. 2015. https://openknowledge

.worldbank.org/handle/10986/24076 (accessed December 18, 2020).

15. R. A. Cooper, T. E. Getzen, P. Laud. Economic expansion is a major determinant of physician supply and utilization. *Health Serv Res* 2003; **38**(2): 675–696.

16. T. E. Getzen. Macro forecasting of national health expenditures. *Adv Health Econ Health Serv Res* 1990; **11**: 27–48.

17. J. P. Newhouse. Medical-care expenditure: a cross-national survey. *J Hum Resour* 1977; **12**(1): 115–125.

18. World Health Organization. Skilled health personnel: data by country. 2021. https://apps.who.int/gho/data/view.main.HWF10v (accessed June 17, 2021).

19. J. X. Liu, Y. Goryakin, A. Maeda, et al. Global health workforce labor market projections for 2030. *Hum Resour Health* 2017; **15**(1): 11.

20. T. Evans, E. C. Araujo, C. H. Herbst, et al. Addressing the challenges of health professional education: opportunities to accelerate progress towards universal health coverage. 2016. https://interprofessional.global/wp-content/uploads/2019/11/WISH-2016-Health-Professional-Education-Report-ADDRESSING-THE-CHALLENGES-OF-HEALTH-PROFESSIONAL-EDUCATION-OPPORTUNITIES-TO-ACCELERATE-PROGRESS-TOWARDS-UNIVERSAL-HEALTH-COVERAGE.pdf (accessed December 14, 2020).

21. N. Bailey, K. L. Mandeville, T. Rhodes, et al. Postgraduate career intentions of medical students and recent graduates in Malawi: a qualitative interview study. *BMC Med Educ* 2012; **12**: 87.

22. K. Krajewski-Siuda, A. Szromek, P. Romaniuk, et al. Emigration preferences and plans among medical students in Poland. *Hum Resour Health* 2012; **10**: 8.

23. S. Kizito, D. Mukunya, J. Nakitende, et al. Career intentions of final year medical students in Uganda after graduating: the burden of brain drain. *BMC Med Educ* 2015; **15**: 122.

24. I. Huntington, S. Shrestha, N. G. Reich, et al. Career intentions of medical students in the setting of Nepal's rapidly expanding private medical education system. *Health Policy Plan* 2012; **27**(5): 417–428.

25. V. C. Burch, D. McKinley, J. van Wyk, et al. Career intentions of medical students trained in six sub-Saharan African countries. *Educ Health (Abingdon)* 2011; **24**(3): 614.

26. P. Serneels, J. G. Montalvo, G. Pettersson, et al. Who wants to work in a rural health post? The role of intrinsic motivation, rural background and faith-based institutions in Ethiopia and Rwanda. *Bull World Health Organ* 2010; **88**(5): 342–349.

27. H. Dossajee, N. Obonyo, S. M. Ahmed. Career preferences of final year medical students at a medical school in Kenya: a cross sectional study. *BMC Med Educ* 2016; **16**: 5.

28. E. A. Akl, N. Maroun, S. Major, et al. Why are you draining your brain? Factors underlying decisions of graduating Lebanese medical students to migrate. *Soc Sci Med* 2007; **64**(6): 1278–1284.

29. M. M. Santric-Milicevic, Z. J. Terzic-Supic, B. R. Matejic, et al. First- and fifth-year medical students' intention for emigration and practice abroad: a case study of Serbia. *Health Policy* 2014; **118**(2): 173–183.

30. T. Lievens, P. Serneels, J. D. Butera, et al. *Diversity in Career Preferences of Future Health Workers in Rwanda: Where, Why, and for How Much?* Washington, DC, World Bank, 2010.

31. M. Sudhinaraset, M. Ingram, H. K. Lofthouse, et al. What is the role of informal healthcare providers in developing countries? A systematic review. *PLoS One* 2013; **8**(2): e54978.

32. X. Scheil-Adlung. Global evidence on inequities in rural health protection: new data on rural deficits in health coverage for 174 countries. 2015. https://reliefweb.int/report/world/global-evidence-inequities-rural-health-protection-new-data-rural-deficits-health (accessed December 28, 2020).

33. R. Strasser, A. J. Neusy. Context counts: training health workers in and for rural and remote areas. *Bull World Health Organ* 2010; **88**: 777–782.

34. I. M. Xierali, R. Maeshiro, S. Johnson, et al. Public health and community medicine instruction and physician practice location. *Am J Prev Med* 2014; **47**(5 Suppl. 3): S297–S300.

35. P. Agyei-Baffour, S. R. Kotha, J. C. Johnson, et al. Willingness to work in rural areas and the role of intrinsic versus extrinsic professional motivations: a survey of medical students in Ghana. *BMC Med Educ* 2011; **11**: 56.

36. W. Jack, J. De Laat, K. Hanson, et al., Incentives and dynamics in the Ethiopian health worker labor market. 2010. https://openknowledge.worldbank.org/handle/10986/5951 (accessed December 22, 2020).

37. P. C. Rockers, W. Jaskiewicz, M. E. Kruk, et al. Differences in preferences for rural job postings between nursing students and practicing nurses: evidence from a discrete choice experiment in Lao People's Democratic Republic. *Hum Resour Health* 2013; **11**: 22.

38. YHEC. Discrete choice experiment (DCE). 2016. https://yhec.co.uk/glossary/discrete-choice-experiment-dce (accessed January 9, 2022).

39. S. Abimbola, L. Baatiema, M. Bigdeli. The impacts of decentralization on health system equity, efficiency and resilience: a realist synthesis of the evidence. *Health Policy Plan* 2019; **34**(8): 605–617.

40. A. N. Kisakye, R. Tweheyo, F. Ssengooba, et al. Regulatory mechanisms for absenteeism in the health sector: a systematic review of strategies and their implementation. *J Healthc Leadersh* 2016; **8**: 81.

41. B. McPake, G. Russo, D. Hipgrave, et al. Implications of dual practice for universal health coverage. *Bull World Health Organ* 2016; **94**(2): 142.

Chapter 7

The Pharmaceutical System and Its Components

Regulation and Management and Associated Challenges

Mohamed R. Ismail, Aukje K. Mantel-Teeuwisse, and Zafar Mirza

Key Messages

- The pharmaceutical system is an integral subset of the health system which must have in place mature regulatory structures and robust supply systems to ensure that it supports national efforts to advance universal health coverage.
- Health technologies are life-enhancing and lifesaving commodities that require the products to be safe, quality-assured, efficacious, and used appropriately to achieve the desired health outcomes.
- Governments are responsible for establishing strong national regulatory authorities (NRAs) that are the gatekeepers of the supply chain of medical products, and are responsible for ensuring the quality, safety, and efficacy of medicines. The World Health Organization (WHO) has developed a global benchmarking tool to facilitate country efforts in strengthening NRAs.
- Managing the supply of health products and technologies has four key areas: selection, procurement, distribution, and use. Each needs to function well to ensure equitable access to health products.
- Pharmaceutical system challenges in low- and middle-income countries (L&MICs) include lack of well-functioning NRAs, inappropriate selection and use of essential medicines, substandard and falsified products, inadequate pharmaceutical workforce, lack of good pharmacy practice, insufficient understanding of intellectual property protection, and innovation processes.

7.1 Introduction

Medicines account for 20–30% of global health spending, more so in L&MICs. They constitute a major part of the budget of whosoever is paying for health services [1]. Their impact on health financing places them in a central position in discussions, strategies, and plans for universal health coverage (UHC) [2]. Currently, the majority of people in L&MICs pay for medicines out-of-pocket, often leading to financial hardship [1]. Unaffordability commonly results in people not taking their medication as prescribed or not at all, which in turn leads to poor health outcomes. With the rise in noncommunicable diseases – many of which are chronic conditions that require long-term treatment – the threat of financial burden has become even greater, as is the need to accelerate progress toward UHC.

> **Box 7.1** Health Technologies
>
> According to WHO, health technology is "the application of organized knowledge and skills in the form of devices, medicines, vaccines, procedures and systems developed to solve a health problem and improve quality of lives" [3]. Health technologies equip health care providers with tools for prevention, diagnosis, treatment and rehabilitation, and attainment of internationally agreed health-related development goals.

This chapter discusses the pharmaceutical system as part of the health system and describes health products and technologies (see Box 7.1). While focused on medicines and vaccines, which are essential for a well-functioning health system, the content also applies to other health products, such as medical devices, health applications and software, wearables, and other durable and nondurable commodities. Table 7.1 gives an overview of definitions of various types of health technologies, specifically health products commonly used in health care. This chapter also highlights the regulatory and management challenges of the pharmaceutical system, while Chapter 21 discusses how to improve health system performance by strengthening the pharmaceutical system.

7.2 The Pharmaceutical System and Its Components

Equitable access to health products is a key condition and an indicator for countries' progress toward UHC [12]. Ensuring access to health products depends on a well-functioning health system, in particular its components of governance, information, financing, workforce, and service delivery. It requires robust regulatory and supply systems which take into account the countries' contexts, address the needs of vulnerable populations, and foster innovation [13]. Access to health care, including essential medicines, is a fundamental human right [14]. Realization of this right involves various combinations of public and private financing and service provision arrangements [15].

A *pharmaceutical system* may be defined as a subset of the health system which "consists of all structures, people, resources, processes, and their interactions within the broader health system that aim to ensure equitable and timely access to safe, effective, quality pharmaceutical products and related services that promote their appropriate and cost-effective use to improve health outcomes" [16].

A pharmaceutical system thus includes, but is not limited to, the NRA or equivalent body, the Central Medical Store or equivalent procurement and purchasing unit(s), and all related agencies or units in charge of financing medicines and their appropriate use. It needs to have functional or collaborative links to other bodies that influence its performance, such as professional orders or associations, social insurance systems, and patent offices. Those in charge of each component of the pharmaceutical system, or related functions (e.g., selection, financing, regulation, quality assurance, services planning, and monitoring) are *collectively* responsible for the system's performance on access to medicines.

A well-functioning pharmaceutical system, as an integral component of the health system, should ensure reliable access to quality-assured, safe, and efficacious essential medicines and health technologies that are available in sufficient quantities and are affordable to the population [17]. This requires effective regulatory and procurement systems, as well as legal provisions for access to medicines, governance arrangements, and efficient

Table 7.1 Common types of health technologies used in health care provision

Product	Description
Medicines	Medicines may be defined as "articles intended for use in the diagnosis, cure, mitigation, treatment, or prevention of disease" and "articles (other than food) intended to affect the structure or any function of the body of man or other animals" [4].
Vaccines	Vaccines are a heterogeneous class of prophylactic medicinal products containing antigenic substances capable of inducing specific, active, and protective host immunity against an infective agent or toxin, or against other important antigenic substances produced by infective agents [5].
Advanced therapy medicinal products (ATMPs)	ATMPs are medicines for human use that are based on genes, tissues, or cells. They offer groundbreaking new opportunities for the treatment of disease and injury [6].
Homeopathic medicines	Products are prepared following a well-defined procedure, starting from substances derived from the mineral, herbal, and animal worlds. The techniques of preparation of these drugs include the dilution of the raw material, in hydroalcoholic solutions or in other excipients, and the potentization of the product into different grades [7].
Traditional and complementary medicines (T&CMs)	T&CM products include herbs, herbal materials, herbal preparations, and finished herbal products that contain parts of plants, other plant materials, or combinations thereof as active ingredients. In some countries herbal medicines may contain, by tradition, natural organic or inorganic active ingredients that are not of plant origin (e.g., animal and mineral materials) [8].
Biological medical products (biotherapeutic medicines)	Biological products are a diverse category of products and are generally large, complex molecules. These products may be produced through biotechnology in a living system, such as a microorganism, plant cell, or animal cell, and are often more difficult to characterize than small-molecule drugs. They may be developed using genetically engineered bacteria, yeast, fungi, cells, or even whole animals and plants [9].
Blood products	Any therapeutic substances derived from human blood, including whole blood, blood components, and plasma-derived medicinal products [10].
Medical devices	An article, instrument, apparatus, or machine that is used in the prevention, diagnosis, or treatment of illness or disease, or for detecting, measuring, restoring, correcting, or modifying the structure or function of the body for some health purpose. Typically, the purpose of a medical device is not achieved by pharmacological, immunological, or metabolic means [11].

management of resources. Weak governance and inefficient practices leave health systems vulnerable to corruption and mismanagement, and can have a detrimental effect on health budgets, patients' health and wellbeing, and trust in public institutions [18].

7.2.1 The Pharmaceutical System as Part of the Health System

Health system strengthening interventions must address interconnections between system components [19]. In particular, complex relationships between medicines and health governance, financing, human resources, health information, and service delivery should be given sufficient consideration. Otherwise, populations' access to medicines is addressed mainly through fragmented, often vertical approaches usually focusing on supply, unrelated to the wider issue of access to health services and interventions [20].

National medicines policies are recommended by WHO to express and prioritize the medium- to long-term goals set by governments for pharmaceutical systems, and to identify the main strategies for attaining them [21]. A holistic approach to the national medicines policy is required to ensure that the elements are interlinked and should be aligned with the national health policy and other related development policies, such as higher education, industry, trade, and others.

In discussing the pharmaceutical system, this chapter focuses on two main areas: regulation and management. The relationship between health technologies and the health system underscores aspects concerning their regulation and management through robust supply systems and policies in order to ensure quality, safety, and efficacy of products. The chapter also highlights major challenges faced by pharmaceutical systems in low- and middle-income countries (L&MICs).

7.3 Regulation of Health Products and Technologies

Governments are responsible for establishing strong NRAs with a clear mission, sound legal basis, realistic objectives, appropriate organizational structure, adequate number of qualified staff, sustainable financing, access to up-to-date, evidence-based technical literature, equipment and information, and capacity to exert effective market control. NRAs must be free of conflicts of interest and accountable to both the government and the public, and their decision-making processes should be transparent. Monitoring and evaluation mechanisms should be built into the regulatory system to assess attainment of established objectives. NRAs can fall into different categories, such as stringent regulatory authority (SRA), WHO listed authority (WLA), and regional regulatory system (RRS), which are elaborated in Box 7.2.

7.3.1 Main Functions and Assessment of NRAs

National regulatory authorities are the gatekeepers of the supply chain of medical products, and are responsible for ensuring the quality, safety, and efficacy of medicines. The range of health products regulated by NRAs varies depending on the level of development of the NRA, local context, and historical factors, but may include medicines, vaccines, blood and blood products, medical devices including diagnostics, traditional or herbal medicines, and veterinary medicines [24].

The WHO has developed a global benchmarking tool (GBT) to facilitate country efforts in strengthening NRAs. The WHO GBT enables WHO and NRAs to identify strengths and areas for improvement; to facilitate the formulation of an institutional development plan (IDP) to build upon strengths and address the identified gaps; to prioritize IDP interventions; and to monitor progress and achievements [25]. The GBT has been considered a game-changer because it is the first globally accepted tool for assessing and strengthening

---

Box 7.2 Key Terms Related to NRAs

Stringent Regulatory Authority

The concept of an SRA was developed by WHO and the Global Fund to Fight AIDS, Tuberculosis and Malaria to guide medicine procurement decisions, and is now widely recognized by the international regulatory and procurement community [22]. An SRA is defined as a regulatory authority which is:

- a member of the International Council for Harmonisation of Technical Requirements for Pharmaceuticals for Human Use (ICH), being the European Commission, the US Food and Drug Administration, and the Ministry of Health, Labour and Welfare of Japan (represented by the Pharmaceuticals and Medical Devices Agency); or an ICH observer, being the European Free Trade Association, as represented by Swissmedic, and Health Canada; or
- a regulatory authority associated with an ICH member through a legally binding, mutual recognition agreement, including Australia, Iceland, Liechtenstein, and Norway.

WHO Listed Authority

The interim definition of a WLA is "A regulatory authority or a regional regulatory system which has been documented to comply with all the indicators and requirements specified by WHO for listing based on an established benchmarking and performance evaluation process" [23].

Regional Regulatory System

An RRS is defined by WHO as "a system composed of individual regulatory authorities, or a regional body composed of individual regulatory authorities, operating under a common regulatory or legal framework." Examples of an RRS include the European Medicines Agency and the African Medicines Regulatory Harmonization Initiative.

NRAs [26]. The tool proposes nine main functions for an NRA and a set of indicators to measure its performance (Table 7.2).

7.3.2 Other Regulatory Functions

Several additional aspects of a pharmaceutical system are regulated by Ministries of Health or other agencies, including pricing/reimbursement, registration/licensing of pharmacy personnel, control of narcotics, psychotropic substances, and precursors, good pharmacy practice, and international cooperation. The modalities and competent authorities for managing these important functions vary among countries. While these important functions may fall outside the scope of an NRA, they have a strong impact on the pharmaceutical sector.

7.4 Managing Supply of Health Products and Technologies

This section presents the four key areas of pharmaceutical management: selection, procurement, distribution, and use (Figure 7.1).

Table 7.2 The WHO nine NRA functions with a summary of each function based on the GBT [25]

NRA function	Description
01– National regulatory system	Provides the framework that supports WHO recommended regulatory functions
02 – Registration and marketing authorization	A procedure for approval of a medical product for marketing after it has undergone a process of evaluation to determine the safety, efficacy, and quality of the product and the appropriateness of the product information
03 – Vigilance	The science and activities relating to the detection, assessment, understanding, and prevention of adverse effects or any other medical product-related problems
04 – Market surveillance and control	Plays a crucial role in ensuring medical products' consumer safety since its objective is to ensure compliance of the products placed on the market with preset criteria for quality, safety, and efficacy (i.e., verify compliance with marketing authorization and good practices guidelines)
05 – Licensing establishments	Premises, facilities, establishments, and companies throughout the supply chain should possess a license to operate, issued by the NRA
06 – Regulatory inspection	Ensures that operations at pharmaceutical establishments are carried out in accordance with approved standards, norms, and guidelines and are in compliance with the national medical products legislation and regulations
07 – Laboratory testing	Ensures that the NRA is able to assess the quality of medical products by performing quality tests on them in certain situations
08 – Clinical trial oversight	Aims at protecting the safety and rights of humans participating in clinical trials, ensuring that trials are adequately designed to meet scientifically sound objectives, and preventing any potential fraud and falsification of data
09 – NRA lot release	Applies for the regulatory release of specified biological products to ensure the quality, safety, and efficacy of biological products through a regulatory release system

7.4.1 Selection

Selection of essential medicines takes into consideration national disease burden and clinical need, thereby improving access through streamlined procurement and distribution of quality-assured medicines, supporting rational or appropriate prescribing and use, and lowering costs for the health care systems and for patients. Since 1977, WHO has regularly provided guidance for the selection of essential medicines [28]. In 2021, WHO published its twenty-second model essential medicines list and eighth model essential medicines list for children. The concept of essential medicines is closely linked with health insurance and essential health services packages. High-cost medicines such as those for the treatment of cancer may also be included in essential medicines to improve access to lifesaving products. Box 7.3 summarizes the main elements of the concept of essential medicines.

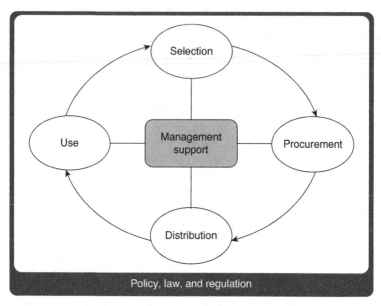

Figure 7.1 Pharmaceutical management framework [27].

7.4.2 Procurement

Procurement practices are a major determinant of availability and cost of pharmaceutical products [27]. Procurement involves efforts to quantify medicines' requirements, selecting appropriate procurement methods, and prequalifying suppliers and products. It also involves managing tenders, establishing contract terms, assuring medicines' quality, obtaining the best prices, and ensuring adherence to contract terms. Procurement methods need to be strengthened to ensure that procurement is linked to national medicines lists and prescribing patterns. Pooled procurement is often considered a valuable option to redress the imbalance in market leverage between supply and demand and to serve public health goals (Box 7.4) [30].

7.4.3 Distribution

A well-managed distribution system focuses on measures that ensure product integrity and quality throughout the distribution chain of the products [27]. The distribution system

---

Box 7.4 Potential Benefits of Pooled Procurement [30]

Existing pooled procurement models that consolidate purchasing across national boundaries have demonstrated the following benefits:

1. reductions in unit purchase prices;
2. improved quality assurance;
3. reduction or elimination of procurement corruption;
4. rationalized choice through better-informed selection and standardization;
5. reduction of operating costs and administrative burden;
6. increased equity between members;
7. augmented practical utility in the role of the host institutions (regional or international) administering the system; and
8. increased access to essential medical products within each participating country.

---

should allow countries to maintain a constant supply of medicines, keep medicines in good condition throughout the process, maintain cold chain where required, minimize medicine loss due to spoilage and expiry, maintain accurate inventory records, rationalize medicine storage points, use available transportation resources efficiently, and reduce theft and fraud.

7.4.4 Use

Medicine use is appropriate when patients receive the medicines they need, in doses that meet their individual requirements, for an adequate period of time, and at the lowest cost both to them and the community [31]. Some of the key interventions advocated for improving use of medicines include establishment of a multidisciplinary national body to coordinate policies on medicine use, use of clinical guidelines, development and use of national essential medicines lists, establishment of drug and therapeutics committees in districts and hospitals, inclusion of problem-based pharmacotherapy training in undergraduate curricula, continuing in-service medical education as a licensure requirement, supervision, audit and feedback, use of independent information on medicines, public education about medicines, avoidance of perverse financial incentives, use of appropriate and enforced regulation, and sufficient government expenditure to ensure availability of medicines and staff [32]. An aspect related to the use of medicines, especially after their authorization, is to monitor long-term efficacy and safety throughout their use in health care practice. This requires the NRA to operate a *pharmacovigilance* system (Box 7.5).

7.4.5 Ensuring Equitable Access to Health Products

The most common causes of death and disability in L&MICs can be prevented, treated, or alleviated with cost-effective essential medicines and health technologies. Still, hundreds of millions of people do not have regular access to essential medicines, despite having developed national essential medicines lists [34]. Among those who do have access, many are given the wrong treatment, receive too little medicine for their treatment, or do not use the medicines correctly. The need to expand access to medicines and health products is highlighted in the Sustainable Development Goals (SDGs) in at least seven targets, including two specific to SDG 3 (3.8 and 3.b) [12].

Box 7.5 Pharmacovigilance System

A *pharmacovigilance system* is the science and activities relating to the detection, assessment, understanding, and prevention of adverse effects or any other medicine-related problem [33]. Before a medicine is authorized for use, evidence of its safety and efficacy is limited to the results from clinical trials, where patients are carefully selected and followed up very closely under controlled conditions. After authorization, the medicine may be used in a large number of patients, for a long period of time, and with other medicines. Also referred to as *postmarketing surveillance*, it is the identification and collection of information regarding medicines after their approval for use in a population.

Several initiatives have been developed to present comprehensive frameworks for access to medicines. Table 7.3 provides a summary of three frameworks. The frameworks overlap on several aspects ("affordability" and "availability") and include components such as "architecture" or "reliable health systems." Limitations of these frameworks have been identified as: adopting a supply-side approach to address demand-side constraints; a focus on products rather than services (except for WHO-MSH 2000); and limitation of the governance of the pharmaceutical sector [20].

7.5 Major Pharmaceutical System Challenges in L&MICs

There are growing concerns about the resilience of health systems and their ability to respond to the challenges of UHC and health emergencies and other emerging threats to health [37]. Efforts to strengthen the resilience of health systems to cope with these challenges should include strengthening of pharmaceutical systems [16].

7.5.1 Lack of Well-Functioning Regulatory Authorities

Many countries still lack a well-functioning regulatory system. According to the WHO regulatory systems strengthening database, among its 194 Member States, only 50 countries (26%) have mature regulatory agencies, while 144 countries have suboptimal regulatory systems. Fifty-one percent of countries are at the lowest level, while 23% are at the second lowest level of maturity [24].

Inappropriate selection of essential medicines may lead to their inappropriate use and inefficiencies in the health system. It may lead to delayed inclusion of new medicines, limitation of physicians' ability to prescribe drugs, a potential impact on new drug research and development programs, and other challenges [38]. Fragmentation in the procurement process for pharmaceuticals and lack of coordination capabilities often result in significant waste of resources. Weak distribution systems may enable product diversion to the black market and proliferation of counterfeit and substandard products [39].

7.5.2 Inappropriate Use of Medicines

Inappropriate use of medicines is a major problem of present-day medical practice, and its consequences include the development of bacterial resistance to antibiotics, ineffective treatment, adverse effects of drugs, and economic burden on the patient and society. Inappropriate use of medicines may take many different forms – for example, polypharmacy, overuse of antibiotics and unnecessary injections, failure to prescribe in accordance

Table 7.3 Domains and determinants covered in existing frameworks for access to medicines

Domains	Specific determinants	Cross-cutting determinant
Access to Medicines Framework 1 – WHO-MSH 2000 (Centre for Pharmaceutical Management 2003)		
Availability	Medicines' supply – type and quantity	Quality of products and services
	Medicines' demand – type and quantity	
Affordability	Prices of medicine products and services	
	User's income and ability to pay	
Acceptability	Characteristics of products and services	
	User's attitudes, expectations of products and services	
Accessibility	Medicines' supply location	
	User location	
Access to Medicines Framework 2 – WHO (2004) [35]		
Rational use	Rational therapeutic choices	Quality of medicines
	Improved medicines' use by consumers	
Affordable prices	Medicines' pricing policies	
Sustainable financing	Resource mobilization	
	Pooling	
	Reduction of OOP expenditures	
Reliable health and supply systems	Medicine procurement and supply	
	Regulation	
	Human resources	
Access to Medicines Framework 3 – Frost and Reich (2010) [36]		
Availability	Manufacturing	Architecture: organization relationships at national and international levels
	Forecasting	
	Procurement	
	Distribution	
	Delivery	
Affordability	Government affordability	
	Nongovernmental agency affordability	
	End-user affordability	
Adoption	Global adoption	
	National adoption	
	Provider adoption	
	End-user adoption and appropriate use	

with clinical guidelines, and inappropriate self-medication. However, despite the global problem of inappropriate use, few countries are monitoring use of medicines or taking sufficient action to correct the situation [40]. It is estimated that over half of all medicines are prescribed, dispensed, or sold inappropriately [31]. Furthermore, half of all patients fail to

> **Box 7.6** Key Definitions Related to Substandard and Falsified Medicines [45]
>
> **Substandard** medical products, also called "out of specification," are authorized medical products that fail to meet either their quality standards or specifications, or both.
>
> **Unregistered/unlicensed** medical products have not undergone evaluation and/or approval by the national or regional regulatory authority for the market in which they are marketed/distributed or used, subject to permitted conditions under national or regional regulation and legislation.
>
> **Falsified** medical products deliberately/fraudulently misrepresent their identity, composition, or source.

take their medication as prescribed or dispensed [41]. In 2012, the Information Medical Statistics Health Institute estimated a global annual loss of US$500 billion that could be avoided by more responsible use of medicines, and identified nine underlying factors, including nonadherence, delayed medicine use, medication errors, antibiotic misuse/overuse, suboptimal generic use, mismanaged polypharmacy, medicine shortages, substandard/counterfeit medicines, and misuse of expensive therapies [42].

7.5.3 Substandard and Falsified Products

Poor access to quality health products is often filled by substandard or falsified products. The growth of e-commerce has also contributed to this trend by making it easier to purchase medicines online, often from unauthorized sources [43]. Box 7.6 highlights the differences between substandard, unregistered/unlicensed, and falsified medical products.

Substandard and falsified medical products are a significant threat to public health, promote drug-resistant infections, and waste valuable resources [44]. NRAs and law enforcement agencies need to be strengthened to comply with international standards in manufacturing and quality assurance of medicines and should collaborate with international agencies to address this important threat to public health.

7.5.4 Weak Collaboration among Stakeholders

The pharmaceutical sector is complex and involves numerous stakeholders, such as the pharmaceutical industry and its shareholders, patients and patient organizations, health professionals, consumer organizations, civil society, wholesalers, hospitals, academia, national and regional competent authorities, and others. Lack of multistakeholder collaboration negatively affects transparency and accountability in the pharmaceutical sector and may hinder progress toward the goal of access to medicines [46]. Global initiatives such as WHO's Good Governance for Medicines program and the Medicines Transparency Alliance have adopted a multisectoral approach in promoting good governance in the pharmaceutical sector [47].

7.5.5 Inadequate Workforce

The shortage of pharmacists and pharmaceutical personnel has implications for the functioning of a health system. The availability of trained human resources in the pharmaceutical sector is of critical importance in meeting national and global health goals, and thus requires special attention [48]. The particular importance of an adequate pharmaceutical workforce is often overlooked by policymakers when addressing the human resources for health needs.

Competent pharmaceutical professionals are required for the development, production, distribution, and appropriate utilization of medicines, as well as supportive functions such as regulation, operational research, and training. Over the period 2006–2012, the density of pharmacists has increased substantially in many low-income countries, but their baseline remains low compared with those of high-income countries [49]. Pharmacy workforce capacity varies considerably between countries and regions and generally correlates with population- and country-level economic indicators. Countries and territories with lower economic indicators tend to have fewer pharmacists and pharmacy technicians, which has implications for inequalities regarding access to medicines and medicine expertise.

7.5.6 Lack of Good Pharmacy Practice

There is increasing recognition that providing consumers with medicines alone is not sufficient to achieve treatment goals. To address medication-related needs, pharmacists should accept greater responsibility for the outcomes of medicines use. Pharmacy practice is evolving to provide patients with enhanced medicines-use services. Good pharmacy practice is the practice of pharmacy that responds to the needs of the people who use the pharmacists' services to provide optimal, evidence-based care [50]. Remuneration of pharmaceutical services is a challenge to achieving good pharmacy practice [51].

7.5.7 Insufficient Understanding of Intellectual Property Protection and Innovation Processes

The current patent protection system under the auspices of the World Trade Organization (WTO) has introduced enhanced global minimum standards for intellectual property protection. The WTO's Trade-Related Aspects of Intellectual Property Rights (TRIPS) agreement has a significant impact on the pharmaceutical sector, and more specifically on medicine prices, and may hamper access to medicines by the poor [52]. Policymakers may sometimes lack a clear understanding of the innovation processes that lead to new technologies and the ways in which these technologies are monopolized and disseminated, which may hinder innovation and equitable access to vital medical technologies. Furthermore, the complex interplay between the distinct policy domains of health, trade, and intellectual property, and of how they affect medical innovation and access to medical technologies, requires a clear understanding, inter-ministerial collaboration, and expertise at the national level in L&MICs [13].

TRIPS flexibilities, including compulsory licensing, are inbuilt public health safeguards that have been further enhanced and affirmed through the Doha Declaration on TRIPS and Public Health and multilateral developments since 1995, and will remain valid until 2033. To maximize the benefits that can be accrued though the use of these flexibilities, a precondition is to have these incorporated in the national legislation, which unfortunately is still not the case in many L&MICs [53]. Box 7.7 defines some of the key related terms.

In light of the high cost of innovative health products, health technology assessment (see Chapter 13) is used by some countries for the systematic evaluation of properties, effects, and/or impacts of health technology, to inform policymaking and selection of health products.

> **Box 7.7** Key Definitions: Innovations and Intellectual Property
>
> **Intellectual property rights** are the rights given to persons over the creations of their minds. They usually give the creator an exclusive right over the use of their creation for a certain period of time [54].
>
> **Compulsory licensing** is the practice of authorizing a third party to make, use, or sell a patented invention without the patentee's consent [55].
>
> **Parallel import** refers to genuine products first put on the market in another country and imported through a channel parallel to the one authorized by the rights holder [13].

7.6 Conclusions

The capacity of many L&MICs to assess and approve health products remains limited, due to inadequate resources, overburdened staff, and incoherent policy frameworks. Innovative strategic approaches are needed globally to increase harmonization among countries and encourage regulatory recognition and reliance. At the time of writing, the COVID-19 pandemic presents a major threat to public health and our way of life. One of the main challenges has been ensuring access to important health products, including treatments, vaccines, personal protective equipment, *in-vitro* diagnostics, and others. The pandemic has highlighted that in both rich and poor countries the pharmaceutical systems may not be fully integrated into health systems or adequately prepared to respond. Stakeholders should continue to collaborate at global and national levels to strengthen pharmaceutical systems and increase preparedness for delivering health technologies where needed in a timely manner.

References

1. World Health Organization. The world medicines situation 2011: medicine expenditures. 2011. www.who.int/health-accounts/documentation/world_medicine_situation.pdf (accessed December 12, 2021).

2. World Health Organization. Public spending on health: a closer look at global trends. 2018. www.who.int/publications/i/item/WHO-HIS-HGF-HFWorkingPaper-18.3 (accessed December 12, 2021).

3. World Health Organization. Health technology assessment: what is a health technology? 2021. www.euro.who.int/en/health-topics/Health-systems/health-technologies-and-medicines/policy-areas/health-technology-assessment#:~:text=The%20definition%20of%20health%20technology,and%20improve%20quality%20of%20life (accessed October 11, 2021).

4. US Food and Drug Administration. Drugs@FDA glossary of terms. 2017. www.fda.gov/drugs/drug-approvals-and-databases/drugsfda-glossary-terms#M (accessed February 17, 2022).

5. World Health Organization. Guidelines on clinical evaluation of vaccines: regulatory expectations. 2016. www.who.int/biologicals/BS2287_Clinical_guidelines_final_LINE_NOs_20_July_2016.pdf (accessed February 17, 2022).

6. European Medicines Agency. Advanced therapy medicinal products: overview. 2022. www.ema.europa.eu/en/human-regulatory/overview/advanced-therapy-medicinal-products-overview (accessed February 17, 2022).

7. World Health Organization. Safety issues in the preparation of homeopathic medicines.

2009. https://apps.who.int/iris/handle/10665/44238 (accessed February 17, 2022).

8. World Health Organization. WHO traditional medicine strategy: 2014–2023. 2013. www.who.int/publications/i/item/9789241506096 (accessed February 17, 2022).

9. US Food and Drug Administration. Biological product definitions. n.d. www.fda.gov/files/drugs/published/Biological-Product-Definitions.pdf (accessed February 17, 2022).

10. World Health Organization. WHO guidelines on good manufacturing practices for blood establishments. 2011. www.who.int/bloodproducts/publications/GMP_Bloodestablishments.pdf (accessed February 17, 2022).

11. World Health Organization. Medical devices. 2022. www.who.int/health-topics/medical-devices#tab=tab_1 (accessed February 17, 2022).

12. United Nations. Sustainable Development Goals. 2021. https://sdgs.un.org/goals/goal3 (accessed October 11, 2021).

13. World Health Organization. Promoting access to medical technologies and innovation: intersections between public health, intellectual property and trade. 2020. www.wto.org/english/res_e/publications_e/who-wipo-wto_2020_e.htm (accessed October 14, 2021).

14. H. V. Hogerzeil, M. Samson, J. V. Casanovas, et al. Is access to essential medicines as part of the fulfilment of the right to health enforceable through the courts? *Lancet* 2006; **368**(9532): 305–311.

15. H. V. Hogerzeil. Essential medicines and human rights: what can they learn from each other? *Bull World Health Organ* 2006; **84**(5): 371–375.

16. T. Hafner, H. Walkowiak, D. Lee, et al. Defining pharmaceutical systems strengthening: concepts to enable measurement. *Health Policy Plan* 2017; **32**(4): 572–584.

17. D. H. Peters, A. Garg, G. Bloom, et al. Poverty and access to health care in developing countries. *Ann N Y Acad Sci* 2008; **1136**: 161–171.

18. World Health Organization. Pharmaceutical system transparency and accountability assessment tool: good governance for medicines – progressing access in the SDG era. 2018. https://apps.who.int/iris/handle/10665/275370 (accessed December 12, 2021).

19. World Health Organization. Systems thinking for health systems strengthening. 2009. https://apps.who.int/iris/bitstream/handle/10665/44204/9789241563895_eng.pdf?sequence=1 (accessed October 12, 2021).

20. M. Bigdeli, B. Jacobs, G. Tomson, et al. Access to medicines from a health system perspective. *Health Policy Plan* 2013; **28**(7): 692–704.

21. World Health Organization. How to develop and implement a national drug policy. 2009. www.who.int/management/background_4b.pdf (accessed October 12, 2021).

22. World Health Organization. List of stringent regulatory authorities. 2021. www.who.int/initiatives/who-listed-authority-reg-authorities/SRAs (accessed October 17, 2021).

23. World Health Organization. Evaluating and publicly designating regulatory authorities as WHO listed authorities: policy document. 2021. www.who.int/publications/i/item/9789240023444 (accessed October 12, 2021).

24. A. Khadem Broojerdi, H. Baran Sillo, R. Ostad Ali Dehaghi, et al. The World Health Organization global benchmarking tool: an instrument to strengthen medical products regulation and promote universal health coverage. *Front Med* 2020; **7**: 457.

25. World Health Organization. WHO Global Benchmarking Tool (GBT) for evaluation of national regulatory systems. 2021. www.who.int/tools/global-benchmarking-tools (accessed October 17, 2021).

26. J. Guzman, E. O'Connell, K. Kikule, et al. The WHO Global Benchmarking Tool: a game changer for strengthening national regulatory capacity. *BMJ Glob Health* 2020; **5**(8): e003181.

27. Management Sciences for Health. MDS-3: managing access to medicines and health technologies. 2012. https://msh.org/wp-content/uploads/2014/01/mds3-jan2014.pdf (accessed October 13, 2021).

28. World Health Organization. Selection of essential medicines at country level: using the WHO model list of essential medicines to update a national essential medicines list. 2020. www.who.int/publications/i/item/9789241515443 (accessed October 11, 2021).

29. World Health Organization. Signpost: WHO essential medicines. 2021. www.who.int/rhem/signpost/essential_medicines/en (accessed October 17, 2021).

30. M. Huff-Rousselle. The logical underpinnings and benefits of pooled pharmaceutical procurement: a pragmatic role for our public institutions? *Soc Sci Med* 2012; **75**(9): 1572–1580.

31. World Health Organization. Promoting rational use of medicines: core components. 2002. www.who.int/medicines/publications/policyperspectives/ppm05en.pdf (accessed October 11, 2021).

32. World Health Organization. Promoting rational use of medicines. 2021. www.who.int/activities/promoting-rational-use-of-medicines/ (accessed October 17, 2021).

33. European Medicines Agency. Pharmacovigilance: overview. 2021. www.ema.europa.eu/en/human-regulatory/overview/pharmacovigilance-overview (accessed December 27, 2021).

34. World Health Organization. Ten years in public health, 2007–2017: report by Dr Margaret Chan, Director-General, World Health Organization. 2017. https://apps.who.int/iris/handle/10665/255355 (accessed October 11, 2021).

35. World Health Organization. Equitable access to essential medicines: a framework for collective action. 2004. https://apps.who.int/iris/handle/10665/68571 (accessed December 27, 2021).

36. L. J. Frost, M. R. Reich. *How Do Good Health Technologies Get to Poor People in Poor Countries*. Boston, MA, Harvard University Press, 2010.

37. A. K. Wagner, J. D. Quick, D. Ross-Degnan. Quality use of medicines within universal health coverage: challenges and opportunities. *BMC Health Serv Res* 2014; **14**: 357.

38. M. M. Reidenberg. Can the selection and use of essential medicines decrease inappropriate drug use? *Clin Pharmacol Ther* 2009; **85**(6): 581–583.

39. M. Tremblay. Medicines counterfeiting is a complex problem: a review of key challenges across the supply chain. *Curr Drug Saf* 2013; **8**(1): 43–55.

40. World Health Organization. Using indicators to measure country pharmaceutical situations: fact book on WHO level I and level II monitoring indicators. 2006. www.who.int/medicines/publications/WHOTCM2006.2A.pdf (accessed October 11, 2021).

41. E. Sabaté, ed., *Adherence to Long-Term Therapies: Evidence for Action*. Geneva, World Health Organization, 2003. https://apps.who.int/iris/bitstream/handle/10665/42682/9241545992.pdf (accessed October 14, 2021).

42. M. Aitken, L. Gorokhovich. Advancing the responsible use of medicines: applying levers for change. 2012. https://ssrn.com/abstract=2222541 (accessed October 17, 2021).

43. World Health Organization. Substandard and falsified medical products. 2021. www.who.int/health-topics/substandard-and-falsified-medical-products#tab=tab_1 (accessed October 17, 2021).

44. World Health Organization. WHO global surveillance and monitoring system for substandard and falsified medical products. 2017. www.who.int/publications/i/item/WHO-MVP-EMP-SAV-2019.04 (accessed October 18, 2021).

45. World Health Organization. Member State mechanism on substandard/spurious/falsely-labelled/falsified/counterfeit medical products. 2017. https://apps.who.int/gb/ebwha/pdf_files/WHA70/A70_23-en.pdf (accessed October 18, 2021).

46. T. Vian, J. C. Kohler, G. Forte, et al. Promoting transparency, accountability, and

access through a multi-stakeholder initiative: lessons from the medicines transparency alliance. *J Pharm Policy Pract* 2017; **10**: 18.

47. Medicines Transparency Alliance. Welcome to MeTA. 2018. www .medicinestransparency.org/ (accessed October 18, 2021).

48. World Health Organization. Pharmaceutical human resources assessment tools. 2011. www.who.int/medicines/areas/coordination/ amrHRToolEnglish.pdf (accessed October 19, 2021).

49. International Pharmaceutical Federation (FIP). Pharmacy workforce intelligence: global trends report. 2018. www.fip.org/ file/2077 (accessed October 12, 2021).

50. World Health Organization. Joint FIP/ WHO guidelines on good pharmacy practice: standards for quality of pharmacy services. 2011. www.who.int/medicines/ services/expertcommittees/pharmprep/ CLEAN-Rev1-GPP-StandardsQ- PharmacyServices-QAS10-352_July2010 .pdf (accessed October 10, 2021).

51. P. Chan, K. A. Grindrod, D. Bougher, et al. A systematic review of remuneration systems for clinical pharmacy care services. *CPJ/RPC* 2008; **141**(2): 102–112.

52. G. Velasquez. The right to health and medicines: the case of recent multilateral negotiations on public health, innovation and intellectual property. *Dev World Bioeth* 2014; **14**(2): 67–74.

53. S. F. Musungu, C. Oh. The use of flexibilities in TRIPS by developing countries: can they promote access to medicines? 2006. https://apps.who.int/iris/ handle/10665/43503 (accessed October 19, 2021).

54. World Trade Organization. What are intellectual property rights? 2021. www.wto.org/english/tratop_e/trips_ e/intel1_e.htm (accessed October 19, 2021).

55. World Trade Organization. TRIPS and public health. 2021. www.wto.org/english/ tratop_e/trips_e/pharmpatent_e.htm (accessed October 20, 2021).

8 Health Information Systems
Data for Decision-Making in Health Systems

Ali H. Mokdad

Key Messages

- Well-functioning health information systems (HIS) are essential for informed decision-making and have four key functions: data generation, compilation, analysis and synthesis, and dissemination and use.
- HIS answer three fundamental questions: What are the health problems in the population? What is the response of the health system? And how could this response be improved?
- HIS include two broad data categories – primary micro-data and aggregated secondary macro-datasets. The primary data sources include vital registration, household interview surveys, health examination surveys, health service registry data, hospital discharge data, census data, budgets and expenditure reports, epidemiological observational studies, and health facility assessments.
- Essential health system metrics include estimating mortality, causes of death, morbidity, functional health status, risk factors, health financing, and burden of diseases, injuries, and risk factors. Tracking individual and population health requires specifying health outcomes to be measured, disaggregating outcomes into causal fractions, tracking time trends, and measuring inequalities.

8.1 Introduction

Health information systems have evolved in an uncoordinated and fragmented manner. These days, with rapid advances in technology, processing, sharing, and managing health information has become easier, as well as faster and cheaper. The HIS provide the underpinnings for decision-making and have four key functions: data generation, compilation, analysis and synthesis, and dissemination and use. The HIS collect data from the health sector and other relevant sectors, analyze the data and ensure its overall quality, relevance, and timeliness, and convert the data into information for health-related decision-making [1]. However, it is important to define the information that a health system should provide to answer three fundamental questions: (1) what are the health problems in the population, (2) what is the response of the health system, and (3) how could this response be improved? It is also important to be aware of common challenges in measuring data, such as controlling quality and making sure that the population coverage is inclusive and representative. These challenges can be met by designing intelligently, optimizing data collection instruments, and collecting and integrating data from multiple systems.

Historically, HIS have been developed to answer questions related to a specific topic or illness and have therefore evolved through a series of independent information systems that function as silos (e.g., malaria programs in many countries). This has often resulted in a complex set of overlapping but incomplete data collection strategies; often with different government departments and levels (local, regional, national) in charge of different parts of the system. The result is extraordinarily inefficient systems that require extensive corrections and adjustments after data has been collected to provide the desired health information.

In this chapter, we provide a brief overview of HIS and an example using the Global Burden of Disease (GBD) Study as a case study of how different sources of HIS are used to estimate the burden of disease to guide policies and programs. The GBD provides detailed information on what is killing (mortality) and ailing (health loss and disability) a population.

8.2 What Are the Key Questions That HIS Should Answer?

8.2.1 What Are People's Health Problems?

Strategic decision-makers are concerned with the overall stewardship and governance of the health system and need information on the burden of disease, how it is distributed in the population, and how it is changing over time. Therefore, a systematic scientific effort to quantify the comparative magnitude of health loss due to diseases, injuries, and risk factors by age, sex, and geographies for specific points in time is needed. There are four aspects to tracking individual and population health: the types of health outcomes that should be measured; disaggregating outcomes into causal fractions by disease, injury, or risk factor; tracking time trends; and measuring inequalities.

Types of outcomes. Tracking the health of individuals and groups of individuals requires information about death (or the risk of death) and about functional health status. Hence, we need information on morbidity, mortality, and disabilities for various diseases, injuries, and risk factors.

Causal attribution. Information systems need to not only detect levels and trends in health outcomes in individuals, but also to provide information on the attribution of these outcomes to diseases, injuries, and risk factors. Relating outcomes such as death to a particular disease, injury, or risk factor requires rigorous information about the related health event and the affected individual.

Time trends. For many decisions, tracking trends in a population's health through individual records is essential. Tracking trends in the incidence of infectious diseases with the potential for rapid spread, such as Asian avian influenza (H5N1) or the current COVID-19 pandemic, requires the capacity of the HIS to detect and track changes over very short time periods, such as days or weeks at the most.

Inequalities. Aggregate information on population health outcomes is not sufficient to guide policy and action. Health outcomes need to be tracked for individuals and groups of individuals defined on the basis of geography, race, ethnicity, or socioeconomic status [2]. Many dimensions of inequalities may be relevant to decision-makers and researchers as they provide insights into reasons for disparities and how to address these.

8.2.2 How Is the Health System Performing?

Decision-makers, including citizens choosing a health care provider, a local program manager allocating supervisory resources, and a minister of health choosing budget priorities, all need information on the performance of factors in the health system or the performance of the health system overall (see Chapter 13).

Coverage of interventions. Coverage is defined as the application of an intervention conditional on needing the intervention [3]. In other words, this is the population that gets the intervention as a proportion of the population that needs the intervention. The need for a given intervention can be extrapolated from simple demographic attributes such as age, sex, or pregnancy status that are clear, easing their collection.

Effective coverage of interventions. The construct of effective coverage [3] was introduced as part of the WHO Health Systems Performance Assessment framework [4]. Effective coverage brings together the constructs of "coverage" of interventions and "quality" to determine the fraction of health gain at the population level that is being delivered by the system (Table 8.1).

Quality of intervention delivery. Receiving an intervention does not mean that it has been delivered with quality. There are many definitions of quality and some use quality as a broad rubric encompassing health outcomes and all performance metrics (see Chapter 26) [5].

Efficiency of public health and health care delivery. Another key dimension of performance is how efficiently public health and health care interventions are being delivered. A simple way to consider efficiency is as the production function, where the y-axis is effective coverage for an intervention or a set of interventions, and the x-axis is resource inputs. Resource inputs can be summarized in terms of dollars (= prices × quantities of inputs) or can be assessed directly as units of input, such as doctors, nurses, or beds. In Figure 8.1, Model 5 would require ~2.9 billion Kenyan shillings (KES; US$29 million) to

Table 8.1 Crude coverage vs. effective coverage: difference in crude and effective coverage of measles immunization in Nicaragua in 2015 [6]

Effective coverage is a measure of health system performance that is intended to combine three aspects of health care delivery or intervention into a single measure: need, use, and quality. Crude coverage has been a standard measure of performance for interventions. It simply represents the fraction of those who need an intervention who use it. Effective coverage adjusts this fraction for the quality or efficacy of the intervention received by a population.		Effective coverage (analyses of direct blood spots)		
		Yes	No	Total
Crude coverage (according to health card)	Yes	46.7%	35.4%	82.2%
	No	3.7%	14.2%	17.8%
	Total	50.4%	49.6%	100%

Adapted from [6].

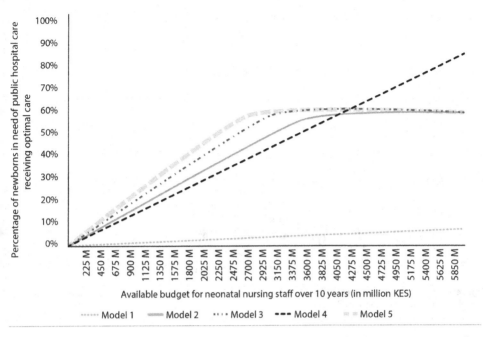

Figure 8.1 Models of effective coverage of newborns by the level of budget in KES for neonatal nursing staff [5].

provide quality care to 59% of all newborns in need of nursing care in public hospitals (i.e., the current level of coverage) over 10 years. If more budget were available, then Model 4 would require ~5.9 billion KES (US$59 million) to provide quality of care to >90% of all newborns [5].

Distributional aspects of performance analysis. For decision-makers, program managers, and the public, there is interest and value in the array of performance metrics at many different levels of disaggregation. Figure 8.2 illustrates the pattern of expenditure associated with surgery by patients treated at central hospitals in Malawi disaggregated by income quintiles [7]. In Q1 (the poorest quintile) the median direct cost of accessing surgery significantly exceeds the median monthly per capita income (by a factor 3.6), while in Q5 (the richest quintile) the median direct cost was 13% of the median per capita income. Similarly, the public may want measurement at the level that relates to their set of individual choices, such as which doctor or hospital to visit.

Decision support pathways. Strategic decision-makers, program managers, and clinicians require detailed information for multiple steps on an intervention pathway. Consider the key drivers of outcomes for acute myocardial infarction (MI) that include risk behaviors such as tobacco use, diet, physical activity, primary care management of risks such as elevated blood pressure, LDL (low-density lipid) cholesterol, and clinical management of the acute MI. Hence, information is needed at every step of the pathway to promote a healthy lifestyle, prevent another MI by controlling behavioral risk factors, or provide appropriate care for effective management in a hospital setting.

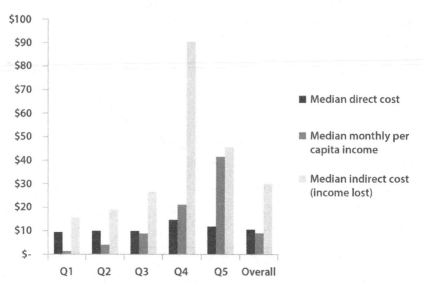

Figure 8.2 Comparison of direct and indirect cost of accessing surgery at district hospitals disaggregated by household income quintiles (*N* = 136).

Risk adjustment methods. Performance metrics constantly evolve. Improved risk adjustment methods or new clinical intervention strategies are just two examples of how the set of performance indicators computed today might be different from those five years hence.

Risk adjustment is a method to offset the cost of providing health insurance for individuals – such as those with chronic health conditions – who represent a relatively high risk to insurers [8]. In the absence of risk adjustment policies, insurers have a financial incentive to deny coverage to higher-risk individuals or to impose unaffordable premiums for individuals with pre-existing medical conditions. Risk adjustment aims to make comprehensive insurance available to all individuals, regardless of risk, and allows insurance organizations to charge similar average premiums, as for relatively healthy populations, when insuring sicker-than-average populations. Risk adjustment models typically use an individual's demographic data (age, sex, etc.) and diagnoses to determine a risk score. The risk score is a relative measure of the probable costs to insure the individual, especially by private insurers.

8.2.3 What Are the Best Options to Improve Outcomes or Reduce Costs?

Strategic decision-makers seek policy options that can improve outcomes and/or reduce costs. Good information about health problems and current performance provides an important basis for choosing the most feasible option. Assessing the expected costs and consequences of a policy that has not yet been implemented anywhere in a system nonetheless requires some type of information to guide decision-making. Information on the efficacy of interventions usually comes from systematic reviews or meta-analyses of published randomized trials or other types of intervention studies. However, in any given health system, the expected costs and benefits will be affected by many factors influencing the behavior of local providers and individual beneficiaries. These factors account for the oft-noted gap between the efficacy (the ability to achieve the desired result in *ideal circumstances*) and effectiveness (the ability to achieve the desired result in *real life*) of an intervention [9].

Three strategies can enhance the ability of a well-designed information system to inform policy choices. First, *linking information on supply and demand of health services* based on provider and individual data can provide guidance for decision-making. Information systems that can link information relating to individual choices for care-seeking or public health intervention uptake, and attributes of providers such as training, location, cost, quality, or medicine availability can provide a much stronger empirical basis for assessing the likely costs and consequences for new policy options. Second, *post-implementation evaluation of effectiveness of interventions* can provide highly contextual information on how well a policy performs. For example, country-specific information on the impact of insecticide-treated bed nets in a real population program can be highly informative, especially when the results are different from those obtained in previously conducted randomized controlled trials. The ability to capture additional information, such as recording in household surveys the use of interventions in children who have died and their exposure to interventions (e.g., bed nets), can enrich the assessment of post-implementation impact. Third, information systems that provide *geospatial information about the distribution of providers and populations* can play an important role in the development of strategies for improving physical access to providers or the expansion of community outreach workers. Taking into consideration the current and likely distribution of public and private providers is an important dimension of this type of analysis.

8.3 Health Data Sources

Health information systems at the global level include two broad data categories: (1) primary micro-data and (2) aggregated secondary macro-datasets. At the national and subnational levels, especially in large countries, HIS often focus on the primary micro-data produced within the health system. There are different sources of health data that are briefly discussed below, while Table 8.2 provides examples of major sources of information from different countries.

8.3.1 Vital Registration

Vital events registration data collects birth and death information and, given their importance, provides some of the most advanced and standardized types of health data across countries. The goal of any complete vital registration system is to accurately record all births and deaths in the whole population.

8.3.2 Household Interview Surveys

Most household interview surveys for health rely on standardized instruments and protocols, beginning with the World Fertility Survey in the 1970s. It is useful to think of them in several different clusters, with each cluster having its own general purpose. They may also include verbal autopsy, an essential and highly specialized survey aimed only at collecting cause-of-death information in particular areas that lack vital registration.

Table 8.2 Major sources of information: examples from different countries

Data source	Country example
Vital registration	**India – *Sample Registration System*** (SRS). This system has functioned since the 1970s as an interim measure to generate vital statistics on the basis of a probability sample. It covers a population of approximately 7.0 million from 7,600 sampling units and records fertility and mortality indicators at national and state levels [12].
Household interview surveys	**90 countries – *Demographic and Health Surveys*** (DHS) are nationally representative household surveys that provide data for a wide range of monitoring and impact evaluation indicators in the areas of population, health, and nutrition. These surveys have sample sizes usually between 5,000 and 30,000 households, and are typically conducted every five years to allow comparisons over time [13].
National health examination surveys	**United States – *National Health and Nutrition Examination Survey*** (NHANES). This survey is designed to assess the health and nutritional status of adults and children. It combines interviews and physical examinations. The NHANES is conducted by the National Center for Health Statistics and has responsibility for producing vital and health statistics for the nation [14].
Health service registry data	**Finland – *Performance, Effectiveness, and Costs of Treatment episodes (PERFECT) Hip Fracture Database*** contains all hip fracture patients identified from the Hospital Discharge Register in Finland since 1999. Register-based data is useful for performance assessment and has helped improve outcomes of hip fracture treatment [15].
Hospital discharge data	**Brazil – *National Database on Health Units (CNES), Public Hospital Information System (SIH), and the Private Hospital Information System (CIH)*** provide basic registration data for hospitals, and most send some information about hospital performance-related outcomes (see Chapter 12).
Census data	**South Africa – *Department of Statistics (Stats SA)*** is responsible for census data. The first population census was conducted in 1996 and subsequently in 2001 and 2011. Census results are used to ensure equity in distribution of government services, allocation of government funds across regions, delineation of electoral districts, and measurement of the impact of industrial development [16].

8.3.3 National Health Examination Surveys

In addition to standardized questions, national health examination surveys also gather physical examination data. They may collect blood samples, administer audiometry or optometry tests, conduct radiological examinations, or administer performance tests for basic functional health status (e.g., motor capabilities). The WHO STEPwise Approach to NCD Risk Factor Surveillance (STEPS) is a simple, standardized method for collecting, analyzing, and disseminating data on key NCD risk factors in countries [10]. Among others, the survey instrument covers key biological risk factors, including excess weight and obesity, elevated blood pressure, elevated blood glucose, and abnormal blood lipids.

8.3.4 Health Service Registry Data

The focus of health service records is typically on subnational information used to manage health services. These records are based on service-generated data derived from health facilities and patient–provider interactions covering care offered, cost and quality of care, treatments administered, and so on. The key role of health service statistics is their use to inform facility management.

8.3.5 Hospital Discharge Data

Hospital discharge data is a specific type of health service registry data. It is widely available and when of good quality is very useful for the quality monitoring of health services. This source almost always includes individual records capturing different dimensions of health care experience, including interactions between health providers and individuals.

8.3.6 Census Data

Where available, population-level census data can serve as the primary information source for determining the size of a population, its geographical distribution, and the social, demographic, and economic characteristics of its people.

8.3.7 Budgets and Expenditure Reports

Expenditure and budget data provide valuable information on financial resources for health. This data comes from national budget documents, expenditure reviews, and auditor reports. Most often, this information is available at the summary level. One source, the National Health Accounts, provides information on overall flow of funds in the health system by tracking health expenditures across multiple financing streams, regardless of the entity or institution that finances and/or manages that spending (see Chapter 13) [11].

8.3.8 Epidemiological Observational Studies

Epidemiological observational studies follow a cohort of individuals over several years and are useful in providing information about disease progression and risk factors for disease and survival. They are generally completely researcher-driven but nonetheless can be useful for assessing population health.

8.3.9 Health Facility Assessments

Health facility assessments are intended to capture the resources and inputs of a specific health center, be it a primary care clinic, community health center, or a specialty clinic. Modules include facility infrastructure, health center budget reviews, pharmaceutical inventories, secondary output review, and services for specific conditions, such as tuberculosis treatment.

8.3.10 Secondary and Macro-Datasets

Aggregate indicators on health, such as those created by international organizations, are those datasets that compile national indicators. They often combine a diverse and often deficient mix of datasets. Two major problems characterize these types of datasets. First, some countries lack data related to a range of specific topics, resulting in incomplete aggregate data which in turn impedes the ability to draw valuable comparisons between countries. Second, those who create these aggregates (WHO, World Bank, UNICEF, UNDP, UNFPA, etc.) do not always detail how the aggregate was generated. One way to improve these indicators is to report the missing data by country and provide details of how the aggregates were created. Providing such information would dramatically improve aggregate reports.

8.4 Essential Health System Metrics

Using the sources of data mentioned above, there is a range of important and useful health indicators that should be generated by all HIS.

8.4.1 Mortality

Mortality data allows us to examine differences in the average age at death and distribution of deaths across age and sex in populations, usually broken down into adult and child mortality. Vital registration systems are the best source of data for this metric; however, the lack of data on deaths for almost half of the countries of the world is an internationally recognized problem.

8.4.2 Causes of Death

This data captures the underlying cause of each death in a population in a way that is comparable. Timely, valid, and reliable information on causes of death by age and sex is a critical input into public health planning, program implementation, and evaluation.

8.4.3 Morbidity

Morbidity is the relative incidence of a particular disease, and health surveys are a good source of morbidity data in a country or community. Self-reported conditions are not often validated against gold standard clinical data but can nonetheless provide a starting point for estimates of the prevalence and incidence of certain conditions at the population level. More robust data can be derived by verifying morbid conditions through health examination surveys.

8.4.4 Functional Health Status

Death rates do not tell the whole story about population health. Functional health status gathers information on an individual's physical ability compared to others. For many conditions such as blindness, mental disorders, or musculoskeletal diseases, the main effects are loss of health function. Years lived with disability (YLDs) is a commonly used metric summarizing functional health status. The combination of YLDs and years of life lost due to premature mortality (YLL) in a population add up to disability-adjusted life years (DALYs; see Section 8.4.7 and Chapter 13).

8.4.5 Risk Factors

A number of risk factors modulate health outcomes. These span a range of categories, including behavioral, environmental, genetic, metabolic, nutritional, reproductive, and occupational. By controlling or at least reducing some of these risk factors, countries can markedly improve the overall health of their populations.

8.4.6 Health Financing

In many countries, local or national surveys can drive and inform health financing. Politicians and local health officials react to their own data and often the data leads to action. It is crucial to have periodic surveys to adequately guide policy and allocate resources. Monitoring health financing indicators has become a critical metric for national governments and, among other things, can inform the percentage of households that incurred catastrophic health expenditure or became impoverished as a result of seeking health care (see Chapters 5 and 16).

8.4.7 Burden of Diseases, Injuries, and Risk Factors

The concept of burden of disease brings together a combination of mortality, causes of death, morbidity, and functional health status by using a summary health measure, the *disability-adjusted life year or DALY*, to compare the impact of different health conditions. DALY and the related concept of *comparative risk assessment*, which compares the impact of different health risks, are two extremely important pieces of evidence for policymakers to understand the health of their populations. The policy relevance and importance of the concept of burden of disease is evident in the myriad national burden of disease studies that have been independently undertaken since the original Global Burden of Disease Study (Box 8.1).

Box 8.1 Case Study: The Institute for Health Metrics and Evaluation's 2019 Global Burden of Disease [4]

The GBD 2019 study provides for the first time an independent estimation of population for each of 204 countries and territories across the globe, using a standardized, replicable approach, as well as a comprehensive update on fertility and migration. GBD 2019 incorporates major data additions and improvements, and methodological refinements. Mortality and life expectancy estimates have expanded to a total of 990 locations at the most detailed level, and new causes have been added to the fatal and nonfatal cause lists, for a total of 369 diseases and injuries. Two new risk factors (high and low non-optimal temperatures) and 54 new risk–outcome pairs have also been added. Produced with the input of over 5,000 collaborators from 152 countries and territories, GBD 2019 also includes estimates at the subnational level for five new countries (Italy, Nigeria, Pakistan, the Philippines, and Poland) in addition to the countries for which subnational estimates have been published in previous editions of the GBD study (Russia, Brazil, China, India, Indonesia, Japan, Kenya, Mexico, South Africa, Sweden, the UK, and the US).

GBD estimates incidence, prevalence, mortality, years of life lost (YLLs), YLDs, and disability-adjusted life years (DALYs) due to diseases and injuries by sex, age, and geography. Input data were extracted from censuses, household surveys, civil registration and vital statistics, disease registries, health service use, air pollution monitors, satellite imaging, disease notifications, and other sources. Cause-specific death rates and cause fractions were calculated using the Cause of Death Ensemble model and spatiotemporal Gaussian process regression. Cause-specific deaths were adjusted to match the total all-cause deaths calculated as part of the GBD population, fertility, and mortality estimates. Deaths were multiplied by standard life expectancy at each age to calculate YLLs. A Bayesian meta-regression modeling tool, DisMod-MR 2.1, was used to ensure consistency between incidence, prevalence, remission, excess mortality, and cause-specific mortality for most causes. Prevalence estimates were multiplied by disability weights for mutually exclusive sequelae of diseases and injuries to calculate YLDs.

GBD uses a hierarchical list of risk factors so that specific risk factors (e.g., sodium intake), and related aggregates (e.g., diet quality), are both evaluated. Relative risks were estimated as a function of exposure based on published systematic reviews, 81 systematic reviews done for GBD 2019, and meta-regression. Levels of exposure in each age–sex–location–year included in the study were estimated based on all available data sources using spatiotemporal Gaussian process regression, DisMod-MR 2.1, a Bayesian meta-regression method, or alternative methods. 30,652 distinct data sources were used in the analysis.

The GBD results are presented in the context of the Socio-demographic Index (SDI), a composite indicator of income per capita, years of schooling, and fertility rate in women younger than 25 years. Uncertainty intervals (UIs) were generated for every metric using the 25th and 975th ordered 1000 draw values of the posterior distribution.

8.5 Conclusion

Health information systems are crucial for guiding sound public health policies and programs. Information systems are complex entities formed of diverse parts with one common plan and purpose. Strong health information systems are paramount for surveillance and response, and for monitoring progress toward the SDGs and national and subnational health priorities. The health information systems should generate timely, reliable, disaggregated, comparable and actionable data to measure and track population health determinants and outcomes along with health inequalities [17].

A critical feature of information systems is that their components have regular interactions and interdependences. The systems should be flexible and adaptable to changes in burden and circumstances. Building HIS should start by complementing what is currently in place and improving existing systems. It should use new technologies and include training for collectors and users. Most importantly, the data and findings should be rigorously analyzed, interpreted, translated, disseminated, and used to inform implementation.

References

1. World Health Organization. Toolkit on monitoring health systems: strengthening, health information systems. 2008. www.who.int/healthinfo/statistics/toolkit_hss/EN_PDF_Toolkit_HSS_Information Systems.pdf (accessed March 12, 2020).

2. Institute of Medicine (US) Committee on Quality of Health Care in America. Crossing the quality chasm: a new health system for the 21st century. 2001. https://pubmed.ncbi.nlm.nih.gov/25057539/ (accessed March 12, 2020).

3. B. Shengelia, A. Tandon, O. B. Adams, et al. Access, utilization, quality, and effective coverage: an integrated conceptual framework and measurement strategy. *Soc Sci Med* 2005; **61**(1): 97–109.

4. Global Burden of Disease. IHME measuring what matters. 2021. www.healthdata.org/gbd/2019 (accessed January 14, 2020).

5. A. Tsiachristas, D. Gathara, J. Aluvaala, et al. Effective coverage and budget implications of skill-mix change to improve neonatal nursing care: an explorative simulation

study in Kenya. *BMJ Glob Health* 2019; **4** (6): e001817.

6. K. E. Colson, P. Zúñiga-Brenes, D. Ríos-Zertuche, et al. Comparative estimates of crude and effective coverage of measles immunization in low-resource settings: findings from Salud Mesoamérica 2015. *PLoS One* 2015; **10**(7): e0130697.

7. L. Bijlmakers, M. Wientjes, G. Mwapasa, et al. Out-of-pocket payments and catastrophic household expenditure to access essential surgery in Malawi: a cross-sectional patient survey. *Ann Med Surg (Lond)* 2019; **43**: 85–90.

8. Advancing the Business of Healthcare. What is risk adjustment. 2021. www.aapc.com/risk-adjustment/risk-adjustment.aspx (accessed March 19, 2020).

9. A. P. Weiss, J. Guidi, M. Fava. Closing the efficacy–effectiveness gap: translating both the what and the how from randomized controlled trials to clinical practice. *J Clin Psychiatry* 2009; **70**(4): 446–449.

10. World Health Organization. STEPwise approach to NCD risk factor surveillance (STEPS). 2021. www.who.int/teams/noncommunicable-diseases/surveillance/systems-tools/steps (accessed November 22, 2021).

11. World Health Organization. Health accounts. 2021. www.who.int/health-topics/health-accounts/#tab=tab_1 (accessed November 22, 2021).

12. P. Mahapatra. An overview of the sample registration system in India. 2017. http://citeseerx.ist.psu.edu/viewdoc/download;jsessionid=A193D503CD99492050B8675082B0BAB4?doi=10.1.1.669.528&rep=rep1&type=pdf (accessed March 11, 2020).

13. USAID. The DHS program, demographic and health surveys. 2021. https://dhsprogram.com/ (accessed March 11, 2020).

14. CDC. National Centre for Health Statistics, National Health and Nutrition Examination Survey. 2021. www.cdc.gov/nchs/nhanes/index.htm (accessed March 11, 2020).

15. R. Sund, M. Juntunen, P. Lüthje, et al. Monitoring the performance of hip fracture treatment in Finland. *Ann Med* 2011; **43**(Suppl. 1): S39–S46.

16. Stats SA. Census. 2021. www.statssa.gov.za/?page_id=3836 (accessed March 19, 2020).

17. S. Pooransingh, R. Abdullah, S. Battersby, et al. COVID-19 highlights a critical need for efficient health information systems for managing epidemics of emerging infectious diseases. *Front Public Health* 2021; **9**: 767835.

The Organization and Management of Health Services

Toby Kasper

Key Messages

- There is no magic solution for organizing health services. Services are organized in remarkably diverse ways and yet manage to produce comparable outcomes, so countries should feel comfortable building on the strengths of their own systems as they consider reforms to improve performance, rather than feeling pressure to adopt models of health service organization that are imported from elsewhere.
- Most countries have both centralized and decentralized elements that coexist, and that generally are embedded in a governance and political economy context that is broader than the health sector.
- Efforts to use decentralization to improve health outcomes are unlikely to succeed unless they build the organizational capacity to exercise newfound decision rights soundly and unless they ensure robust accountability systems.
- The private sector encompasses a diverse set of actors that together play a critical role in delivering health services but that are often inappropriately neglected in public sector policy and planning efforts.
- There is no one perfect model of care that will work in all places; instead, the best models of care are ones that are adaptable and can evolve to address shifting epidemiological patterns and emerging threats such as pandemics and climate change.
- Addressing the organization and management of health services inevitably involves a focus on supply-side factors, but demand-side considerations play a critical role in the success or failure of efforts to improve health outcomes and so cannot be ignored.

9.1 Introduction

The diversity in how health services are organized is remarkable. Countries with roughly equivalent health outcomes provide health care in entirely different ways, from being tightly managed from the central level to very decentralized, from being largely publicly provided to mostly privately run, and from being heavily reliant on hospitals to delivering services largely at primary care facilities and/or through community health workers.

This chapter explores three key elements of how health services are organized and managed:

- decentralization;
- the relationship between public and private sectors; and
- models of care.

These three areas – particularly the first two – influence health systems well beyond the delivery of health services. These broader considerations are largely beyond the scope of this chapter and, with regard to the relationship between public and private sectors, are touched upon elsewhere in this volume (see Chapters 27 and 28). The chapter concludes by examining several themes that are shaping the debate about how the organization and management of health services should evolve in the coming decades.

9.2 Key Elements of How Health Services Are Organized and Managed

9.2.1 Decentralization

The question of where decision-making power rests – whether it is concentrated at the national level or whether some authority is exercised at peripheral levels – is one of the most important decisions about the organization of a health system. Decentralization has implications for many aspects of a health system and is rarely a reform focused solely on service delivery. It is addressed here because it has such an important impact on how health services are organized and managed.

The process of shifting decision-making authority from higher to lower levels of government has been perhaps the most common organizational reform of the past 40 years, estimated to have occurred in more than 80% of countries [1]. This has been driven by a number of factors, the most prominent of which is a push for efficiency (both technical and allocative), often shaped by the New Public Management philosophy that emerged in the United Kingdom, United States, Australia, and New Zealand in the 1970s and 1980s. Other rationales for decentralization include improving accountability (e.g., because decision-makers at local levels are more closely tied to the communities for which they are making decisions) and increasing equity (e.g., because local decision-makers are better able to target resources to the least advantaged).

The concept of decentralization comes from the field of public administration, and its use in public health has not always been straightforward. The range of actions covered under the rubric of decentralization is enormous and the term can obscure as much as it reveals. As Anne Mills puts it in a seminal book on the subject, "[de]centralization is therefore not only an important theme in health management but also a confused one" [2].

Decentralization plays out on two main axes: the types of functions decentralized and the form and extent to which decision-making is decentralized. The first category is typically grouped into three main types:

- **Political decentralization:** the process of broadening the involvement of citizens or their representatives in decision-making and/or in determining the leadership of local entities (i.e., rather than those being appointed by the central level).
- **Administrative decentralization:** the transfer of authority for planning and managing the provision of service delivery, potentially including areas such as running health facilities, managing human resources, and maintaining adequate stocks of medicines and commodities.
- **Fiscal decentralization:** the transfer of authority for financial management, which can include the authority to generate and retain revenue (e.g., user fees, local taxes) and/or

make local decisions about budgetary and expenditure management (e.g., control over resources that are provided by a central government).

Frequently, these different types of decentralization are used in tandem. For example, administrative decentralization frequently occurs in the context of political decentralization, and a lower level of government (e.g., a province or a district) could have decision-making authority over both the management of human resources in health facilities and the budgets for them.

With regard to the form and extent of decentralization, four main forms of decentralization have been described in the literature. The first three involve shifts of decision-making across different levels of government, whereas the fourth involves a move to an external actor.[1] From least to most transfer of power, the four forms are (Figure 9.1):

- **Deconcentration:** moving decision-making from higher to lower levels of a government body, such as from Ministry of Health officials in a capital city to ministry officials based in regional hubs, typically within existing laws. The officials remain accountable to the central government.

- **Delegation:** transferring authority (typically via a contractual arrangement) from a central body to an autonomous entity, which could be a public–private partnership, an "authority" with its own board of directors, or a hospital corporation such as a university teaching hospital that typically has considerable decision-making discretion.

- **Devolution:** shifting decision-making authority from central government to lower levels of government (e.g., province/state, district), with considerable independent power to act.

- **Privatization:** transferring responsibility and, typically, ownership from the government to a private entity (which can be for-profit or not-for-profit).

Another important dimension is the level of government to which power is shifted: authority can be transferred from central level to provincial/state, district, municipal, or facility level. In practice, decentralization efforts often involve a blend, with some decisions being shifted to provincial/state level while others are pushed to districts or even facilities. Clearly outlined responsibilities and accountability at all levels is essential regardless of the specific model of decentralization [3].

These different aspects of decentralization mean that it is rarely useful to think of a health system as either simply centralized or decentralized. Instead, most systems sit on a spectrum between the two extremes, with a wide range of possible permutations for which functions are handled at which levels. Areas such as service delivery and human resource management may be decentralized, while policy formulation remains the preserve of the national government. Within the broader trend toward decentralization, recent years have seen a number of countries embracing the value of maintaining central control – or even recentralizing control – over certain functions, such as around procurement of medicines and/or data and information. The roll-out of systems such as DHIS2 has standardized data collection and facilitated much more rapid analysis of trends at national and regional levels

---

[1] The fourth form listed – privatization – is not always considered a form of decentralization, both because it does not involve the transfer of authority from a higher level to a more peripheral one and because it often involves a permanent divestment of government interests or assets in an area rather than an ongoing engagement as in the other forms of decentralization (although a privatized entity may still be subject to government regulation).

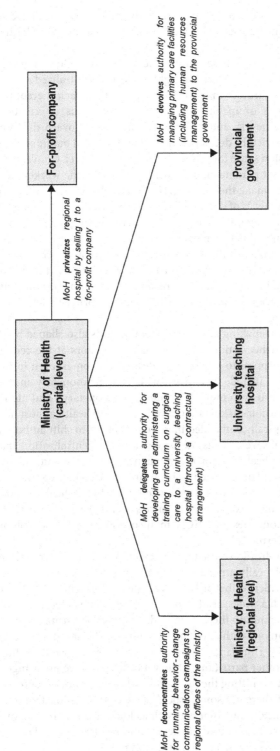

Figure 9.1 Hypothetical examples of the different forms of decentralization as they could impact the organization and management of health services.

than is possible with decentralized systems. Similarly, many countries have adopted centrally defined essential benefits packages that provide a measure of standardization across the country.

A useful concept for analyzing these complexities is that of the "decision space" afforded to actors at the peripheral level [4]. Decision rights may be decentralized as a matter of law, policy, regulation, or even through managerial practice or the lack thereof (e.g., a central government's unwillingness or inability to enforce a law ends up creating additional decision space at the local level), and different regimes may govern different functions. For example, a law may restrict the decision space around firing of public sector workers and so leave only narrow decision space for actors at the peripheral level. Conversely, in the same country, regulations may set parameters for salaries of these same workers but allow local authorities wide latitude to make the final determination on each individual's pay.

Table 9.1 presents an analysis of decision space in four countries. Although it reflects the situation a number of years ago, it is nonetheless useful for highlighting the diversity of decision space both within and between countries.

It is important to recognize that the decision space created on paper – de jure decentralization through laws or policies – may be considerably wider than the de facto decision space that can be exercised in reality. This can result in shifting the responsibility to deliver without a corresponding transfer in decision-making authority, which runs the risk of yielding limited benefits [6].

The practice of decision-making at the peripheral level is also shaped by the efforts of central authorities to influence actions at the local level. Actors at the central level have a range of tools at their disposal to secure their desired outcomes, even in fully devolved systems. These mechanisms include incentives (which can be monetary and/or nonmonetary), punitive measures (also both monetary and/or nonmonetary), and monitoring.

Decentralization of decision-making on matters related to health almost never occurs in a vacuum, but rather is typically embedded in a broader effort to shift authority and power from central to peripheral levels. Thus, decisions about decentralization that may have significant impacts on the health sector are frequently driven by considerations entirely unrelated to health. Health planners need to be aware of this wider context, as they rarely have the freedom to design a system that is optimized solely for the health sector, but instead must situate their efforts within existing governance systems. This is particularly relevant in low- and middle-income countries (L&MICs), many of which are former colonies that have legacies of centralized governance.

The idea that decentralization is a natural evolution as a country develops – and therefore that it is unequivocally a positive reform – has been taken for granted in some quarters. However, the evidence that it improves the performance of a health system is surprisingly mixed for such a widespread reform [1, 6–9]. Some heterogeneity in outcomes is perhaps inevitable. By definition there is more diversity in performance in a system with thousands of actors than in one with a unitary decision-maker, so it is not surprising when decentralization improves performance in some parts of a country while leading to drops in outputs and outcomes in other parts (and while yet other parts see no change) [10].

This has led to interest in shifting the focus from whether or not decentralization works to trying to understand if there are some aspects of decentralization that are particularly important for improving health outcomes, as well as looking at the impact on key characteristics of health systems such as equity, efficiency, and resilience [11]. This is a promising area of research but to date the evidence base is still limited.

Table 9.1 Comparative decision space in Ghana, the Philippines, Uganda, and Zambia

	Decision space		
	Narrow	**Moderate**	**Wide**
Financing			
Sources of revenue	Zambia	Ghana, Uganda	Philippines
Expenditures		All four	
Income from fees		Ghana, Uganda, Zambia	Philippines
Service organization			
Hospital autonomy	Ghana, Zambia	Uganda	Philippines
Insurance plans	Ghana, Uganda		Philippines, Zambia
Payment mechanisms	Ghana, Uganda	Philippines	Zambia
Contracts with private providers		Ghana, Philippines, Zambia	Uganda
Human resources			
Salaries	All four		
Contracts	Ghana	Philippines	Uganda, Zambia
Civil service	Ghana	Philippines, Uganda, Zambia	
Access rules (targeting of populations)	Ghana	Philippines, Uganda, Zambia	
Governance			
Local government	Ghana, Zambia		Philippines, Uganda
Facility boards	All four		
Health offices	Ghana, Philippines	Uganda, Zambia	
Community participation	Ghana, Uganda	Philippines, Zambia	
Total by country			
Ghana	11	4	0
Philippines	3	7	5
Uganda	5	7	3
Zambia	5	7	3

Source: [5].

There is some evidence about the success factors for decentralization initiatives. The manner in which decentralization is carried out – including whether decision-making authority is actually transferred and whether the decentralization process is well managed and clearly communicated by those handling the decentralization – plays a key role in the success or failure of the reform. In addition, two determinants of whether decentralization works are organizational capacity and accountability systems [3].

A range of organizational capacities – administrative, managerial, financial, technical, and human resources – is needed at the peripheral level to make sound use of the authority being transferred. However, capacity-building is not always included in reform processes, which can result in responsibilities being transferred to parts of the system that are not capable of delivering successfully [12, 13]. Capacity at the central level is also required to make a decentralization effort successful, as the skills needed to guide, oversee, and hold accountable other actors in a decentralized system are different from the skills required to centrally manage a health system.

Several types of accountability play roles in decentralization: within the bureaucracy of a health system (e.g., monitoring and supportive supervision provided by the central level); between local health officials and representatives of local government at the corresponding level (e.g., between district health management teams and district administrators or municipal leaders); and through the engagement of community members and media (e.g., through community health boards and the public release of information about health facility performance). Each of these three is important and makes distinct contributions to improving health system performance, so ideally all three are addressed in any decentralization effort.

9.2.2 The Relationship between Public and Private Sectors

It is obvious that any effort to improve health outcomes must be grounded in an accurate understanding of how health services are organized. However, documents such as national health plans and health sector strategies neglect a key component of service delivery surprisingly frequently: the private sector. This is despite the fact that the private sector plays a significant role in delivering health care in most L&MICs, particularly for primary care services such as family planning and basic care for sick children. In many countries, the private sector's share of these services exceeds 50% [14–17]. The private sector is particularly prominent in urban areas, so as urbanization increases globally it is likely that the private sector's share will also grow.

This section focuses specifically on the role of the private sector in service delivery, but it is important to recognize that the private sector's engagement with health systems extends beyond service delivery into areas such as the development and distribution of medicines and other health technologies, health financing (e.g., health insurance), health workforce production and training, information and communications technology, and infrastructure development, all of which are beyond the scope of this chapter.

Numerous types of private sector actors are involved in providing health care. As shown in Table 9.2, these can be categorized into for-profit and not-for-profit and by size. In most L&MICs, these different forms coexist and individual providers may practice in multiple sites.

Similarly, it is important to recognize that public and private sectors operate in relation to each other, rather than as completely separate spheres. This is true on both the supply and

Table 9.2 Different types of private sector providers

	Small	Large
For-profit	• Qualified sole providers (doctors, nurses, midwives) operating independently • Traditional healers • Trained pharmacists (dispensing medicines but also often providing medical advice) • Informal drug sellers (e.g., at small shops or markets)	• Networks of private providers (e.g., group practices, franchised networks) • Private hospitals (sometimes organized into chains)
Not-for-profit	• Community-based organizations offering medical services	• Nongovernmental organizations (national or international) operating health facilities • Mission hospitals and other faith-based facilities (sometimes organized into networks)

the demand sides. On the supply side, in many countries providers work both for public facilities and privately, and public facilities that have inadequate stocks of medicines or other supplies may send patients to private pharmacies. On the demand side, patients routinely shop around, seeking medical advice or diagnoses from both public and private providers, or adjust their behavior based on their perceptions of the quality of care and the conditions in one or the other type of facility.

These interactions highlight the importance of engagement between public and private sectors. This includes both at the policy level (e.g., involving private sector representatives in policy formulation) and at the service delivery level. One framework [18] identifies four approaches for engaging the private sector around service delivery:

- **prohibition:** banning some or all forms of private provision of services;
- **constraint:** regulating private practice, whether through self-regulation or statutory rules/controls (e.g., accreditation, licensing, registration);
- **encouragement and subsidization:** attempting to improve private provision of services (e.g., quality of care) through incentives, subsidies, social franchising, social marketing, and/or the provision of training (see Chapter 30); and
- **purchasing:** buying services or goods, contracting private providers (e.g., to address capacity constraints in the public sector or to tap specialized expertise), or providing vouchers to address demand-side constraints and/or encourage the utilization of specific services (e.g., family planning, maternal and child health).

Most L&MICs mix these approaches, although outright prohibitions are rare, in part because they are very difficult to enforce. Almost all countries have some form of constraint on private practitioners, although the capacity to implement regulations varies widely and is often suboptimal, which has resulted in numerous scandals around substandard or fraudulent medicines and practitioners who had no qualifications but routinely offered services to patients in need. Building regulatory quality is an area that frequently does not receive the attention or support that it deserves, given its importance in improving health outcomes.

Contracting out is another common form of engagement, particularly in settings when governments have inadequate capacity to deliver essential services, such as in fragile and conflict-affected situations (see Chapters 22 and 30). It is closely tied to the organization of health financing functions in a country, especially whether the "provider" and "purchaser" roles are split or unitary (see Chapters 17 and 18 for more on health financing and purchaser–provider splits). The evidence base around the impact of contracting out is weak [19], but one important lesson is that the process of managing contracts itself requires some capacity on the part of government. The stewardship function of governments is another area that has not received much investment but that could pay significant dividends if properly resourced.

9.2.3 Models of Care

Low- and middle-income countries use a wide range of models of care to organize, manage, and deliver health services. These can be understood as having four main dimensions:

- **where** (at which level) the services are being delivered;
- **who** is delivering services;
- **how** services are provided; and
- **what** conditions are included.

Perhaps the most controversial of these is **where** services are delivered, which has been characterized by pendulum swings over time between a focus on hospital-based service delivery and on the delivery of services at the primary care level and/or at the community level. This debate can be fiercely contested and often has important implications for the allocation of resources; given the interests involved it is unlikely to be resolved purely by evidence. However, there are some areas of consensus. This includes that it is generally preferable for the first and most regular point of contact for a patient to be at the primary care level, and that robust care coordination systems are essential for connecting the different levels, including referral systems that operate smoothly in reality rather than merely existing on paper.

In practice, even these basics are not widely implemented successfully. Patients may vote with their feet and opt for hospital care over services from primary care facilities if they perceive the latter to be of inadequate quality or insufficiently patient-centered. Referral networks may be beset with problems that stem from governance (e.g., referral hospitals may be under the jurisdiction of the central level or provinces/states, while primary care facilities are controlled by districts, leading to difficulties in communication and coordination) and from financial or operational difficulties (e.g., insufficient numbers of functioning ambulances).

With regard to **who** is delivering services, a key area of emphasis in recent years is delivering care through a team-based approach that enables patients to receive multidisciplinary support that addresses their needs in a comprehensive manner. There is not a single model for these teams, but they often include general practitioners/family doctors, nurses, community health workers, pharmacists, and managerial/administrative staff. This approach is commonly paired with empanelment, in which patients in a defined geographical area are assigned to an "accredited"/quality-recognized provider/team.

How services are delivered is covered in detail in Chapter 10, but one element that is particularly relevant for understanding the organization and management of health services is the distinction between vertical (disease-specific) and horizontal (integrated/systems-oriented) approaches to service delivery. Although vertical programs have been around for decades, the rise of global health initiatives in the early 2000s brought considerable resources and political attention to bear on HIV, TB, malaria, and vaccines and immunizations. The accompanying emphasis on a rapid response and on the accountable use of resources contributed to the establishment of management systems that were frequently verticalized, with parallel human resources, supply chains, and monitoring and evaluation. These mechanisms have generally been considered successful in improving health outcomes for the targeted conditions, but the impacts on health systems have been more controversial, with concerns having been raised that they cause fragmentation and make governing the system as a whole more challenging [20]. This has given rise to considerable efforts to ensure that these initiatives strengthen health systems while continuing to focus on their priority areas and, more generally, to efforts to develop synergies between vertical and horizontal efforts (sometimes termed a "diagonal" approach [21]).

The final issue that shapes discussions of models of care is **what** services must be provided. This is driven primarily by the shifting burden of disease, as most L&MICs are seeing noncommunicable diseases increase their share of the disease burden due to a combination of successful efforts to address communicable diseases and larger demographic and societal factors that increase the risk of noncommunicable diseases (e.g., aging populations, urbanization, changing patterns of consumption leading to increases in obesity and other risk factors). In many L&MICs this is posing a significant challenge for health systems, which need to be able to deliver services simultaneously to address the unfinished (and at times re-emerging) agenda on communicable diseases, which are often of a time-limited but time-sensitive nature, and noncommunicable diseases, which often require chronic care. This shift is playing out at both the population level and for individual patients, necessitating attention to multimorbidity, which is one of the drivers behind the increased emphasis on multidisciplinary teams that can deliver comprehensive care.

The COVID-19 pandemic is creating interest in another aspect of what services health systems must provide: essential public health functions (see Chapter 32). Even prior to the pandemic, the Global Conference on Primary Health Care in Astana, Kazakhstan in 2018 highlighted the importance of integrating public health functions and primary care [22], and identified six models for doing so [23]:

1. public health professionals integrated into primary care;
2. public health services and primary care providers working together;
3. comprehensive and proactive benefit packages that include public health;
4. primary care services within public health settings;
5. building public health incentives in primary care; and
6. multidisciplinary training of primary care staff in public health.

COVID-19 has shone an unpleasant light on the failure to integrate public health into the basic management of health systems, as well as on the longstanding underinvestment in public health, even in a number of high-income countries. There is little doubt that this crisis will spur new models for how to integrate public health into routine health services.

9.3 Emerging Directions on How Health Systems Are Organized and Managed

The plethora of different approaches for organizing and managing health services described above is a double-edged sword. On the one hand, this diversity is an important factor behind the surprisingly thin evidence base on the best ways to organize service delivery. On the other hand, it means that L&MICs should not feel pressure to adopt models of health service organization that are imported from elsewhere and instead should feel comfortable building on the strengths of their own systems as they consider reforms to improve performance.

There are inevitably multiple ways that the organization of service delivery can be changed to improve performance, but reform efforts are more likely to succeed if they appreciate the inherent complexity of health systems and the history that shapes this complexity, rather than succumbing to the trap of "isomorphic mimicry" [24], the habit of governments to imitate the approaches of other countries despite critical differences in context and capacity.

The early history of the COVID-19 pandemic has highlighted the perils of ignoring this lesson. L&MICs that attempted to follow the path adopted by highly resourced countries and employ a high-tech model of care ended up spending considerable time and resources trying to procure ventilators at the cost of neglecting more basic but ultimately more important management challenges, such as the distribution of personal protective equipment and oxygen supplies.

COVID-19 has also brought renewed attention to an important but often ignored dimension to the management of health services: the trust of a population is a critical factor in delivering services successfully. Across income classifications, the countries that managed the pandemic better were those in which populations had trust in their governments and so responded more supportively to their government's actions [25].

This underscores the importance of strengthening community engagement and local accountability as part of efforts to improve the management of health services. It also connects with another important recent theme in the management of health services: the shift from treating patients as passive recipients of health services to active co-creators of health outcomes. This requires empowering individuals and communities to jointly design the health services that they want to use. It also recognizes that – particularly with the development and rapid dissemination of new digital technologies – individuals are increasingly able to be active participants in improving their own health, learning about the health conditions they have and the treatment options available, as well as monitoring their own health.

The final trend that is shaping the management of health services is the need to build resilience into the heart of systems. COVID-19 has highlighted the importance of having health systems that are resilient to shocks, and this attribute is only likely to become more critical in the face of more frequent disruptions caused by climate change and threats such as antimicrobial resistance and emerging pathogens.

References

1. A. Dwicaksono, A. Fox. Does decentralization improve health system performance and outcomes in low- and middle-income countries? A systematic review of evidence from quantitative studies. *Milbank Q* 2018; **96**(2): 323–368.

2. A. Mills, Decentralization concepts and issues: a review. In A. Mills, J. P. Vaughan,

D. L. Smith, et al., eds., *Health System Decentralization: Concepts, Issues and Country Experience*. Washington, DC, WHO, 1990. https://apps.who.int/iris/bitstream/handle/10665/39053/9241561378.pdf?sequence=1&isAllowed=y (accessed June 14, 2020).

3. B. Adhikari, S. R. Mishra, R. Schwarz. Transforming Nepal's primary health care delivery system in global health era: addressing historical and current implementation challenges. *Global Health* 2022; **18**(8). doi: 10.1186/s12992-022-00798-5.

4. T. Bossert. Analyzing the decentralization of health systems in developing countries: decision space, innovation and performance. *Soc Sci Med* 1998; **47**(10): 1513–1527.

5. T. Bossert, J. Beauvais. Decentralization of health systems in Ghana, Zambia, Uganda, and the Philippines: a comparative analysis of decision space. *Health Policy Plan* 2002; **17**(1): 14–31.

6. J. Mohammed, N. North, T. Ashton. Decentralisation of health services in Fiji: a decision space analysis. *Int J Health Policy Manag* 2016; **5**(3): 173–181.

7. A. M. Sumah, L. Baatiema, S. Abimbol. The impacts of decentralisation on health-related equity: a systematic review of the evidence. *Health Policy* 2016; **120** (10): 1183–1192.

8. D. C. Muñoz, P. M. Amador, L. M. Llamas, et al. Decentralization of health systems in low and middle income countries: a systematic review. *Int J Public Health* 2017; **62**(2): 219–229.

9. A. Channa and J. P. Faguet. Decentralization of health and education in developing countries: a quality-adjusted review of the empirical literature. *World Bank Res Observ* 2016; **31**: 199–241. https://openknowledge.worldbank.org/bitstream/handle/10986/29307/wbro_31_2_199.pdf?sequence=1 (accessed November 14, 2020).

10. J. P. Faguet. Low decision space means no decentralization in Fiji: comment on "Decentralisation of health services in Fiji:

a decision space analysis". *Int J Health Policy Manag* 2016; **5**(11): 663–665.

11. S. Abimbola, L. Baatiema, M. Bigdeli. The impacts of decentralization on health system equity, efficiency and resilience: a realist synthesis of the evidence. *Health Policy Plan* 2019; **34**(8): 605–617.

12. T. E. Roman, S. Cleary, D. McIntyre. Exploring the functioning of decision space: a review of the available health systems literature. *Int J Health Policy Manag* 2017; **6**(7): 365–376.

13. T. J. Bossert, A. D. Mitchell, M. A. Janjua. Improving health system performance in a decentralized health system: capacity building in Pakistan. *Health Syst Reform* 2015; **1**(4): 276–284.

14. M. Mackintosh, A. Channon, A. Karan, et al. What is the private sector? Understanding private provision in the health systems of low-income and middle-income countries. *Lancet* 2016; **388** (10044): 596–605.

15. K. Grépin. Private sector an important but not dominant provider of key health services in low- and middle-income countries. *Health Aff (Millwood)* 2016; **35** (7): 1214–1221.

16. T. Powell-Jackson, D. Macleod, L. Benova, et al. The role of the private sector in the provision of antenatal care: a study of Demographic and Health Surveys from 46 low- and middle-income countries. *Trop Med Int Health* 2015; **20**(2): 230–239.

17. SHOPS Plus, USAID. Private sector counts. www.privatesectorcounts.org (accessed November 18, 2020).

18. D. Montagu, C. Goodman. Prohibit, constrain, encourage, or purchase: how should we engage with the private health-care sector? *Lancet* 2016; **388** (10044): 613–621.

19. W. A. Odendaal, K. Ward, J. Uneke, et al. Contracting out to improve the use of clinical health services and health outcomes in low- and middle-income countries. *Cochrane Database Syst Rev* 2018; **4**(4): CD008133.

20. R. G. Biesma, R. Brugha, A. Harmer, et al. The effects of global health initiatives on country health systems: a review of the evidence from HIV/AIDS control. *Health Policy Plan* 2009; **24**(4): 239–252.

21. J. Frenk. Bridging the divide: comprehensive reform to improve health in Mexico. Lecture for WHO Commission on Social Determinants of Health, Nairobi. 2006. www.who.int/social_determinants/resources/frenk.pdf (accessed November 25, 2020).

22. World Health Organization. Declaration of Astana. Global Conference on Primary Health Care, Astana, Kazakhstan. 2018. https://apps.who.int/iris/bitstream/handle/10665/328123/WHO-HIS-SDS-2018.61-eng.pdf (accessed December 24, 2020).

23. World Health Organization. Primary health care: closing the gap between public health and primary care through integration. https://apps.who.int/iris/rest/bitstreams/1242113/retrieve (accessed December 25, 2020).

24. M. Andrews, L. Pritchett, M. Woolcock. Looking like a state: the seduction of isomorphic mimicry. In M. Andrews, L. Pritchett, M. Woolcock, *Building State Capability: Evidence, Analysis, Action.* Oxford, Oxford University Press, 2017, pp. 29–52.

25. COVID-19 National Preparedness Collaborators. Pandemic preparedness and COVID-19: an exploratory analysis of infection and fatality rates, and contextual factors associated with preparedness in 177 countries, from Jan 1, 2020, to Sept 30, 2021. *Lancet* 2022. https://doi.org/10.1016/S0140-6736(22)00172-6.

Health Services Delivery
Key Concepts and Characteristics

Delanyo Dovlo, Sharon Ametepeh, and Koku
Awoonor-Williams

Key Messages

- Evidence-based policies and strategies should inform the delivery of services and the investment of resources in the hardware and software inputs required for effective coverage.
- Demand generation is essential as services are only useful if utilized by the people who need them and should therefore be considered when designing health services.
- Needs-driven essential packages and continuity of services along the life course should be established based on disease burden and risk assessment that addresses the majority of health conditions affecting the population and vulnerable groups.
- Health services are much more likely to influence outcomes when they adhere to the key characteristics of accessibility, coverage, quality, efficiency, person-centeredness, coordination, comprehensiveness, continuity, and accountability.
- Quality of care is essential for coverage and utilization to result in good health. "Effective coverage" translates the inputs into health gains.
- Equity in the provision of health services is a fundamental value for any low- or middle-income country aspiring to achieve universal health coverage.
- Information and monitoring systems are key to generating baseline data and to measure progress, as well as to support research and knowledge platforms.

10.1 Introduction

Health services are the interface between the health system and the population, and are commonly understood by people and many decision-makers as the primary purpose of health systems. The delivery of health services translates health policies, plans, and strategies into specific interventions to address the health needs of individuals and collectives. Along with biological, social, and environmental determinants of health, health services are critical in shaping health outcomes. Fundamental considerations regarding the delivery of health services include: (1) how services should be *organized* and resources allocated to serve as many people as possible; (2) how to ensure that the services *reach* the people who need them; and (3) whether services are *effective* in meeting the needs of the population [1].

Building on the previous chapter on the organizational and management aspects of health services, this chapter describes the norms, enablers, and challenges associated with effective service delivery with a focus on low- and middle-income countries (L&MICs). The chapter considers key concepts and definitions, the organization of services, the characteristics and enablers of high-quality services, assessing the needs and demand for services, and key considerations in the composition of health services packages.

10.2 Concepts and Definitions

"Service delivery" is one of the six building blocks of health systems (see Chapter 1, Figure 1.4) [2]. This chapter uses the terms *delivery* and *provision* interchangeably. Health services include information (e.g., public campaigns to encourage handwashing), assistance (e.g., ambulance services and pharmacies), and direct technical and clinical maneuvers (e.g., diagnostic history taking, psychotherapy, or surgery) carried out to address specific health needs. The full spectrum of essential health services includes promotion, prevention, treatment, rehabilitation, and palliation. Some services represent a single element of the spectrum (e.g., a vaccine to prevent measles), but most simultaneously include several interventions (e.g., the use of antiretrovirals for HIV treatment and prevention).

The selected services and interventions that are ultimately available, accessible, and acceptable, together with utilization constitute the dimension of coverage, which is central to progress toward universal health coverage (UHC). A more comprehensive discussion of coverage is provided in Chapter 3. Given the indissociable relation between social determinants and health, the term *health and social services* is increasingly used to refer to the continuum of interventions that directly affect the biology and physiology of health, and those that provide social support and protection. In this chapter, the term *health services* is understood to include social services. The term *population* refers to individuals and groups, and to those actively seeking and receiving care as well as those who benefit passively from promotive and preventive services.

The *provision* of effective health services involves the purposeful orchestration of complex resources and processes [3]. Resources or *inputs* include physical structures, supplies, funding, technology, and service infrastructure and information systems – sometimes termed *hardware inputs* – as well as less tangible factors such as skills, ideas, professional relations and interactions, power structures, values and norms influencing community engagement, transparency, and accountability – sometimes called *software inputs* [4]. *Processes* shape the transformation of hardware and software inputs into competence, capacity, distribution of services, reliable supply, and effective communication, which in turn influence access, equity, acceptability, overall demand, and ultimately the utilization of services. Optimal orchestration of resources and processes enhances supply as well as demand, mobilizing people to accept and utilize services and adopt positive health-seeking behaviors [5].

10.3 Organization of Health Service Delivery

The organization of health services has been described according to a variety of dimensions and frameworks, each with a particular purpose, advantages, and challenges. Any given health system typically uses a number of these frameworks concurrently. We review here some of the common ways in which health services are organized, including the levels of care, location and platforms/facilities, vertical and horizontal modes of integration, and personal or nonpersonal services (also called individual or population-based).

10.3.1 Levels of Care

Health services are commonly organized according to *levels of care*, including primary, secondary, tertiary, and in some cases quaternary super-specialized care. While the specific services, human resources, and facilities included in each level vary widely among jurisdictions, the "levels" generally reflect increasing degrees of specialization. In well-functioning health systems, secondary and tertiary levels deliver services that require more specialized expertise and often more elaborate and expensive technology. However, all levels are expected to be adequately resourced with the required skills, technology, facilities, and processes to allow them to deliver high-quality services and to fulfill their expected roles in the overall system. This includes a well-resourced and well-performing primary (care) level able to address the majority of people's health concerns, which is essential to optimize the performance of secondary and tertiary levels. The services delivered at this primary level include primary care, which further needs to meet certain characteristics in order to deliver optimal outcomes. Primary care is described further in Chapter 2.

10.3.2 Service Delivery Platforms

Service delivery can also be organized according to location, which is also referred to as the "platform" and includes the community (meaning a facility not primarily dedicated to health services, such as a school, community center, or the workplace), a range of outpatient and ambulatory clinics and facilities of various sizes and ranges of services, and hospitals. In some countries, "levels" are associated with specific types of facilities. In primary health care (PHC) oriented health systems, primary care services strive to address the majority of essential health needs close to where people live and work, which may include community-based services delivered in fixed settings, or through mobile outreach, either at home, at school, at work, or in other community-based facilities. For example, in L&MICs, immunization services and health-promotion activities are often provided through outreach services delivered in the community (schools, public spaces). An increasingly wide range of services is delivered at home, including treatment for HIV and tuberculosis, palliative care, and rehabilitation services. An example of community-based services is provided in Box 10.1.

Whereas limited resources and skills are best concentrated in referral centers to optimize administrative and clinical efficiency in the delivery of specialized services (for example, in many L&MICs highly specialized cardiac services or cancer care are not available at primary or even secondary care levels), clear referral and counter-referral pathways can be established between such specialized centers and the network of primary care facilities to enable access.

Historically, health services have commonly been delivered either in clinical settings organized around the expertise of the providers and the infrastructure and equipment required to treat or diagnose a particular condition (e.g., infectious diseases hospital, TB hospital, mental health facility), around the unique needs of a population (e.g., pediatric hospital, rehabilitation center), or according to a specific model of care (e.g., child and maternity services, which combine obstetrics and pediatrics). Regardless of location, in a PHC approach, services need to be centered on the person rather than a given condition [7] and are integrated to address the comprehensive needs of the user with optimal effectiveness and efficiency (see Chapter 24).

10.3.3 Vertical vs. Horizontal Integration of Services

The organization of health services as vertical (integrated around a disease) or horizontal (integrated around the comprehensive needs of people) is discussed in Chapter 24. In either

Box 10.1 Community-Based Health Planning Services (CHPS) in Ghana

An example of a community-based service delivery model is the CHPS initiative in Ghana, which was created to reduce geographic and financial barriers to accessing health care in rural communities. CHPS involves the mobilization of community leadership, decision-making systems, and resources in a defined catchment area (zone), the placement of reoriented frontline health staff with logistic support, and community volunteer systems to provide services within the communities. The core CHPS workforce comprises community-deployed professional nurses, termed "community health officers" (CHOs), who are responsible for primary care service delivery that includes provision of integrated management of childhood illnesses (IMCI), antenatal and postnatal care, immunizations, treatment of minor ailments, family planning, referral, and home visitation services. The CHO together with the local community creates service operational "zones" involving 3–5 contiguous communities. CHOs are trained to liaise with the village health volunteers (VHV), who are part of the traditional system of governance and are trained to provide health education, prevention, and promotion through community mobilization activities, as well as with the community health management committee (CHMC) involved in marshaling traditional social structures for supporting supervision and resources for service delivery. CHPS is therefore a "close-to-client" service delivery system [6].

case, integration can apply to any or all of the following: funding, organization, management, and delivery. These include (1) a vertically funded, managed, delivered, and monitored program such as HIV care in many L&MICs; (2) services with dedicated funding, organization, and management but delivered through a functionally integrated platform, such as immunization or tuberculosis services delivered through primary care clinics; and (3) services fully integrated horizontally, such as comprehensive primary care services in some settings [8].

Extensive efforts have been made in the past 20 years to better integrate health services. New models of integrated care in high-income countries have been linked to improved patient satisfaction, improved access, and a perceived improvement in quality, but their link to other outcomes is less clear. A systematic review conducted in 2006 did not show that integrating vertical programs into primary care in L&MICs improved service delivery or people's health status, although the study did not control for levels of training and funding, which are typically more concentrated in vertical programs [9]. Vertical programs may be desirable as a temporary measure if the health system (and primary care) is weak, a rapid response is needed, or to address the needs of specific target groups. In practice, most health services combine vertically and horizontally integrated elements, with varying degrees of balance between them. A recent review examined integration of health services during the COVID-19 pandemic and emphasized that integrated approaches are potentially viable to improve health systems resilience during health emergencies in L&MICs [10]. Furthermore, the integration of health services is far more complex than is captured by the vertical–horizontal spectrum, and is more fully explored in Chapter 24.

10.3.4 Personal vs. Nonpersonal Services

Health services can also be organized according to their types of outputs, into personal (individual) and nonpersonal (population-level) health services. Personal health services are delivered individually, and may include promotive, preventive, treatment, rehabilitative, and palliative care. Nonpersonal health services are actions applied to collectives. They can be promotive, such as mass health education campaigns, preventive, such as mass immunizations, or they can target nonhuman components of the environment to mitigate risk or improve health outcomes, such as basic sanitation and water purification [1].

10.4 Characteristics and Enablers of High-Quality Health Services

The planning of health services typically includes the two closely related elements of "what" services are to be included and "how" they are to be organized for optimal delivery. There is no universally accepted list of what constitutes "essential health services" as countries need to determine what is deemed essential based on their specific circumstances. The organization of services will also vary according to the context, including the prevailing epidemiology, service readiness, and the priorities identified in each jurisdiction. The WHO considers nine characteristics of health services: comprehensiveness, accessibility, coverage, continuity, quality, person-centeredness, coordination, accountability, and efficiency [11].

A framework of service delivery characteristics (Figure 10.1) has been proposed, outlining factors that translate health services into favorable outcomes. The depiction of these characteristics as layers does not mean they are independent of one another. The figure illustrates that achieving the ultimate dual goal of *health* and *responsiveness* requires health services to be appropriately *covered, utilized,* and *equitable*. For this to happen, the services should be *accessible, available, acceptable,* and *affordable* to the users, as proposed by Tanahashi in 1978 [12], and of high *quality,* including in the attributes of *safety, timeliness, efficiency,* and *effectiveness*. In addition, their organization should result in health services that enable *first contact* and are *comprehensive, coordinated, continuous,* and *person-centered* (sometimes referred to as the 5Cs). Finally, from a broader systems perspective, service should be *resilient, sustainable,* and *accountable* to its users. Presented in the following is a brief summary of these characteristics; a detailed discussion of each is beyond the scope of this chapter.

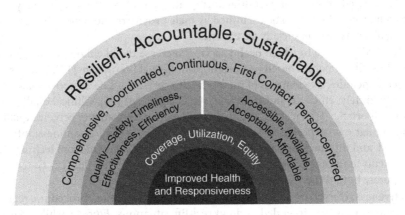

Figure 10.1 Framework for the characteristics of health services.
Source: Siddiqi S; Rouleau KD, Mataria A, Iqbal M

10.4.1 Service Outcome-Related Characteristics

- **Coverage:** Service coverage (also sometimes called crude coverage) refers to the percentage of people who receive the health interventions, whether they produce a health benefit or not. *Effective coverage* is the proportion of the population that receives an intervention and gains health benefits.
- **Utilization** is the use of health services by a population for the purpose of promoting health, preventing disease, obtaining relief for an illness or through rehabilitation or palliative care [13]. Utilization rates can be measured through different methods: (1) the number of service units used over a period divided by a population denominator (e.g., visits/person/year); (2) the percentage of persons who use a certain service over individuals eligible for that service in a period, which is the same as service coverage (e.g., immunization coverage; antenatal care attendance), or, less accurately, the number of visits per day or the number of consultations per provider per day.
- **Equity** is the absence of avoidable or remediable differences among groups of people, whether those groups are defined socially, economically, demographically, or geographically [14]. An equity lens can be applied to both service provision and financing. *Equitable care* means giving people the care they need when they need it. Equity in service provision means that those in greater need of health services should receive the services they need without reference to their social or economic ability, while equity in financing means that those with lower ability to pay contribute less irrespective of the level of their health needs.

10.4.2 Service Delivery-Related Characteristics

- **Availability** of health services implies the presence of service inputs and processes such as infrastructure, workforce, essential medicines, and supplies that are required to provide a service.
- **Accessibility** implies that the service is reasonably reachable, and access is not obstructed by physical distance, or social, cultural, financial, and other barriers for people who are expected to benefit from it.
- **Acceptability** denotes the willingness of people to use services that are available and accessible based on social and cultural norms and values. For example, in many cultures, women may be reluctant to be examined by male providers and hence the services, even if available, may not be socially acceptable.
- **Quality** is the degree to which health services increase the likelihood of achieving the desired health outcomes based on current professional knowledge [15]. The Institute of Medicine includes six elements of quality health services – safe, effective, patient-centered, timely, efficient, and equitable (see Chapter 26) [16]. Clinical quality and patient experience are facets of the quality of health care. Patients perceive quality through their own experiences such as reception, waiting time, cleanliness, information provided, and interpersonal attention received, which is different from technical quality assessments in terms of clinical processes and outcomes. Service delivery systems should incorporate both dimensions of quality of care [17].
- **Effectiveness** refers to the extent to which a specific intervention, procedure, regimen, or service does what it is intended to do in real-life situations. *Efficacy*, while related to

effectiveness, refers to the extent to which a specific intervention, procedure, regimen, or service produces the intended result under ideal conditions, such as in a laboratory.

- **Efficiency**: An intervention is said to be *efficient* if it obtains the maximum output from a given set of inputs or achieves the desired output from a minimum input. Interventions can be effective (produce results), but not efficient in terms of cost per unit of health produced. *Allocative efficiency* refers to when resources are applied to the most effective use among a number of competing needs. *Technical efficiency* refers to the extent to which the choice and utilization of input resources produce a specific health output or a service at the lowest cost.

10.4.3 Key Characteristics of High-Quality Primary Care

Evidence has clearly shown that PHC-oriented health systems with high-quality primary care and integrated essential public health function as their core lead to better outcomes, better equity, and better cost effectiveness [18]. Evidence has further shown that to achieve these outcomes, primary care services need to be organized to achieve a number of key characteristics described here. These characteristics are not meant to diminish the crucial role of secondary and tertiary care (for which these characteristics can apply), but rather outline how to optimize the performance of primary care and its link to other levels of care in order to achieve the best clinical outcomes and patient experience.

- **Comprehensiveness** refers to the range of services that address the health needs of a target population and includes health promotive, preventive, curative, rehabilitative, and palliative services, in addition to personal and population-based interventions. A comprehensive set of services should address health needs for all age groups and across the life course, from birth to death. This attribute is particularly relevant and should be considered in the development of essential packages of health services.
- **Continuity** of care refers to "the extent to which a series of discrete health care events is experienced by people as coherent and interconnected over time and is consistent with their health needs and preferences"[8]. It presupposes mutual intent to establish an ongoing relationship between the provider(s) and the user. It is related to, and enabled when the primary care provider (or team) is able to coordinate care between different levels and types of services through effective referrals and counter-referrals, minimizing fragmentation and care gaps that ultimately lead to poor health outcomes and low patient satisfaction. It reflects intentional provision of care over time and for various needs, and underpins the development of personal relationships that are central to effective primary care. It has been associated with better outcomes as well as seen as valuable in its own right [19]. Continuity ensures that individuals and families can access services for various conditions at various levels of care, and over their life course as a thread, with past experiences and encounters informing subsequent ones. It has been described as having five dimensions, namely chronological, geographical, interdisciplinary, interpersonal, and informational [20], which means that continuity can exist between a person and a single provider, a team, and a particular clinic, and is enabled by proper documentation. Continuity of services has also become important in the context of major outbreaks (e.g., Ebola and COVID-19) and/or natural disasters that disrupt routine services (e.g., for TB or maternal health). An aspect of continuity of services, therefore, calls for the ability to maintain a certain amount of accessible essential services even during such disruptions.

- **Person-centeredness** ensures that services are organized around an individual's unique needs and wants, and not primarily around a disease or a particular program. It acknowledges the individual and their circumstances as the legitimate and primary guide and beneficiary for the delivery of services. A person-centered approach generates actual and perceived responsiveness and a continuity of care for different health needs. It can improve participation of target populations and engage individuals as partners in their own health care [21]. Person-centeredness is distinct from patient-centeredness in that it acknowledges that people's entire human experience defines their needs and preferences, and not only their illness experience where they assume the role of "patient." In the context of comprehensive primary care, where promotion and prevention services are delivered to people who are well, identifying the central actors (also called users) as persons rather than patients is particularly appropriate. The term *people-centered services* offers yet another nuance and captures the broader, collective dimension of key health actors. Typically used in the context of health systems planning rather than individual service delivery, people-centeredness is often synonymous with *community-centered* or *community-informed* to underscore the central role of people as actors and creators of health, as opposed to providers, diseases, or facilities [22].

- **Coordination** among members of a multidisciplinary team, across health and social services, between facilities and the community and between providers across levels of care is critical to the delivery of effective health services. It is especially so where vertically integrated services abound and when comprehensiveness requires the engagement of other sectors in order to influence the social determinants of health. Coordination, which is a process more than a characteristic, can enable efficiency by enabling integration of care and by minimizing duplicated use of resources across platforms, providers, and episodes of care.

10.4.4 Service Organization-Related Characteristics

- **Sustainability** implies the continued provision of health services at the same level of effort over time for as long as it is needed. It is best understood by what undermines sustainability, such as the absence of guaranteed funding over the timeline of need; available skills and capacity to continue to deliver the service; and continued availability of infrastructure, logistics, and processes and procedures. Changes in ownership or in sources of resources are other factors that affect sustainability, which is frequently a challenge in L&MICs when pilot projects, special programs, or NGO-led initiatives rely on external financing.

- **Accountability** refers to the demonstrated ability to meet one's obligations. In the context of health services, these obligations include ensuring efficiency and reducing wastage of resources while achieving core objectives. Managers and providers must be held accountable for resources and results and must respond to the target population's demands. An important aspect of accountability rests with the empowerment of service users and beneficiary communities to whom health systems are ultimately accountable [23].

- **Resilience:** Health services can effectively prevent, prepare for, detect, adapt to, respond to, and recover from public health threats while ensuring the maintenance of quality essential and routine health services in all contexts, including in fragile, conflict, and violent settings [24].

10.5 Assessing the "Demand" and "Need" for Health Services

A community's demands for health services can be different from its needs as determined from disease burden assessments and from community health profiles. "Assessed needs" derived from technical processes do not readily translate into a community's "felt needs" or "revealed demand" for services [25]. There is often a hierarchy of priorities and urgent technical needs, but overlooking the preferences of the community can undermine trust. Community engagement can help identify, understand, and prioritize needs and demands. Health needs evolve and are influenced by changes in culture, education (including health education), environment, climate change, economic activities, wealth, and other influences of health-seeking behaviors (Box 10.2) [26].

10.6 Essential Package of Health Services

An essential package of health services (EPHS) is a detailed list of interventions/ services (preventive, promotive, curative, rehabilitative, and palliative) selected by the government, communities, individuals, and other stakeholders to be delivered across different platforms of care to address the health care needs of the population. Within the UHC context, the set of prioritized health services that are publicly financed has sometimes been termed a health benefits package [28]. EPHS should be need-based, available to all, be safe and effective, high quality, and people-centered. Services should be provided without user fees, especially at the primary care level, to the maximum possible extent, in a manner that ensures financial protection without deterring use [29]. In the past, there have also been successful experiences of implementing benefit packages in post-conflict countries such as Afghanistan that offer several lessons [30].

The concept of an EPHS for L&MICs was first introduced in 1993 as a means to tackle major public health problems and achieve substantial health gains at modest cost [31] followed by subsequent efforts [32, 33]. The third edition of *Disease Control Priorities* (DCP3) was published in 2017 and provides evidence on cost-effective interventions to

---

Box 10.2 Understanding Community Perceptions and Cultural Norms during the Ebola Outbreak

Community perceptions and cultural understanding of the causes and effects of ill-health were key lessons for service providers during the Ebola outbreak in West Africa in 2014–2015. Social anthropologists played key roles in understanding the cultural practices that facilitated the outbreak. Lessons derived helped design measures that allow burial parties to perform and handle remains with dignity and in line with local customs, while still observing the strict infection-prevention protocols [27]. This encouraged reluctant communities to permit the bodies of their family members to be handled by these external teams. Continuous community engagement helps health service managers to understand factors that can create more efficient and responsive interventions and better acceptance and utilization.

address the burden of disease in low-resource settings. DCP3 proposes 218 essential interventions for UHC that L&MICs can choose from to develop their national or subnational EPHS, along with a high-priority package comprising 108 health interventions for highly resource-constrained settings (see Chapter 15). The WHO has also developed a UHC Compendium, which is a database of health services and intersectoral interventions designed to assist countries in making progress toward UHC. It provides a strategic way to organize and present information and creates a framework that offers the full spectrum of promotive, preventive, diagnostic, resuscitative, curative, rehabilitative, and palliative services, as well as a full complement of intersectoral interventions [34].

10.6.1 Guiding Principles for Designing an Essential Package of Health Services

The decision to include an intervention in a service package must be evidence-informed and not driven by the preferences of decision-makers or interest groups. Inclusion of an intervention should be based on consideration of a range of criteria: (1) burden of disease or risk in the population; (2) cost-effectiveness of interventions; (3) budgetary impact; (4) feasibility of implementation; (5) social acceptability; (6) financial risk protection; and (7) equity concerns. Selection always includes an element of judgment and compromise. A major hurdle in designing evidence-based EPHS in L&MICs is the absence of data and inadequate analyses of data and costs. Countries may find it useful to start with a "foundational" package and plan toward an "optimal" package as more resources become available.

The determination of a national EPHS requires significant efforts to design, cost, and implement essential services, and to monitor progress toward UHC. There is no blueprint for developing an EPHS, and every country must chart its own course, possibly learning from countries with similar health challenges (Box 10.3). Packages should be reviewed at regular intervals to adapt to evolving needs, available resources, emerging technologies, and innovations. Once developed, effective delivery of a package requires a gap analysis and health system strengthening that includes capacity development of staff, upgrading of infrastructure, providing essential equipment and medicines, establishing referral mechanisms, strengthening information systems, and enhancing the use of digital and other technologies. A mechanism for monitoring coverage, access, and effectiveness of the package as part of the information system is as essential as the package itself.

10.7 Conclusion

Primary health care should be the foundational approach to strengthening health services in L&MICs. Health systems should aim at delivering services that translate inputs into population health outcomes. Culture and societal norms impede service uptake and utilization, especially in the most vulnerable segments of communities. Engaging communities and populations is a critical investment toward having robust, resilient, and result-oriented health services (see Chapter 12).

Box 10.3 UHC Benefit Package: The Case of Pakistan, 2020 [35]

The government of Pakistan has committed to UHC in its National Health Vision Pakistan 2016–2025 document. Despite this commitment, its *UHC Service Coverage Index* was estimated at 40 in 2015, against a target of 80. The Federal Ministry of Health in partnership with academic institutions and funded by the Bill & Melinda Gates Foundation (B&MGF) embarked on developing a UHC benefit package (UHC BP), which was endorsed by the government in October 2020. The UHC BP has been adapted from the EUHC package of DCP3.

Process: A core group of partner institutions along with four technical working groups (TWGs), one each for RMNCAH,* communicable diseases, noncommunicable diseases, and health services including surgical care were established to review the 218 EUHC interventions and the most relevant were proposed for inclusion in UHC BP. These interventions were assessed for the best available local evidence and costed by the core group. Subsequently, these were presented to the National Advisory Committee, an International Advisory Group, and finally recommended to the National Steering Committee for endorsement. The process went through several iterations based on predefined criteria and actual voting in the TWGs while choosing interventions.

Prioritization criteria: These included (1) burden of disease or risk; (2) cost-effectiveness of intervention; (3) budgetary impact; (4) feasibility of implementation; (5) social acceptability; (6) financial risk protection; and (7) equity. The first four were used as the primary criteria for selecting interventions. A specially designed software was used to prioritize interventions.

Costing: Each intervention was costed based on inputs that comprised, among others, workforce requirements, equipment, medicines, supplies, and laboratory support. Cost per capita was calculated for each intervention using the estimates of population in need and the total population of the country.

Package: The district-level package shown in Table 10.1 was developed at the end of the process.

Table 10.1 The district-level package

Platform	Finally selected services	Distribution by clusters					DALYs averted (in millions)
		RMNCAH* related	Infectious diseases	NCD and injury	Health services	Cost per capita (USD)	
Community level	19	15	3	1	0	2.9	6.8
PHC center level	37	13	7	9	8	4.4	21.5
First level hospital	32	14	2	3	13	5.7	12.1
District UHC BP	**88**	**42**	**12**	**13**	**21**	**13.0**	**40.4**

* Reproductive, maternal, neonatal, child, and adolescent health.

References

1. O. Adams, B. Shengelia, B. Stilwell, et al., Provision of personal and non-personal health services: proposal for monitoring. In C. J. L. Murray, D. B. Evans, ed. *Health Systems Performance Assessment: Debates, Methods and Empiricism*. Ginebra: Organización Mundial de la Salud, 2003, pp. 235–250.

2. World Health Organization. *Monitoring the Building Blocks of Health Systems: A Handbook of Indicators and Their Measurement Strategies*. Geneva, World Health Organization, 2010.

3. W. D. Arinah, J. Musheer, M. H Juni. Health care provision and equity. *IJPHCS* 2016; 3(4).

4. K. Sheikh, L. Gilson, I. A. Agyepong, et al. Building the field of health policy and systems research: framing the questions. *PLoS Med* 2011; 8(8): e1001073.

5. World Health Organization. Working Paper on the use of essential package health services in protracted emergencies.2018. www.who.int/health-cluster/about/work/t ask-teams/EPHS-working-paper.pdf?ua=1 (accessed October 18, 2021).

6. F. K. Nyonator, J. K. Awoonor-Williams, J. F. Phillips, et al. The Ghana community-based health planning and services initiative for scaling up service delivery innovation. *Health Policy Plan* 2005; 20(1): 25–34.

7. M. Kidd, C. Haq, J. de Maeseneer, et al., eds. *The Contribution of Family Medicine to Improving Health Systems*, 2nd ed. London, Radcliffe Publishing, 2013.

8. World Health Organization. *Continuity and Coordination of Care: A Practice Brief to Support Implementation of the WHO Framework on Integrated People-Centred Health Services*. Geneva, World Health Organization, 2018. http://apps.who.int/iris/bitstream/handle/10665/274628/97892 41514033-eng.pdf (accessed December 24, 2021).

9. C. J. Briggs, P. Garner. Strategies for integrating primary health services in middle- and low-income countries at the point of delivery. *Cochrane Database Syst Rev* 2006; 2: CD003318.

10. M. Z. Hasan, R. Neill, P. Das, et al. Integrated health service delivery during COVID-19: a scoping review of published evidence from low-income and lower-middle-income countries. *BMJ Glob Health* 2021; 6(6): e005667.

11. World Health Organization. Health service delivery. 2010. www.who.int/healthinfo/systems/WHO_MBHSS_2010_section1_web.pdf (accessed February 12, 2022).

12. T. Tanahashi. Health service coverage and its evaluation. *Bull World Health Organ* 1978; 56(2): 295–303.

13. M. Donaldson, K. D. Yordy, N. A. Vanselow. *Defining Primary Care: An Interim Report*. Washington, DC, National Academy Press, 1994.

14. World Health Organization. Health equity. 2020. www.who.int/health-topics/health-equity#tab=tab_1 (accessed January 19, 2021).

15. K. I. Hower, V. Vennedey, H. A. Hillen, et al. Implementation of patient-centred care: which organisational determinants matter from decision maker's perspective? Results from a qualitative interview study across various health and social care organisations. *BMJ Open* 2019; 9(4): e027591.

16. T. J. Foley, L. Vale. What role for learning health systems in quality improvement within healthcare providers? *Learn Health Syst* 2017; 1(4): e10025.

17. N. R. Llanwarne, G. A. Abel, M. N. Elliott, et al. Relationship between clinical quality and patient experience: analysis of data from the English quality and outcomes framework and the National GP Patient Survey. *Ann Fam Med* 2013; 11(5): 467–472.

18. World Health Organization, United Nations Children's Fund (UNICEF). A vision for primary health care in the 21st century: towards universal health coverage and the Sustainable Development Goals.

2018. https://apps.who.int/iris/handle/10665/328065 (accessed February 12, 2022).

19. G. van Servellen, M. Fongwa, E. Mockus D'Errico. Continuity of care and quality care outcomes for people experiencing chronic conditions: a literature review. *Nurs Health Sci* 2006; **8**(3): 185–195.

20. E. M. Wall. Continuity of care and family medicine: definition, determinants, and relationship to outcome. *J Fam Pract* 1981; **13**(5): 655–664.

21. J. M. Virdis, M. Lobo, M. E. Elorza, et al. Economic impact of the use of hospital services of aged people affiliated to the INSSJYP: the case of a municipal public hospital (Argentina). 2019. https://repositoriodigital.uns.edu.ar/xmlui/bitstream/handle/123456789/5113/Tesis%20Virdis,%20Juan%20Marcelo.pdf?sequence=1 (accessed February 12, 2022).

22. A. Edward, K. Osei-Bonsu, C. Branchini, et al. Enhancing governance and health system accountability for people centered healthcare: an exploratory study of community scorecards in Afghanistan. *BMC Health Serv Res* 2015; **15**: 299.

23. E. J. Emanuel, L. L. Emanuel. What is accountability in health care? *Ann Intern Med* 1996; **124**(2):229–239.

24. World Health Organization. WHO community engagement framework for quality, people-centred and resilient health services. 2017. https://apps.who.int/iris/bitstream/handle/10665/259280/WHO-HIS-SDS-2017.15-eng.pdf (accessed February 12, 2022).

25. T. Wellay, M. Gebreslassie, M. Mesele, et al. Demand for health care service and associated factors among patients in the community of Tsegedie District, Northern Ethiopia. *BMC Health Serv Res* 2018; **18**(1): 697.

26. L. Anselmi, M. Lagarde, K. Hanson. Health service availability and health seeking behaviour in resource poor settings: evidence from Mozambique. *Health Econ Rev* 2015; **5**(1): 26.

27. A. Wilkinson, M. Parker, F. Martineau, et al. Engaging "communities":

anthropological insights from the West African Ebola epidemic. *Philos Trans R Soc Lond B Biol Sci* 2017; **372**(1721): 20160305.

28. A. Glassman, U. Giedion, Y. Sakuma, et al. Defining a health benefits package: what are the necessary processes? *Health Syst Reform* 2016; **2**(1): 39–50.

29. World Bank. *World Development Report 1993: Investing in Health*. Washington, DC, World Bank, 1993. https://openknowledge.worldbank.org/handle/10986/5976 (accessed January 19, 2021).

30. W. Newbrander, P. Ickx, F. Feroz, et al. Afghanistan's basic package of health services: its development and effects on rebuilding the health system. *Glob Public Health* 2014; **9**(Suppl. 1): S6–S28.

31. G. Le, R. Morgan, J. Bestal, et al. The impact of universal health coverage, people centered care and integrated service delivery on key health system outcomes 2014. 2014. www.researchgate.net/project/The-Impact-of-Universal-Health-Coverage-People-Centred-Care-and-Integrated-Service-Delivery-on-Key-Health-System-Outcomes-2014 (accessed January 11, 2021).

32. L. Dudley, P. Garner. Strategies for integrating primary health services in low- and middle-income countries at the point of delivery. *Cochrane Database Syst Rev* 2011; **7**: CD003318.

33. M. E. Kruk, D. Porignon, P. C. Rockers, et al. The contribution of primary care to health and health systems in low- and middle-income countries: a critical review of major primary care initiatives. *Soc Sci Med* 2010; **70**(6): 904–911.

34. World Health Organization. UHC Compendium: health interventions for universal health coverage. 2022. www.who.int/universal-health-coverage/compendium (accessed January 25, 2022).

35. World Health Organization. People-centred and integrated health services: an overview of the evidence – interim report. 2015. https://apps.who.int/iris/bitstream/handle/10665/155004/WHO_HIS_SDS_2015.7_eng.pdf (accessed January 10, 2021).

Role and Contribution of the Community in Health System Strengthening

Amirhossein Takian, Haniye Sadat Sajadi, Naima Nasir, and Katherine Rouleau

Key Messages

- Communities are integral parts of health systems and their engagement in defining health needs, priorities, and solutions, and in the delivery of services, is essential to improving health and wellbeing.
- All communities, regardless of how they are defined, include individuals or subgroups who, for a host of reasons, are marginalized and/or disadvantaged and consequently experience a disproportionate burden of ill-health. Identifying, understanding, and engaging such individuals and groups is both essential and challenging, and should be prioritized.
- Trust and accountability across various levels of governance within communities and between communities and various levels of leadership is essential to effective engagement.
- Community engagement can be seen as a continuum of community involvement from informing to empowering.

11.1 Introduction

The engagement of the community in identifying its health needs, setting priorities, and developing solutions, and in the provision of care, is widely acknowledged to lead to improved health outcomes. Yet, how to foster, implement, and sustain community engagement to impact health outcomes remains challenging, particularly within low- and middle-income countries (L&MICs), and as pertains to those who are marginalized based on gender, poverty, ethnicity, and other social determinants of health in all countries [1–3].

Over the past 50 years our understanding of the relation between the community and health systems has evolved. In an earlier paradigm, health systems primarily focused on treating diseases. Hospitals occupied a central role in defining health problems and their solutions. The community was conceived as a social or geographical "space" located "outside the hospital." A more recent paradigm considers the community as integral to an effective health system and as a central actor and stakeholder in defining health priorities, rather than as a passive recipient. This paradigm shift was expressed in the Declaration of Alma-Ata in 1978 [4] and reinforced in the renewed global commitment to primary health care (PHC) in the Declaration of Astana in 2018 [4], where "Engaged people as communities and individuals" is highlighted as one of the essential components of PHC. Community is also integral to universal health coverage (UHC), which entails that all individuals and *communities* receive the health services they need – in good quality to be effective – and without suffering financial hardship (see Chapter 3) [5]. PHC is acknowledged as the approach to health systems necessary to achieve the Sustainable Development Goal (SDG) target of UHC (SDG 3.8) and other health-related SDG targets [6]. Community engagement is also one of the 14 levers of the WHO PHC Operational Framework [7].

In this chapter, we explore the concepts of community and community engagement and consider their roles in health systems. We examine the concept of health, the changing health needs of communities, and the influence of community in defining health issues and informing solutions, including the delivery of services. Finally, we discuss the modalities of community engagement for health systems, particularly within L&MICs.

11.2 The Concepts of Community and Community Engagement

11.2.1 The Concept of Community: Who and What Is It?

The concept of community is complex and subject to various definitions [8, 9]. Communities are often defined in geographical terms (relating to human settlement or people within a location or geographical place) [10]. However, this understanding of community is generally agreed to be limited [8, 10, 11]. "Communities" are increasingly recognized as collectives comprising individuals, groups, and organizations with a variety of characteristics, interactions, and relationships (within and outside the community) [9, 11]. Furthermore, the concept of community is not static but dynamic, shaped and reshaped as the needs, actions, values, and relationships of the community and its members change [12].

Although there is no consensus on a standard definition of community, several core dimensions and characteristics have been identified [9, 12–14]. In the context of health systems, we highlight some of these key dimensions:

- **Geographical:** an entity that can be located and described in terms of a geographical area or boundaries, such as a neighborhood or catchment area, county, state, or an area under local governance.
- **Social:** ties, interactions, interpersonal relations, and connections for communication, sharing information, knowledge, resources, and experiences. A community may exist among individuals who are scattered geographically but who share values, traditions, cultures, knowledge, and resources.
- **Political:** a sense of cohesion and joint action, ability to set priorities, legitimate political authority, social and political responsibility, and accountability. May have representative groups/individuals.
- **Community of practice:** a collaborative framework for public health (or other) professionals working together to identify and leverage best practices and standards. Through these evolving collaborative efforts and sharing lessons learned in the community-building process, the community of practice approach is being implemented in many public health areas as a model of how public health partners work together [14].

The extent to which communities reflect these features will vary and may overlap. Most communities include a degree of diversity and complexities that need to be taken into consideration in the engagement process, including in the assessment of needs (regardless of who is assessing), the building of trust, the development of partnerships for action, and in ensuring accountability of both health system users and providers.

In the context of PHC, achieving Health for All requires that priority be given to engaging those who are most difficult to reach, often those most marginalized and disenfranchised by formal societal structures, including gender, income, and other determinants of health.

11.2.2 Community Engagement

The terms "community engagement" and "public participation" are often used interchangeably [15]. For this chapter, we use the term "community engagement" (CE) to align with WHO terminology, particularly in the context of the renewed global commitment toward PHC [2].

One of the most quoted definitions of CE is: "a process of working collaboratively with and through groups of people affiliated by geographic proximity, special interest, or similar situations to address issues affecting the well-being of those people"[16]. Within health systems, CE can occur "for" and "through" any of the building blocks (see Figure 11.1) to enrich the processes and improve outcomes [17]. For example, communities may be engaged in policymaking, health service planning, organization and delivery, health promotion, and research.

While there are several perspectives to the rationale and need for CE, at least three are noteworthy here. First is a *moral perspective* that maintains that people should have a say in the planning, organization, and delivery of health services that affect them, and that planners, managers, and providers are accountable to the beneficiaries of health care. The second is a *utilitarian perspective*, which presumes that engaging the community will improve health-related behavior and ultimately lead to better health outcomes [18]. Lastly, a third and emerging perspective highlights the *relational imperative of CE* and proposes that to achieve health, engagement needs to be anchored in trusting and sustained relationships among stakeholders [19].

11.3 The Conceptual Models of Health and Their Relevance to CE

It is useful to consider different *conceptual models of health* that range from biomedical to biodevelopmental, and at the same time recognize that these are not the same as the *health system models and frameworks* presented in Chapter 1 and in other chapters of the book. Figure 11.2 summarizes three well-recognized conceptual models of health [20–22] that have relevance to the ways in which communities can play a role in health systems.

How these models are understood can have implications for the practice of CE. In the *biomedical model*, the individual is understood primarily as a patient who "flows through" health services as the potentially passive recipient of services and interventions. In the context of the biomedical model, engagement is presented as patient engagement in the context of a doctor– or provider–patient relationship, an important but limited aspect of the concept. The *biopsychosocial model* has a more complex notion of health that takes into consideration the full circumstances of individuals and communities and therefore entails engagement not only as patients, but as people and citizens who can identify health needs, inform strategies, help prioritize, and choose solutions that account for the complex interplay of determinants in their own lives and communities. Lastly, the

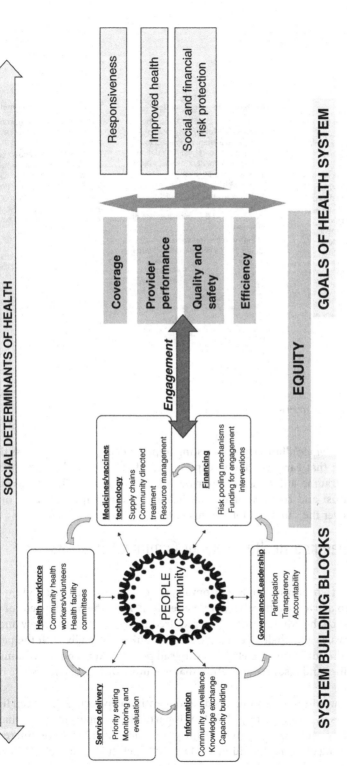

Figure 11.1 CE and the health system building blocks by WHO.

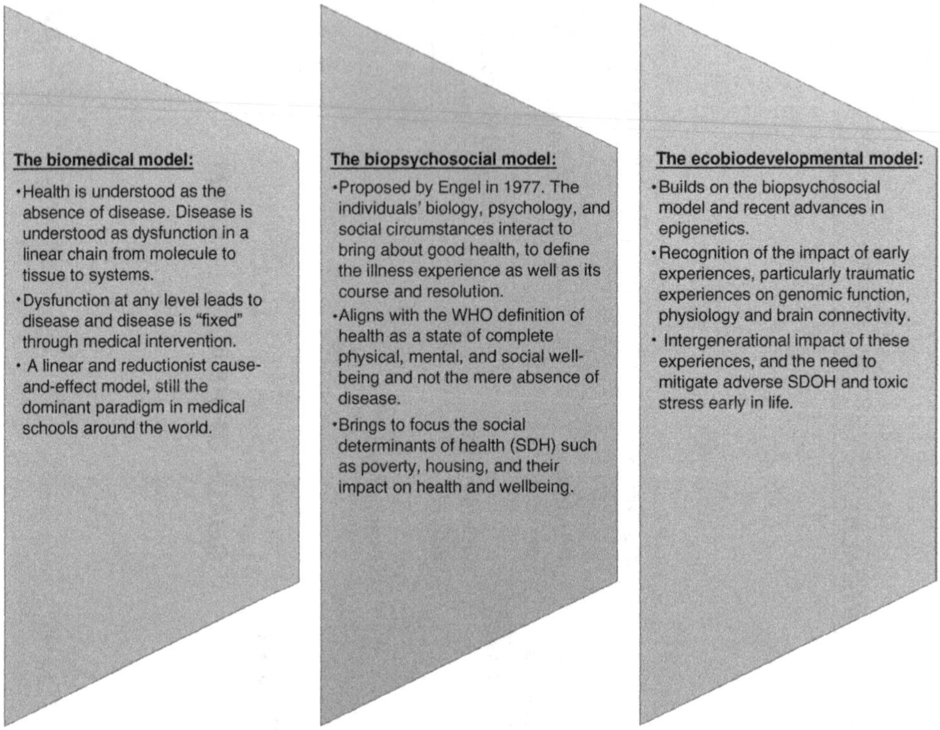

The biomedical model:
- Health is understood as the absence of disease. Disease is understood as dysfunction in a linear chain from molecule to tissue to systems.
- Dysfunction at any level leads to disease and disease is "fixed" through medical intervention.
- A linear and reductionist cause-and-effect model, still the dominant paradigm in medical schools around the world.

The biopsychosocial model:
- Proposed by Engel in 1977. The individuals' biology, psychology, and social circumstances interact to bring about good health, to define the illness experience as well as its course and resolution.
- Aligns with the WHO definition of health as a state of complete physical, mental, and social well-being and not the mere absence of disease.
- Brings to focus the social determinants of health (SDH) such as poverty, housing, and their impact on health and wellbeing.

The ecobiodevelopmental model:
- Builds on the biopsychosocial model and recent advances in epigenetics.
- Recognition of the impact of early experiences, particularly traumatic experiences on genomic function, physiology and brain connectivity.
- Intergenerational impact of these experiences, and the need to mitigate adverse SDOH and toxic stress early in life.

Figure 11.2 The conceptual models of health [19–22].

ecobiodevelopmental model illuminates the lasting impact of circumstances across time and generations, noting that early childhood experiences of "toxic stress" can translate into transgenerational trauma and cycles of poor health. In this model CE is focused on the development of trust and compassionate and healing relationships that drive improved health outcomes over the short and long terms [20, 22].

11.3.1 The Changing Health Needs of Communities across the Lifespan

The ultimate aim of a health system is to promote, restore, or maintain health [23]. To this end, it is crucial to deliver health services that effectively meet the health needs of defined populations. As such, health authorities are required to systematically review and determine the health issues and challenges facing a community, optimally with the participation and voice of the community itself. This will lead policymakers and the community to agree upon priorities and resource allocation that will improve health and reduce inequalities [24].

Engaging communities in defining needs and identifying priorities has been linked to improved outcomes in several settings [2]. This is particularly important given that health needs are constantly evolving, such that health priorities today (2022) are different from those at the beginning of the millennium, let alone 100 or even 50 years ago. The evolution of health needs is partly due to rapid demographic and epidemiological changes/transitions, which are themselves a result of health-related behaviors and their various determinants.

Since the beginning of the third millennium, noncommunicable diseases (NCDs) such as cardiovascular diseases, diabetes, and cancers, as well as accidents, have become the leading causes of death [25]. In L&MICs, the epidemiological transition is progressing differently than in high-income countries (HICs) and at different rates among countries. L&MICs are witnessing reduced mortality rates due to infectious diseases within shorter periods than the HICs, leaving a much shorter time to adjust the health system to respond adequately to the needs of adults and the elderly, while simultaneously needing to maintain efforts to reduce the burden of infectious diseases in children, as well as adolescent and reproductive health problems. As such, many L&MICs suffer from significant dual burdens of communicable and noncommunicable diseases, with the epidemics of AIDS, tuberculosis, malaria, and neglected tropical diseases adding complexity to the process of epidemiological transition [26–28].

In recent decades, pandemics, epidemics, and outbreaks – most notably COVID-19 in 2020, as well as MERS, SARS, and to some extent Zika – have affected HICs as well as L&MICs, highlighting the disproportionate vulnerability of some communities to a double burden of disease, affecting notably the elderly and those most socially marginalized. The evolving health needs related to the epidemiological transition highlight the requirement for improved health system accountability and greater engagement by communities. Changes in patterns of diseases and their related risk factors have presented many challenges to health systems, particularly in L&MICs, and CE initiatives can act as "critical enablers" to pave the way toward meeting the health needs of communities. Such initiatives may be particularly important in settings where health systems are under-resourced, and the collective capacity of communities represents a key resource in effecting behavioral change and delivering health outcomes.

11.3.2 The Modalities of Community Engagement: From Information to Engagement

Community engagement or "engaged people as individuals and communities" is the process of working collaboratively with and through groups of people affiliated by geographic proximity, special interest, or similar situations to address issues affecting the wellbeing of those people [16]. It allows people to actively play a role in identifying and interpreting the issues, weighing options and solutions, and prioritizing actions. Since the Alma-Ata Declaration in 1978, there has been a call for greater participation along the full spectrum of engagement described below [29, 30], which has recently transformed into a broader inclusion in health policy development and implementation [31].

Community engagement can be implemented in formal, semi-formal, and informal ways. This includes the use of community/lay health workers, women's groups, community advisory panels, participatory learning, use of volunteers/peers, use of local leaders, and involvement of family members [2]. Table 11.1 illustrates a spectrum of public participation derived from Arnstein's ladder of citizen participation [32], with increasing levels of participation from informing (with no or little influence) to empowering (when the public has the highest possible degree of influence in health policy and implementation) [33].

Table 11.1 Community engagement spectrum

Increasing impact on decision →

	Inform	Consult	Involve	Collaborate	Empower
Public participation goal	To provide the public with information to assist them in understanding the problem and/or solutions	To obtain public feedback on analysis, alternatives, and/or decisions	To work directly with the public throughout the process to ensure that public concerns and aspirations are consistently understood and considered	To partner with the public in each aspect of the decision, including the development of alternatives and the identification of the preferred solution	To place final decision-making in the hands of the public
Promise to the public	We will keep you informed.	We will keep you informed, listen to and acknowledge concerns and aspirations, and provide feedback on how public input influenced the decision	We will work with you to ensure that your concerns and aspirations are directly reflected in the alternatives developed and provide feedback on how public input influenced the decision	We will look to you for advice and innovation in formulating solutions and incorporate your advice and recommendations into the decisions to the maximum extent possible	We will implement what you decide
Example techniques	Fact sheets Websites Open houses	Public comment Focus groups Surveys Public meetings	Workshops Deliberative polling	Citizen advisory committees Consensus-building Participatory decision-making	Citizen juries Ballots Delegated decisions Public participation, e.g., people health assemblies

Source: [33].

Informing: Policymakers provide the public with information to assist them in understanding the health issues, advantages, and disadvantages of different options to address an issue, and considerations of solutions. For instance, during the COVID-19 outbreak in many L&MICs (e.g., Iran, Lebanon), several websites were launched to inform the public about the latest news and guidelines [34, 35]. Informing the public is a necessary starting point both as an expression of accountability and to build trust, which are essential to effective CE. It is also necessary to allow people to effectively engage in self-care. However, only providing information to people does not engage them in the decision-making process.

Consulting: Obtaining public opinion and feedback using different techniques, including public comments, focus groups, surveys, and public meetings. These have been used to listen to and acknowledge concerns and provide feedback on how their input influenced the decision. For instance, in India a lack of interest in neonatal care among adult males in a given community resulted in a fatalistic outlook toward the survival of newborns among their families. To address this shortcoming, a wider consultation process with community members, including men and women, was carried out and has led to increase male support regarding the values and traditions around the time of childbirth [36].

Involving: Working directly with the community or communities through a defined process to ensure that their opinions and concerns are taken into consideration, particularly during the development of decision criteria and options. Workshops and deliberative polling are examples of techniques used to engage the public. The establishment of the National Health Assembly (NHA) in Thailand is a good example in this category. For over a decade, the Thai NHA has brought together people from government agencies, academia, civil society, professional health care, and the private sector to discuss and prioritize critical health issues and produce resolutions to guide policymaking [37]. Similarly, since 2016 Iran has implemented assemblies at the local, provincial, and national levels to engage with community representatives in decision-making for health, while attempting to enhance public awareness about social determinants of health [38].

Collaborating: Partnering with the public in each aspect of the decision-making process, including developing the decision criteria and alternatives and identifying the preferred solutions to challenges. Meaningful collaboration can be built through the establishment of citizens' advisory committees, consensus-building, and participatory decision-making. Although collaborating with communities in health policymaking is common in some HICs, it is less common within the context of L&MICs. One example is the citizen's jury, the first of its kind in Brazil, which allowed poor citizens to have a say in the decision to reject the introduction of genetically modified organisms in Brazil [39]. This technique was recently used in Tunisia as part of the "dialogue societale" on the health and future of the health system following the political changes in the country [40, 41].

Empowering: This seeks to place final decision-making authority in the hands of the community, meaning that what the community decides will be implemented. While informing does not always transform the community, empowering does. The empowerment of communities, particularly women and girls, has been receiving much attention over the years and is the focus of SDG 5 [42]. Evidence has shown that the empowerment of women and girls not only improves health outcomes, but yields benefits that extend beyond themselves and their families, leading to empowered communities and sustainable development [43]. Despite the progress that has been made toward achieving gender equality and the empowerment of women and girls, particularly in the Middle East and North Africa, evidence shows that gender disparities remain persistent in most countries, with many women facing social, cultural, and economic barriers and exclusions that limit their ability to make informed choices about their health and act on them [43]. Therefore, health-related policies should address inequalities in women's empowerment, education, and economic status. Community engagement efforts should explicitly seek to integrate the perspectives of women.

Many HICs have established and institutionalized CE practices in their decision-making process, albeit with varying degrees of fulsome representation and leadership [44]. However, many L&MICs are still struggling to incorporate meaningful processes of CE in health policy and implementation [3]. Still, some examples exist. A well-recognized example of CE in many L&MICs is to engage community health workers (CHWs) to deliver health services. CHWs are typically selected from their own community (in both urban and rural environments) and are either paid or volunteer to work in association with the local health care system.

Although CHW programs vary by country and context, CHWs have been very effective in providing primary care services in several L&MICs [45–47]. For instance, *behvarzes*, the Iranian CHWs, are fulltime health system employees who are recruited from the communities they serve and work in the most peripheral health delivery facilities within rural areas. These CHWs mainly focus on responding to the health needs of the rural population who may suffer from inadequate health care services, compared to their urban counterparts. In the case of Iran, hiring CHWs from their own communities has improved the equity in access to health care services, and also serves to effectively engage the community in the delivery of health services [48]. A systematic review reported that communities in the L&MICs have engaged or participated in a range of interventions to improve maternal and child health, HIV care, and management of other diseases, as well as in various health promotion activities, including the use of community/lay health workers [2].

11.4 The Role and Influence of the Community in Enhancing the Accountability of Health Systems

In the context of health systems, communities are expected to engage in defining and prioritizing their needs, outlining the solutions and in delivering care. Communities also play an important role in holding the health workforce accountable. The way in which a given community is defined, based on geography, social factors, or political alignment, has implications for the way in which needs and solutions are defined and how the community can be engaged.

11.4.1 Geographically Defined Communities

Communities determined by geographic boundaries are often defined as such by external stakeholders. The inclusion of every individual in a geographical area (sometimes called a catchment area) can facilitate the logistics of service planning and delivery, and enable consistency, accountability, and equity. On the other hand, people living in a given catchment area, particularly in dense and diverse urban areas with rapid population turnover, cannot be assumed to all share the same values and health priorities, nor to favor the same solutions, with implications for CE (Box 11.1). For example, while the involvement of CHWs can enhance uptake and improve outcomes in some settings, in others the use of CHWs to visit homes can feel invasive and may

Box 11.1 CE in Geographically Defined Communities

Brazil's family health model is organized around geographically defined communities. Geographic areas of people are attached to a family health team located in a nearby health center. Each health center houses several teams. The number of teams attached to a given health center depends on the density of the population and distance to the health center. A typical team includes one physician, one nurse, one nursing assistant, at least four CHWs, and a dental professional, each looking after roughly 4,000 people. The CHWs visit all families regularly, enquiring about health needs and capturing key data such as the immunization status of children and blood pressure. The data can be used to inform what and how health services are delivered. At the entrance of each health center is a large board summarizing some of the community's key health indicators, enabling accountability on the part of the clinic toward the citizens it serves.

Box 11.2 CE in Socially Defined Communities

- Some indigenous communities in North America and Australia offer good examples of CE and culturally safe and responsive health services. The postcolonial era, in some countries, has offered greater opportunities for thoughtful engagement of communities through their own governance and leadership structures, which has led to innovations in the models of care and care spaces, and effective integration of traditional healing practices.
- In the early 2000s clinical trials of a promising HIV drug were hindered by a limited approach to engagement with sex workers and other vulnerable groups. Protests led by activists and sex worker advocacy groups resulted in the discontinuation of trials in Cambodia, Nigeria, and Cameroon. Activists argued that sex workers' rights and opinions were not adequately considered in the planning and design of trials.

fail to deliver the expected results [49]. Thus, even equity-enabling definitions of a community as a catchment area requires attention to ensure that those most marginalized are given authentic voice and representation to express their needs and priorities [50].

11.4.2 Socially Defined Communities

Socially defined communities are those defined by shared culture, language, or values, and are typically defined by the members of the community itself. They may be geographically clustered or dispersed, such that a given geographic area may include a number of overlapping social communities, each with its own needs, priorities, and preferred solutions. Because health-related behavior is influenced by culture, values, and language, it is important for planners and providers to take these elements into consideration (Box 11.2).

Engagement of community members across diverse social groups is essential and can be challenging, particularly the involvement of those socially most marginalized or vulnerable. This includes, for example, strategies to engage and empower women to make decisions related to childbearing and the ability to seek health care as they see fit. Strategies for CE with marginalized and "hard-to-reach" communities need to be holistic, utilize people-centered [51, 52] and bottom-up approaches, addressing the sociopolitical, structural, and cultural issues that underpin exclusion and present barriers to participation and engagement [53, 54]. This includes efforts to understand the historical and current contexts of disadvantages and vulnerabilities within the community, and working together for a coordinated, relevant, and sustainable response to the needs of the community [53, 54].

11.4.3 Politically Defined Communities

There is overlap between communities defined through social and political structures. While all communities are subject to political forces, some can be defined, explicitly or implicitly, in terms of their ability to fully engage in governance, in decision-making structures, and by the relative power of their members compared to and over others. Feudal systems, hierarchical and caste systems, some tribal traditions, structurally racist and colonial systems, and other exclusionary and oppressive political systems deliberately enable the dominance of some over others. These formal and informal political forces create and compound adverse social determinants of health, including gender where women and girls are commonly disempowered, excluded, and actively silenced. Thus, entire communities can be disenfranchised or oppressed, as is the case for refugees or some ethnic minorities in certain parts of the world. In other cases, within a given community, some clearly have more power and voice than others – for example, between racial groups. Identifying the needs of the whole community and the specific health needs of the least powerful and therefore most vulnerable is essential to the health of all. It requires a balance between engaging the existing formal and informal leadership and taking steps to purposefully include the perspectives of those with the least power, working through existing governance structures such as traditional chiefs, elders, and other formal and informal leaders to engage the community [55, 56]. However, since power differentials can hinder progress toward better health outcomes, health system improvement in such communities may require novel governance mechanisms (such as the health assemblies and committees used in many L&MICs) to increase collaboration and promote social accountability (Box 11.3).

The ways in which communities are engaged can therefore vary depending in part on the ways in which they are defined. In all cases, several factors can either enable or hinder CE. Some of those factors are summarized in Box 11.4 [3].

Box 11.3 CE in Politically Defined Communities

Decades of political conflict and economic instability in Myanmar have driven large communities of refugees, migrants, and displaced people along the Thailand–Myanmar border. The Tak Province Community Ethics Advisory Board (T-CAB) was established in 2009 to formalize CE between humanitarian/research groups working along the border and community members. T-CAB provides the communities with a means to express views on proposed research, and a voice to influence and direct research, based on their needs.

Box 11.4 Enablers and Barriers of Community Engagement

Enablers of Community Engagement
- The presence of partnerships and existing structures for CE
- Having a prepared workforce and technical support for CE
- Encouraging dialog and transparent communication, including among those most affected and responsible
- Understanding the culture, religious beliefs, social norms, and traditional beliefs and practices
- Having knowledge about factors/approaches affecting CE and systems improvement
- Being willing to share power and decision-making
- CE activities being adequately financed
- Sustained trusting relationships

Barriers to Community Engagement
- Unclear mandates and turf issues
- Authoritarian, top-down approaches and perceived abuses of power
- Lack of trust at the community level

11.5 Conclusion

Community engagement is a process integral to effective health systems. The ways in which communities engage vary according to the characteristics of the context and of the communities themselves. The spectrum of CE is wide, from informing citizens about their rights to empowering them to contribute to key decisions in the health system. Among the many factors that can enable or hinder CE, trust and the strength of relationships is central and needs to be cultivated over time.

References

1. H. Waddington, A. Sonnenfeld, J. Finetti, et al. Citizen engagement in public services in low-and middle-income countries: a mixed-methods systematic review of participation, inclusion, transparency and accountability (PITA) initiatives. *Campbell Syst Rev* 2019; 15(1–2): e1025.

2. G. Pilkington, S. Panday, N. K. Mahalaqua, et al. The effectiveness of community engagement and participation approaches in low and middle income countries: a review of systematic reviews with particular reference to the countries of South Asia. 2017. http://eppi.ioe.ac.uk (accessed May 21, 2021).

3. K. B. Alderman, D. Hipgrave, E. Jimenez-Soto. Public engagement in health priority setting in low- and middle-income countries: current trends and considerations for policy. *PLoS Med* 2013; 10(8): e1001495.

4. World Health Organization, United Nations Children's Fund. Declaration of Astana. Global Conference on Primary Health Care. 2018. www.who.int/docs/default-source/primary-health/declaration/gcphc-declaration.pdf (accessed May 23, 2021).

5. World Health Organization. Universal health coverage. 2021. www.who.int/news-room/fact-sheets/detail/universal-health-coverage-(uhc) (accessed December 10, 2021).

6. World Health Organization. Goal 3: Sustainable Development Goals. WHO SDGS progress, targets and indicators. 2018. https://sustainabledevelopment.un.org/sdg3 (accessed May 27, 2021).

7. World Health Organization, United Nations Children's Fund. Operational framework for primary health care: transforming vision into action. 2020. www.who.int/publications/i/item/9789240017832 (accessed February 14, 2022).

8. A. S. George, V. Mehra, K. Scott, et al. Community participation in health systems research: a systematic review assessing the state of research, the nature of interventions involved and the features of engagement with communities. *PLoS One* 2015; **10**(10): e0141091.

9. K. M. MacQueen, E. McLellan, D. S. Metzger, et al. What is community? An evidence-based definition for participatory public health. *Am J Public Health* 2001; **91** (12): 1929–1938.

10. R. K. Sharma. Putting the community back in community health assessment: a process and outcome approach with a review of some major issues for public health professionals. *J Heal Soc Policy* 2003; **16**(3): 19–33.

11. M. Ruderman. Resource guide to concepts and methods for community-based and collaborative problem solving. 2000. https://citeseerx.ist.psu.edu/viewdoc/download?doi=10.1.1.127.9401&rep=rep1&type=pdf (accessed May 22, 2021).

12. P. O. Tindana, J. A. Singh, C. S. Tracy, et al. Grand challenges in global health: community engagement in research in developing countries. *PLoS Med* 2007; **4**(9): 1451–1455.

13. C. Weijer, E. J. Emanuel. Ethics: protecting communities in biomedical research. *Science* 2000; **289**(5482): 1142–1144.

14. R. A. Goodman, R. Bunnell, S. F. Posner. What is "community health"? Examining the meaning of an evolving field in public health. *Prev Med (Baltim)* 2014; **67**(S1): S58–S61.

15. H. Ross, C. Baldwin, R. W. Carter. Subtle implications: public participation versus community engagement in environmental decision-making. *Australas J Environ Manag* 2016; **23**: 123–129.

16. Clinical and Translational Science Awards Consortium Community Engagement Key Function Committee Task Force on the Principles of Community Engagement. Principles of community engagement, 2nd ed. 2011. www.atsdr.cdc.gov/community engagement/pdf/PCE_Report_508_FINAL.pdf (accessed February 12, 2022).

17. World Health Organization. Everybody's business: strengthening health systems to improve health outcomes. WHO's Framework for Action. 2007. www.who.int/healthsystems/strategy/everybodys_business.pdf (accessed February 14, 2022).

18. S. B. Rifkin. Examining the links between community participation and health outcomes: a review of the literature. *Health Policy Plan* 2014; **29**(Suppl. 2): ii98–ii106.

19. A. Odugleh-Kolev, J. Parrish-Sprowl. Universal health coverage and community engagement. *Bull World Health Organ* 2018; **96**(9): 660–661.

20. B. S. Siegel, M. I. Dobbins, M. F. Earls, et al. Early childhood adversity, toxic stress, and the role of the pediatrician: translating developmental science into lifelong health. *Pediatrics* 2012; **129**(1): e224–e231.

21. A. Farre, T. Rapley. The new old (and old new) medical model: four decades navigating the biomedical and psychosocial understandings of health and illness. *Healthcare* 2017; **5**(4): 88.

22. W. T. Boyce. The lifelong effects of early childhood adversity and toxic stress. *Pediatr Dent* 2014; **36**(2): 102–108.

23. World Health Organization. *The World Health Report 2000 Health Systems: Improving Performance.* Washington, DC, WHO, 2000. www.who.int/whr/2000/en/whr00_en.pdf (accessed May 13, 2021).

24. S. Cavanagh, K. Chadwick. Health needs assessment: a practical guide. National Institute for Clinical Excellence. 2005. www.nice.org.uk (accessed May 18, 2021).

25. A. Omran. The epidemiologic transition: a theory of the epidemiology of population

change. *Bull World Health Organ* 2001; **79** (2): 161–170.

26. J. Frenk, J. L. Bobadilla, J. Sepuúlveda, et al. Health transition in middle-income countries: new challenges for health care. *Health Policy Plan* 1989; **4**(1): 29–39.

27. A. Santosa, S. Wall, E. Fottrel, et al. The development and experience of epidemiological transition theory over four decades: a systematic review. *Glob Health Action* 2014; **7**(Supp. 1): 23574.

28. A. Santosa, P. Byass. Diverse empirical evidence on epidemiological transition in low- and middle-income countries: population-based findings from INDEPTH network data. *PLoS One* 2016; **11**(5): e0155753.

29. E. R. Cohen, H. Masum, K. Berndtson, et al. Public engagement on global health challenges. *BMC Public Health* 2008; **8**: 168.

30. E. Stewart. What is the point of citizen participation in health care? *J Health Serv Res Policy* 2013; **18**(2): 124–126.

31. W. E. Thurston, G. MacKean, A. Vollman, et al. Public participation in regional health policy: a theoretical framework. *Health Policy* 2005; **73**(3): 237–252.

32. S. R. Arnstein. A ladder of citizen participation. *J Am Plan Assoc* 1969; **35**(4): 216–224.

33. Tamarack Institute. TOOL | IAP2's public participation spectrum. 2021. www.tamar ackcommunity.ca/library/iap2s-public-participation-spectrum (accessed January 11, 2021).

34. American University of Beirut. K2P COVID-19 response. 2021. www.aub.edu .lb/k2p/Pages/K2PCOVID19.aspx (accessed January 15, 2021).

35. Ministry of Health and Medical Education, Iran. Second step guides to combat COVID-19. 2021. https://behdasht.gov.ir/ step2corona (accessed May 23, 2021).

36. A. T. Bang, R. A. Bang, H. M. Reddy. Home-based neonatal care: summary and applications of the field trial in rural Gadchiroli, India (1993 to 2003). *J Perinatol* 2005; **25**(Suppl. 1): S108–S122.

37. K. Rasanathan, T. Posayanonda, M. Birmingham, et al. Innovation and participation for healthy public policy: the first National Health Assembly in Thailand. *Heal Expect* 2012; **15**(1): 87–96.

38. J. Hsu, R. Majdzadeh, I. Harirchi, et al, eds. Health system transformation in the Islamic Republic of Iran: an assessment of key health financing and governance issues. 2019. www.who.int/publications/i/item/ health-systems-transformation-in-the-islamic-republic-of-iran-an-assessment-of-key-health-financing-and-governance-issues (accessed May 23, 2021).

39. A. Toni, J. von Braun. Poor citizens decide on the introduction of GMOs in Brazil. *Biotechnol Dev Monit* 2001; **47**: 7–9.

40. H. Ben Mesmia, R. Chtioui, M. Ben Rejeb. The Tunisian societal dialogue for health reform (a qualitative study). *Eur J Public Health* 2020; **30**(Suppl. 5): ckaa166-1393.

41. World Health Organization. Tunisia citizens and civil society engage in health policy. https://extranet.who.int/country planningcycles/sites/default/files/ planning_cycle_repository/tunisia/stories_ from_the_field_issue1_tunisia.pdf (accessed February 12, 2022).

42. United Nations. Goal 5: Sustainable Development Knowledge Platform. 2015. https://sustainabledevelopment.un.org/ sdg5 (accessed May 19, 2021).

43. D. T. Doku, Z. A. Bhutta, S. Neupane. Associations of women's empowerment with neonatal, infant and under-5 mortality in low- and/middle-income countries: meta-analysis of individual participant data from 59 countries. *BMJ Glob Health* 2020; **5**(1): e00158.

44. M. Ellen, R. Shach, M. Kok, et al. There is much to learn when you listen: exploring citizen engagement in high- and low-income countries. *World Health Popul* 2017; **17**(3): 31–42.

45. J. B. Christopher, A. Le May, S. Lewin, et al. Thirty years after Alma-Ata: a systematic review of the impact of community health workers delivering curative interventions against malaria, pneumonia and diarrhoea on child mortality and

morbidity in sub-Saharan Africa. *Hum Resour Health* 2011; 9(27).

46. B. Gilmore, E. McAuliffe. Effectiveness of community health workers delivering preventive interventions for maternal and child health in low- and middle-income countries: a systematic review. *BMC Public Health* 2013; 13(847).

47. S. M. Swider. Outcome effectiveness of community health workers: an integrative literature review. *Public Health Nurs* 2002; 19(1): 11–20.

48. S. Javanparast, F. Baum, R. Labonte, et al. Community health workers' perspectives on their contribution to rural health and well-being in Iran. *Am J Public Health* 2011; 101(12): 2287–2292.

49. C. Wayland, J. Crowder. Disparate views of community in primary health care: understanding how perceptions influence success. *Med Anthropol Q* 2002; 16(2): 230–247.

50. D. C. Malta, M. A. Santos, S. R. Stopa, et al. Family health strategy coverage in Brazil, according to the National Health Survey, 2013. *Cien Saude Colet* 2016; 21(2): 327–338.

51. A. Durey, S. McEvoy, V. Swift-Otero, et al. Improving healthcare for Aboriginal Australians through effective engagement between community and health services. *BMC Health Serv Res* 2016; 16: 224.

52. E. Mills, B. Rachlis, P. Wu, et al. Media reporting of tenofovir trials in Cambodia and Cameroon. *BMC Int Health Hum Rights* 2005; 5: 6.

53. D. Tangseefa, K. Monthathip, N. Tuenpakdee, et al. "Nine dimensions": a multidisciplinary approach for community engagement in a complex postwar border region as part of the targeted malaria elimination in Karen/Kayin State, Myanmar. *Wellcome Open Res* 2019; 3: 116.

54. H. N. Thanh, P. Y. Cheah, M. Chambers. Identifying "hard-to-reach" groups and strategies to engage them in biomedical research: perspectives from engagement practitioners in Southeast Asia. *Wellcome Open Res* 2019; 4: 102.

55. P. Y. Cheah, K. M. Lwin, L. Phaiphun, et al. Community engagement on the Thai–Burmese border: rationale, experience and lessons learnt. *Int Health* 2010; 2(2): 123–129.

56. S. Wali, S. Superina, A. Mashford-Pringle, et al. What do you mean by engagement? Evaluating the use of community engagement in the design and implementation of chronic disease-based interventions for Indigenous populations – scoping review. *Int J Equity Health* 2021;20: 8.

Chapter 2

Performing Health Systems
Attributes and Approaches to Assessment

Viroj Tangcharoensathien, Walaiporn Patcharanarumol,
Titiporn Tuangratananon, Nattadhanai Rajatanavin, and
Shaheda Viriyathorn

Key Messages

- There is currently neither a universally accepted definition of a high-performing health system, consensus on attributes, nor quantitative scoring to aid health system performance assessment (HSPA).
- HSPA acknowledges the determinants that impact health but does not explicitly assess them. Operationally, HSPA is "a system-wide exercise whose aim is to appraise the health system as a whole."
- Key characteristics of HSPA include being regular, systematic, transparent, comprehensive, and analytical. Choice of appropriate HSPA indicators according to local needs should be based on importance, relevance, feasibility, reliability, and validity.
- Measuring hospital performance is an important subset of HSPA and commonly includes indicators such as average length of stay, bed occupancy rates, and bed turnover rates. Other measures include the rates of unplanned or prolonged admission, discharge, antibiotic prescription, mortality, health care associated infection, readmission, staff turnover and burnout, and patient satisfaction.
- Progress toward universal health coverage (UHC) is an important measure of health system performance. Two indicators have been designated to monitor progress toward achieving UHC under the Sustainable Development 2030 Agenda: coverage of essential health services (Indicator 3.8.1) and assessment of financial risk protection (Indicator 3.8.2).

12.1 Background

In its wider definition, the health system means all activities and structures that determine or influence health in its broadest sense within a given society; this includes social, environmental, and economic determinants of health (Chapter 1). The importance of health systems strengthening (HSS) had been highlighted before the COVID-19 pandemic, but is even more clearly acknowledged and prioritized at present. HSS is the foundation for achieving the health-related SDGs, including UHC (Chapter 3). Effective HSS efforts should be guided by HSPA, which offers stakeholders a potent instrument to inform priorities while enhancing equity, improving efficiency, and enhancing quality.

This chapter reviews (1) the attributes of a well-performing health system; (2) the principles, frameworks, and approaches for HSPA; (3) the indicators of inputs, processes, outputs, outcomes, and impacts and their data sources; and (4) a special case related to hospital performance assessment. The chapter further highlights the significance of HSPA for monitoring UHC achievement and presents a case of a well-performing health system in the context of the COVID-19 pandemic.

12.2 Well-Performing Health Systems

Recalling the six building blocks of health systems (Chapter 1), the World Health Organization (WHO) defines a *well-functioning health system* in relation to "its capacity to improve the health status of the population, defending the population against the social determinants of ill health and from use of health services, protecting people against the financial consequences of ill-health and from use of health services, providing equitable access to people-centred care, and enabling people to fully participate in decisions affecting their health and health system" [1].

A well-performing health system can be achieved with goal-oriented leadership and good governance, the mobilization of adequate resources and the use of strategic purchasing, evidence-informed policy guided by functional health information systems, investment in training and retention of the health workforce – in particular at the primary care level, which is the point of first contact by individuals – and equitable access to essential medicines and medical products with proper referral between the lower and higher levels of care.

12.3 Health Systems Performance Assessment

Health systems performance is a broad concept that considers the full range of determinants of population health, either positive or negative. It recognizes that the health status of a population is only partly influenced by the quality of the available and accessible health services, and that there are many other social, cultural, political, economic, environmental, educational, and demographic factors that influence population health [2]. A well-performing health system is expected to improve health outcomes by addressing the chain of events that minimize adverse outcomes, including the underlying proximal and distal causes. Proximal factors act directly or almost directly to cause disease, and distal factors are more remote from adverse outcomes along the causal chain and act via a number of intermediary causes [3]. Addressing distal, also called structural determinants, requires multisectoral actions for health [4] and citizens' empowerment [5] – two of the three components of primary health care (PHC) enshrined in the 2018 Astana Declaration (Chapter 2) [6].

Thus, HSPA needs to cover the proximal and distal determinants of health. In practice, common approaches of HSPA follow the scope and boundaries of health systems as mentioned in the landmark WHO *World Health Report* of 2000: "health actions whose primary intent is to improve, maintain or restore health"[7]. In keeping with this definition, HSPA as it is currently commonly carried out acknowledges the overall determinants of health, but does not explicitly and specifically assess them.

Health system performance assessment refers to the process of monitoring, evaluating, and communicating the extent to which various aspects of a health system meet key objectives. Operationally, HSPA is considered as *a system-wide exercise whose aim is to appraise the health system as a whole*. The goal of HSPA is to assess whether progress has been made toward desired goals and whether appropriate policy actions are undertaken to promote the achievement of those goals. Actors across the globe use varied terminologies for HSPA, including but not limited to "health sector situation analysis," "health system monitoring," "health system analysis," and "health sector profile," highlighting its wide scope and diversity in purpose and objectives. It is thus crucial to clearly define and outline the goals and objectives of a health system in order to carry out HSPA.

12.3.1 Frameworks for HSPA

Over the last three decades there has been a growing body of literature and frameworks for HSPA. Despite the diversity of tools and frameworks for HSPA, there is relative consensus on health systems' intermediate and final outcomes. In 1999, Murray and Frenk introduced an HSPA framework that consists of three health system goals – health of the population, responsiveness, and fairness in financing – and three health system attributes – equity, efficiency, and quality [8]. WHO in 2000 modified the HSPA framework by adding the four functions of stewardship, creating resources, service delivery, and financing to the three goals (health, responsiveness, and financial protection) [7]. Further, in 2007, WHO introduced six building blocks and added the goal of improved efficiency to health, responsiveness, and financial protection. It also incorporated intermediary goals: improved access, coverage, quality, and safety (see Chapter 1) [9]. In short, the current HSPA framework, tools, and methods were progressively developed by adding foundational elements of health systems and outcomes of interest to the WHO framework of 2000. A recent WHO publication presents the HSPA framework for UHC, which while not novel, depicts the health system functions, their corresponding subfunctions, the assessment areas used to evaluate their performance, and the intermediate objectives and final goals of the health system [10].

The repertoire of health systems performance assessment tools and frameworks is by no means exhaustive. Although the many tools differ in scope and structure, they generally incorporate measures of the health of people, responsiveness, efficiency, equity, and financial risk protection as an intermediary or final goal. Regardless of which approach and framework is chosen for HSPA, it is essential that the boundaries of the given health system are clearly defined, its structural and organizational components are outlined, its goals and objectives are laid out, and the assessment is carried out in the broader context addressing external influences [11].

12.3.2 Key Characteristics of HSPA

The European Public Health online platform proposes five key characteristics for successful implementation of HSPA [12]. These are:

- **Regular:** HSPA should be a continuous and iterative process;
- **Systematic:** the approach should be structured and consistent;
- **Transparent:** the assessment should be unambiguous and accessible to all;
- **Comprehensive:** the whole system should be considered, while recognizing that performance of a system is more than the sum of the performance of its various components; and
- **Analytical:** complementary sources of information, including qualitative and quantitative components, should be included and analyzed to have a well-founded view of the health system's performance.

The HSPA in low- and middle-income countries (L&MICs) should **engage multistakeholders** in identifying indicators that are relevant and feasible to measure to enhance ownership and implementation, and to change courses of actions after the assessment

[13]. Stakeholders may include all relevant agencies of public and private sectors, communities, and funders. Individuals responsible for HSPA should be equipped with a thorough understanding of the breadth and depth of health systems and possess skills such as communication, data collection, analysis, interpretation, and dissemination of results.

12.3.3 Measuring Health Systems Performance

A systematic review [14] of 57 articles could not identify a consistent definition, homogeneous organization, and uniform attributes of high-performing health systems. Rather, it highlighted various intermediate goals such as quality, cost, access, equity, patient experience, and safety. Comparing quality with cost was commonly used to assess health system performance. This systematic review suggested that HSPA should be guided by: (1) context-specific health system goals; (2) data availability; and (3) policy preferences. Furthermore, the lack of universal and reliable indicators of health system performance precludes meaningful cross-national comparison, which could differentiate good and poor performers. This in turn prevents health payers from providing financial or nonfinancial incentives for the better performers.

The WHO European Regional Office worked with some of its Member States, including Estonia [15] and Georgia [16], on HSPA. A full report of HSPA in seven European countries is available [17]. Drawing from Estonia's experience, the HSPA used a descriptive approach of how different attributes of the health system were achieved – the greater the achievement, the higher the performance of the health system. The Estonian HSPA seeks to address eight policy questions:

1. How healthy are Estonians?
2. How well is the health system performing in keeping people healthy?
3. What is the impact of broader determinants of health in Estonia?
4. How responsive is the health system to the needs and expectations of Estonians?
5. Is the way the health system funded fair and equitable?
6. Does the health system provide good and equitable access to health care services?
7. In their interaction with health care services, are Estonians receiving safe and high-quality care?
8. Is the health system effective and efficient?

Table 12.1 has been adapted from the Estonia HSPA and proposes performance indicators and their sources to respond to the eight policy questions above. HSPA has also been reported for L&MICs. For example, a holistic HSPA tool that includes 6 objectives and 54 indicators was developed by Ghana's Ministry of Health [18].

Recent work by Papanicolas et al. [11] suggests that all HSPAs should first address the following four considerations: (1) define the boundaries of the health system; (2) identify the organizational and structural components that constitute the health system; (3) state the objectives of the health system; and (4) describe the impact of external influences on the objectives and functions of the health system. The actions and actors whose *primary* intent is to improve health, as proposed by Murray and Frenk [8], can serve as a useful benchmark to delineate the scope of HSPAs. Further, identifying the components of health systems could be based on various available frameworks, such as the building blocks outlined by WHO. While some of the objectives of health systems will necessarily reflect contextual factors, improving the health of people, responsiveness, and financial risk

Table 12.1 Key health system attributes and performance indicators used in the Estonia HSPA, 2009

Performance indicators	Data sources
1. Health status: level and distribution	
Change in life expectancy (LE) at birth	Most indicators are drawn from
Male and female LE at birth	• civil registration and vital statistics
Changes in LE 2000 vs. 2008 attributable to different disease groups	• life tables
Potential gains in LE if mortality were avoided in 2008	
Infant and child mortality rate	
Main disease groups causing burden of disease (BOD)	Burden of disease study including for disability-free LE
Regional levels of BOD (DALYs/per 1,000 population)	
Disability-free LE	
Self-assessed health	Self-assessed health from surveys of sample population
2. Health behavior and health promotion	
Immunization rates of two-year-olds with national immunization schedule	Routine immunization statistics WHO/UNICEF joint reporting form [19] UNICEF multi-indicator cluster surveys (MICS)
Proportion of daily smokers aged 15+ years	Nationally representative household surveys
Annual consumption of pure alcohol per person	
Prevalence of overweight and obesity	
Physical activity	
3. Broader determinants of health	
Level of education	Census
Unemployment rate	Labor force surveys
Percentage of population having access to clean drinking water	Household survey on access to WASH (MICS)
Average concentration of small particles in the air in cities	Surveillance/sentinel sites for $PM_{2.5}$
Incidence of occupational diseases	Routine statistical records on workplace safety
Deaths from work-related accidents	
4. Responsiveness of the health system	
Satisfaction with quality and access to health care services, hospital care, primary care during the last visit, health care benefit package	National representative household surveys
5. Equitable financing, financial protection, resource allocation, and coverage	
Government spending on health as a percentage of	Treasury records on GDP
• Overall spending	
• GDP	
Out-of-pocket payments (OOPs) as a percentage of GDP	

Table 12.1 (cont.)

Performance indicators	Data sources
OOP as a percentage of total health expenditure (THE)	National Health Accounts National representative household income and expenditure survey
Sources of health care financing as a percentage of THE	
Total household OOPs as a percentage of total household expenditure by income quintile	
Proportion of households impoverished due to OOPs	
Total population health service coverage	National household survey on service coverage

6. Health system efficiency

Technical efficiency	Routine hospital statistics in the MoH
Hospital beds per 1,000,000 population	
Average length of stay, all hospitals	
Bed occupancy rate (%), acute care hospitals only	
Physicians per 100 hospital beds	
Allocative efficiency	Routine financial reports from health care facilities
PHC and inpatient care expenditure compared with THE	MoH budgetary report
GPs and specialist physicians per 100,000 population	Routine hospital statistics on utilization
Ratio of nurses to physicians	
GP utilization versus hospitalization rate	

7. Access to health care services

Rates of inpatient admissions and outpatient contacts	Routine health care statistics
Relationship between standardized mortality rates compared with hospitalization rates, and GP contacts	
Average hospital waiting times for inpatient, outpatient, ambulatory care	Sample survey of patient waiting times
Reported waiting times for specialist services and access to GPs	
Percentage of population reporting problems accessing dental care by income quintile	Nationally representative household survey on unmet needs of dental health services

8. Quality and safety of health care services

Hospital readmission rates for acute myocardial infarction and asthma	Hospital statistics with patient personal ID number for track and trace

Adapted from [16].

protection are fundamental objectives for all health systems. In addition, two cross-cutting aims of health systems should also be assessed – efficiency and equity. Lastly, health systems do not work in silos, but are embedded in their economic, social, cultural, environmental, and political contexts, which need to be given due consideration in an HSPA. This is well illustrated in the case study from Thailand on managing the COVID-19 pandemic, presented later in the chapter.

12.3.4 Choosing Indicators

An important process of HSPA is choosing the appropriate indicators for assessment. There are five proposed criteria [20] that make an indicator suitable for inclusion in an HSPA. First, **importance**: the indicator should reflect critical aspects of health system functions. Second, **relevance**: the indicator should provide information that is useful for monitoring and measuring health system performance for an extended period. Third, **feasibility** is critical for a successful HSPA: the required data should be readily available or can be obtained with reasonable efforts – unavailability of key data should be addressed by improving health information systems or through regular surveys. Fourth, **reliability** means the indicator produces consistent results. And finally, **validity** means the indicator reflects the dimension it is supposed to represent.

Carrying out HSPA is a cumbersome task that presents challenges that need to be overcome to produce reliable findings for the informed policy decision on HSS. Effective HSPA requires measuring indicators that capture health outcomes (e.g., improved health, system responsiveness, equity, and efficiency) rather than only process and input measures (e.g., number of beds, health workforce size, etc.). Progress should be monitored using reliable metrics, and HSPA should be a consistent process embedded in health policy development. Governments are responsible and accountable to citizens for a well-performing health system and consequently for conducting HSPA and using results for further improving health system performance.

12.4 Hospital Performance Assessment

Hospitals have a central role in achieving the goals of improving health, increasing responsiveness, and ensuring fairness in financing. It is estimated that hospitals generally consume more than half of the overall health care budget [21]. They are an integral component of health systems, although they sometimes work in isolation. Hospitals can produce discrete and quantifiable outputs such as the number of hospitalizations and surgeries, and measurable quality of care such as mortality and readmissions of certain conditions. The published literature is abundant on hospital performance assessment [22, 23].

12.4.1 Measuring Hospital Performance

Measuring hospital performance as a subset of health systems can be a complex exercise. A systematic review [24] reported that process indicators are commonly used, such as average length of stay (ALS), bed occupancy rates (BOR), and bed turnover rates (BTR) (Box 12.1). Other measures include rates of unplanned admission, prolonged admissions, and number of discharge and readmission; maintenance of medical records, timeliness of hospitalization reports; blood pressure measurement by health care workers; patient to staff ratio, rates of staff turnover, staff burnout rates; patients' satisfaction rates; antibiotic prescription rates, health care-associated infection rates, pressure ulcer rates, and mortality rates.

Box 12.1 Definition of Key Parameters in a Pabon Lasso Graph

1. Bed occupancy rate (BOR)

   a. BOR is the average number of days for which hospital beds were occupied as a percentage of the available 365 days. It shows how many hospital beds have been utilized, or in another words, the crowdedness of a hospital.
   b. Calculation: utilized bed-days in a year × 100/available bed-days during the calendar year.[1]

2. Average inpatient length of stay (ALS)

   a. ALS represents the average number of days for which patients occupy a hospital bed. It either reflects the severity of the disease as more complicated cases require longer stays, or hospital performance as better care should lead to a shorter stay period.
   b. Calculation: total number of days stayed by all inpatients/total number of admissions or discharges.

3. Bed turnover rate (BTR)

   a. BTR is the number of times there is a change of occupant for a bed during a given period. This reflects the dynamicity of inpatient change. Higher BTR with quality care means the hospital can serve more patients with its available resources while maintaining quality. On the other hand, high BTR with low quality of care means patients are receiving inadequate care prior to discharge, which may result in high mortality outcomes.
   b. Calculation: number of admissions or discharges in one year/available beds during the calendar year.

These indicators have been used to develop a balanced scorecard for measuring and improving hospital performance in Maghreb countries (Algeria, Libya, Mauritania, Morocco, and Tunisia). Similarly, studies from Nigeria [25] and Myanmar [26] applied hospital BTR, BOR, and ALS to assess hospital performance in terms of efficiency in resource utilization. A "Pabon Lasso graph" [27] (Figure 12.1) is a graphical representation that combines the three indicators of BTR, BOR, and ALS into four quadrants to demonstrate relative efficiency across a set of similar types of hospitals. Box 12.1 explains the key parameters used in the Pabon Lasso graph.

Quadrant 1 (left lower quadrant): These are poorly performing hospitals that have surplus hospital beds relative to hospital demand by the people; or patients do not utilize the hospitals due to geographic, socioeconomic, or cultural barriers, or lack of trust and confidence.

Quadrant 2 (left upper quadrant): This includes hospitals that may have unnecessary hospitalizations, oversupply of beds, or the use of beds for simply observing patients.

Quadrant 3 (right upper quadrant): Hospitals here are characterized by high BTR and BOR with a short stay. These are efficient hospitals with relatively few vacant beds at any time.

---

[1] One bed-day is equal to one bed occupied by a patient overnight.

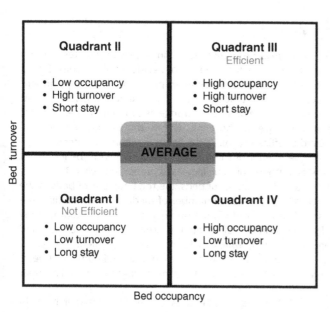

Figure 12.1 Pabon Lasso graph, assessing hospital performance. Adapted from [28].

Quadrant 4 (right lower quadrant): Hospitals here are characterized by high BOR, low bed turnover (BTO), and long stay. These hospitals serve a large number of complicated or chronically ill patients who require continuous care. The hospitals may also offer unnecessarily long stays for patients who could be discharged for intermediate or home care [29].

In the middle of the four quadrants is the average box. Hospitals with average indicator results will be grouped around here, illustrating a good comparison with other hospitals. To prevent misinterpretation, hospitals with a similar case mix or technical capacity should be plotted in the same category in the Pabon Lasso graph. Also, hospitals that fall in quadrants 3 and 4 in the graph do not imply adherence to standards and high-quality care. When applied to Iranian hospitals, the Pabon Lasso graph showed that 60.9% of the studied hospitals had low performance in terms of either BOR, BTO, or both, making a strong case for enhanced performance in the future [30].

A scoping review of hospital performance assessment [30] comprising 42 studies showed that 9 had applied data envelopment analysis (Box 12.2), 6 used the Pabon Lasso graph, 3 used balanced scorecards, another 3 used organizational excellence models, and the remainder used key performance indicators to evaluate hospital performance. Key indicators under input, process, output, and outcome have been identified by Rasi et al. and can be used in hospital performance assessment in L&MICs (Table 12.2) [30].

12.5 Progress Toward UHC: A Measure of Performing Health Systems

Progress toward UHC is an important measure of health system performance, as target 3.8 of the SDGs entails achieving UHC for all by 2030 (Box 12.3). Two indicators have been designated to monitor progress toward target 3.8 within the SDG framework. SDG indicator 3.8.1 monitors coverage of essential health services, and SDG indicator 3.8.2 assesses

---

Box 12.2 Data Envelopment Analysis

Data envelopment analysis (DEA) is a linear programming technique that estimates the relationship between inputs and multiple outputs for a sample of decision-making units (DMUs) such as hospitals. By solving a series of linear programming problems, this nonparametric approach constructs a "best practice frontier" that estimates the maximum possible outputs for a set quantities of inputs among DMUs. The production frontier is considered a best practice as it relies on the relative performance of hospitals within the sample rather than a predetermined absolute standard of efficiency. All DMUs lie on or within the interior of the frontier. The DMUs that lie within the interior of the frontier are considered to be inefficient since, given these levels of inputs, all outputs could be increased proportionately [31].

Examples of **input variables** include: (1) number of beds, the total number of beds in the health facility; (2) number of medical staff, the total number of medical staff, including the number of physicians and nurses; (3) number of CT, the number of computed tomography (CT) devices; (4) number of MR, the number of magnetic resonance (MR) devices; and (5) number of medical equipment together, which is the number of all medical devices. **Output variables** include: (1) BOR, which is the percentage use of the total number of beds; and (2) average nursing time in days, which is the ratio of treatment days to the total number of hospitalized patients [31].

For a comprehensive review of DEA in health care, please refer to the paper by Kohl et al. [32].

---

health expenditure as a share of total household income, to recognize financial distress (Chapter 3).

WHO and World Bank developed the UHC Service Coverage Index (SCI) to monitor progress on coverage of essential services toward UHC as committed in the SDG indicator 3.8.1. It is defined as "coverage of essential services based on tracer interventions that include reproductive, maternal, newborn and child health, infectious diseases, non-communicable diseases and service capacity and access, among the general and the most disadvantaged population" [33]. SDG indicator 3.8.2 relates to financial protection while using health care services. Globally, many people suffer from financial hardship as a result of paying for the health services they need. Two indicators of UHC focus on this issue: "catastrophic spending on health" and "impoverishing spending on health" (see Chapter 3 for a detailed discussion on UHC monitoring).

12.6 Health System Performance in the Context of the COVID-19 Pandemic

In addition to the ongoing monitoring of health system performance described above, the performance of health systems in response to unusual, rapid, changing, and surging demand can provide important information about their strengths and weaknesses. This was clearly demonstrated for all health systems of the world during the successive waves of the COVID-19 pandemic, which persisted at the time of writing this chapter. Box 12.4 presents the initial experience of interventions related to the health system approach to contain COVID-19 in Thailand [34].

Table 12.2 Indicators commonly used in hospital performance assessment

Input	Process	Output	Impact
Number of:	Number of:	Number of deaths:	Patient satisfaction
• inpatient beds	• hospitalization days	• after admission	Relocation of staff
• outpatient beds	• outpatient visits	• in outpatient	Absence of staff
• physicians	• emergency patients	• after surgery	Employee sick leave rates
• nurses	• emergency visits to outpatient visits	Incidence of nosocomial infections	Hospital success in obtaining credentials in quality management
• other clinical team staff	• correct diagnoses to total diagnoses to each specialist	Number of falling patients	Legal complaint rate from the hospital during the year
Total number of employees equivalent to fulltime	• patients referred to the hospital to admitted patients	Percentage of:	Staff satisfaction percentage
Cost of human and other resources	• patients admitted per day	• readmission for the same diagnosis	Complaint patient percentage
Ratio of number of administrative staff to total staff	• minor surgeries	• repeat surgical procedures	
Physician to nurse ratio	• major surgeries	• medical errors	
Physician to bed ratio	Proportion of patients who have to use expensive medical equipment to total patients	• postoperative hematomas and hemorrhages	
Nurse to bed ratio	Hospital survival rate	• agreement between diagnosis at the time of admission and at discharge	
Ratio of number of employees to the number of active beds	Combined index of hospitalization adjusted days	Mortality rate in intensive care unit	
Day-case rates	Total number of nonemergency outpatient visits	Needlestick	
	Patient admitted ratio	Unplanned readmissions to the intensive care unit within 48 h after discharge	
	Ratio of perfect nursing documentation	Prevalence of smoking among staff	
		Readmission rate per active bed	

Source: [30].

Box 12.3 SDG Goal 3: Ensure Healthy Lives and Promote Wellbeing for All at All Ages

Target 3.8: Achieve UHC, including financial risk protection, access to quality essential health care services, and access to safe, effective, quality, and affordable essential medicines and vaccines for all.

- Indicator 3.8.1: Coverage of essential health services
  - Measured through the Service Coverage Index (SCI)

- Indicator 3.8.2: Proportion of the population with large household expenditures on health as a share of the total household expenditure or income
  - catastrophic health expenditure
  - impoverishing spending on health

Box 12.4 Application of the Health System Approach during the First Wave of COVID-19 in Thailand

The first COVID-19 case in Thailand was detected on January 8, 2020. Thailand's early epidemic curve was categorized by three stages: the first stage was a few imported cases (January 2020); the second stage was limited local transmission (late January to late March 2020); and the third stage was widespread clustered transmissions (late March to April 2020).

Governance and immediate multisectoral actions. The government took important measures to contain the local transmission, including national lockdown. It declared a state of emergency on March 25, 2020 as the cases approached 1,000 and established a center for COVID-19 situation administration (CCSA), led by the prime minister, and emergency operating centers (EOC) in all ministries. Provincial governors were entrusted to manage COVID-19 in their provinces.

Public health measures. Measures introduced included hand and food hygiene, physical distancing, and refraining from touching the mouth, nose, and eyes. Although face mask use was not mandatory at that point, its coverage was 95% [35]. People gained trust as the government disseminated daily situational updates. All international travelers were tested, and 14-day mandatory quarantine was enforced.

The International Health Policy Program, a research arm of the Ministry of Public Health, monitored citizens' adherence to personal preventive behaviors through weekly and later biweekly national online surveys. Findings from surveys were fed back to the CCSA and EOC for policy decisions and were made publicly available.

Mobilizing the workforce. A conventional approach of test, trace, and quarantine was applied through contributions of more than 1,000 surveillance and rapid responses teams (SRRTs) at subdistrict, district, provincial, and ministerial levels. Trained epidemiologists formed the corpus of SRRTs; nurses and public health officers were also mobilized for support. Village health volunteers (VHVs) monitored outsiders who traveled from affected areas into their communities and informed SRRTs for investigation.

Clinical services. All tertiary care public and private hospitals having ventilators and ICUs were requested to treat serious COVID-19 cases. Cohort wards for mild and moderate cases were scaled up, including plans for field hospitals by the Ministry of Defence. Pressure on critical resources, such as ICU and ventilators in Greater Bangkok, at the peak of the epidemic triggered the development of a "rationing protocol" [36].

Acute respiratory infection clinics were relocated outside outpatient buildings to prevent COVID-19 droplet infection inside the hospitals. All patients/visitors were liable for thermo-scanning, handwashing, and mask-wearing prior to entry. Health facilities had a separate entry and exit. Noncommunicable disease-related consultations were provided through telemedicine using the LINE application; medicines were delivered at home by post or VHVs to avoid the risk of COVID-19 infection.

Financial subsidies. All COVID-19 public health measures (tests, PPE, quarantine, treatment) were fully subsidized through the three public health insurance funds. Additional cost for community-based test, trace, or quarantine was subsidized by the government for Thais and non-Thais.

Health technology support. Certified PCR test laboratories were scaled up from 80 to 222, which covered all 77 provinces. The private sector constructed a factory for manufacturing N95 face masks for free distribution to all public health care facilities. Other PPE, such as surgical gloves, gowns, and ventilators, were mobilized and prepared for the worst-case scenario. Stock and flows of PPE were monitored through a dashboard and reported daily to the EOC.

With the **health sector and multisectoral** efforts through a whole-of-government approach, the COVID-19 epidemic curve was brought down to fewer than 10 cases per day, and local transmission stopped by May 25, 2020. The low active caseload did not overwhelm the health system.

12.7 Conclusion

Health system performance assessment is a promising approach to evaluate a health system's capacity in achieving its goals and informing policy for HSS. This chapter has highlighted the evolution of HSPA frameworks, which follow the scope and boundaries of health systems. HSPA should be regularly carried out, and should be transparent and comprehensive to track progress toward health-related SDGs, including UHC. Hospital performance assessment is a vital subset of HSPA as it consumes a significant portion of health resources. Hospital performance can be monitored by applying balanced scorecards, Pabon Lasso graphs, DEA, or organizational excellence models, depending upon the nature and context of assessment.

References

1. World Health Organization. Key components of a well functioning health system. 2010. www.who.int/healthsystems/EN_HSSkeycomponents.pdf?ua=1 (accessed August 18, 2020).

2. European Public Health. Health system performance assessment. 2016. www.europeanpublichealth.com/health-systems/health-system-performance-assessment (accessed September 30, 2020).

3. World Health Organization. A conceptual framework for action on the social determinants of health. Social Determinants of Health Discussion Paper 2. 2010. https://apps.who.int/iris/bitstream/handle/10665/44489/9789241500852_eng.pdf (accessed June 30, 2020).

4. S. Bennett, D. Glandon, K. Rasanathan. Governing multisectoral action for health in low-income and middle-income countries: unpacking the problem and rising to the challenge. *BMJ Glob Health* 2018; **10**: 3.

5. World Health Organization. A vision for primary health care in the 21st century: towards universal health coverage and the Sustainable Development Goals. 2018. https://apps.who.int/iris/handle/10665/328065 (accessed July 30, 2020).

6. World Health Organization. Declaration of Astana. Global Conference on Primary

Health Care. 2018. www.who.int/docs/
default-source/primary-health/
declaration/gcphc-declaration.pdf
(accessed July 15, 2020).

7. World Health Organization. *The World Health Report 2000, Health Systems: Improving Performance*. Geneva, World Health Organization, 2000.

8. C. J. Murray, J. Frenk. A WHO framework for health system performance assessment. 1999. https://pdfs.semanticscholar.org/9ac0/3257fcffff670c40a2b9868c201742a30b4a.pdf (accessed March 19, 2021).

9. World Health Organization. Everybody's business: strengthening health systems to improve health outcomes: WHO's Framework for Action. 2007. www.who.int/healthsystems/strategy/everybodys_business.pdf (accessed March 19, 2021).

10. World Health Organization. *Health System Performance Assessment: A Framework for Policy Analysis*. Geneva, World Health Organization, 2022.

11. I. Papanicolas, D. Rajan, M. Karanikolos, et al. Health system performance assessment: a framework for policy analysis. World Health Organization, 2021.

12. European Public Health. Health system performance assessment. 2016. www.europeanpublichealth.com/health-systems/health-system-performance-assessment (accessed August 18, 2021).

13. C. K. Tashobya, V. C. da Silveira, F. Ssengooba, et al. Health systems performance assessment in low-income countries: learning from international experiences. *Glob Health* 2014; **10**: 5.

14. S. C. Ahluwalia, C. L. Damberg, M. Silverman, et al. What defines a high-performing health care delivery system: a systematic review. *Jt Comm J Qual Saf* 2017; **43**(9): 450–459.

15. World Health Organization. Estonia health system performance assessment. 2009. www.euro.who.int/__data/assets/pdf_file/0015/115260/E93979.pdf (accessed September 30, 2020).

16. World Health Organization. Georgia health system performance assessment. 2009.

https://reliefweb.int/sites/reliefweb.int/files/resources/900DCDCC6D22843C C1257671004774F2-Full_Report.pdf (accessed September 30, 2020).

17. World Health Organization. Case study on health system performance assessment: a long-standing development in Europe. 2012. www.euro.who.int/__data/assets/pdf_file/0008/168875/Case-Studies-for-HSPA-ENG.pdf (accessed September 30, 2020).

18. E. Kumah, S. E. Ankomah, A. Fusheini, et al. Frameworks for health systems performance assessment: how comprehensive is Ghana's holistic assessment tool? *Glob Health Res Policy* 2020; **5**(1): 1–2.

19. WHO, UNICEF. Immunization, vaccines and biologicals: data, statistics and graphics. 2020. www.who.int/immunization/monitoring_surveillance/data/en/ (accessed September 30, 2020).

20. J. Veillard, T. Huynh, S. Ardal, et al. Making health system performance measurement useful to policy makers: aligning strategies, measurement and local health system accountability in Ontario. *Healthcare Policy* 2010; **5** (3): 49.

21. M. McKee, J. Healy. *Pressures for Change: In Hospitals in a Changing Europe*. Milton Keynes, Open University, 2002.

22. World Health Organization Europe. How can hospital performance be measured and monitored? 2003. www.euro.who.int/__data/assets/pdf_file/0009/74718/E82975.pdf (accessed January 9, 2020).

23. O. Groene, J. K. Skau, A. Frølich. An international review of projects on hospital performance assessment. *Int J Qual Health Care* 2008; **20**(3): 162–171.

24. S. Rouis, H. Nouira, M. Khelil, et al. Development of a balanced scorecard for the monitoring of hospital performance in the countries of the Greater Maghreb: systematic review. *Tunis Med* 2018; **96**(10–11): 774–788.

25. H. E. Aloh, O. E. Onwujekwe, O. G. Aloh, et al. Is bed turnover rate a good metric for hospital scale efficiency? A measure of resource utilization rate for hospitals in

Southeast Nigeria. *Cost Eff Resour Alloc* 2020; **18**: 21.

26. World Health Organization. The Republic of the Union of Myanmar health system review. 2014. https://iris.wpro.who.int/handle/10665.1/11354 (accessed October 15, 2020).

27. A. Goshtasebi, M. Vahdaninia, R. Gorgipour, et al. Assessing hospital performance by the Pabon Lasso model. *Iranian J Public Health* 2009; **2**: 119–124.

28. P. Lasso. Evaluating hospital performance through simultaneous application of several indicators. *Bull Pan Am Health Organ* 1986; **20**(4): 341–357.

29. B. Mohammadkarim, S. Jamil, H. Pejman, et al. Combining multiple indicators to assess hospital performance in Iran using the Pabon Lasso model. *Australas Medical J* 2011; **4**(4): 175.

30. V. Rasi, B. Delgoshaee, M. Maleki. Identification of common indicators of hospital performance evaluation models: a scoping review. *JEHP* 2020; **9**.

31. R. Stefko, B. Gavurova, K. Kocisova. Healthcare efficiency assessment using DEA analysis in the Slovak Republic. *Health Econ Rev* 2018; **8**(1): 6.

32. S. Kohl, J. Schoenfelder, A. Fügener, et al. The use of data envelopment analysis (DEA) in healthcare with a focus on hospitals. *Health Care Manag Sci* 2018; **22**(2): 245–286.

33. World Health Organization. The Global Health Observatory: UHC service coverage index. www.who.int/data/gho/indicator-metadata-registry/imr-details/4834 (accessed July 8, 2021).

34. W. Patcharanaruamol, A. Issac, N. Asgari-Jirhandeh, et al. COVID-19 health system response monitor: Thailand. 2020. www.searo.who.int/entity/asia_pacific_observatory/publications/covid_thailand/en/ (accessed August 18, 2021).

35. YouGov. Thais most likely to wear facemasks in ASEAN. 2020. https://th.yougov.com/en-th/news/2020/05/19/thais-most-likely-wear-facemasks-asean/ (accessed September 29, 2020).

36. A. Marshall, R. Archer, W. Witthayapipopsakul, et al. Developing a Thai national critical care allocation guideline during the COVID-19 pandemic: a rapid review and stakeholder consultation. *Health Res Policy Syst* 2021; **19**(1): 1–5.

Decision-Making Tools for Informed Decisions by Health Policymakers and Managers

Meesha Iqbal, Hiba Sameen, Mohammad Abu-Zaineh, Awad Mataria, and Sameen Siddiqi

Key Messages

- The global response to COVID-19 has underscored the inadequate preparedness of health systems and emphasized that countries should systematically evaluate and disseminate evidence about what works and what does not, to implement and scale up innovations to improve people's lives.
- Decision-making tools, such as burden of disease analysis, health technology assessment, cost-effectiveness analysis, health equity analysis, national health accounts, and stakeholder analysis, can help policymakers make informed decisions.
- The process of decision-making is not linear and is affected by multiple factors beyond the availability of evidence, such as the political context, personal over public interests, decision-makers' accountability, relationships with stakeholders, recognition of familiar experiences in the past, and how people construct the narrative. Furthermore, cultural context shapes the degree to which these factors affect decisions and influence how people make sense of events.

13.1 Introduction

Decision-making is an act of processing information related to a problem or situation to arrive at a judgment. The information to be processed is based on what is salient and objectively presented, as well as the context in which the information is extracted [1]. Health policymakers in all countries are required to make decisions that have implications for health systems, health outcomes, and the costs involved in achieving these. Policymakers can take decisions intuitively or be informed by evidence. While decision-making in many situations can be a political choice, presenting evidence makes it less likely for policymakers to overlook it.

Evidence-informed decisions positively influence access, quality, efficiency, equity, and sustainability of health services, and improve transparency and accountability, thereby reducing opportunities for wastage, abuse, and corruption in the health system [2]. A rational decision-making process involves identifying the problem at hand, collecting the needed information, looking at options, considering evidence, choosing the best option, taking the required actions, and reviewing the decision. Decision-making can be quite complex at every step, notwithstanding the personal over public interests that can influence decisions under varying circumstances.

There are several tools available to help health policymakers make informed decisions. This chapter presents a repertoire of such tools to help answer fundamental questions: What are the major causes of disease, disability, and death in a population? How amenable are these to interventions and at what cost? What is the feasibility of implementing these interventions? To what extent do these protect the vulnerable and poor segments of the population? What is the public and private expenditure on health, and how can it be rationalized? What different constituencies can influence these decisions?

Policymakers are not expected to know the methodological aspects of these tools; rather, they should know what tools are available, their purpose and application, strengths and limitations, and how to interpret the results in the local context. This chapter presents six decision-making tools that can help policymakers and managers take evidence-informed decisions: burden of disease analysis; health technology assessment; cost-effectiveness analysis; health equity analysis; national health accounts analysis; and stakeholder analysis.

13.2 Decision-Making Tools for Informed Decisions

13.2.1 Burden of Disease Analysis

The burden of disease (BOD) analysis, whether global or local, aims to: (1) incorporate the burden of nonfatal conditions along with mortality into assessments of health status; (2) produce an independent and demographically plausible assessment of the burden of certain conditions and diseases; and (3) measure disease and injury burden in a metric that can be used to assess the cost-effectiveness of interventions [3]. BOD analysis allows policymakers to appreciate the importance of nonfatal conditions such as mental health problems, to compare the cost-effectiveness of different interventions, and to make rational allocation of scarce resources.

The disability-adjusted life year (DALY) is a time-based unit for measuring the BOD. Hence, *time* is the common metric that allows estimation of *years of life lost due to premature death* (YLL) and *years of life lost due to disability* (YLD) [4]. One DALY is one year lost of "healthy" life. Calculating DALYs requires estimating YLL and YLD for specific conditions in the population (Figure 13.1). BOD analysis is a value-laden approach and requires answering two fundamental questions.

1. *How long should people live?* The Global Burden of Disease (GBD) Study assumes a standard life expectancy at birth for all populations, irrespective of geography, education, or socioeconomic status, fixed at 86 years for women and 84 years for men [5]. This allows deaths in all communities at the same age to contribute equally to the BOD. Hence, a child dying at the age of four in Sierra Leone, Syria, or Serbia will contribute the same number of YLL.

2. *How should we compare years of life lost due to premature death with years of life lost while living with disabilities of differing severities?* Nonfatal health outcomes of diseases are different from one another in their causes, nature, and impact on the individual. The time lived with disabilities must be defined, measured, and valued in a clear framework. For example, a year lived with blindness appears to cause more severe disability than a year lived with dermatitis, while quadriplegia is regarded as more severe than blindness. Two methods commonly used to put a value on different states of health involve asking people their preference between the quantity and quality of life: time trade-off[1] and person trade-off.[2] Using such techniques with participants from diverse

---

[1] How many years lived with a given disability would you trade for a fixed period of perfect health?
[2] Would you prefer to save one life year for 1,000 perfectly healthy individuals as opposed to saving one life year for 2,000 individuals in a worse health state?

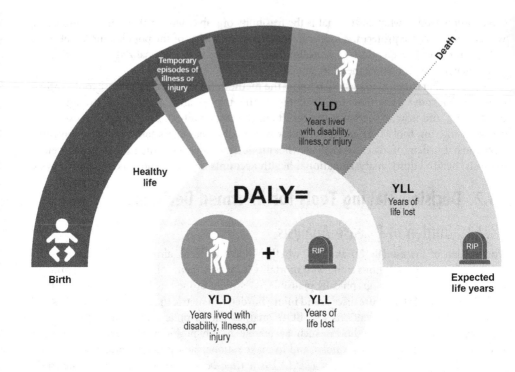

Figure 13.1 The concept underpinning burden of disease estimation [6].

cultural backgrounds, a consensus has been developed on disability weights for different disease states that vary between 0 (perfect health with no disability) and 1 (equivalent to death), which are used in BOD analysis (Table 13.1). Once both can be measured in terms of time lost, it is easy to add YLL with YLD to get the DALY estimate.

The BOD analysis has high *policy relevance* for countries as it: (1) allows comparison of population health across regions (Table 13.2); (2) captures changes in population health over time; (3) identifies and quantifies health inequalities; (4) gives appropriate attention to nonfatal outcomes; and (5) informs debates on priorities for health planning.

13.2.2 Health Technology Assessment

Health policymakers are frequently confronted with decisions about how to allocate finite budgetary resources while providing maximum health benefits to the population. Health technology assessment (HTA) is one of the tools available to inform this decision. *HTA is an interdisciplinary process that assesses all relevant aspects of technology, including effectiveness and safety, as well as its economic, social, and ethical implications* [9]. It assesses both the direct, intended consequences of technologies and their indirect, unintended consequences in the short and long terms.

Health technology assessment informs policymaking by prioritizing technologies that are identified to be safe, efficacious, and effective while considering economic, social, and ethical considerations. It needs to be conducted in an impartial, transparent, and robust

Table 13.1 The conceptual basis for measuring DALYs as the metric of burden of disease estimation

$DALY = YLL + YLD$	$YLL = N \times L$	$YLD = I \times DW \times L$
where:	where:	where:
YLL = years of life lost due to premature mortality	N = number of deaths	I = the number of incident cases
YLD = years lived with disability	L = the average difference in standard life expectancy and age at death (years)	DW = disability weight
		L = the average duration of disability (years)

Measuring the burden of a specific disease in a hypothetical population

$YLL = 15{,}750$	$N = 450$	$I = 7{,}000$
$YLD = 31{,}500$	$L = 35$ years	$DW = 0.3$
		$L = 15$ years
$DALY = 15{,}750 + 31{,}500 = 47{,}250$ years	$YLL = 450 \times 35 = 15{,}750$	$YLD = 7{,}000 \times 0.3 \times 15 = 31{,}500$

Source: [7].

Table 13.2 Distribution of DALYs per 100,000 population by three major disease groups for 2019

Major disease groups	Pakistan	India	Afghanistan	Iran
Noncommunicable diseases	18,708 (48%)	19,227 (56%)	21,120 (42%)	18,868 (76%)
Communicable, maternal, neonatal, and nutritional diseases	17,062 (43%)	11,564 (34%)	22,217 (45%)	2,614 (11%)
Injuries	3,577 (9%)	3,547 (10%)	6,229 (13%)	3,307 (13%)
Total	39,348 (100%)	34,338 (100%)	49,566 (100%)	24,789 (100%)

Source: [8].

manner as it feeds into the process of health prioritization, which can benefit some groups at the expense of others. In some countries, cost-effectiveness analysis (CEA) is included as part of the HTA process, while in other countries it is undertaken separately. The two are presented separately in this chapter.

Clinical trials conducted as part of the development of new technologies form the basis of HTA, though its wider scope also includes economic, social, and ethical aspects. While the purpose of clinical trials (e.g., vaccine trials) is to test the efficacy and identify the side-effects of diagnostic and therapeutic medical interventions, HTA aims to demonstrate how the interventions work in the real world, taking other aspects into consideration.

Health technology assessment considers a health technology when integrated into the health system setting and, as such, requires consideration of the specific contexts (e.g., system structure, resource availability) in which the technology will be used, as well as societal factors (e.g., population health state, inequalities, people's preferences). For example, HTA considers the resource requirements of implementing an intervention, which clinical trials do not. In principle, HTA explores all dimensions of the value of a technology, not only those that can be demonstrated in clinical trials [10].

Who Uses HTAs and When?

Health technology assessments are used to inform decisions by various professionals, institutions, and organizations working in diverse settings:

- regulatory authorities, to permit the commercial use (e.g., marketing) of medicines, devices, or other regulated technology;
- payers and insurers (health care authorities, health planners, drug formularies developers, employers, etc.), to determine which interventions to enlist and/or cover;
- clinicians, to identify the appropriate health care interventions for a particular patient's clinical needs and circumstances;
- health professional associations, to outline the role of technology in clinical protocols or practice guidelines;
- hospitals, health care networks, group purchasing, and other health care organizations, to inform decisions regarding technology acquisition and management;
- standards-setting and health care delivery organizations, to ascertain the manufacture, performance, appropriate use, and other aspects of health care technologies; and
- government health department officials, to develop public health programs (e.g., immunization, screening, and environmental protection programs).

13.2.3 Cost-Effectiveness Analysis

Cost-effectiveness analysis is another tool used by policymakers to help allocate resources most efficiently, by informing which health intervention(s) should be provided compared to others. CEA does that by comparing the costs and consequences – that is, "health outcomes" (effectiveness) – of an alternate course of action using limited resources for a defined population, during a defined period of time, and from a pre-identified perspective. The alternate course of action could be another active intervention addressing the same health condition (or other conditions) or no intervention, labeled as the "do nothing" option. This type of analysis can either be part of a HTA process or a standalone analysis. *Generally, the process of HTA begins by defining the overall scope of assessment followed by choosing an appropriate type of health economic evaluation, such as CEA.*[3]

"Health outcomes" are measured and valued using a standardized health unit, such as DALYs averted (see Section 13.2.1) or quality-adjusted life years (QALYs) gained, where a QALY is a function of *duration* adjusted to *quality of life*. One QALY is one life-year in perfect health [11]. Practically, the net costs of an intervention relative to that of an alternate course of action are first quantified. These net costs are *incremental* and should include all implementation costs (such as labor, materials, transportation, education, administration,

---

[3] Precisely different forms of health economic evaluation are distinguished based on the way health outcomes are valued. This leads to a spectrum of techniques, including cost–consequences analysis, cost-effectiveness analysis, cost–utility analysis, cost-minimization analysis, and cost–benefit analysis. This chapter uses CEA.

training, and others) that are estimated net of costs averted due to the intervention (such as averted health costs from reduced hospitalization or further treatment).

The incremental net costs (input) are then compared to the health outcomes of the intervention (in QALYs or DALYs) relative to the alternative course of action. A ratio of cost to a standardized health unit is calculated. This is known as the *incremental cost-effectiveness ratio (ICER)* and is measured as cost per DALY averted or cost per QALY gained. The lower the cost per DALY or QALY, the more cost-effective the specific intervention is. The ICER metric can then be used to inform decisions about which intervention, programs, and/or strategy to prioritize for funding:

$$ICER = \Delta \text{ Net costs}/\Delta \text{ Health outcomes (measured in DALYs averted or QALYs gained)}$$

There are some limitations to using standardized methods of CEA when working with aggregated data and secondary sources. Effectiveness data is not always derived from systematic reviews, and interventions may have different effectiveness in different populations and settings. Additionally, comparisons at an aggregate level are often more difficult to justify as there may be significant variation in current practice across geographies.

Implementing CEA: A Simple Example

Consider two therapies for acute diarrhea with mild to moderate dehydration: supervised *oral rehydration therapy* (ORT) and *intravenous rehydration therapy* (IVT). Supervised ORT is less costly to administer than IVT, but IVT generates marginally better health outcomes relative to ORT [12]. The question for the policymaker is to determine which treatment is more cost-effective.

To do a CEA, we undertake the following (simplified) steps (Table 13.3):

1. We estimate the health benefits from each treatment based on predetermined data.
2. We calculate the total net cost for each treatment, including the costs averted from future hospitalizations, pharmaceutical costs, and other costs. It is worth noting that we can also have cost-saving interventions, where the costs averted completely offset the costs of administrating and implementing the intervention. For this exercise, we assume that the net costs are positive.
3. We calculate the cost-effectiveness ratio relative to the "do nothing" option.

Using information from the 2019 GBD Study, we select data on the burden of diarrhea in DALYs averted for under-fives in Pakistan that provides the following figures (rounded to the nearest thousand) [8]: YLLs, 1,215,000; YLDs, 63,000; DALYs, 1,278,000; number of incident cases, 36,000,000; and number of deaths, 14,000.

We determine, based on a systematic review of various clinical trials, that ORT reduces mortality (YLL) by 20% and IVT reduces mortality (YLL) by 25%. For simplicity, we assume that neither ORT nor IVT has any impact on morbidity (YLD). We also determine from a systematic review that 1% of all cases of diarrheal diseases result in severe dehydration, and identify this as a proxy of avertable adverse outcomes.

This example shows that ORT is more cost-effective than IVT since averting one DALY costs US$740, compared to $5,925 using IVT. Given this, and all else being equal, a policymaker would likely choose to fund ORT over IVT.

In a setting where ORT is already available and funded, the decision to use public funds to provide a more expensive but more effective treatment, such as IVT, depends on whether the added expenses result in significantly greater health gains. The ICER measures the

Table 13.3 Cost-effectiveness analysis of ORT vs. IVT in diarrhea treatment of children under five years old in Pakistan

Step	Measuring benefits and cost	ORT	IVT
1	Estimating health benefits	DALYs = YLL + YLD = YLLs × 1% × 20% + 0 = 1,215,000 × 1% × 20% = 2,430 DALYs	DALYs = YLL + YLD = YLLs × 1% × 25% + 0 = 1,215,000 × 1% × 25% = 3,038 DALYs
2	Net costs to administer intervention	$5 per patient	$50 per patient
	Total net costs to administer intervention	$5 × 1% × 36,000,000 = $1.8m	$50 × 1% × 36,000,000 = $18m
3	Cost-effectiveness ratio	$1.8m/2,430 DALYs ≈ $740/ DALY	$18m/3,038 DALYs ≈ $5,925/ DALY

additional cost of a more expensive intervention compared to a less costly one for each additional DALY averted. To calculate the ICER, the difference between the net costs for each intervention is divided by the difference between the health benefits of each treatment:

$$ICER = \frac{\text{Net cost of IVT} - \text{Net cost of ORT}}{\text{Health benefits from IVT} - \text{Health benefits from ORT}}$$

$$= \frac{\$18m - \$1.8m}{3{,}038 \text{ DALYs} - 2{,}430 \text{ DALYs}}$$

$$= \$26{,}645 \text{ per DALY}$$

This measure tells us the extra cost per extra unit of health effect for the more expensive therapy, in this case IVT, relative to the alternative (ORT). In this case, using IVT rather than ORT costs an additional $26,645 per DALY averted.

However, this metric is not enough by itself to determine whether a new treatment should be funded or not. Determining whether to fund such a new treatment requires consideration of the *maximum threshold* or *willingness to pay* per DALY averted. Interventions with favorable ICERs that remain below that threshold suggest that their added costs are justified by commensurate health gains and should be implemented. Conversely, ICERs above the threshold represent interventions whose additional health gains do not justify the sizable additional resources required to implement them.

Decision Rules for Maximizing Population Health

An ICER helps us decide which interventions to fund (and which not to fund) in order to maximize population health. Once all feasible interventions are ranked according to their DALYs per dollar (the inverse of the cost-effectiveness ratio), funding can be ascribed to

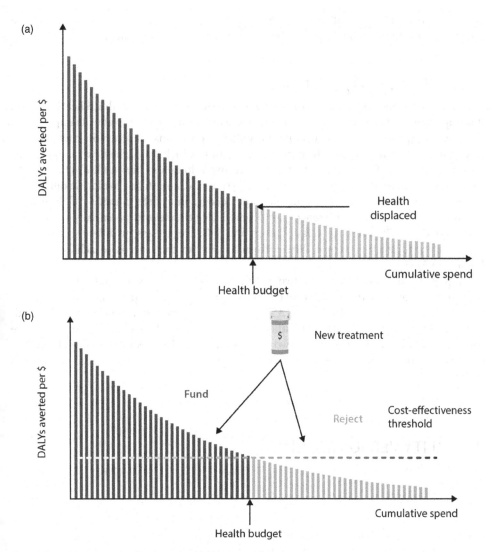

Figure 13.2 (a) Maximizing population health; (b) decision rule for a new intervention.

those highest on the list, progressing through interventions with decreasing DALYs per cost until the allocated budget is exhausted, as demonstrated in Figure 13.2.

Given limited budgets, some interventions cannot be funded (light gray bars). As a result, health is said to be "displaced," meaning that the burden of illness shifts to those conditions for which treatment is not funded. However, if we have evaluated the costs and benefits of each intervention correctly, and we have rank-ordered the treatments by cost-effectiveness when choosing which to fund, then we can be confident that the interventions that have been funded will maximize DALYs averted for a given budget.

There are, however, significant uncertainties in determining the costs and benefits associated with a particular intervention and in determining the costs and benefits across disease areas in a consistent manner. Policymakers should see these tools as a guide to informing decisions, though given the uncertainty, expert judgment will need to be exercised.

13.2.4 Health Equity and Equality

Equity is a core value of public health and reflects the level of fairness within a health system. It is important that decision-makers understand what health equity is, value its importance, and use an equity lens when formulating policies, programs, and health interventions. A fundamental premise of health equity is the extent to which people have equal opportunities to attain their full health potential (i.e., to live a long and healthy life) [13]. Health inequities are health disparities that arise from systematic, unjust, and avoidable differences in the social, economic, demographic, and geographic determinants of health of a population [14]. These differences are deemed illegitimate and potentially remediable [15]. While *equality* refers to treating everyone alike, regardless of differences in need, equity refers to treating people differently according to their needs to achieve fairness (Figure 13.3) [16, 17].

Applied to health care there are two distinct, but related, views of equity. The first view starts with the premise that health care ought to be allocated according to individuals' health needs rather than their ability to pay (ATP). The second view requires payments for health care to be linked to individuals' ATP rather than their needs and use of health care. These are commonly described in terms of the two egalitarian principles of equity: *horizontal equity* – equal treatment of equals – and *vertical equity* – appropriate unequal treatment of unequals (Table 13.4).

EQUALITY VERSUS EQUITY

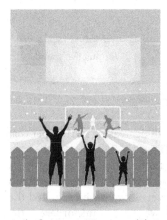

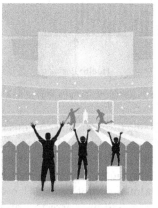

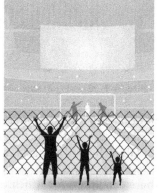

In the first image, it is assumed that everyone will benefit from the same supports. They are being treated equally.

In the second image, individuals are given different supports to make it possible for them to have equal access to the game. They are being treated equitably.

In the third image, all three can see the game without any supports or accommodations because the cause of the inequity was addressed. The systemic barrier has been removed.

Figure 13.3 Concept of equality, equity, and justice [18].

Table 13.4 Horizontal and vertical equity in the provision and financing of health care

	Health equity	
	Horizontal	**Vertical**
Provision of health care	Equal provision of care for those with equal health care needs	Unequal treatment for those with unequal medical needs
Financing of health care	Equal payment by those with the same ATP (irrespective of needs)	Greater payment by those with greater ATP (irrespective of needs)

In empirical research, most attention has been given to horizontal equity, defined as *equal treatment for equal medical need, irrespective of other characteristics such as income, race, residence, etc.* [16], while the notion of vertical equity has often been applied to assess equity in health care financing. For a proper assessment of equity performance of health care systems, a simultaneous examination of the distribution of health care use/need and the distribution of health care payments is essential.

Measuring Health Inequality and Inequity

Measuring health equity is an essential first step to assess and address the health needs and priorities of vulnerable segments of the population. Decision-makers and managers need to be able to use and interpret the different tools and techniques commonly used to measure health equity and inequality.

Equity can be assessed in terms of the distribution of health in a population (e.g., the Gini index and the index of dissimilarity), or using various measures of socioeconomic inequalities in health. While the latter uses measures of association (e.g., odds ratio, regression coefficients), the former is based on ranking of socioeconomic variables (e.g., concentration index, slope and relative indices of inequality) and measures of potential impact (e.g., population attributable risk) [19]. There is no straightforward way to decide which measure to choose. Choosing the appropriate measure of inequality depends on the type of health variable under consideration and the purpose of the analysis (Figure 13.4). It is important to consider the advantages and limitations of each measure. Some of the commonly used measures are explained below.

The Range

Range is the most widely used measure of concentration in a distribution. It is a rudimentary measure of inequality that is very simple to calculate and interpret. It is computed as the difference between the values of the health variable of the most and least advantaged groups in the population: $R(h) = \max(h) - \min(h)$. Where individual data is grouped, such as by socioeconomic status (SES), the range compares average values between the best-off and the worst-off SES groups, $R(h) = \bar{\mu}_g - \underline{\mu}_g$, where $\bar{\mu}_g$ and $\underline{\mu}_g$ are the means of the health variable of the best-off and worst-off SES groups, respectively. The range can also be expressed in relative terms as the proportion of the mean. This gives the relative range $(RR(h) = [\max(h) - \min(h)]/\mu_h)$. Another related simple measure is the ratio of maximum to minimum health $(\text{Ratio}(h) = \max(h)/\min(h))$. For grouped data the ratio can be defined as $\text{Ratio}(h) = \bar{\mu}_g / \underline{\mu}_g$.

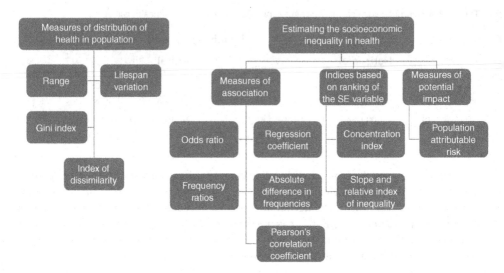

Figure 13.4 Typology of measures in health inequality [20].

We now provide an example illustrating how these measures can be computed and compared for different distributions of the self-assessed health (SAH) variable. The example also illustrates their interpretations and limitations. Table 13.5 reports three hypothetical distributions of SAH (individuals reporting good health status): $n^1 = n^2 = 4,523$ and $n^3 = 4,878$ individuals.

Despite their simplicity, there are two drawbacks to using range and ratio as measures of inequalities. First, both measures look only at the two extreme groups of the distribution; thus, they overlook any variations elsewhere in the distribution. For instance, comparing distributions 1 and 2, both measures do not capture the pro-poor change in distribution 2. As shown in Table 13.5, the gap between the top and bottom groups remains unchanged, although the extent of inequality between the intermediate groups decreases. Second, the range does not consider the size of the groups being compared. A careful look at Table 13.5 illustrates these limitations. For instance, distribution 3 reflects changes in the size of the poorest and richest groups. Although the number of individuals reporting good health in both groups does not change, the values of the three range measures significantly change due to the changes in the sizes of the two extreme groups. This may be misleading when comparisons are held across countries or over time.

The Relative Lorenz Curve and the Associated Gini Coefficient

The relative Lorenz curve and the associated Gini coefficient can be used to measure total (*pure*) health inequality (not linked to SES). Unlike simple measures, they allow incorporating value judgments vis-à-vis the degree of inequality aversion by attributing weights to individuals based on their SES rank. The Lorenz curve allows scrutinizing inequality over the entire distribution, while the Gini coefficient provides a summary measure of the degree of inequality of the distribution, and hence facilitates comparisons across countries and over time. The Gini index is a summary measure of inequality. It is calculated with reference to the Lorenz curve, where inequality is measured by departure of the Lorenz curve from the perfect equality line. Geometrically, the Gini index is defined as the area of the concentration (A) over the area of the triangle (A + B) (Figure 13.5). For a continuous cardinal

Table 13.5 Distribution of SAH across SES groups (%)

SES	Distribution 1			Distribution 2			Distribution 3		
	n_g	h	μ_g	n_g	h	h	n_g	h	μ_g
Poorest 20%	1,650	295	17.88	1,650	295	17.88	2,000	300	15.00
2nd quintile	1,230	283	23.01	1,230	283	23.01	1,230	283	23.01
3rd quintile	998	300	30.06	998	350	35.07	998	300	30.06
4th quintile	365	106	29.04	365	120	32.88	365	106	29.04
Richest 20%	280	198	70.71	280	198	70.71	285	200	70.18
n	4,523	1,182		4,523	1,246		4,878	1,189	
μ			26.13			27.55			24.37
R			52.84			52.84			55.18
RR			2.02			1.92			2.26
Ratio			3.96			3.96			4.68

n = number, μ = mean, R = range, RR = relative ratio.

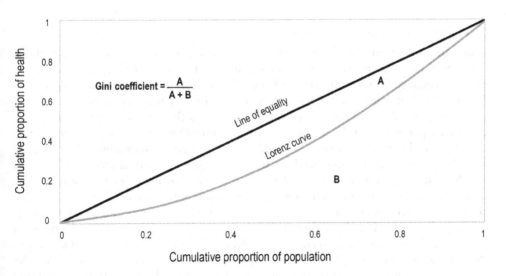

Figure 13.5 Relative Lorenz curve and Gini coefficient of health distribution.

measure of health, the relative Lorenz curve, $L(h)$, plots the cumulative proportions of health (y-axis) against the cumulative proportions of the population (x-axis, ranked from the sickest person to the healthiest). Note that individuals are ranked by their health rather than by SES. If health is equally distributed, $L(h)$ coincides with the diagonal. Otherwise it lies beneath the diagonal [21]. The Gini coefficient is twice the area between the Lorenz curve and the diagonal. A higher Gini coefficient indicates greater inequality.

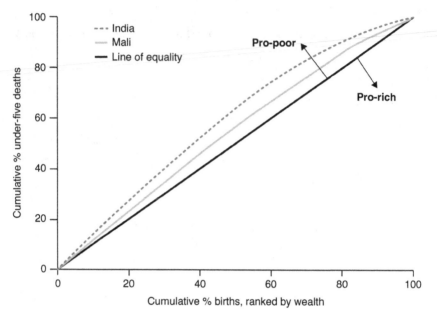

Figure 13.6 Concentration curve for under-five deaths in India and Mali (1982–1992) [25].

Concentration Curve and Concentration Index

Unlike the Lorenz curve and Gini coefficient, the concentration curve and the associated concentration index are bivariate measures of inequality that enable measuring socioeconomic inequality in a health variable (where individuals are ranked according to SES rather than their health status). The concentration curve for a given health variable, $CC(h)$, displays the cumulative percentage of the health variable (y-axis) against the cumulative percentage of the population (x-axis) ranked by SES, starting with the worst-off. The main difference between $CC(h)$ and $L(h)$ is that in the latter individuals are ranked according to a health variable, while in the former they are ranked according to a SES variable. The $CC(h)$ can lie below or above the diagonal. The interpretation depends thus on whether the health variable under consideration is a good or a bad result. A $CC(h)$ above the perfect equality line reflects a pro-poor inequality and vice versa. The concentration index, $C(h)$, is defined with reference to the concentration curve. Like the Gini coefficient, the value of the $C(h)$ equals twice the area between the $CC(h)$ and the diagonal (the line of perfect equality). It takes a negative value when the $CC(h)$ lies above the diagonal, indicating disproportionate concentration of the health variable among the poor, and a positive value when it lies below the diagonal (Figure 13.6). If the health variable is a "bad" outcome, such as ill-health, a negative value of the index means that ill-health is higher among the poor [22–24].

13.2.5 National Health Accounts Analysis

National health accounts (NHA) are a diagnostic tool used to describe and evaluate the overall flow of funds through a health system by tracking health expenditures across multiple financing streams, regardless of the source of funding [26]. NHA uses a series of

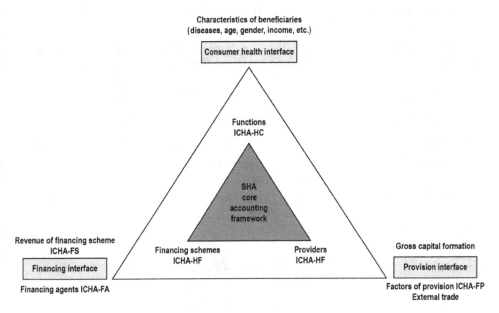

Figure 13.7 System of Health Accounts 2011 Framework [27].

interlinked tables and classifications to follow the flow of funds from their original sources to their final use. It is based on the premise that what is consumed in the health system is hence provided and has been financed.

Figure 13.7 depicts the structure of health accounts as employed by the System of Health Accounts 2011 (SHA 2011) [27]. SHA 2011 is the most up-to-date reference for performing health accounts worldwide. It describes a triaxial relation between consumption, provision, and financing in the health system and summarizes the key classifications in relation to each of the three pillars. This approach to health accounting is well aligned with the three health financing functions of revenue raising, pooling, and purchasing (Chapter 5). In addition, NHA describes the magnitude of revenues, outputs, and expenditures in the health system relative to the overall economy. Table 13.6 presents the classification of health care functions with an application to the case of Sri Lanka.

NHA Definitions and Purposes

National health accounts provide standardized definitions for all levels of the health accounting system. *Health expenditure* refers to any expenditure that fulfills the following criteria, regardless of who pays or who provides: (1) the *primary purpose* of the expenditure is to promote health, prevent diseases or cure illness, care for chronic conditions or persons with disabilities, or administer public health, health insurance, and others; (2) a transaction is taking place; (3) the expenditure is benefiting a resident in a country; and (4) the provider of health care has some formally recognized medical qualification. *Accordingly, most spending on social determinants of health and indirect expenditures are excluded from NHA.*

Table 13.6 Classification of health care functions (first-digit level) and curative care classification (second- and third-digit levels) with example from Sri Lanka NHA 2013

Classification at the first-digit level	Curative care classification (second- and third-digit levels)	Sri Lanka – curative care expenditure	
		Million LKR*	CHE %*
HC.1 Curative care	HC.1 – Curative care	237,532.52	91
HC.2 Rehabilitative care	HC.1.1 – Inpatient curative care	145,433.25	55.9
HC.3 Long-term care (health)	HC.1.1.1 – General inpatient curative care	10,415.26	4.0
HC.4 Ancillary services (nonspecified by function)	HC.1.1.2 – Specialized inpatient curative care	135,017.99	51.9
HC.5 Medical goods (nonspecified by function)	HC.1.2 – Day curative care	–	–
HC.6 Preventive care	HC.1.2.1 – General day curative care	–	–
HC.7 Governance and health system and financing administration	HC.1.2.2 – Specialized day curative care		
HC.9 Other health care services not elsewhere classified (n.e.c.)[4]	HC.1.3 – Outpatient curative care	84,615.95	32.5
Memorandum items: reporting items	HC.1.3.1 – General outpatient curative care	48,841.50	18.8
HC.RI.1 Total pharmaceutical expenditure	HC.1.3.2 – Dental outpatient curative care	–	–
HC.RI.2 Traditional complementary alternative medicines	HC.1.3.3 – Specialized outpatient curative care	11,692.49	4.5
HC.RI.3 Prevention and public health services (according to SHA 1.0)	HC.1.4 – Home-based curative care	–	–
Memorandum items: health care related			
HCR.1 Long-term care (social)			
HCR.2 Health promotion with a multisectoral approach			

CHE %, percentage of current health expenditure; LKR, Sri Lankan rupee (130 LKR = 1 USD [2013]). *Source:* [28].

---

[4] The classification ends at HC.7; HC.9 is for services not classified elsewhere.

National health accounts examine the *financial health* of the health system and are an appealing tool for policymakers interested in assessing health care financing, the impact of health reforms, or health system performance. Concretely, NHA helps answer questions such as:

- Who pays for health services at the national and subnational levels and what is their respective share of total health spending?
- Who manages the health-related budgets and their relative size in the overall health system?
- Who provides health care and what is their respective market share?
- What services are being provided and how much do they cost to the overall health system?
- Who uses health care and how much do they benefit from the overall health system?

System of Health Accounts 2011: Methods and Tools

The above questions are answered using a standardized set of tables that allow estimation of key macro- and micro-level indicators based on a standardized methodology that proposes nine classifications (Figure 13.7) and six cross-tables (Table 13.7) as the core for building a cohesive system of health accounts. These tables are important for policymakers and managers to comprehend and interpret, though their construction requires a team of expert accountants and economists. Each table links two classifications, describing a specific financial flow. The classifications are identified to be exhaustive, mutually exclusive, complete, consistent, policy relevant, and compatible with other related systems.

In addition, a set of "memorandum items" are estimated as aggregates of other expenditures, from within or outside the boundaries of the health accounting system. When all the aggregated amounts comply with the definition of health expenditure – that is, fall within the boundaries of what constitutes a health expenditure, often described as "above the line" – the memorandum item is referred to as a "reporting item"; this includes things such as total expenditure on pharmaceuticals. If one or more of the aggregated items fall outside the boundaries of a health expenditure, the memorandum item is referred to as a "related item"; this might be the social part of long-term care or areas involving cross-sectoral health promotion. It is worth noting that while research and development and education and

Table 13.7 The six basic tables of NHA analysis

1. Health expenditure by type of financing scheme and by function (HCxHF).
2. Health expenditure by type of provider and by function (HCxHP).
3. Health expenditure by financing scheme and by type of provider (HPxHF).
4. Types of revenues by revenues of the financing scheme (HFxFS).
5. Health expenditure by financing agent and by financing scheme (HFxFA).
6. Factors of provision by type of provider (HPxFP), by type of function (HCxFP), and by financing scheme (HFxFP).

HC, functions; HP, providers; HF, financing schemes: FA, financing agents; FS, revenues of financing scheme; FP, factors of provision.
Source: [29].

Table 13.8 Selected indicators available from NHA analysis

General	Providers
Total current health expenditure (CHE)	Hospital health spending
Total CHE plus capital spending	Ambulatory health spending
Health functions	Externally funded expenditure on health
Preventive spending	Privately funded expenditure on health
Curative spending	Beneficiaries
Inpatient spending	Expenditure on health on NCDs
Outpatient spending	Expenditure on health on injuries
Financing schemes	Expenditure on health age 65 and over
Government health schemes	Capital formation
Compulsory contributory health insurance schemes	Total public spending on capital formation
Voluntary health insurance schemes	Total private spending on capital formation
Out-of-pocket expenditure on health	Spending on capital formation by hospitals

Source: [29].

training, are key to ensuring effective delivery of the needed care, they mostly fall outside the boundaries of the system of health accounts and are hence classified as "related items." Structurally, NHA builds on a health system's revenues, schemes, providers, and functions.

The SHA 2011 [30] provides detailed descriptions of all related classifications and tables, including decision trees to help categorize health spending. There is an accompanying Health Accounts Production Tool [31] and a Health Accounts Analysis Tool [31] that can be used by experts to undertake and institutionalize health accounting exercises. Most countries now use SHA 2011 classifications as the standardized approach for reporting on health expenditure indicators (Table 13.8) as part of the Global Health Expenditure Database (https://apps.who.int/nha/database).

13.2.6 Stakeholder Analysis

Stakeholders are parties who can affect or be affected by an activity. They are parties that have a *stake*, meaning that they stand to gain or lose as a result of a decision or activity. Stakeholders can be individuals, groups, institutions, or communities with common interests.

Stakeholder analysis is an approach to exploring the roles, interests, intentions, behaviors, and interrelations of actors (individuals or organizations), to understand the resources and influence they bring to implementation processes and decision-making. It is used in research, management, planning and decision-making for planning, policy analysis, and program implementation.

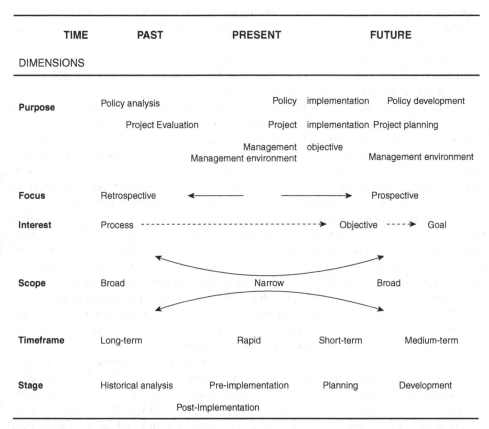

Figure 13.8 Time focus (past, present, or future) by key dimensions to be considered in a stakeholder analysis. Adapted from [32].

Identifying the purpose of stakeholder analysis helps to outline its scope and time dimension (Figure 13.8) [32]. Its scope can be broad in the policy domain, *retrospectively* assessing the engagement and perception of stakeholders as the policy evolves in terms of its context, content, and processes for a policy such as one on mental health; and for delineating a roadmap for future directions. Stakeholder analysis follows a *prospective* timeframe in program planning, implementation, and decision-making by engaging stakeholders, drawing out their interests, understanding relationships, identifying conflicts of interest, and building alliances for enhanced collaboration. It is essential to relate the analysis with the stage of design or implementation of the initiative. The focus can be *narrow* if analysis is conducted to aid the implementation of a specific policy/project as part of a political mapping process, or *broad* in policy development and strategic planning.

Conducting Stakeholder Analysis

Stakeholder analysis is initiated by defining the elements of a policy issue or program under consideration and mapping relevant actors in relation to each element and to one another by experienced analysts. This can involve brainstorming with policymakers, reviewing existing information about the issue, consulting experts in the field, and identifying potential stakeholders by snowballing. Stakeholder identification can be straightforward when the context is stable and the issues are circumscribed. It can also be a complex and complicated process when the issues are multifaceted and involve local and international actors. Stakeholders can usually be identified from the public sector (Ministries of Health, finance, planning), unions and associations of health workers, for-profit private sector, nongovernmental organizations, academia, media, development partners, civil society, and communities.

The next step is to collect data regarding stakeholder involvement, knowledge, and interests in relation to the policy in question: ascertain their position for or against the issue (supporters, neutral, or opponents); gauge their power to influence the issue; and determine their potential alliances with other stakeholders, their resourcefulness, and the best approaches to engage them. This can be done through in-person interviews or self-administered questionnaires. Additional information can also be gathered by scrutinizing newspapers, social media, institutional reports, speeches, and political platforms.

To avoid individual bias, data is best organized and analyzed by a team. Literature offers many models of charts, matrices, network maps, position maps, and other illustrations to present data [33–35]. The stakeholders can also be classified according to their power and interest in the issue (Figure 13.9) [36]. This prioritization grid is particularly useful when the analysis is carried out to guide decision-making related to policy or program implementation. Strong coalitions need to be built with stakeholders having high interest and influence over the policy or program to summon their support. People or organizations with high influence but little interest also warrant attention to seek their resources. Strategies need to be devised for those having strong opposition but high influence.

Stakeholder analysis has been used as a research tool to help understand how policies have been formulated in the past and to guide future policy directions. It has been utilized as a management and strategic tool for crafting optimal strategies to manage other stakeholders, build meaningful alliances, identify opportunities and threats and the means to handle them, to facilitate the implementation of programs and policies, and to achieve organizational objectives. The findings of the analysis can inform strategic planning, policy analyses, organizational assessment, development of coalitions and action plans, and can

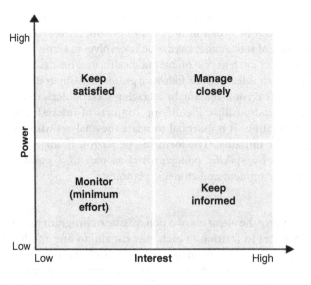

Figure 13.9 Power–interest grid for stakeholder prioritization. Adapted from [36].

guide participatory consensus-building. Stakeholder analysis, if carried out at the planning stage, can be critical for, though is not a guarantee of, success during implementation.

Nonetheless, stakeholder analysis has its limitations. The power, associations, influence, and interests of stakeholders change over time, impacting the reliability of results, especially over time. The context of policymaking also evolves; one actor changing position can change the position of others. Stakeholders' views can be influenced by the *Hawthorne effect* [37], where the individuals tend to alter their opinions and behaviors in response to their awareness of being observed. These uncertainties and inherent biases necessitate a cautious approach in using stakeholder analysis as a decision-making tool and in interpreting its results.

13.3 Conclusion

With the recent COVID-19 pandemic, health policymakers are now increasingly expected to use research evidence in making informed decisions. The tools described in this chapter are available to aid the process and to adopt a more rigorous, rational, and systematic approach while making decisions that impact population health. The list of described tools is not exhaustive, and additional tools can be explored to respond to the context and nature of public health concern.

References

1. S. Glazer, T. Karpati. The role of culture in decision making. *Cut IT J* 2014; 27(9): 23–29.

2. R. Gaitonde, A. D. Oxman, P. O. Okebukola, et al. Interventions to reduce corruption in the health sector (Review). *Cochrane Database Syst Rev* 2016; 8: CD008856.

3. C. J. Murray, A. D. Lopez; World Health Organization. The global burden of disease: a comprehensive assessment of mortality and disability from diseases, injuries, and risk factors in 1990 and projected to 2020: summary. 1996. https://apps.who.int/iris/handle/10665/41864 (accessed November 11, 2020).

4. World Health Organization. Disability-adjusted life years (DALYs). 2022. www.who.int/data/gho/indicator-metadata-registry/imr-details/158 (accessed January 9, 2022).

5. Global Burden of Disease Collaborative Network. Global burden of disease study 2019 (GBD 2019): life expectancy and healthy life expectancy 1990–2019. 2020. https://doi.org/10.6069/5R23-RQ49 (accessed June 17, 2021).

6. Public Health England. The burden of disease and what it means in England. https://publichealthmatters.blog.gov.uk/2015/09/15/the-burden-of-disease-and-what-it-means-in-england/ (accessed March 19, 2021).

7. World Health Organization. Burden of disease concepts, introduction and methods: assessing the environmental burden of disease at national and local levels. 2003. www.who.int/quantifying_ehimpacts/publications/9241546204/en/ (accessed December 11, 2020).

8. IHME. Measuring what matters: global burden of disease (GBD). 2020. www.healthdata.org/gbd/2019 (accessed October 25, 2021).

9. International Network of Agencies for Health Technology Assessment (INAHTA). Homepage. www.inahta.org/HTA (accessed March 19, 2021).

10. M. F. Drummond, J. S. Schwartz, B. Jönsson, et al. Key principles for the improved conduct of health technology assessments for resource allocation decisions. *Int J Technol Assess Health Care* 2008; 24(3): 244.

11. L. Prieto, J. A. Sacristán. Problems and solutions in calculating quality-adjusted life years (QALYs). *Health Qual Life Outcomes* 2003; 1: 80.

12. NICE Clinical Guidelines. Cost-effectiveness of IVT versus ORT for children with dehydration. 2009. www.ncbi.nlm.nih.gov/books/NBK63840/ (accessed March 19, 2021).

13. M. Fleurbaey, E. Schokkaert. Equity in health and health care. In A. J. Culyer, J. Newhouse, eds., *Handbook of Health Economics*. Amsterdam, Elsevier, 2011, vol. 2, pp. 1003–1092.

14. P. Braveman, S. Gruskin. Defining equity in health. *J Epidemiol Community Health* 2003; **57**(4): 254–258.

15. M. Fleurbaey, E. Schokkaert. Unfair inequalities in health and health care. *J Health Econ* 2009; **28**(1): 73–90.

16. Daisy. Equality and equity. 2019. https://social-change.co.uk/blog/2019-03-29-equality-and-equity#:~:text=Although%20both%20promote%20fairness%2C%20equality,people%20differently%20dependent%20on%20need.&text=Referring%20back%20to%20the%20student,the%20same%20level%20of%20support (accessed March 19, 2021).

17. Interaction Institute for Social Change. Illustrating equality vs. equity. 2016. https://interactioninstitute.org/illustrating-equality-vs-equity/ (accessed March 19, 2021).

18. CAWI. Advancing equity and inclusion a guide for municipalities. 2015. www.cawi-ivtf.org/sites/default/files/publications/advancing-equity-inclusion-web_0.pdf (accessed October 25, 2021).

19. E. Regidor. Measures of health inequalities: part 1. *J Epidemiol Community Health* 2004; **58**(10): 858.

20. Scottish Public Health Observatory. Measuring health inequalities. 2021. www.scotpho.org.uk/comparative-health/measuring-inequalities (accessed October 25, 2021).

21. Y. Tao, K. Henry, Q. Zou, et al. Methods for measuring horizontal equity in health resource allocation: a comparative study. *Health Econ Rev* 2014; **4**(1): 10.

22. O. Alonge, D. H. Peters. Utility and limitations of measures of health inequities: a theoretical perspective. *Glob Health Action* 2015; **8**(1): 27591.

23. M. Abu-Zaineh, R. H. Abul Naga. Bread and social justice: measurement of social welfare and inequality using anthropometrics. *Rev Income Wealth* 2021. doi-org.lama.univ-amu.fr/10.1111/roiw.12545.

24. M. Abu-Zaineh, R. H. Naga. Wealth, health, and the measurement of multidimensional inequality: evidence from the Middle East and North Africa. In *Health and Inequality*. Bingley, Emerald Group Publishing, pp. 421–439.

25. World Bank. Concentration curves. 2007. www.worldbank.org/content/dam/Worldbank/document/HDN/Health/HealthEquityCh7.pdf (accessed June 18, 2021).

26. World Health Organization. Health accounts. www.who.int/health-topics/health-accounts/#tab=tab_1 (accessed July 11, 2021).

27. OECD. A system of health accounts 2011. 2011. www.oecd.org/publications/a-system-of-health-accounts-2011-9789264270985-en.htm (accessed July 15, 2021).

28. Ministry of Health, Nutrition and Indigenous Medicine. Sri Lanka national health accounts 2013. 2016. www.health.gov.lk/moh_final/english/public/elfinder/files/publications/NHA/Sri%20Lanka%20National%20Health%20Accounts%202013.pdf (accessed June 17, 2021).

29. OECD. A system of health accounts 2011. 2017. www.oecd.org/publications/a-system-of-health-accounts-2011-9789264270985-en.htm (accessed October 25, 2021).

30. OECD, Eurostat, WHO. A system of health accounts 2011 edition. 2011. www.who.int/health-accounts/methodology/sha2011.pdf (accessed July 13, 2021).

31. World Health Organization. NHA production tool. User Guide, Version 1.0. www.who.int/health-accounts/tools/NHAPT_User_Guide_2.5.12.pdf (accessed July 14, 2021).

32. Z. Varvasovszky, R. Brugha. A stakeholder analysis. *Health Policy Plan* 2000; **15**(3): 338–345.

33. J. D. Blair, M. D. Fottler, C. J. Whitehead. Diagnosing the stakeholder bottom line for medical group practices: key stakeholders' potential to threaten and/or cooperate. *Med Group Manage J* 1996; **43** (2): 40–42.

34. K. Schmeer. Stakeholder analysis guidelines: policy toolkit for strengthening health sector reform. 2000. www.paho .org/hq/dmdocuments/2010/47-Policy_Toolkit_Strengthening_HSR.pdf (accessed December 11, 2020).

35. M. Reich. *Political Mapping of Health Policy: A Guide for Managing the Political Dimension of Health Policy.* Boston, MA, Harvard School of Public Health, 1994.

36. A. L. Mendelow. Environmental scanning: the impact of the stakeholder concept. 1981. http://aisel.aisnet.org/icis1981/20 (accessed February 7, 2022).

37. K. Cherry. The Hawthorne effect and behavioral studies. 2020. www .verywellmind.com/what-is-the-hawthorne-effect-2795234 (accessed October 23, 2021).

Health Policy and Systems Research: The Role of Implementation Research

David H. Peters and Olakunle Alonge

Key Messages

- Implementation research offers a way to understand and address implementation challenges and contribute to building stronger health systems within specific and changing contexts.
- Implementation research is used to assess how and why interventions work, including the feasibility, adoption, and acceptance of interventions and their coverage, quality, equity, efficiency, scale, and sustainability.
- A well-designed research question is critical to successful implementation research, provides the basis for choosing the research methods, and impacts the likelihood that research outcomes will influence policy and practice.
- The theories, approaches, and tools of implementation research are well suited to addressing the mandate for universal health coverage and the Sustainable Development Goals to address interdependent problems to improve people's wellbeing.

14.1 Introduction

Every health system around the world – whether at community, national, or international level – needs information and evidence to achieve its goals. Information and evidence are also critical drivers for continuous adaptation, innovation, improvement, and sustainability of health systems. Research plays many critical roles in society, with health policy and systems research (HPSR) playing a particular role: to inform and influence health systems so they are better able to pursue health goals [1]. Many challenges remain for health systems, particularly in low- and middle-income countries (L&MICs), which face greater economic constraints in a wide variety of social, institutional, and political contexts. Although L&MICs have benefited from many lower-cost health technologies (e.g., medicines, vaccines, and diagnostics), learning how to deliver health goods and services to those who need them (e.g., changing provider behavior, adapting program logistics or financing), how to change people's demand for health products, services or their health-related behaviors (e.g., diet, smoking), or how to address the underlying structural determinants that undermine people's health (e.g., poverty, discrimination, educational opportunities, lack of accountability) requires both adoption of appropriate policies and an ability to problem-solve during implementation.

Every health system faces problems with implementation – that is, how to carry out interventions (i.e., policies, programs, health practices, and technologies) in ways that improve people's health, reduce health impoverishment, and provide equitable, efficient, transparent, and sustainable opportunities and processes for all in society. Experience shows that problems with the implementation of interventions in health systems are widespread [2]. Studying these problems to improve implementation is what implementation research is all about.

The SDGs reflect a change in how people understand health and human development. It is a paradigm that moves away from a siloed approach to building up core sectors in a country, such as the health sector, to one that seeks convergence across sectors that influence and depend on each other. The SDG approach should influence the choice of implementation research topics and how implementation research is conducted, particularly to address underlying issues that extend beyond the traditional boundaries of the health care system, and to be more engaged with wider sets of stakeholders. Issues related to inequity and social justice are at the core of such problems, but also how to address interconnected problems around environmental degradation, conflict, urbanization, population movements, access to technology, and expectations around political participation and public institutions. Implementation research provides a set of theories, approaches, and tools that are well suited to addressing these complex and changing conditions.

14.1.1 Conceptual Clarification

Implementation research can be conceptualized as a type of HPSR that is organized around tackling problems of implementation within defined health systems, and has overlapping and complementary concerns with other types of research, as well as with policy and implementation processes. Until recently, much of the research in global health was focused on developing interventions and then demonstrating that they are efficacious and safe in controlled settings, or on how cost-effective they can be in the particular field situations (Figure 14.1). Implementation research shifts attention to focusing on understanding the real-world contexts in which the implementation of interventions occurs, the role of key stakeholders, the complex interactions and strategies involved in the implementation

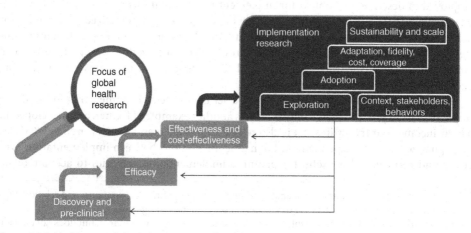

Figure 14.1 Health research from discovery to implementation. Adapted from [3].

process, and the outcome of these processes (adaptation, fidelity, costs, coverage, sustainability, and scale).

Implementation research is neither defined nor constrained by a single set of disciplinary theories and methods, but around the application of relevant theories and research methods toward the common denominator of implementation problems. Although it is an emerging area of study in the health sciences fields, implementation research has a history in multiple research traditions based in different disciplines that started outside the health sciences, but are all applicable to health issues (Table 14.1). Each tradition has focused on different types of research questions and audiences, and used different methodologies and languages, adding richness and multiple perspectives to the field of implementation studies [4, 5]. This has also resulted in a wide variety of definitions and terms [5, 6]. Although particular groups who practice and fund implementation research have continued to follow their disciplinary origins, there is also a growing convergence around a broader and more inclusive view of implementation research that includes the full range of research traditions and has some common characteristics and language (Table 14.2).

14.2 Implementation Frameworks and Theories

Theories and frameworks[1] are helpful to understand implementation problems and outcomes, identify variables that can be studied, and guide and evaluate implementation processes [8]. Over the years implementation research has acquired a sound theoretical basis that provides better *a priori* understanding of the associated enablers and barriers that determine the success of interventions. Given that implementation research is not constrained by a single set of disciplinary theories and methods, diverse theories and frameworks have been employed to understand implementation problems (Table 14.3).

In most health systems, implementation problems arise from the context or from complex interactions between the context and interventions. Hence, theories and frameworks that help to understand context, and how interventions may be adapted, or strategies developed to address facilitators and barriers, are particularly relevant to conducting implementation research conceptualized as HPSR. The consolidated framework on implementation research (CFIR) [19] is an example of such frameworks, and has been widely employed to describe the context for implementing interventions more completely within health systems. The CFIR identifies concepts that can be operationalized as variables for conducting implementation research and studying the intervention, implementation process, outer setting (e.g., sociopolitical environment), inner setting (e.g., organizational culture of the implementing agencies), and the individuals within those implementing agencies.

The active implementation frameworks, a set of interrelated frameworks for studying implementation processes and context [14], is another example of frameworks developed in a high-income country setting that is also relevant for implementation research in L&MICs. It emphasizes the interdependent and dynamic interactions between implementation processes and context and is useful for planning implementation activities to accommodate

---

[1] Nilsen [8] defines a theory as a set of analytical principles (e.g., variables, domains, and relationships between variables) designed to structure observation, understanding, and explanation, whereas a framework is a structure of descriptive categories and relations between them, but does not provide explanations. There is much overlap between theories and frameworks.

Table 14.1 Implementation research traditions, audiences, research questions, and core disciplines

Implementation research tradition (and related names)	Typical primary audience for research	Typical research questions	Disciplinary origins
Management improvement (performance management; quality improvement; continuous quality improvement; total quality management)	Managers and teams using improvement strategies	How are the right services delivered to the right clients while meeting the right standards for quality?	Engineering, management
Operational research (operations research; decision science; management science)	Executive decision-makers (executive bodies, policymakers)	Which solution provides the most rational basis for a decision concerning the optimal performance of a system?	Mathematics, engineering, management
Policy implementation research	Top-down: central-level policymakers Bottom-up: "street-level" program implementers	Top-down: How was a policy/program implemented, and what contributed to its outcomes? Bottom-up: Which actors are involved in program delivery in specific locations, how do they understand the problem of implementation, and what influences their behavior?	Political science, public policy, public administration
Program evaluation (formative evaluation; needs assessment; process evaluation; outcome/effectiveness/summative evaluation; impact evaluation)	Stakeholders of a program (e.g., funders, implementers, and/or intended beneficiary)	Is the program producing intended effects? How is it designed, implemented, used, fit to context and problems, with what results and program changes?	Sociology, public policy, economics, social work, psychology
Dissemination and implementation of evidence-based medicine (implementation science; knowledge translation)	Practitioners, health organization managers, policymakers not using evidence-based interventions	What promotes the integration of research findings and evidence on interventions into health care practice?	Behavior change (psychology, sociology, education), epidemiology
Participatory action research (action research)	Research participants, community members	How can we (community members as research participants) learn and be empowered to take action?	Nondisciplinary or transdisciplinary, but largely influenced by social psychology, education, and anthropology

Adapted from [7].

Table 14.2 The defining characteristics of implementation research applied in L&MICs

Characteristic	Description	Implications
Context-specific	The details of context are made explicit, alongside level of analysis and action, e.g., community, district, national.	Focus on what can be learned and acted on in a particular setting, and the role that the setting plays in implementation. Often this requires specifying the health and equity issues for different population groups, the role of key stakeholders in the health system, and the location where the health intervention occurs.
Purpose: relevant and agenda setting	Identify and address challenges related to any implementation decisions or processes at any level.	There is a need to identify relevant health problems, and involve those with a stake in the problem and influence over decisions (e.g., communities, providers, policymakers).
Methods fit for purpose	Research design responsive to an implementation problem or question; typically a range of data sources and methods are used as appropriate for the implementation questions, decision context, and community or patient characteristics, being sensitive to gender and other social stratifiers.	Ensure the ways to collect and analyze data will answer the prioritized research question (see Table 14.5) and how it will be used, and does not simply represent what the researcher can do.
Demand-driven	Research questions are framed or based on needs identified by implementers, intended beneficiaries, and/or policymakers and research consumers in the health system.	Ensure that one or more key stakeholders in the health system (e.g., community organizations, health providers, Ministry of Health) are able to identify the priority and use of the research.
Multistakeholder and multidisciplinary	Implementers, policymakers, and researchers (and often also communities, including the most marginalized) are involved in co-producing the research, co-creating solutions, and using the results together, drawing on multiple disciplines.	Try to involve a range of key stakeholders (e.g., community organizations, health providers, Ministry of Health) in the oversight or conduct of the research, and employ researchers who are able to use different methods and perspectives to address a health problem.
Real world	Not usually under controlled trial conditions, and usually working within the reality of implementing organizations, communities, and financing systems, and within the context of health systems that are changing and adaptive.	Try to use routine management systems and usual level of resources to implement the "solution," and where possible take advantage of existing data sources.
Real time	Implementation research is designed to provide evidence or solutions through short feedback loops that can be used for real-time improvements and course corrections.	Make sure that the research is conducted in a timely way, so that the results can support relevant decision-making opportunities. Some research will need to be short term to make quick improvements, but some research questions will require a longer timeframe to get the type of evidence that is needed.
Focuses on processes as well as outcomes/impacts	Implementation research is focused on processes and engages implementers, documenting how interventions are implemented and delivered to assess acceptability, fidelity, adoption, scale-up, and impact. Tacit knowledge is used and acknowledged.	Make sure the research has a framework that involves those who are implementing health interventions and that it makes sense to them, so that they can see the causes and consequences of the intervention.

Source: [4]

Table 14.3 Examples of theories and frameworks used in implementation research

Category	Description	Examples particularly relevant for L&MICs
Process models	Process models identify or describe steps in the process of translating research into practice, including the implementation and use of research. An action model is a type of process model that provides practical guidance of activities.	The CIHR model of knowledge translation (CIHR), active implementation frameworks – implementation stages [9], the Ottawa model [10, 11]
Determinant frameworks	Determinant frameworks specify factors which act as facilitators and barriers that influence implementation outcomes (dependent variables). These factors may be grouped into classes or domains or by socioecological levels (e.g., individual, organizational, community, external policy environment).	PARIHS [12, 13], active implementation frameworks [14, 15], understanding-user-context framework [16], framework by Grol et al.[17], ecological framework by Durlak and DuPre [18], CFIR [19], theoretical domains framework [20]
Classical/implementation theories	Classical/implementation theories are theories that originate from fields external to implementation science, e.g., psychology, sociology, and organizational theory, or are developed by implementation researchers, and which can be applied to provide understanding and/or explanation of aspects of implementation.	Theory of diffusion [21], social network theories [22], social capital theories, communities of practice [23], organizational readiness [24], normalization process theory [25]
Evaluation frameworks	Evaluation frameworks describe aspects and pathways of implementation that could be evaluated to determine implementation success.	RE-AIM [26]; PRECEDE-PROCEED [27]; framework by Proctor et al. [28]

Adapted from [8].

these interactions. It specifies frameworks for organizing stage-appropriate implementation activities, and infrastructure and supports needed to sustain these activities in a defined context. These supports include creating implementation teams, facilitating policy–practice feedback, and identifying strategies that address key contextual barriers.

Although theories and frameworks may be used to study any aspect of implementation, the CFIR and active implementation frameworks are highlighted here as examples of frameworks relevant for studying contexts as part of implementation research. While both frameworks have been applied in different L&MICs to varying degrees, there is still opportunity to further adapt them to different settings and to generate new theories and frameworks for understanding implementation in L&MICs.

14.3 Definition of Essential Terms

14.3.1 Implementation Variables

Implementation research is about the "how to" of implementation, including issues around feasibility, adoption, acceptance, the degree to which interventions are delivered as designed (fidelity), or how they are adapted in response to local conditions and new information. Implementation research also attempts to answer questions around quality, equity, efficiency, scale, sustainability, and ensuring coverage to all, even the marginalized, with the ultimate goal of strengthening health systems to improve health outcomes. These characteristics are described as implementation variables and are typically the focus of implementation research (Table 14.4).

14.3.2 Evidence-Based Interventions and Implementation Strategies

Ideally, every intervention (e.g., policy, program, practice, or technology) in a health system should be grounded in evidence. The tradition of "evidence-based medicine" focuses on providing guidance based on the strength of evidence that a medicine, technology, or practice is sufficiently effective. This is based on assessments that are driven by a hierarchy of research designs that emphasize experimental approaches, statistical comparison, and internal validity [29]. The field of clinical epidemiology has developed a range of guidelines and tools to promote and assess such evidence and to guide the development of evidence, such as the GRADE framework [30] or Cochrane collaboration [31]. When more broadly applied in public health or other social, behavioral, and educational fields, an evidence-based intervention (EBI) is one that is informed by the explicit use of scientific research and evaluation to demonstrate that the intervention produces the desired outcomes [32]. But often evidence that is produced in one setting does not have the same result in another setting. This may occur because the population involved is not the same, the intervention is not identical, or because there are other contextual factors that influence whether an intervention will produce the same outcome. Implementation research is often needed to unpack these differences in contexts and populations, paying particular attention to how interventions are implemented.

The more complex the intervention, such as when they have multiple components, the more difficult it is to replicate and obtain consistent results across settings. It is often helpful to try to identify the core element(s) of an intervention that should be replicated with fidelity, in contrast to those elements that may need to be adapted to fit a particular context, population, or individual. Although somewhat arbitrary, it is often useful to distinguish core

Table 14.4 Definitions of implementation variables

Implementation variable	Definition
Acceptability	The perception among stakeholders (e.g., consumers, providers, managers, policymakers) that an intervention is agreeable
Appropriateness	The perceived fit or relevance of the intervention in a particular setting or for a particular target audience (e.g., provider or consumer) or issue
Adoption	The intention, initial decision, or action to try to employ a new intervention
Feasibility	The extent to which an intervention can be carried out in a particular setting or organization
Fidelity	The degree to which an intervention was implemented as it was designed in an original protocol, plan, or policy
Adaptation	The degree to which an intervention is modified in the process of implementation, often in response to the needs of a population or new information
Implementation cost	The incremental (or total) cost of the implementation strategy (e.g., how the services are delivered in a particular setting)
Coverage	The degree to which the population that is eligible to benefit from an intervention actually receives it
Sustainability	The extent to which an intervention is maintained or institutionalized in a given setting

Adapted from [7].

EBIs, traditionally understood as "evidence-based practice," from "implementation strategies." Both are informed by evidence, but the core EBIs are expected to be strictly replicable or have very little variation across settings. They may also be considered as the core ingredient of a complex intervention that should not change. Typically, these types of EBIs consistently lead to a given health outcome (at least with a reliable probability), and do not substantially depend on other intervenable steps to achieve their intended effects. Nonetheless, one would still expect some variation in outcomes even with a completely identical intervention, just as the same dosage of a given medicine may have a range of results in different patients. Medicines, vaccines, and diagnostic tests are types of EBIs that best fit the characteristics of core EBIs. They are expected to have more predictable effects despite slight variation, and often do not differ greatly when studied in similar populations. Implementation strategies, on the other hand, are interventions designed to support how EBIs can work. They present a greater degree of variation, and may need to be modified to fit local contexts and populations. Interventions such as patient educational materials, digital reminders, health provider job aids, community engagement strategies, or continuous quality improvement practices in an organization are examples of implementation strategies. Techniques such as intervention mapping approaches are helpful to assess the fit of

EBIs and implementation strategies with the population needs, health problem, and the organizational capacity, and to plan for adaptations, evaluation, and learning [29].

14.4 The Central Role of the Research Question

Implementation research often begins with an implementation problem that prompts a research process to develop a solid understanding of how filling a knowledge gap will help address that problem. An early step in that process involves translating the problem into a research question (or questions) that can inform the selection of an appropriate scientific method of inquiry. The development of a research question can be done by researchers themselves, or by engaging with key stakeholders, such as those who "own" the problem or are affected by it. Even when a research team develops the question, it is important to involve other stakeholders to ensure they are asking the right questions, and to frame the research in a way that the results can be interpreted and used. The PO-PICO formulation describes a structured way to develop good implementation research questions by systematically answering questions about the problem, objectives, people, implementation, comparisons, and outcomes (Box 14.1). There are other similar formulations to the PO-PICO that add additional dimensions, (e.g., environment and stakeholders' perspectives) to systematically structure complex implementation research questions [13].

Using the answers to the questions in the PO-PICO guidance, the next step is to draft a simple and clear research question. Usually, two short sentences are sufficient. If drafting this as an individual or research team, it may help to also write why this question is important to the researcher personally, whom it affects, and how the researcher hopes the research will make a positive change for the people identified. It is also useful to think about how other people will read the question. These include policymakers, other researchers, and people who make decisions about what research to fund or publish and who needs to understand how your question could be turned into a study. A structured way of assessing

---

Box 14.1 Developing the Research Question: PO-PICO

PO-PICO is a mnemonic that can be used to create a good research question by addressing the following issues.

Problem: What is the implementation problem you would like to study? Who has defined the problem (e.g., policymaker, implementer, intended beneficiary, researcher)? Will the research results be relevant to them? Is it considered an important problem?

Objective: What is the purpose of your study – What knowledge gap will you fill? Will it provide information that is not already known?

People: Who are the people (or population) you are to study? Are they people affected by the problem? Are they people at risk or otherwise vulnerable? Are they those who are providing services?

Implementation: What is the implementation strategy you are interested in?

Comparisons: What comparisons do you want to make? Differences in the implementation strategies? For different people? At different places or times?

Outcome: What outcome measure(s) are you interested in (e.g., implementation outcomes, benefits, harms)? Will those who define the problem be able to make an informed choice based on the outcomes and comparisons?

Box 14.2 A Checklist for Relevance of Implementation Research Questions

- Is the research question relevant to the primary audience of the research?
- Is there potential for application of results?
- Is it timely to the needs of the decision-maker, and when decisions need to be made?
- Is the research ethically acceptable?
- Is the research itself acceptable (to policymakers, implementers, beneficiaries)?
- Is the research feasible, given the time, financial, and personnel constraints?

Adapted from [33].

whether your research question will serve its intended purpose in terms of actionable change is shown in Box 14.2.

14.4.1 Engaging Stakeholders in Co-creating Research Design

There are a number of ways for researchers to engage with policymakers to enhance the implementation of their findings. These include deliberative dialogs between researchers and policymakers [34], implementer-led research [35], or other research processes embedded within an organization. For example, research can be embedded in Ministries of Health through institutional processes or by assigning formal roles to researchers within the ministry to facilitate productive and ongoing exchanges between researchers, policymakers, and other stakeholders toward the development and implementation of evidence-informed strategies [36]. Specific events can also be organized to serve this purpose. In Kenya, for example, a symposium was held to bring together policymakers, implementing organizations, researchers, and funding groups to identify and prioritize implementation research that could improve noncommunicable disease policies [37]. Regardless of the process used to generate the implementation research question, it is useful to validate the theory underlying how the intervention is expected to work in consultation with stakeholder groups. These processes should provide a systematic approach to assess the problem that is being addressed by the research question across the range of possible implementation concerns about barriers and facilitators, and implementation variables [33].

14.4.2 What Methods Should You Use?

Once you have a well-defined research question, it is important to use research methods that are designed to answer it. No single set of implementation research methods can answer all the possible questions and the full range of qualitative, quantitative, and mixed methods approaches can be used to respond to the problem being studied and the research question in a given context [5]. The more complex the implementation problem or question, the more likely it is that multiple methods or hybrid approaches will be required, or that the research study will need to be conducted in phases. In any case, the choice of methods should fit the purpose, be congruent with the research question and nature of the implementation problem, as well as time and funding constraints, the availability of data, and the concerns of key stakeholders. Table 14.5 summarizes some examples of research questions commonly found in implementation research, and the broad categories of research designs that are most appropriate for them.

Table 14.5 What type of research design is best for the type of question?

Research question	In-depth interviews and focus groups	Surveys	Case–control studies	Cohort studies	RCTs	Pragmatic RCTs	Quasi–experimental studies	Nonexperimental evaluation	Mixed methods & hybrid designs	Systematic reviews
Effectiveness: Does this work? Does doing this work better than doing that?	**			*	**	**	*		**	***
Process of service delivery: How does it work?	*	*						*	**	**
Salience: Does it matter?	**	**							**	**
Safety: Will it do more good than harm?	*		*	*	*	**	*	*	**	***
Acceptability: Will patients want to take up the service offered?	***	*			**	**		*	**	**
Cost-effectiveness: Is it worth buying the service?					**	**			**	**

Research question	In-depth interviews and focus groups	Surveys	Case–control studies	Cohort studies	RCTs	Pragmatic RCTs	Quasi-experimental studies	Nonexperimental evaluation	Mixed methods & hybrid designs	Systematic reviews
Appropriateness: Is this the right service for these clients?					**	**			**	**
Satisfaction: Are users, providers, and other stakeholders satisfied with the service?	**	**	*	*		**			**	*

Stars signify the relevance or appropriateness of the research design to the research question. RCT, randomized controlled trials.
Adapted from [38].

14.5 Challenges and Opportunities

There are many challenges to conducting implementation research in L&MICs [39]. For example, it is a major challenge to conduct research under real-world conditions in most L&MICs. The problems of implementation in such settings often originate from the context, and their implementation during the study. Implementation research requires external resources, management support, and other control measures, which limit the external validity of study findings and the ability to scale-up or sustain the identified solutions once the study ends. As a result, very few implementation research studies have shown how to widely and reliably scale and sustain promising solutions. Moreover, producing large-scale impact implementation research requires multistakeholder collaboration and partnerships across various areas of influence. This can be challenging to accomplish and sustain when negotiating different views, interests, and incentives during a time-limited study. Implementation research studies that involve multiple stakeholders and are successfully carried out under real-world conditions often require significant deviation from the original research protocol. The complexity of the original processes may be difficult to replicate, and results may therefore vary.

These challenges also present opportunities for advancing implementation research in addressing health system challenges in L&MICs [39]. A common thread to these challenges revolves around the issue of how to study complexities (i.e., either to understand the context more completely or to accommodate adaptations to conducting the study under real-world conditions while working with multiple stakeholders). This calls for increased use of implementation variables, adaptive designs that account for changes in context, intervention, and implementation strategies (e.g., mixed methods and hybrid designs), and systems thinking tools and methods in conducting implementation research [39].

In addition to knowledge of the theories and methods that are relevant to implementation research, training and capacity-building activities for researchers and practitioners conducting implementation research in L&MICs should enhance competencies in areas that are not traditionally emphasized in research training, such as stakeholder engagement, communication, and advocacy [39]. Moreover, there is an opportunity to adapt existing research designs and develop new methods to study the critical questions of scale-up and sustainability of health system initiatives in L&MICs.

14.6 Debates

Similar to other fields that involve multiple disciplines, implementation research frequently stimulates debate over research methods and the interpretation of data. This can be valuable as it helps to make assumptions explicit and allows for a fuller understanding of the problems and solutions. The acceptability of trade-offs to address different contexts and multistakeholder interests can also be a subject of debate. Understanding and addressing these trade-offs is particularly important during the design of implementation research as they have the potential to influence the research outcomes (Table 14.6) [4].

The nature of what is to be studied through implementation research is yet another subject of debate [7]. The boundaries of health care delivery are changing as information technologies enable greater self-care and nontraditional care. But the relatively neglected prevention and public health approaches that are needed to promote and maintain good health often require collective action beyond the usual services delivered in clinics, hospitals, and health departments. These include the so-called "common goods for health," which take the form of policies, financing, information, regulatory activities, or population-

Table 14.6 Implementation research trade-offs that influence research design

Generalizable knowledge	Context-specific problem-solving
Methodological rigor	Timeliness and usefulness
Fidelity of intervention implementation	Adaptation of intervention to changes
Internally embedded approaches – "building quality in"	Externally "objective" approaches – "speak truth to power"
Researcher reward through potential application of research	Risk of low academic recognition
Implementer reward through strengthened programs	Risk of exposure through research highlighting poor performance

Adapted from [4].

based services that impact human health and wellbeing, and are either public goods or have large social externalities beyond individual private benefit [40]. Finally, the challenges of the SDGs – to address the complex and interdependent factors that affect human development – will require broadening of stakeholders, data from other relevant sectors, and innovations in analytic methods than are typically involved in research in the health sector. Implementation research provides a set of approaches and tools that can serve to bridge and shape the debates needed to address the SDGs.

References

1. World Health Organization. *World Report on Health Policy and Systems Research.* Geneva, World Health Organization, 2017. www.who.int/alliance-hpsr/resources/publications/worldreport-hpsr/en/ (accessed November 28, 2020).

2. World Bank. Improving health services in developing countries: from evidence to action. 2009. https://openknowledge.worldbank.org/bitstream/handle/10986/12335/48790.pdf?sequence=1&isAllowed=y (accessed September 11, 2020).

3. J. Landsverk, C. H. Brown, P. Chamberlain, et al. Design and analysis in dissemination and implementation research. In R. C. Brownson, G. A. Colditz, E. K. Proctor, eds., *Dissemination and Implementation Research in Health: Translating Science to Practice.* Oxford, Oxford University Press, 2012.

4. S. Theobald, N. Brandes, M. Gyapong, et al. Implementation research: new imperatives and opportunities in global health. *Lancet* 2018; **392**(10160): 2214–2228.

5. World Health Organization. Implementation research in health: a practical guide. 2013. www.who.int/alliance-hpsr/resources/implementationresearchguide/en/ (accessed December 11, 2020).

6. B. A. Rabin, R. C. Brownson, D. Haire-Joshu, et al. A glossary for dissemination and implementation research in health. *J Public Health Manag Pract* 2008; **14**: 117–123.

7. D. H. Peters, T. Adam, O. Alonge, et al. Implementation research: what it is and how to do it. *BMJ* 2013; **347**: f6753.

8. P. Nilsen. Making sense of implementation theories, models and frameworks. *Implement Sci* 2015; **10**(1): 53.

9. Active Implementation Research Network. Implementation stages. 2021. www.activeimplementation.org/frameworks/mplementation-stages/ (accessed September 14, 2020).

10. J. Logan, I. Graham. Toward a comprehensive interdisciplinary model

of health care research use. *Sci Commun* 1998; **20**: 227–246.

11. J. Logan, I. Graham. The Ottawa model of research use. In J. Rycroft-Malone, T. Bucknall, eds., *Models and Frameworks for Implementing Evidence-Based Practice: Linking Evidence to Action*. Oxford, Wiley-Blackwell, 2010.

12. A. L. Kitson, G. Harvey, B. McCormack. Enabling the implementation of evidence-based practice: a conceptual framework. *Qual Health Care* 1998; **7**: 149–158.

13. J. Rycroft-Malone. Promoting action on research implementation in health services (PARIHS). In J. Rycroft-Malone, T. Bucknall, eds., *Models and Frameworks for Implementing Evidence-Based Practice: Linking Evidence to Action*. Oxford, Wiley-Blackwell, 2010.

14. D. L. Fixsen, S. F. Naoom, K. A. Blase, et al. Implementation research: a synthesis of the literature. 2005. http://citeseerx.ist.psu.edu/viewdoc/download;jsessionid=B2848 E493952A6F47A4EBB48A67CB4C5?doi= 10.1.1.610.6226&rep=rep1&type=pdf (accessed June 14, 2020).

15. K. A. Blase, M. Van Dyke, D. L. Fixsen, et al. Implementation science: key concepts, themes and evidence for practitioners in educational psychology. In B. Kelly, D. F. Perkins, eds., *Handbook of Implementation Science for Psychology in Education*. Cambridge, Cambridge University Press, 2012.

16. N. Jacobson, D. Butterill, P. Goering. Development of a framework for knowledge translation: understanding user context. *J Health Serv Res Policy* 2003; **8**: 94–99.

17. R. Grol, M. Wensing, M. Eccles. *Improving Patient Care: The Implementation of Change in Clinical Practice*. Edinburgh, Elsevier, 2005.

18. J. A. Durlak, E. P. DuPre. Implementation matters: a review of research on the influence of implementation on program outcomes and the factors affecting implementation. *Am J Community Psychol* 2008; **41**: 327–350.

19. L. J. Damschroder, D. C. Aron, R. E. Keith, et al. Fostering implementation of health services research findings into practice: a consolidated framework for advancing implementation science. *Implement Sci* 2009; **4**(1): 1–5.

20. L. Atkins, J. Francis, R Islam, et al. A guide to using the theoretical domains framework of behaviour change to investigate implementation problems. *Implement Sci* 2017; **12**(1): 1–8.

21. E. M. Rogers. *Diffusion of Innovations*, 5th ed. New York, Free Press, 2003.

22. C. Kadushin. *Understanding Social Networks: Theories, Concepts, and Findings*. New York, Oxford University Press, 2012.

23. E. Wenger, R. A. McDermott, W. Snyder. *Cultivating Communities of Practice: A Guide to Managing Knowledge*. Cambridge, MA, Harvard Business Press, 2002.

24. B. J. Weiner. A theory of organizational readiness for change. *Implement Sci* 2009; **4**: 67.

25. C. May, T. Finch. Implementing, embedding, and integrating practices: an outline of normalization process theory. *Sociology* 2009; **43**(3): 535–554.

26. R. E. Glasgow, T. M. Vogt, S. M. Boles. Evaluating the public health impact of health promotion interventions: the RE-AIM framework. *Am J Public Health* 1999; **89**: 1322–1327.

27. L. W. Green, M. W. Kreuter. *Health Program Planning: An Educational and Ecological Approach*. New York, McGraw-Hill, 2005.

28. E. Proctor, H. Silmere, R. RaghaVan, et al. Outcomes for implementation research: conceptual distinctions, measurement challenges, and research agenda. *Admin Policy Mental Health* 2011; **38**: 65–76.

29. L. K. Bartholomew, C. M. Markham, R. A. C. Ruiter, et al. *Planning Health Promotion Programs: An Intervention Mapping Approach*, 4th ed. San Francisco, 2016.

30. BMJ Best Practice. What is GRADE? 2020. https://bestpractice.bmj.com/info/us/tool kit/learn-ebm/what-is-grade/ (accessed March 3, 2021).

31. Cochrane Methods. Methodological expectations of Cochrane intervention reviews. 2020. https://methods .cochrane.org/methodological-expectations-cochrane-intervention-reviews (accessed March 19, 2021).

32. L. Rychetnik, P. Hawe, E. Waters, et al. A glossary for evidence based public health. *J Epidemiol Community Health* 2004; **58**(7): 538–545.

33. D. H. Peters, M. A. Peters, K. Wickramasinghe, et al. Asking the right question: implementation research to accelerate national non-communicable disease responses. *BMJ* 2019; **20**(365): l1868.

34. J. A. Boyko, J. N. Lavis, J. Abelson, et al. Deliberative dialogues as a mechanism for knowledge translation and exchange in health systems decision-making. *Soc Sci Med* 2012; **75**: 1938–1945.

35. N. Tran, E. V. Langlois, L. Reveiz, et al. Embedding research to improve program implementation in Latin America and the Caribbean. *Rev Panam Salud Publica* 2017; **41**: e75.

36. A. Ghaffar, E. V. Langlois, K. Rasanathan, et al. Strengthening health systems through embedded research. *Bull World Health Organ* 2017; **95**: 87.

37. S. Subramanian, J. Kibachio, S. Hoover, et al. Research for actionable policies: implementation science priorities to scale up non–communicable disease interventions in Kenya. *J Glob Health* 2017; **7**: 010204.

38. M. Petticrew, H. Roberts. Evidence, hierarchies, and typologies: horses for courses. *J Epidemiol Community Health* 2003; **57**: 527–529.

39. O. Alonge, D. C. Rodriguez, N. Brandes, et al. How is implementation research applied to advance health in low-income and middle-income countries? *BMJ Glob Health* 2019; **4**(2): e001257.

40. A. S. Yazbeck, A. Soucat. When both markets and governments fail health. *Health Syst Reform* 2019; **5**(4): 268–279.

Chapter

15

Universal Health Coverage and Beyond

Health System Interventions and Intersectoral Policies

Ala Alwan, Arian Hatefi, and Dean T. Jamison

Key Messages

- Universal health coverage (UHC) is about bridging the gap between what a health system should be doing and what it does.
- The way countries translate UHC in practice focuses on two questions: (1) what services and policies should be covered and implemented; and (2) what the key challenges are in country implementation capacity that need to be addressed for effective implementation.
- The services and policies to be covered under UHC include both health sector interventions and intersectoral policies. The health sector interventions are distributed across four clusters: age-related, noncommunicable disease and injury, infectious diseases, and health services. The intersectoral interventions and policies fall under four domains: fiscal, regulatory, information and education, and built environment. Both health sector interventions and intersectoral policies were prioritized in the *Disease Control Priorities* third edition (DCP3) packages.
- There are some generalizable themes of how countries can adapt the above packages as they progress toward UHC and the health-related Sustainable Development Goals (SDGs).

15.1 Introduction

Health systems around the world share common goals, but attainment is widely variable. UHC has emerged as a consolidated response to bridge the gap between what a health system should be doing and what it does. This chapter introduces and draws its approach from key sources like the *World Development Report* of 1993 [1], the World Health Organization's *World Health Reports* [2–4], the 2013 Lancet Commission on Investing in Health [5], and the Disease Control Priorities third edition [6]. It explores how countries in practice could translate and achieve UHC, focusing on two central questions: first, what services and policies should be covered and implemented; and second, how can health financing meet the UHC requirements? The chapter then looks at the key challenge of country-level implementation capacity. Finally, it concludes by drawing out generalizable themes of country responses to the UHC SDG target to inform the way forward.

15.1.1 The UHC Concept

Universal health coverage simply means that all people and communities have access to the quality health services they need (spanning health promotion, prevention, treatment, rehabilitation, and palliation) without financial hardship (see Chapter 3). UHC is now an overarching health target of the SDGs that all countries strive to reach by 2030 [7]. SDG target 3.8 aims to "achieve UHC, including financial risk protection, access to quality essential health care services and access to safe, effective, quality and affordable essential medicines and vaccines for all." The Sustainable Development Agenda has thus challenged all countries to achieve UHC by 2030.

Universal health coverage is not a new concept, even though it has gained momentum in recent years. Two of the most important historical milestones for UHC occurred in 1948, when both the constitution of WHO and the Universal Declaration of Human Rights (adopted by the United Nations General Assembly) unequivocally articulated the human right to health [8, 9]. The WHO constitution states that "the enjoyment of the highest attainable standard of health is one of the fundamental rights of every human being without distinction of race, religion, political beliefs, economic and social condition" [10]. The World Health Assembly endorsed the modern concept of UHC as an aspiration for all countries, and subsequent *World Health Reports* expanded on various technical aspects of UHC [4].

More recently, UHC became a priority for heads of state and governments when a high-level meeting on UHC was convened by the UN General Assembly in September 2019 [8]. In the political declaration that emerged from the meeting, heads of state recognized that UHC is fundamental in achieving the SDGs related not only to health and wellbeing but also to eradicating poverty in all its forms, ensuring quality education, and achieving gender equality and women's empowerment. They committed to scaling up their efforts toward the attainment of UHC by 2030 and implementing the most effective, evidence-based, high-impact, and quality-assured interventions to meet the needs of all, and in particular those who are vulnerable or in vulnerable situations.

Primary health care (PHC) is the cornerstone of a sustainable health system for achieving UHC and other health-related SDGs [8]. Accordingly, the Declaration of Alma-Ata in 1978 and that of Astana in 2018 on PHC further underscored the importance of UHC [11, 12].

15.1.2 The Mismatch between UHC Goal and Health System Attainment

Acknowledging the trade-offs forced by scarcity and choice, the aspiration to UHC bridges the gap between what a health system aims to do and what it achieves. The WHO has defined goals, objectives, and means to inform the evolution of health systems in a series of *World Health Reports* [2–4]. Beginning in the *World Health Report 1999*, WHO suggested a core list of goals for health system development likely to elicit broad agreement: improving health status; reducing health inequalities; enhancing responsiveness to legitimate expectations; increasing efficiency; protecting individuals, families, and communities from financial loss; and enhancing fairness in the finance and delivery of health services. *World Health Reports 2000* and *2010* continued the analysis of focusing on the means to achieve these goals. Related efforts explored similar themes [13].

Scarcity of health resources requires decisions on difficult choices – across and within health system goals. The world collectively spends about 10% of its gross domestic product (GDP) on health, yet public funds account for only 60% of the nearly US$8 trillion, with wide variability among countries [14]. All health systems must confront scarcity, but it particularly undermines the ability of low- and middle-income countries (L&MICs) to deliver a modest but essential basket of quality health services to all individuals and communities without imposing the risk of impoverishment. Illustrating this, L&MICs together account for 46% of the global population but only 3.5% of global health spending [15, 16]. High-income countries (HICs) account for about 80% of global health spending, with an average spending of US$2,937 per person in 2017 compared to US$41 in low-income countries (LICs) [16].

In the absence of rational, evidence-informed policies, scarcity results in trade-offs among population, service, and cost coverage – the three axes of UHC (Figure 15.1). In these situations, countries contend with some combination of the exclusion of some vulnerable population groups; limited service availability and access, and/or high out-of-pocket expenditures. Greater than half of the global population does not currently receive all of the essential health services they need [17], while health spending impoverishes about 500 million people and almost 1 billion people spend at least 10% of their household budgets on health care [18]. At the current pace, almost one-third of the global population will continue to be underserved by 2030 [18].

Stemming from and compounding the challenge of scarce financial resources for health is the limited capacity in L&MICs to respond to people's health needs because of major gaps across the health system building blocks – spanning financing, human resources, health information systems, access to essential medicines and health technologies, service delivery, and leadership and governance. Shortcomings beget more shortcomings, limiting access, coverage, quality, and safety. Together, these factors limit health system performance and exacerbate the mismatch between health system goals and attainment.

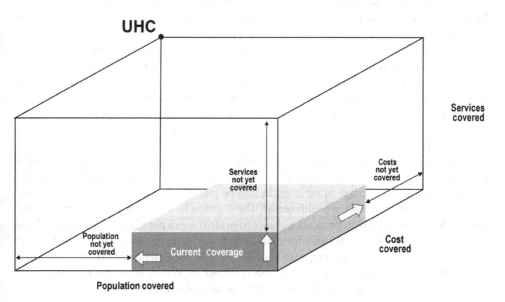

Figure 15.1 The three axes of UHC. Adapted from [5].

In addressing the mismatch, two important questions are raised in countries aiming to achieve UHC: (1) Which health services should be considered for full population access and eventually full cost coverage? (2) How can health planners expand the size or power of pooled funds such that they can achieve UHC? These important questions will be the focus of the remainder of this chapter.

15.2 UHC, Essential Health Services, and Intersectoral Interventions

There are three fundamental dimensions to health coverage: population, services, and cost coverage. The box model in Figure 15.1 illustrates this [4]. The outer box represents full coverage in the three dimensions, while the inner box represents the current coverage, indicating what remains in terms of population missed, services excluded, and cost unfunded under various national coverage mechanisms.

Countries with unlimited resources for health and strong health systems can theoretically provide their whole populations with full coverage of all needed services with full quality and financial protection; but this is not the reality even in HICs. An approach of *progressive universalism* is introduced, whereby pooled funds are progressively expanded toward ensuring that UHC leaves no one behind by ensuring full population coverage by a predefined – even if limited – set of interventions [5, 19]. The *World Health Report 1999* advocates this approach. In the WHO director-general's message of this report, Gro Harlem Brundtland states that the "new universalism" "recognizes government's limits but retains government's responsibility for leadership, regulation and finance of health systems . . . it recognizes that if services are to be provided for all then not all services can be provided. The most cost-effective services should be provided first." Here, WHO explicitly points to a version of universalism that acknowledges the implications of budget constraints.

There are two fundamental approaches to easing the scarcity of pooled resources for health. The more obvious of the two is to expand the pool of health resources. This can be accomplished through two approaches. The first approach involves employing various streams of revenue raising and pooling mechanisms (e.g., taxation, innovative financing approaches, social insurance schemes, private voluntary insurance schemes, or external assistance), prioritizing the health sector in national budgets, or merging risk pools to further distribute the financial risk – all of these mechanisms aim to get *more money for health*. The second approach concerns extracting more value out of currently available funds by targeting resources toward their most effective and efficient use – that is, getting *more health for the money*.

Health policymakers and planners must make decisions about the extent of coverage in each of the three dimensions of UHC. One conception of UHC is focused on the appropriate content of a benefits package of interventions to be publicly financed for the entire population, typically delivered by the health sector. The decision to take a progressive universalism approach to achieve UHC represents a choice to prioritize full population coverage and cost coverage through prepayment arrangements, but leaves open the question of which health services can be prioritized in a stepwise approach within the timeline of the SDG 3.8 target. Put another way, the central question of this approach is: Which health services should all people receive in good quality and with full financial protection?

Starting with an affordable publicly financed essential package of health services,[1] the package can be progressively expanded when resources and health system capacity allow. Smaller health financing envelopes, as in L&MICs, force more difficult choices than do the much larger envelopes of HICs. To help inform the decision-making process, the *Making Fair Choices* report recommended that the most cost-effective interventions that prioritize the health of the worst-off and provide financial risk protection should be focused on to progress toward UHC [19].

15.2.1 DCP3: Pathway to UHC

Among the several strategic frameworks that countries are implementing to address UHC is the approach adopted by DCP3 and its model packages [6].

Health Sector Interventions: Toward UHC Benefit Package

DCP3 provides the critical evidence needed for strategic health policy and for laying out an approach to support countries in expanding coverage. It conducted a comprehensive review of the efficacy and cost-effectiveness of priority health interventions across 21 health areas (Table 15.1), through a structured process of systematic appraisal of evidence, economic evaluation, and expert judgment to support decision-making on resource allocations, particularly in resource-constrained contexts.

What makes DCP3 unique is not only the focus on service packages, but also the fact that it provides a strategic approach that covers the three UHC dimensions. Assessing the evidence and recommendations presented on a wide range of health conditions in the

Table 15.1 Health areas covered by the DCP3 packages

Age-related cluster (packages 1–5)	Noncommunicable disease and injury cluster (packages 11–17)
1 Maternal and newborn health	11 Cardiovascular, respiratory, and related disorders
2 Child health	
3 School-age health and development	12 Cancer
4 Adolescent health and development	13 Mental, neurological, and substance-use disorders
5 Reproductive health and contraception	
Infectious diseases cluster (packages 6–10)	14 Musculoskeletal disorders
6 HIV and sexually transmitted infections	15 Congenital and genetic disorders
7 Tuberculosis	16 Injury prevention
8 Malaria and adult febrile illness	17 Environmental improvements
9 Neglected tropical diseases	**Health services cluster (packages 18–21)**
10 Pandemic and emergency preparedness	18 Surgery
	19 Rehabilitation
	20 Palliative care and pain control
	21 Pathology

---

[1] The health benefits package (HBP) and essential package of health services (EPHS) are used interchangeably in this chapter.

first eight volumes has been reoriented toward UHC by developing packages of health interventions that formed the major content of a ninth volume: two packages focusing on essential health services and a package of intersectoral health policies [20]. No package – neither for health services nor intersectoral policies – can be applied "off-the-shelf" to any given context; rather, the DCP3 packages offer guidance or an option set that can be adapted by a country based on its disease burden, needs, health system capacity, available financing, and local circumstances.

Beyond the Health Sector: Intersectoral Policies for Health

Health is determined by a complex set of interrelated factors and measures (Figure 15.2). It hence cannot be confined to the health sector alone [5]. Working together across sectors to promote health is often referred to as intersectoral action for health.

Advancing UHC would hence require an inclusive approach that includes a priority suite of health-enhancing intersectoral interventions and policies that would typically be financed and implemented by other nonhealth sectors. In this respect preventive and health promotion services provided through intersectoral action are instrumental to advancing UHC. Intersectoral health-promoting policies are therefore critical components of national health policy and are essential in addressing common risk factors like tobacco use, micronutrient deficiencies, other forms of malnutrition and unhealthy diet, physical inactivity, harmful use of alcohol, injuries, and air pollution and other environmental risks. Intersectoral health policies were a key message of the political declaration of the United Nations high-level meeting on UHC in 2019, and prior to it the political declaration on the prevention and control of noncommunicable diseases in 2011 [8, 21].

Accordingly, due consideration should be given to the intersectoral agenda in any strategy to advance UHC. It is an important function of the Ministry of Health to be actively engaged with the relevant sectors and serve as an informed advocate for

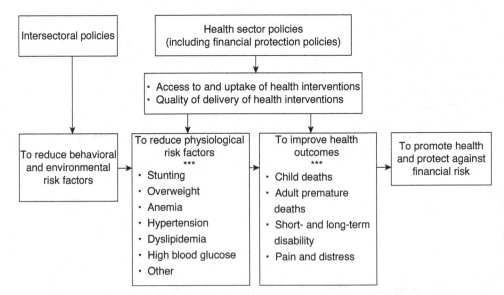

Figure 15.2 Interactions between health sector and intersectoral policies. Adapted from [6].

developing and monitoring the implementation of these intersectoral priorities. Hence, we include in this chapter one recent assessment of what those priorities are likely to include.

The key risk factors prioritized for inclusion in the DCP3 package of intersectoral policies and interventions include: addictive substance use, tobacco and the harmful use of alcohol, dietary risk factors covering both inadequate and excessive nutrient intake, environmental risks – mainly air pollution, occupational hazards, poor access to safe water and sanitation, environmental toxins, road traffic accidents, and common injuries – and other risks like high-risk sex and antimicrobial resistance. The policies included in the package fall under four main policy instruments: legislative and regulatory, fiscal, built environment, and communication and information. Initially, 71 intersectoral policies were included, but further prioritization resulted in a core early implementation package of 29 policies for consideration by L&MICs. The content of the DCP3 package of core intersectoral policies is included in Table 15.2,

Effective actions to prevent or correct behavioral and environmental risk factors will require full commitment of nonhealth sectors. Like health care services, a wide range of intersectoral policies are required to achieve UHC and have to be prioritized through systematic consideration of health concerns and disease burden. Planning and implementing intersectoral policies require high-level government support, motivated engagement of the relevant sectors, and joint work with the health sector based on mutual benefits, pooled resources, and a climate of trust.

Developing Packages of Health Services and Intersectoral Policies

To achieve UHC, the health system should be able to provide full access to a package of publicly financed services designed to meet the essential health care needs of the population. Such a package is referred to as the health benefits package (HBP) or essential package of health services (EPHS) [22]. Needless to say, there is no universal package. The DCP3 essential UHC package (EUHC) provides an option set of high-priority health services for L&MICs that is grounded in economic reality and is determined by the extended cost-effectiveness analysis (ECEA) approach [23]. Nested within that EUHC is a subset in part of highest-priority interventions, known as the highest-priority package (HPP), which is proposed to guide the development of the UHC essential package in LICs where EUHC is not affordable.

Whereas standard cost-effectiveness analysis assesses only health outcomes relative to costs (see Chapter 13), the DCP3 used the ECEA approach to include nonhealth benefits like financial risk protection and distributional consequences (e.g., equity) in its analysis to provide a richer comparison of the value of interventions [23]. Both methods aim to capture the relative value of an intervention to support decision-making and prioritization.

The process of developing the DCP3 packages of essential health services and the priority intersectoral policies is depicted in Figure 15.3. The recommendations made in 21 health areas (Table 15.1) were subjected to a further review through a set of criteria covering disease burden, evidence impact, cost-effectiveness, financial risk protection, equity, and feasibility of implementation to select a set of essential interventions in each of these areas which collectively form the EUHC package of 218 health interventions and the more affordable HPP of 108 interventions proposed for LICs. Further prioritization of

Table 15.2 DCP3 package of core intersectoral policies

Key health risk	Policy	Instrument
Air pollution	1. Indoor air pollution: subsidize other clean household energy sources, including liquid propane gas (LPG), for the poor and other key populations	Fiscal
	2. Indoor air pollution: halt the use of unprocessed coal and kerosene as a household fuel	Regulatory
	3. Indoor air pollution: promote the use of low-emission household devices	Information and education
	4. Emissions: tax emissions and/or auction off transferable emissions permits	Fiscal
	5. Emissions: regulate transport, industrial, and power generation emissions	Regulatory
	6. Fossil fuel subsidies: dismantle subsidies for and increase taxation of fossil fuels (except LPG)	Fiscal
	7. Public transportation: build and strengthen affordable public transportation systems in urban areas	Built environment
Addictive substance use	8. Substance use: impose large excise taxes on tobacco, alcohol, and other addictive substances	Fiscal
	9. Substance use: impose strict regulation of advertising, promotion, packaging, and availability of tobacco, alcohol, and other addictive substances, with enforcement	Regulatory
	10. Smoking in public places: ban smoking in public spaces	Regulatory
Inadequate nutrient intake	11. School feeding: finance school feeding for all schools and students in selected geographical areas	Fiscal
	12. Food quality: ensure that subsidized foods and school feeding programs have adequate nutritional quality	Regulatory
	13. Iron and folic acid: fortify food	Regulatory
	14. Iodine: fortify salt	Regulatory
Excessive nutrient intake	15. Trans fats: ban and replace with polyunsaturated fats	Regulatory
	16. Salt: impose regulations to reduce salt in manufactured food products	Regulatory
	17. Sugar-sweetened beverages: tax to discourage use	Fiscal
	18. Salt and sugar: provide consumer education against excess use, including product labeling	Information and education
Road traffic injuries	19. Vehicle safety: enact legislation and enforcement of personal transport safety measures, including seatbelts in vehicles and helmets for motorcycle users	Regulatory
	20. Traffic safety: set and enforce speed limits on roads	Regulatory
	21. Traffic safety: include traffic calming mechanisms in road construction	Built environment

Table 15.2 (cont.)

Key health risk	Policy	Instrument
Other risks	22. Pesticides: enact strict control and move to selective bans on highly hazardous pesticides	Regulatory
	23. Water and sanitation: enact national standards for safe drinking water, sanitation, and hygienic behavior within and outside households and institutions	Regulatory
	24. Hazardous waste: enact legislation and enforcement of standards for hazardous waste disposal	Regulatory
	25. Lead exposure: take actions to reduce human exposure to lead, including bans on leaded fuels and lead in paint, cookware, water pipes, cosmetics, drugs, and food supplements	Regulatory
	26. Agricultural antibiotic use: reduce and eventually phase out subtherapeutic antibiotic use in agriculture	Regulatory
	27. Emergency response: create and exercise multisectoral responses and supply stockpiles to respond to pandemics and other emergencies	Regulatory
	28. Safe sex: remove duties and taxes on condoms, then introduce subsidies in brothels and for key at-risk populations	Fiscal
	29. Exercise: take initial steps to develop infrastructure enabling safe walking and cycling	Built environment

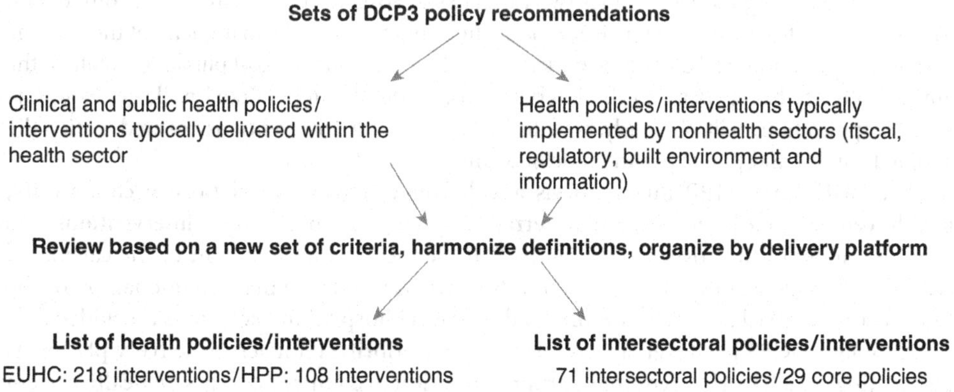

Sets of DCP3 policy recommendations

Clinical and public health policies/interventions typically delivered within the health sector

Health policies/interventions typically implemented by nonhealth sectors (fiscal, regulatory, built environment and information)

Review based on a new set of criteria, harmonize definitions, organize by delivery platform

List of health policies/interventions
EUHC: 218 interventions/HPP: 108 interventions

List of intersectoral policies/interventions
71 intersectoral policies/29 core policies

Figure 15.3 Process for translating DCP3 evidence and recommendations into model UHC packages [23, 24].

EUHC into HPP focused on value for money, priority to the most disadvantaged populations, and financial risk protection afforded.

While countries are expected to consider the same or similar criteria for selecting interventions, their interpretation and application will obviously have to be localized.

Translating the DCP3 packages into a national or subnational EPHS for a country will involve data collection, evidence generation and assessment, and analysis of demographics, disease burden, and costs. The process will require considerable capacity-building in priority-setting, decision-making, and design and revision of essential packages. Sustainability with changes of policies or fiscal space will depend on how capacities in these areas are developed and maintained.

Costing of UHC Packages

It is worth emphasizing the importance of understanding the cost of the EUHC and HPP packages in the local context. DCP3 presented these packages with estimates of costs and mortality impacts. Countries would then have an option of adapting these packages according to their own needs and available fiscal space, and strive to implement them with progressively increasing coverage to achieve the SDG target 3.8 on UHC and other health-related targets by 2030. Costing and budgeting of UHC packages is challenged by limited transferability between contexts and validity over time, although it does nonetheless seem to capture the order of magnitude and relative balance of costs. The DCP3 has published a detailed costing methodology for the EUHC and HPP, which will not be detailed further here [25].

The DCP3 EUHC and HPP costs are detailed in Table 15.3. EUHC costs are driven by health system costs (40% of total costs at full coverage), with noncommunicable diseases representing the highest service delivery costs [25]. The per capita cost of the HPP and EUHC at full coverage were US$42 and US$76, respectively, in LICs, and US$58 and US$110, respectively, in lower middle-income countries (LMICs). These cost estimates exceed current per capita health expenditure in many countries, presenting a significant financing gap [26, 27]. This point highlights the importance of countries designing, prioritizing, and costing their own UHC packages in a more realistic way, based on available resources and fiscal space.

The packages were costed on the basis that 80% coverage is achieved for most interventions by 2030. The costing model provides two estimates of costs for the health system component. The first is an estimate of how much additional funding it would take to implement the package and the second is the total cost of the package defined as incremental cost plus an estimate of the amount already being spent on the interventions. In developing national packages, country-specific applications will obviously have to be based on the interventions covered, nationally adopted clinical and public health guidelines, and local cost structures.

The EUHC and HPP interventions are delivered across five platforms: community, health center, first-level hospital, referral hospital, and population interventions. As expected, most of the costs are related to PHC services. More than half of the calculated costs occur at the health center level, and this increases to more than three-quarters of the total cost of the package if community and first-level hospital interventions are added.

Although DCP3 has taken a step forward with prioritization across delivery platforms and costing, much work is required during translation to country packages on health system assessment and the capacity needed to bridge bottlenecks and gaps for implementation. Costs of implementing the package will depend on population coverage rates. Although the aim is to achieve 80% coverage of the interventions in the EUHC package by 2030, because of health system capacity and fiscal space, some countries may decide to start with what is achievable and progressively increase coverage along the timeline for attainment of the target coverage in 2030.

Table 15.3 Total and incremental costs of EUHC and HPP in 2015

	Low-income countries		Lower middle-income countries	
	HPP	EUHC	HPP	EUHC
1. Incremental annual cost (US$ billions)[a]	23 (9.2–51)	48 (20–100)	82 (32–180)	160 (66–350)
2. Incremental annual cost per person (US$)	26 (10–57)	53 (22–110)	31 (12–67)	61 (25–130)
3. Total annual cost (US$ billions)[a]	38 (19–71)	68 (34–130)	160 (81–280)	280 (150–500)
4. Total annual cost per person (US$)	42 (21–79)	76 (37–140)	58 (30–100)	110 (54–190)
5. Incremental annual cost as a share of current GNI (%)[b]	3.1 (1.2–6.9)	6.4 (2.6–13)	1.5 (0.57–3.2)	2.9 (1.2–6.2)
6. Total annual cost as a share of current GNI (%)[b]	5.1 (2.5–9.5)	9.1 (4.5–17)	2.8 (1.4–4.8)	5.2 (2.6–9.1)

EUHC, essential health coverage; GNI, gross national income; UHC, universal health coverage. Incremental annual cost is the estimated cost of going from current to full implementation (80% population coverage) of the EUHC and HPP interventions. The total annual cost is the incremental cost plus current spending assuming the same cost structure for current and incremental investments. Estimated costs are inclusive of estimates for (large) health system strengthening cost and are steady-state (or long-run average) costs in that investments to achieve higher levels of coverage and to cover depreciation are included.
[a] The 2015 population of LICs was 0.90 billion. For LMICs it was 2.7 billion. Population sizes are estimated using 2017 data from UN DESA.
[b] The 2015 GNI of LICs was US$0.75 trillion and for LMICs it was US$5.4 trillion. Aggregate GNI figures were estimated using data from the World Bank.
Source: [26].

15.3 Financing and Budgeting

Although the cost estimates may be feasible for some countries, not all countries will find them affordable. Either the health financing envelope needs to expand in order to reasonably attain the package, or the scope of interventions needs to be reduced [28, 29]. Fiscal space assessment is a critical component to ground cost assessments in reality. In Pakistan, for example, two packages were endorsed: a full package of 107 interventions that is currently unaffordable, and a more prioritized package of 88 interventions for immediate implementation until the government conducts a fiscal space analysis to guide increased health allocations (see Chapter 10, Box 10.3) [30]. In this case, the journey to UHC will start with a smaller package with a plan to implement the full package when the fiscal space for public financing increases.

15.3.1 Funding, Pooling, and Purchasing to Achieve UHC

Addressing financial gaps is the objective of the three core functions of health financing: expanding health resources by collecting more revenues, pooling more effectively, and strategically purchasing services to greater effect (see Chapters 5, 16–18 for a more detailed discussion on health financing functions).

The proposal of the Commission on Investing in Health to raise revenues to meet the needs of the grand convergence package can guide UHC financing. The Commission estimated that the principal funding sources to close the convergence cost gap would be economic growth (with proportional health sector growth), increased mobilization of domestic resources through broadened and more efficient taxation, intersectoral reallocations and efficiency gains (primarily through the transfer of harmful subsidies such as for fossil fuels), and the roles of both private finance and external assistance [5]. Notably, the Commission estimated that the cost of convergence would be just 3% of the anticipated economic growth in LICs and less than 1% of the anticipated economic growth in LMICs over the period to 2035. These projections provide an option to raise revenues, assuming country health spending keeps pace with GDP growth and those funds are pooled and distributed equitably and efficiently.

Pooling is typically regarded as the insurance function of health financing because it ensures a system of cross-subsidization whereby the financial risk of health service demand is shared among the population (also known as redistributive capacity) [31]. The pooling function is especially useful for health services that are costly or needed unexpectedly; however, pooling can also provide a mechanism to ensure equity even for services of relatively low cost or predictable demand, such that the better-off cross-finance the disadvantaged to some degree. Work is now beginning to quantify the benefits of financial risk protection, but at present the value of financial risk protection or insurance remains only partially estimated for HBP packages [22, 23, 32].

Finally, strategic purchasing can have a powerful influence over the rules and incentives governing health service provision. It actively links information on aspects of provider behavior and performance with the way the providers are paid. This linkage can extract value by improving outputs or outcomes and/or limiting costs, or by prioritizing equity through the targeting of vulnerable groups. And a strong purchaser will have significant monopsony (a market in which there is only one buyer) power to negotiate industry prices, as well as to conduct or interpret health intervention assessments [33, 34]. In recognition of the vital roles of a strategic purchasing authority, there are many successful examples of purchasing reforms to support UHC (see Chapter 18) [35].

Revenue collection helps expand the resource envelope in pursuit of UHC, while strategic purchasing improves the efficiency of how existing funds are spent. Health financing strategies that maximize *both* revenue and value can meet the costs of HBPs like the EUHC or HPP.

15.4 Implementing UHC: Challenges and Capacity Needs

This chapter has so far described the dimensions of UHC, how essential services are prioritized in the context of limited resources, and the critical service coverage and financing choices of a progressive universalism approach to UHC. Resource scarcity is a critical constraint to UHC attainment; however, even a well-resourced system cannot achieve, iterate, and sustain UHC without adequate health system capacity. What follows is a sample of pressing country capacity needs.

15.4.1 Institutionalizing Priority-Setting and Informed Decision-Making

Benefits package design is an exercise in priority-setting that should be performed by the informed application of epidemiological, economic, financial, ethical, and legal tools to arrive at an EPHS that meets the goals of the health system and the values of a society. Without an informed, objective, transparent, and multicriteria decision-making process, health priorities are subject to sociopolitical forces and distortions, among other factors, that can lead to inefficiency and inequity [36]. Also, elements of the package will require the capacity for periodic review and refinement beyond the timeline of a project. However, most L&MICs do not yet have institutions with adequate capacity to deliver and maintain this valuable priority-setting function. Therefore, an essential requirement is to pursue a capacity-building component to ensure that national expertise exists to implement, monitor, and revise the package and move it into the future.

15.4.2 Strategic Purchasing

Anemic health budgets challenge L&MICs to meet UHC funding gaps by mobilizing financial resources for health while using existing resources to greater effect. However, if scarcity is a central challenge to meeting UHC, then capacity within the health sector to manage the core financing functions is of critical importance. Among those functions, strategic purchasing is a powerful lever to shape health system architecture and influence providers' behavior. Strategic purchasing requires complex linkages of varied payment mechanisms with information on providers' behavior, health outputs, and health outcomes to shape the rules and incentives of the health system. The primary reason why so few L&MICs have well-established strategic purchasers is because its complexity requires significant organizational and institutional capacity that is often not found in resource-poor environments.

15.5 Conclusions

Countries around the world are challenged to improve the performance of their national health systems and to achieve UHC by 2030. The COVID-19 crisis has not only demonstrated that health systems in most countries are not prepared, but has also exacerbated inequities and major gaps in capacity and performance leading to considerable disruptions of health services. L&MICs therefore need to reinforce their commitment to UHC and scale up their efforts in designing, updating, and implementing evidence-based packages of essential health interventions that meet the needs of their population [37].

Several strategic frameworks are being adopted by countries to accelerate progress toward UHC. Among these, the DCP3 approach presented in this chapter provides an entry point and a roadmap to provide background for national visions and initiatives on UHC. This includes estimates not only of cost but of mortality reduction as well [24]. The DCP3 packages serve as a model to guide policymakers to design their own national or subnational packages based on their needs and contexts, health system capacity, available resources, and other local circumstances.

Current experience, in the DCP3 model packages and also in countries, demonstrates the complex challenge of designing an affordable UHC package that can be implemented within the available fiscal space and health system capacity. Affordability of the UHC package and feasibility of implementation determine the success of the HBP design. By implementing a publicly financed package starting with the highest-priority services followed by stepwise expansion in coverage and services, countries can address the gaps in the three dimensions of UHC. The decision to take a progressive universalism approach to achieve UHC represents a choice to prioritize full population and financial protection, but leaves open the question of which health services can be prioritized in a gradual approach within the timeline of the SDG 3.8 target.

Universal health coverage attainment implies a change process – often of the care delivery model and the financing system, or both simultaneously [38]. The UHC reform process prioritizes and redistributes health resources to promote coverage across three dimensions, thereby forcing both economic and political trade-offs [39].

The change required to strengthen health systems and promote unimpeded access to essential health services is challenging for many countries. Commitment to invest in UHC at the highest level is a prerequisite, and visionary leadership can generate solidarity and buy-in, reconcile political trade-offs, interface with other sectors for intersectoral health policy development, and develop a theory of change for system transformation. Health resources are scarce, and the careful stewardship of each building block of the health system requires strong management, accountability, and feedback systems, and regulatory or incentive mechanisms to shape the health ecosystem across public and private sectors.

Finally, progress toward UHC will require considerable capacity-building in priority-setting, decision-making, design, and revision of essential packages, and action to address health system gaps. Sustainability with changes of policies or fiscal space will depend on how capacities in these areas are developed and maintained. In short, health systems require institutionalized leadership and stewardship to cultivate a system based on UHC that performs to its goals.

References

1. World Bank. *World Development Report 1993: Investing in Health*. Washington, DC, World Bank, 1993. https://openknowledge .worldbank.org/handle/10986/5976 (accessed January 28, 2022).

2. World Health Organization. *The World Health Report:1999, Making a Difference*. Geneva, World Health Organization, 1999. https://apps.who.int/iris/handle/10665/ 42167 (accessed December 13, 2020).

3. World Health Organization. *The World Health Report 2000*. Geneva, World Health Organization, 2000. www.who.int/whr/ 2000/en/whr00_en.pdf?ua=1 (accessed January 31, 2022).

4. World Health Organization. *The World Health Report: Health Systems Financing – the Path to Universal Coverage*. Geneva, World Health Organization, 2010. https:// apps.who.int/iris/handle/10665/44371 (accessed December 10, 2020).

5. D. T. Jamison, L. H. Summers, G. Alleyne, et al. Global health 2035: a world converging within a generation. *Lancet* 2013; **382**(9908): 1898–1955.

6. D. T. Jamison, H. Gelband, S. Horton, et al., eds., *Disease Control Priorities: Improving Health and Reducing Poverty*. Washington, DC, International Bank for Reconstruction and Development and World Bank, 2017.

7. United Nations. Resolution adopted by the General Assembly on 25 September 2015: Transforming our world: the 2030 Agenda for Sustainable Development. 2015. www .un.org/ga/search/view_doc.asp?symbol=A/ RES/70/1&Lang=E (accessed December 12, 2020).

8. United Nations. UN High-Level Meeting (UN HLM) on Universal Health Coverage, 23 September 2019, New York. 2019. www .uhc2030.org/un-hlm-2019/ (accessed December 11, 2020).

9. United Nations. Universal Declaration of Human Rights. www.un.org/en/about-us/universal-declaration-of-human-rights (accessed February 6, 2022).

10. World Health Organization. Constitution of the World Health Organization. 1946. https://apps.who.int/gb/bd/PDF/bd47/EN/constitution-en.pdf?ua=1 (accessed December 11, 2020).

11. World Health Organization. Declaration of Alma-Ata. 1978. https://cdn.who.int/media/docs/default-source/documents/almaata-declaration-en.pdf?sfvrsn=7b3c2167_2 (accessed December 12, 2020).

12. World Health Organization and the UNICEF. Global Conference on Primary Health Care: Declaration of Astana. 2018. www.who.int/docs/default-source/primary-health/declaration/gcphc-declaration.pdf (accessed February 6, 2022).

13. M. Roberts, W. Hsiao, P. Berman, et al. *Getting Health Reform Right: A Guide to Improving Performance and Equity.* Oxford, Oxford University Press, 2003.

14. World Health Organization. Global spending on health: a world in transition. Working Paper. 2019. www.who.int/publications/i/item/WHO-HIS-HGF-HFWorkingPaper-19.4 (accessed December 10, 2020).

15. IHME. Financing global health data visualization. https://vizhub.healthdata.org/fgh/ (accessed December 11, 2020).

16. World Bank Group. Population, total: low income, lower middle income. 2020. https://data.worldbank.org/indicator/SP.POP.TOTL?end=2017&locations=XM-XN&start=1960 (accessed December 11, 2020).

17. World Health Organization. *Tracking Universal Health Coverage: 2017 Global Monitoring Report.* Geneva, World Health Organization, 2017. https://apps.who.int/iris/bitstream/handle/10665/259817/9789241513555-eng.pdf (accessed December 10, 2020).

18. World Health Organization. *Tracking Universal Health Coverage: 2021 Global Monitoring Report.* Geneva, World Health Organization, 2021. www.who.int/publications/i/item/9789240040618 (accessed January 27, 2022).

19. World Health Organization. Making fair choices on the path to universal health coverage: final report of the WHO consultative group on equity and universal health coverage. 2014. https://apps.who.int/iris/handle/10665/112671 (accessed December 10, 2020).

20. Department of Global Health, University of Washington. DCP3 country translation. 2021. http://dcp-3.org (accessed January 27, 2022).

21. United Nations. Prevention and control of non-communicable diseases: report of the Secretary-General. 2011. https://undocs.org/en/A/66/83 (accessed December 18, 2020).

22. A. Glassman, U. Giedion, Y. Sakuma, et al. Defining a health benefits package: what are the necessary processes? *Health Syst Reform* 2016; 2(1): 39–50.

23. S. Verguet, D. T. Jamison. Health policy assessment: applications of extended cost-effectiveness analysis methodology. In: D. T. Jamison, H. Gelband, S. Horton, et al., eds., *Disease Control Priorities: Improving Health and Reducing Poverty.* Washington, DC: International Bank for Reconstruction and Development and World Bank, 2017, pp. 157–166.

24. D. Watkins, O. F. Norheim, P. Jha, et al. Mortality impact of achieving essential universal health coverage in low- and lower-middle-income countries. Working Paper 21 for Disease Control Priorities (3rd ed.). Department of Global Health, University of Washington.

25. D. A. Watkins, J. Qi, Y. Kawakatsu, et al. Resource requirements for essential universal health coverage: a modelling study based on findings from Disease Control Priorities, 3rd edition. *Lancet Glob Health* 2020; 8(6): e829–e839.

26. D. A. Watkins, D. T. Jamison, T. Mills, et al. Universal health coverage and essential packages of care. In D. T. Jamison, H. Gelband, S. Horton, et al., eds., *Disease Control Priorities: Improving Health and Reducing Poverty.* Washington, DC,

International Bank for Reconstruction and Development and World Bank, 2017, pp. 43–65.

27. World Health Organization. Global Health Observatory database. 2020. www.who.int/data/gho (accessed December 11, 2020).

28. D. Mcintyre, F. Meheus, J. A. Røttingen. What level of domestic government health expenditure should we aspire to for universal health coverage? *Health Econ Policy Law* 2017; **12**(2): 125–137.

29. K. Stenberg, O. Hanssen, T. T. Edejer, et al. Financing transformative health systems towards achievement of the health Sustainable Development Goals: a model for projected resource needs in 67 low-income and middle-income countries. *Lancet Glob Health* 2017; **5**(9): e875–e887.

30. Pakistan Ministry of National Health Services, Regulations, and Coordination. UHC essential package of health services. 2020. https://phkh.nhsrc.pk/sites/default/files/2020-10/Essential%20Package%20of%20Health%20Services%20with%20Localized%20Evidence%20Pakistan%20WHO%202020.pdf (accessed December 10, 2020).

31. I. Mathauer, L. Vinyals Torres, J. Kutzin, et al. Pooling financial resources for universal health coverage: options for reform. *Bull World Health Organ* 2020; **98** (2): 132–139.

32. J. Skinner, K. Chalkidou, D. T. Jamison. Valuing protection against health-related financial risks. *J Benefit Cost Anal* 2019; **10** (Suppl. 1): 106–131.

33. D. Nicholson, R. Yates, W. Warburton, et al. Delivering universal health coverage: a guide for policymakers. 2015. www.imperial.ac.uk/media/imperial-college/institute-of-global-health-innovation/public/Universal-health-coverage.pdf (accessed December 12, 2020).

34. M. Daher. Overview of the World Health Report 2000 health systems: improving performance. *J Med Liban* 2001; **49**(1): 22–24.

35. D. Cotlear, S. Nagpal, O. Smith, et al. *Going Universal: How 24 Developing Countries Are Implementing Universal Health Coverage from the Bottom up.* Washington, DC, World Bank Publications, 2015.

36. K. Kieslich, J. B. Bump, O. F. Norheim, et al. Accounting for technical, ethical, and political factors in priority setting. *Health Syst Reform* 2016; **2**(1): 51–60.

37. UHC2030. State of commitment to universal health coverage: synthesis, 2020. 2020. www.uhc2030.org/fileadmin/uploads/uhc2030/Documents/Key_Issues/State_of_UHC/SoUHCC_synthesis_2020_final_web.pdf (accessed December 11, 2020).

38. World Health Organization. Stewardship and governance toward universal health. www.paho.org/salud-en-las-americas-2017/?p=47 (accessed December 11, 2020).

39. M. R. Reich, J. Harris, N. Ikegami, et al. Moving towards universal health coverage: lessons from 11 country studies. *Lancet* 2016; **387**(10020): 811–816.

Chapter 6

Pro-Poor Expansion of Universal Health Coverage

Health Financing Strategies and Options

Daniel Cotlear and Ajay Tandon

Key Messages

- As national incomes rise, countries undergo a health financing transition, increasing total levels of health expenditure while increasing the publicly financed share of health spending and reducing the external – and out-of-pocket (OOP) – financed share of spending.
- Increases in public financing in low- and middle-income countries (L&MICs) have historically been associated with economic growth and increased *total* government revenue/spending; for these countries, it has rarely resulted from a greater priority assigned to health in the government budget.
- While most countries initially offer a basic package of services focused on communicable diseases and maternal and child care, they diverge in what interventions to add as a next step. Few countries opt for making small increments to the basic universal benefits – more common is to expand the benefits significantly, but only for selected subpopulations.
- Two pro-poor paths are common for the expansion of health coverage. Many countries implement health insurance schemes for the poor. Others expand platforms of public providers that are mostly used by the poor, often focusing on community and primary care services.
- Countries choosing the pro-poor health insurance path develop targeting and enrolment instruments. Targeting tends to be stricter with social security purchasers compared with ministerial purchasers.
- Fragmented systems, while suboptimal, can sometimes be more pro-poor than integrated systems.

16.1 Introduction

Universal health coverage (UHC) – a policy commitment that is part of the United Nation's Sustainable Development Goals for 2030 – is about ensuring that all people can use essential health services they need, of sufficient quality to be effective, while ensuring their use does not expose the individuals to financial hardship (see Chapter 3). The focus on both effective service coverage and financial risk protection under UHC implies that not only how much a country spends on health is important but also the way a health system is financed (see Chapter 5). Hallmarks of "high-performing" health financing systems for UHC can be characterized as those (1) where financing levels are adequate; (2) prepaid funds are pooled in an effective way to spread the financial risks of ill-health; and (3) spending is efficient and equitable to ensure desired levels of effective service coverage and financial risk protection for all people, both with resilience and sustainability [1].

The journey to UHC is long and there are many paths to get there; but which path countries take matters. In its conceptualization, equity is intrinsic to the very notion of UHC: *everyone* should have access to the services they need, which should be based on need and not on one's ability to pay for health services. In addition, given that UHC is at least as much a direction as a destination, equity concerns have led many to emphasize the notion of "progressive universalism" (see Chapters 3 and 15) – that is, that the poor and vulnerable ought to gain at least as much (if not more) while countries are progressing on the path toward UHC [2].

While each country requires a unique set of policies for UHC advancement, the systematic comparison of many countries allows the identification of common patterns or areas of *policy convergence*. It also enables the identification of areas of *policy divergence*, where countries choose between different options. In this chapter we discuss both patterns, with a focus on financing the pro-poor expansion of UHC in recent decades, highlighting some common challenges faced by many countries. The data sources for this are described in Box 16.1.

The chapter is organized as follows – the next section describes the status of health financing in L&MICs and their health financing transition over the past two decades. Advancing UHC requires an expansion of coverage over three dimensions: (1) health care benefits, (2) population coverage, and (3) cost coverage using prepaid/pooled funds; these are addressed in Sections 16.3, 16.4, and 16.5, respectively. The chapter closes with a summary of the main conclusions.

16.2 Current Status and Trends in Health Expenditure and Financing

Levels and composition of financing for health vary significantly across countries. In 2019 [3], the levels of per capita current health spending ranged from lower than US$25 in Madagascar, Burundi, the Democratic Republic of the Congo (DRC), and South Sudan to higher than US$8,000 in Norway, Switzerland, and the United States. Although these differences do not correct for variations in purchasing power of currencies across countries

---

Box 16.1 Data Sources for this Chapter

- Quantitative data is from the WHO's Global Health Expenditure Database [3].
- Qualitative data relies on a review of 39 country case studies (Figure 16.1) using a common methodology that drills down into instruments to steer the expansion of coverage in a pro-poor direction. All studies were published by the World Bank under the *UHC study series* between 2013 and 2019 [4].

Included case studies: **Africa** – Ethiopia, Gabon, Ghana, Kenya, Malawi, Nigeria, Senegal, South Africa, Tanzania; **South and East Asia** – Bangladesh, China, India, Indonesia, Lao PDR, Malaysia, Philippines, Sri Lanka, Thailand, Vietnam; **Europe and Central Asia** – Armenia, Azerbaijan, Croatia, Georgia, Kyrgyz Republic, Russia, Turkey; **Latin America and the Caribbean** – Argentina, Brazil, Chile, Colombia, Costa Rica, Dominican Republic, Guatemala, Jamaica, Mexico, Peru, Uruguay; **Middle East and North Africa** – Morocco, Tunisia.

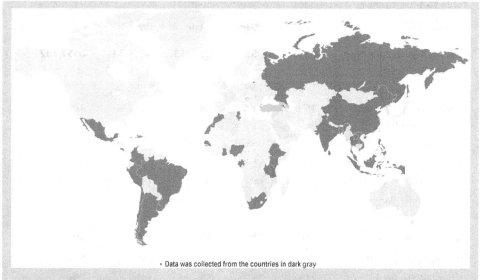

• Data was collected from the countries in dark gray

Figure 16.1 Country case studies used as source of qualitative data in this chapter.

(e.g., US$1 buys more in low-income settings than it does in high-income countries [HICs] due to cheaper labor and other costs), the contrast in levels of health spending across countries is staggering. Differences are less stark when comparing current health spending as a share of GDP. In 2019, current health spending among low-income countries (LICs) averaged 5.2% of GDP (US$34 in per capita terms) relative to 11.5% (US$5,741 per capita) among HICs (Table 16.1). The corresponding shares among lower middle-income countries (LMICs) and upper middle-income countries (UMICs) were 3.6% and 5.9% of GDP, respectively – lower in LMICs than in LICs due to a larger share of external financing among the latter.

Not only are levels of health spending different across income classifications, the way the health sector is financed also differs significantly: private OOP spending dominates among LICs and LMICs, accounting for >40% of current health spending on average in 2019. External financing represents one-third of public spending on health among LICs (33% in 2019, increasing from 17% in 2000), decreasing to 5% among LMICs. Additional external financing flowing from outside of the government budget is included in the "other" category. Public financing for health – via general taxation or social health insurance (SHI) contributions or both – predominates among UMICs and HICs. Voluntary health insurance is not a significant source, accounting for only 6% of country-averaged resources for health globally.

Economic growth and development are usually accompanied by many different and significant transitions related to health. For instance, countries tend to undergo a *demographic transition* as national incomes rise: a decline from high mortality and fertility rates to relatively low mortality and fertility rates that result in aging of the population. Related in part to the demographic transition, countries also undergo an *epidemiological*

Table 16.1 Health financing profiles across income groupings, 2019

Indicators	LICs	LMICs	UMICs	HICs	All countries
Current health spending per capita	US$34	US$95	US$553	US$5,741	*US$1,132*
Share of GDP	5.2%	3.6%	5.9%	11.5%	5.7%
Public share of current health spending	36%	36%	56%	67%	48%
Per capita	US$12	US$38	US$307	US$3,545	US$678
Share from general taxation	64%	83%	60%	66%	71%
Share from social health insurance contributions	2%	11%	40%	34%	24%
Share from external sources	33%	5%	0%	0%	5%
OOP share of current	41%	52%	32%	16%	39%
VHI share of current	2%	5%	9%	3%	6%
Other (NGOs, etc.)	21%	7%	3%	14%	7%

Averages are population weighted; "general taxation" includes borrowing.
Authors' estimates based on [3].

transition: a decline in the overall burden of disease but also a change in patterns – from maternal and child health problems and communicable diseases toward predominance of chronic noncommunicable diseases (NCDs). Furthermore, countries also undergo a *nutrition transition* which typically refers to a move away from problems related to undernutrition toward those attributable to being overweight and obese. In parallel to lifestyle-related transitions, there is also what some have called a *health financing transition*: the tendency for the levels of health expenditure to increase, accompanied by an increase in the domestic publicly financed share of health spending; the flip side is a decline in the external- and OOP-financed share of health spending as national incomes rise [5].

There is strong empirical evidence of a steady increase in resources for health over time: for example, per capita spending levels on health have increased globally from US$706 in 2000 to US$1,132 in 2019, from 5.1% to 5.7% of GDP, respectively, implying that spending levels grew higher than the rate of economic growth over the same period. The average annual increase in per capita current health spending among LICs, LMICs, and UMICs over this period was higher than among HICs, indicating some degree of convergence. Higher levels of current health spending – and a changing composition of financing away from OOP spending and external sources toward a greater share coming from public sources, is also notable, driven by nominal trends in economic growth (Figure 16.2). These trends in health financing are driven by a range of factors, such as institutional development, technological advancements, aging, and changing population preferences.

High levels of OOP spending are correlated with low levels of public financing for health across countries, the latter being a second co-equal challenge facing LMICs (Figure 16.3). High levels of OOP spending are often a result of payments for medicines and diagnostics that are not covered or not available in the public sector due to underfinanced public provision of health

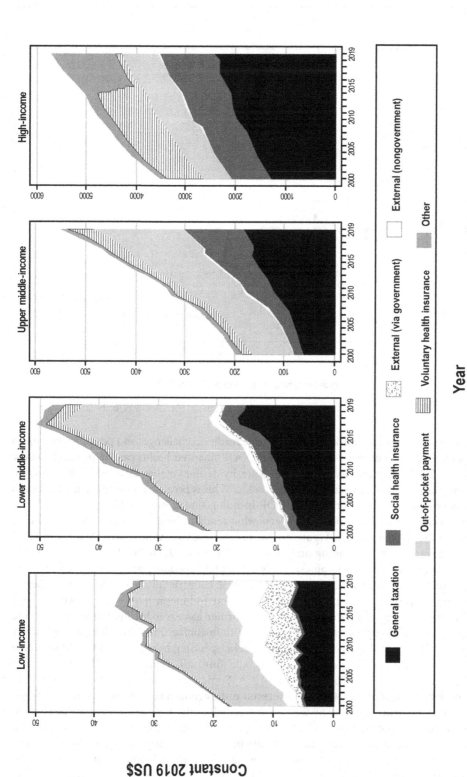

Figure 16.2 Trends in level and composition of health revenues across income groupings, 2000–2019.

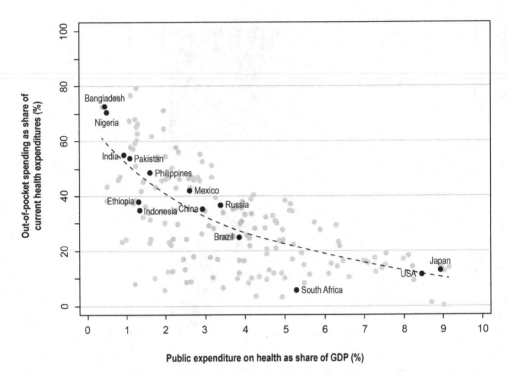

Figure 16.3 Shares of OOP health funding are negatively correlated with public spending on health. Data from 2019.

care, as well as due to other forms of supply-side readiness challenges and poor responsiveness of public facilities that drive people to utilize OOP-financed health care at private facilities. Additionally, the external financing share generally declines earlier than the decline in OOP spending as countries move up the income ladder. This is because public financing for health does not increase enough to crowd out OOP spending among most L&MICs.

The health financing transition reflects what tends to happen on average as countries move up the income ladder. Figure 16.4 compares average annual growth rates in OOP spending versus public spending on health over the period 2000–2019. In many countries, such as Bangladesh, the Philippines, and Nigeria, OOP spending has grown at a faster rate than public spending on health, implying that these countries are regressing in their health financing transition. Countries such as China and Indonesia have seen growth in both public and OOP spending for health, but the former has exceeded the latter; hence, these countries are making progress toward their health financing transition albeit at a relatively slow rate. Finally, we have countries where public spending has grown and OOP spending has declined; these countries – which include Burundi, Kenya, and Thailand – have undergone a rapid health financing transition. Some care in interpretation is needed to ensure that the decline in OOP is not a result of foregone care and that the rise in public spending is not being captured by the rich. Nevertheless, this kind of landscaping can help to monitor the composition of health financing across countries over time. It also makes it clear that the level of public spending in health influences not only total expenditure but also its structure and, with it, the incentives faced by populations and by providers. Understanding the drivers of public spending is key to guiding advocacy efforts.

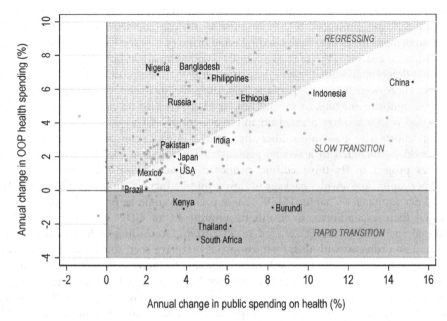

Figure 16.4 Comparing growth rates of OOP vs. public spending for health, 2000–2019.

The following section discusses the three dimensions of the expansion of health coverage: services, population, and cost, and how this could be done in a manner to ensure pro-poor strategies (see the UHC cube in Chapter 3).

16.3 Expanding Service Coverage

The notion of UHC includes the idea of providing a core set of good-quality health services to which all citizens and residents are entitled, regardless of their circumstances [6]. The journey to UHC is long, and at every step countries must decide how to expand the benefits offered to these individuals. In this section we describe the benefits package (BP) that L&MICs are promising as an entitlement to these individuals, and we discuss how much consensus there is across countries regarding what benefits to add to the package at each step (see also Chapter 15). We find that there is much policy convergence regarding the initial composition of the BP, but there is no consensus and much policy divergence regarding the expansion of the package beyond the initial step.

Two studies that sought to compare BPs across countries defined it as the list of benefits for which government policy is to make them available (1) to all individuals; and (2) at no cost at the point of use. Using this definition, a study of 46 African countries found a high degree of policy convergence in that region in 2018: over 85% of African countries offered a BP that included child immunizations and interventions to fight HIV/AIDs, malaria, and tuberculosis [7]. It also found a lower but still significant degree of consensus regarding the inclusion of reproductive and child care interventions (60%). Another study comparing 24 L&MICs found that a similar consensus had been reached by countries from all world regions: 19 of these countries had a BP that included interventions to fight communicable diseases and reproductive, maternal, and child health care [8].

In all these countries, the debate about advancing UHC refers to expanding the benefits beyond the existing universal BP. Among the 46 African countries studied, 10 countries expanded benefits for all citizens by adding other primary care services to the list of services provided at no charge to the user. Six countries added inpatient hospital services, and the rest chose different combinations of outpatient, inpatient, diagnostic, and pharmaceutical benefits. There were no clear patterns regarding the inclusion of emergency services, surgery, diagnostic imaging, or mental health. There are also no clear patterns regarding how to deal with secondary prevention and treatment of NCDs.

Many efforts have gone into studies attempting to create a consensus about the benefits that should be included in a second-generation BP. For example, the Disease Control Priorities project in its third edition proposed a package for LICs that would cost US$42 per capita, and a wider package for lower middle-income countries (LMICs) costing US$110 per capita (see Chapter 15) [9]. These packages could be financed if governments increased their expenditures in health by around 3% of GDP and channeled all the additional spending to the BP offered to all citizens. According to historical evidence, there are two problems with this. First, countries that have been able to suddenly increase health expenditures rapidly have still only been able to increase it by a fraction of that; and second, only a fraction of government spending is allocated to the basic package as governments face strong pressure to allocate additional resources to politically expedient uses. Governments that increase their expenditure by less than such an amount, say by "only" 20%, are left with no guidance regarding what benefits to increase next in the BP.

What the empirical studies have shown is that countries choose a path that involves much smaller increments in public health expenditures. Given this constraint, instead of expanding the BP for the entire population, they are channeling the incremental funds to the creation of systems that provide broader benefits to subsets of the population. Often, this is done by creating contributory health insurance schemes. In Africa in 2017, 60% of countries had created a contributory SHI system providing mandatory coverage for civil servants, and in some cases also for private sector payroll workers. In addition to the creation of contributory schemes, 80% of countries had implemented schemes that exempted vulnerable groups from the payment of user fees for broader benefit packages than those offered by the BP. While these programs are often criticized for adding to the fragmentation of the health system, it is important to recognize that they are now an important part of the landscape of health systems in the African context.

16.4 Expanding Population Coverage

At the onset of UHC reforms, many countries became aware that public health spending was significantly pro-rich, with countries spending more public funds on the better-off than on lower income populations. The studies also showed an important caveat: some service platforms were more utilized by the poor than others. Specifically, in country after country the evidence showed that services provided by community and primary care clinics were more accessible to low-income populations and were often not utilized by the better-off [10]. By contrast, higher-complexity hospitals in urban areas tended to serve the better-off to a larger extent than they served the poor [11]. Faced with this information, countries chose from two pro-poor paths: some chose to introduce reforms that would make hospitals and higher-complexity services more accessible to low-income populations; this required what is known in the field as "separating financing and provision" by creating health insurance schemes for low-income populations (see Chapter 17). The second group chose to expand and improve the service platforms that already served low-income populations; these countries continued to operate with "integrated health systems" (i.e., systems that do not separate financing and provision).

One-quarter of the countries in Figure 16.1, including most of the LICs studied, but also countries such as Brazil and Malaysia, decided to expand the platforms that were already serving low-income populations. Typically, they chose a path that expanded community and primary care services to rural and peri-urban populations. In some cases, these programs also included low-complexity urban hospitals. Financing for these programs uses the classic model of Ministries of Health allocating inputs to public facilities that are essentially budgetary units of the ministry itself. These countries aimed to expand the capacity of health care providers to increase the volume and quality of services. In 80% of the countries studied there were reforms that introduced health insurance for low-income populations. A key objective of these reforms was to overcome the economic barrier that limits the access of low-income populations to hospitals and other high-complexity services. Low income populations have little access to them because of the existence of a cost at the point of use. The solution chosen by these countries consists of the implementation of an insurance scheme that pays health care providers for services delivered to the low-income populations. While in conventional SHI revenues are obtained from payroll contributions, health insurance schemes for these populations are almost always fully financed by the government through general taxes.

Typically, health insurance provides coverage for an enrolled population. Pro-poor health insurance reforms require identifying and enrolling low-income populations. In the last 30 years, many L&MICs have developed "social registries" [12]; these are systems typically managed by social assistance agencies that identify and maintain lists of poor households or individuals for use by anti-poverty programs, such as cash transfers. Typically, these registries initially use simple systems to identify the poor; the most common are: (1) community-based targeting which uses a group of community leaders to decide who in the community is eligible; (2) demographic targeting which uses age and gender as a proxy for vulnerability; (3) proxy means tests which generate a score for households based on easily observable household characteristics; and (4) means-test targeting which seeks to collect nearly complete information on household income and wealth [12].

An area of policy divergence across countries implementing pro-poor health insurance is with regards to what subpopulations should receive a subsidy, and what subpopulations should fully pay the cost of their insurance. Most countries studied require that the costs of insurance for the families of civil servants and formal sector wage earners be fully financed with payroll taxes (see Chapter 17). At the other end of the income pyramid, all countries studied fully subsidize health coverage for the poor. There is, however, a fierce debate regarding the fairness and sustainability of subsidizing coverage for "the missing middle," an income group that combines the near-poor and the nonpoor informal sector workers. Many countries initially created schemes exclusively for the poor, including Georgia, India (RSBY, later PMJAY), Indonesia, Peru, Tunisia, the Philippines, and Vietnam. Most of these countries later expanded eligibility of the subsidized schemes to include the near-poor – a population that is close to but above the poverty line and who are at high risk of being pushed below the poverty line by a medical emergency. Expanding coverage to the near-poor may seem uncontroversial, but this step is often politically challenging even in HICs. For example, in the United States the Medicaid scheme provided insurance for the poor for many decades; its mandate was expanded by "Obamacare" to cover the near-poor only recently, and while this change benefited tens of millions of people, it was subject to huge political controversy.

The debate surrounding coverage of the nonpoor is even fiercer. Most L&MICs have not been able to cover the nonpoor informal sector population to date. Among those that have are Argentina, Colombia, Mexico, and Thailand, which opted to tax-subsidize their coverage. Other countries, including Chile, Costa Rica, Turkey, and China, made significant progress at covering these populations by developing capabilities to make it possible to collect contributions from these nonpoor populations. The studies identified the existence of a pattern linking subsidy policy with the placement of a scheme in relation to the SHI agency: in countries where there is an autonomous agency (Table 16.2) managing the scheme for low-income populations, the coverage of the fully subsidized schemes is often rapidly extended to all populations not covered by the SHI, including the nonpoor. By contrast, in countries where the scheme is embedded with SHI (Table 16.2), it is politically harder to fully subsidize the nonpoor because this creates a feeling of unfairness with the formal sector populations. Instead, in these countries, the nonpoor are offered partial subsidies and SHI makes a stronger effort to develop capacities to charge a premium to the nonpoor.

The use of different systems to finance health insurance for different groups sometimes leads to fragmentation. Although theoretically the benefits of single risk pools should outweigh those of fragmented systems (see Chapters 5 and 17), the empirical evidence about the impact of fragmentation is mixed. Countries with single pools (funds covering health services for the entire population of the country) sometimes redistribute toward the poor, while others redistribute toward the rich. Costa Rica pooled revenues from contributory and subsidized populations and spent them in pro-poor ways: the poorest 20% of the population received over 30% of pooled expenditure benefits. Ghana and Jamaica pooled contributory and noncontributory revenues and the incidence of benefits was generally pro-rich [8]. Furthermore, anecdotal evidence suggests that many of the new SHI schemes recently created in sub-Saharan Africa collect small contributions from civil servants and combine them with large subsidies theoretically directed to vulnerable populations, but that in practice are directed to civil servants. Also, some countries with fragmented pools, including Mexico, Colombia, and Thailand, expanded coverage and improved health system outcomes. Some of these countries, including Colombia and Tunisia, explicitly cross-subsidized the lower income pools with transfers financed by the higher income pools.

Fragmentation can also occur because of the existence of myriad financing flows – private OOP, domestically financed public financing, external financing that is channeled outside of the government budget, etc. In addition, within public financing there are often

Table 16.2 Publicly financed health insurance schemes for low-income populations

New and existing schemes	Country examples
▪ Managed by autonomous agencies	▪ Argentina, Colombia, Mexico, Thailand, and Peru
▪ Embedded within existing SHI agencies	▪ Ghana, Kyrgyzstan, the Philippines, Vietnam, Chile, and Costa Rica

different streams for covering vertical programs such as immunization and HIV and TB treatments, separate schemes for coverage for the poor and the formal sector, and a general lack of integration and complementarity of public and private financing. Whereas in the short term some of this fragmentation may be necessary to ensure that funds are used as intended for specific programs, sustained levels of fragmentation contribute to inefficiencies, resulting in duplication and unnecessary administrative burdens, and can present barriers to planning and accountability at the systems level.

16.5 Expanding Financial Protection

All UHC-related reforms in recent decades aim to reduce OOP payments at the time and place of seeking care. In general, one type of policy convergence that has been observed across countries has been exemptions for any cost-sharing for the poor and, in some cases, small payments made to the poor to offset transport and other costs of seeking care. Some L&MICs, including Indonesia, Bhutan, and Sri Lanka, do not levy any copayments for publicly financed services regardless of beneficiary income status.

Nevertheless, despite attempts at expanding publicly financed coverage, one of the biggest challenges that continues to be faced by L&MICs is that private OOP financing remains the largest source of financing for health. OOP financing is both inequitable and inefficient and implies that risks are not pooled, exposing individuals or households to large and often unanticipated financial shocks by enhancing the risk of impoverishment when someone utilizes health services in the event of illness. OOP payments can also deter and delay seeking necessary utilization, especially among the poor, at the same time exacerbating existing inequalities. Foregone care, especially among the poor, is a key consequence of OOP-financed health systems. Furthermore, OOP payments, if associated with a fee-for-service modality for provider payments, inherently incentivize overutilization and reduce the potential for using monopsony power of the purchaser (a market condition in which there is only one buyer) to contain costs and improve system efficiency. In addition, OOP payments constrain the redistributive capacity of health financing systems – from the healthy to the sick and from the well-off to the poor.

At the country level there is a strong correlation between the extent to which health systems are financed from OOP and the extent of financial risk protection: the incidence of both catastrophic and impoverishing OOP expenditures. Catastrophic OOP expenditures are typically defined as occurring when households spend more than 10% (or 25%) of their budget on health, resulting in different estimates of financial hardship; impoverishing OOP expenditures are those that push households either below or further below a defined poverty line (see Chapter 3). The latest estimates for 2017 indicate that, globally, almost one billion individuals experienced catastrophic OOP expenditures exceeding 10% of their budget, with more than one-quarter of that number experiencing OOP expenditures that exceeded 25% of their budget (290 million) [13]. Countries with some of the greatest incidence of catastrophic spending include India, Nepal, Afghanistan, Egypt, Cambodia, Uganda, and Tajikistan. Countries that have made the most progress toward UHC have OOP spending levels that are usually less than 15–20% of total health spending, a threshold benchmark recommended by WHO [14] (e.g., as is the case in high-income OECD countries) or where OOP spending – despite being higher than the 15–20% threshold – is largely incident on well-off segments of the population and therefore is no longer a significant risk factor for impoverishment (e.g., Malaysia and Sri Lanka) [15, 16].

Low levels of public financing for health are typically a function of three key factors: (1) the overall size of the economy; (2) the revenue-raising capacity and the size of the governments within the economy; and (3) the prioritization of health within the government budgets (see Box 16.2). Levels of public financing for health are strongly correlated with the size of the economy and with levels of national income across countries (Figure 16.5). Countries that have experienced high levels of economic growth generally

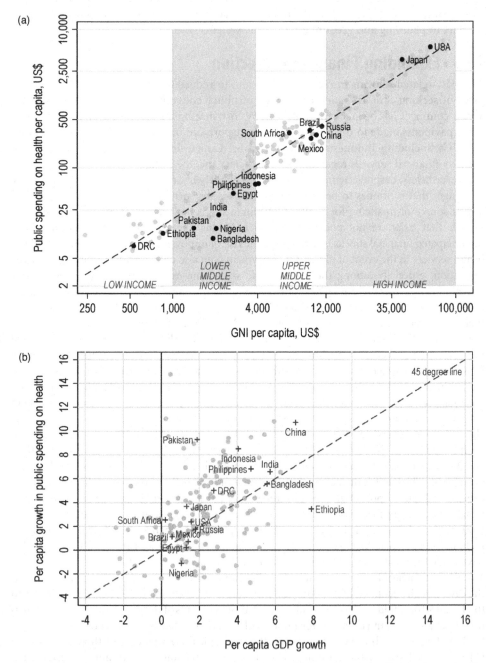

Figure 16.5 The strong relationship between the size and growth of the economy and public spending on health.

see levels of public financing for health increase at faster rates. India is a case in point: although levels of public financing for health remain far below those expected for its income level, and have remained stagnant at roughly 1% of GDP, relatively high economic growth rates have resulted in a doubling of real public financing for health in per capita terms since 2009 – from roughly US$11 to US$21 in 2019 [17]. On the flip side, L&MICs on a lower-growth trajectory (e.g., Nigeria, Mexico, Russia, and Brazil) have faced a more constrained environment for increasing public financing for health. Per capita public spending for health in Nigeria declined from US$15 in 2009 to US$13 in 2019, partly because of the negative economic growth that the country experienced during this period.

A second factor that impacts levels and growth of public financing for health (and, in fact, for all other sectors) is the revenue-generating capacity of governments. Lower income countries tend to have lower levels of economic activity but also raise lower levels of government revenues as a share of their economies, in part due to higher levels of poverty and informality and lower institutional and other capacities to collect "direct" taxes (i.e., taxes on income, profits, property, or wealth). Whereas in HICs, general government revenue is more than 35% of GDP, it is less than 20% in LICs (Figure 16.7a). Even within country income groups (Figure 16.7b) there are large variations; at <10% of GDP, government revenues are especially low in countries such as Nigeria and Bangladesh, constraining their ability to publicly finance spending across all sectors, including health. Even though deficit financing can offset some of

---

Box 16.2 Decomposition of Changes in Levels and Composition of Per Capita Public Spending on Health, 2000–2019

Drivers of public spending for health can be assessed by looking at decompositions in terms of changes in:

1. the *levels* due to three macro-fiscal drivers: (a) economic growth, (b) total public spending, and (c) priority to health; and
2. the *structure* in terms of the shares of: (a) on-budget external financing for health, (b) SHI contributions, and (c) financing from domestic government budgetary sources.

Accordingly, per capita public spending on health in any country for a given year t (P_t) must equal:

$$P_t = H_t \cdot G_t \cdot Y_t = E_t + S_t + D_t,$$

where H_t is the share of total government spending going to health; G_t is the total government spending share of GDP; Y_t is the per capita GDP; E_t is the external financing for health channeled via the government budget; S_t is the SHI contributions; and D_t is the domestic government budgetary spending for health.

Using decomposition methods elaborated by Das Gupta [18], Figure 16.6 shows the annual growth rate in per capita public spending on health decomposed into macro-fiscal drivers (left-hand side) and changes in composition (right-hand side). Annual growth rates exceed 3% for LICs, LMICs, and UMICs, which is higher than the annual growth rates for HICs. Economic growth was the biggest contributor, and together with changes in total public spending were the predominant drivers of increases in per capita public spending for health in all the groups. Reprioritization for health played a relatively minor role, except among HICs. While most of the increase came from domestic budgetary financing for health, there were significant differences between country groups. For LICs, external financing was dominant in driving the increase in spending. For UMICs, SHI contributions played a large role.

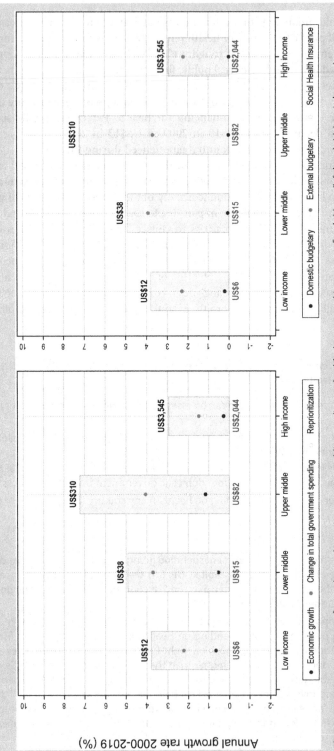

Figure 16.6 Decomposition of annual growth rate in per capita public spending on health decomposed into macro-fiscal drivers (left-hand side) and changes in composition (right-hand side).

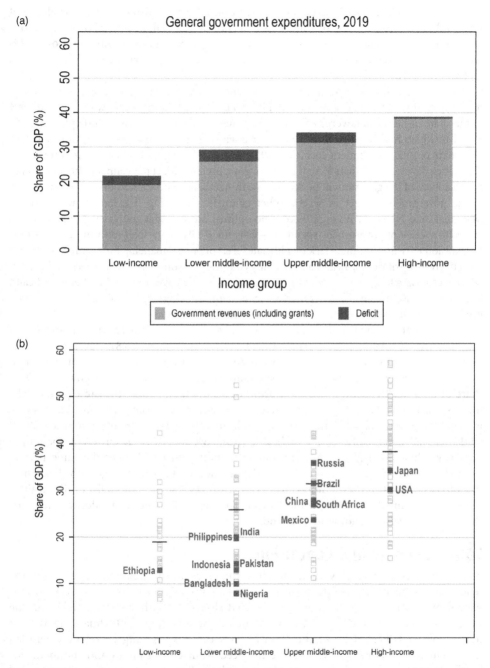

Figure 16.7 Share of general government expenditures in GDP (a) across income groups and (b) for selected countries.

the challenges of low revenues in the short run, longer-term constraints will re-emerge from future debt servicing needs. Sustained improvements in revenue generation will be necessary for some countries to enable additional public financing.

Challenges related to persistent and large informal sectors also constrain the ability of LICs and LMICs to use SHI contributions as a core source of financing: SHI contributions from those insured stand at only 2% of total health spending among LICs and only 11% among LMICs; this is a sharp contrast with UMICs, where the contribution of SHI increases to 40% (Table 16.1).

Finally, low priority for health in government spending is another reason why levels of public spending on health is low in many LICs and LMICs. Countries vary widely with respect to the share of health in government budgets, a metric that can serve as a crude proxy for the extent to which health is prioritized by governments. Globally, on average health receives an 11% share of total government spending [19]. However, there is a huge range across countries: Costa Rica devotes more than 25% of its entire government budget to health; on the other hand, health's share of the government budget is <3% in Azerbaijan and Cameroon, and receives <5% of the government budget in several other countries, including Bangladesh, Egypt, India, Myanmar, and Nigeria. Although there is no optimal number that countries should aspire to as health's share of government spending – calls for a 15% share for health under the Abuja Declaration notwithstanding – lack of adequate levels of public financing for health results from a relatively low priority for health across many countries. In some cases this is because health is not perceived as a long-term investment in human capital by governments; in other cases health loses out because of expenditure pressures from debt servicing needs, military spending, and pro-rich fossil fuel subsidies, among other competing demands.

The cases of China and Thailand are instructive examples of the relative importance of the different drivers of public expenditures for health (Figure 16.8). Per capita public spending on health in China grew more than 10-fold over 2000–2019 (from US$21 to US$300) following a tripling of public spending share from 1% to 3% of GDP; the OOP share of total health spending declined from over 60% to 35% over the same period. The increase in public financing was facilitated not only by economic growth, but also by increases in government revenues and expenditures (the latter grew from 16% to 34% of GDP) as well as reprioritization of health (from 6% to 9% of government spending). Similarly, Thailand tripled per capita public spending on health over the same period: from US$71 to US$212; 1.7% to 2.7% of GDP. In addition to economic growth, Thailand's size of government in the economy also grew (from 19% to 22% of GDP) as did health's share of government spending (from 13% to 14%). The OOP spending has declined to <10% share of total health spending in Thailand.

16.6 Summary and Conclusion

As incomes rise, countries tend to go through a health financing transition: the tendency for health expenditure to increase as a proportion of the economy accompanied by an increase in the publicly financed share of health spending and a decline in the external- and OOP-financed share of health spending. OOP financing is both inequitable and inefficient. At the country level there is a strong correlation between the extent to which health systems are financed from OOP sources and the incidence both of catastrophic and impoverishing spending. Policy can shape the timing and magnitude of the transition.

Levels of public financing for health are typically a function of three key factors: the overall size of the economy; the size of governments within the economy; and the prioritization of health within government budgets. Using decomposition methods, it has been

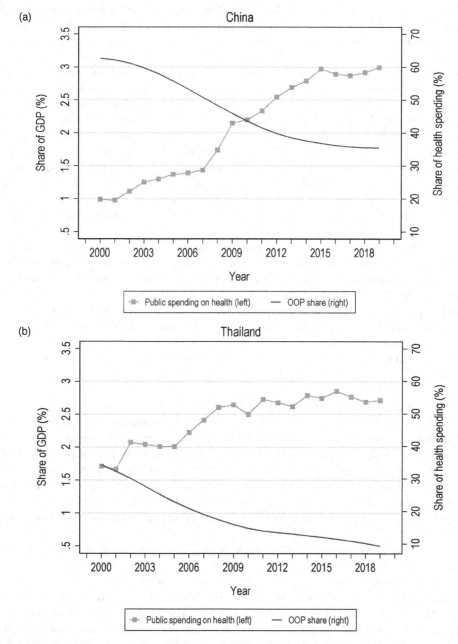

Figure 16.8 Health financing transitions in (a) China and (b) Thailand were facilitated by conducive macroeconomics and reprioritization for health.

shown that the predominant drivers of increases in per capita public spending for health for L&MICs during 2000–2018 were economic growth combined with changes in total public spending. Reprioritization for health played a relatively minor role, except for among HICs.

Regarding health care benefits, most countries have adopted a benefit package that is provided to all citizens at no cost to the user. Across countries there is much convergence about the initial composition of the BP, related to reproductive, maternal, and child health, as well as communicable diseases such as malaria, HIV, and TB. Countries diverge, however, on how to expand benefits beyond this initial package. The recommended packages of benefits for promotive, preventive, curative, rehabilitative, and palliative health services have been estimated to require an increase in health expenditures in LICs equivalent to about 3% of GDP. Countries cannot make such an increase abruptly. Some choose incremental routes for the expansion of benefits for all citizens and diverge in what benefits to include next. Other countries expand widely the list of benefits covered at no cost to the user, but can only do it for fragments of the population. This is usually done by creating contributory and noncontributory health insurance systems that provide broad packages of benefits to specific subpopulations of contributors or of vulnerable people; this choice expands benefits for them but creates fragmentation of the health system.

Regarding population, the pro-poor expansion of coverage involves two paths. Some countries aiming to provide hospital services to the poor implement demand-side reforms separating financing from the delivery of service with the creation of pro-poor health insurance schemes. These systems need to identify and enroll low income populations, and this is usually done with the help of "social or poverty registries" which now exist in most L&MICs after being developed for the use of social assistance programs. Other countries operate on the supply side, expanding platforms and services commonly used by low-income populations; these tend to include the expansion of public providers of community and primary care services.

Some countries implementing health insurance for low-income populations create new agencies, often linked to the Ministry of Health, to manage the scheme; others outsource the management of these schemes to existing SHI agencies originally created to provide insurance to the formal sector. This choice is consequential for the expansion of population coverage to the "missing middle": countries with insurance agencies managed by Ministries of Health tend to rapidly expand tax-financed coverage to the nonpoor in the informal sector. By contrast, countries with schemes embedded in SHI agencies tend to make bigger efforts to collect contributions from the nonpoor.

The use of different systems to finance health insurance for different groups often leads to the fragmentation of the insurance pool. The empirical evidence about the impact of fragmentation is mixed. Some countries with single pools redistribute toward the poor while others redistribute toward the better-off. There are indications that many of the SHI schemes recently created in sub-Saharan Africa to pool civil servants with vulnerable populations have a design that results in large subsidies for civil servants. Also, many countries with fragmented pools successfully channeled subsidies to the poor, expanding their coverage and improving health system outcomes.

It is important to end the chapter by reiterating the message that it is not just that levels of public financing need to increase across many L&MICs, it is also that these resources need to be allocated in ways to improve effective service coverage while reducing or realigning OOP spending so that financial risk protection improves, especially for the poor. Increasing levels of public financing – but also improving efficiency and equity – are core strategies for helping countries accelerate progress toward UHC. Countries cannot just spend their way to UHC.

References

1. World Bank Group. High-performance health financing for universal health coverage: driving sustainable, inclusive growth in the 21st century. 2019. www.worldbank.org/en/topic/universalhealthcoverage/publication/high-performance-health-financing-for-universal-health-coverage-driving-sustainable-inclusive-growth-in-the-21st-century (accessed October 17, 2020).

2. D. R. Gwatkin, A. Ergo. Universal health coverage: friend or foe of health equity? *Lancet* 2011; **377**(9784): 2160–2161.

3. World Health Organization. Global Health Expenditure Database. 2020. https:/apps.who.int/nha/database/Select/Indicators/en (accessed October 18, 2020).

4. World Bank Group. Universal health coverage study series: 2013 through 2019. https://openknowledge.worldbank.org/handle/10986/13083/discover?filtertype_1=title&filter_relational_operator_1=contains&filter_1=&rpp=10 (accessed November 10, 2021).

5. V. Y. Fan, W. D. Savedoff. The health financing transition: a conceptual framework and empirical evidence. *Soc Sci Med* 2014; **105**: 112–121.

6. A. Glassman, U. Giedion, P. C. Smith. What's in, what's out: designing benefits for universal health coverage – key messages for donors and advocates. 2017. https://f1000research.com/documents/6-1864 (accessed October 15, 2020).

7. D. Cotlear, N. Rosemberg. Going universal in Africa: how 46 African countries reformed user fees and implemented health care priorities. Universal Health Coverage Studies 26. 2018. https://openknowledge.worldbank.org/handle/10986/29177 (accessed October 12, 2020).

8. D. Cotlear, S. Nagpal, O. Smith, et al. Going universal: how 24 developing countries are implementing universal health coverage

from the bottom up. 2015. https://openknowledge.worldbank.org/bitstream/handle/10986/22011/9781464806100.pdf (accessed October 11, 2020).

9. D. T. Jamison, H. Gelband, S. Horton, et al., eds., *Disease Control Priorities*, 3rd ed. Washington, DC, World Bank, 2018.

10. A. Asante, J. Price, A. Hayen, et al. Equity in health care financing in low- and middle-income countries: a systematic review of evidence from studies using benefit and financing incidence analyses. *PLoS One* 2016; **11**(4): e0152866.

11. A. Wagstaff, M. Bilger, L. Buisman, et al. Who benefits from government health spending and why? A global assessment. 2014. https://openknowledge.worldbank.org/handle/10986/20376 (accessed October 16, 2020).

12. P. Leite, T. George, C. Sun, et al. Social registries for social assistance and beyond: a guidance note and assessment tool. 2017. https://openknowledge.worldbank.org/handle/10986/28284 (accessed October 14, 2020).

13. World Health Organization, World Bank. Tracking universal health coverage: 2021 Global monitoring report: conference edition. 2021. https://cdn.who.int/media/docs/default-source/world-health-data-platform/events/tracking-universal-health-coverage-2021-global-monitoring-report_uhc-day.pdf?sfvrsn=fd5c65c6_5&download=true (accessed January 29, 2022).

14. World Health Organization. *The World Health Report 2010: Health Systems Financing, the Path to Universal Coverage*. Geneva, World Health Organization, 2010. www.who.int/publications/i/item/9789241564021 (accessed January 29, 2022).

15. W. A. Yap, I. Razif, S. Nagpal. Malaysia: a new public clinic built every four days. 2019. https://openknowledge

.worldbank.org/handle/10986/34668 (accessed January 29, 2022).

16. O. Smith. Sri Lanka: achieving pro-poor universal health coverage without health financing reforms. 2018. https://open knowledge.worldbank.org/handle/10986/29175 (accessed January 29, 2022).

17. A. Tandon, J. Cain, C. Kurowski, et al. From slippery slopes to steep hills: contrasting landscapes of economic growth and public spending for health. *Soc Sci Med* 2020; **259**: 113171.

18. P. D. Gupta. Standardization and decomposition of rates: a user's manual. 1993. www2.census.gov/library/publica tions/1993/demographics/p23-186.pdf (accessed January 29, 2022).

19. World Health Organization. *Global Expenditure on Health: Public Spending on the Rise?* Geneva, World Health Organization, 2021. https://apps.who.int/iris/bitstream/handle/10665/350560/97892 40041219-eng.pdf (accessed January 4, 2022).

Health Insurance for Advancing Universal Health Coverage

Disentangling Its Complexities

Eduardo Banzon

Key Messages

- Prepayment arrangements are a prerequisite to ensure the financial protection goal of universal health coverage (UHC). Prepayment could be implemented using alternative institutional arrangements, including social and national health insurance.

- Many high-income countries (HICs) have implemented social health insurance (SHI) to achieve UHC, and several low- and middle-income countries (L&MICs) are exploring context-relevant modalities of SHI as they reform their health financing systems toward UHC.

- Initial forms of SHI implemented in L&MICs were linked to employment and financed by employer and employee contributions/premiums, similar to what had been practiced in HICs. Nevertheless, the prevalent informal sector and the significant number of people in poverty compromised the capacity of SHI to cover the whole population and advance UHC.

- In response, many L&MICs use tax revenues to subsidize health services for their informal sector workers and their dependents, as well as those who are unable to contribute to the formal SHI arrangement. We refer to such advanced mixed form of SHI as national health insurance (NHI).

- Today, many countries are designing and implementing NHI schemes as their primary mechanism to pursue and achieve UHC.

- NHI arrangements have many advantages, but countries need to build up capacities to implement their functions.

17.1 UHC and the Power of Pooled Funds

Universal health coverage means that all people and communities can use the promotive, preventive, curative, rehabilitative, and palliative health services they need, of sufficient quality to be effective, while also ensuring that the use of these services does not expose the user to financial hardship [1]. Pursuing and achieving UHC means fulfilling the three key objectives of ensuring: (1) equity in access to health services, wherein everyone who needs services gets them, not only those who can pay for them; (2) quality of the health services provided; and (3) financial protection for those who are using health services (Chapter 3).

Universal health coverage is essentially a reiteration of how health systems have been keeping people healthy, treating the sick, and protecting families against financial ruin from medical bills. Countries have designed their health systems in different ways, but aim to keep their populations healthy and provide accessible and affordable treatment to all those who need care, irrespective of their cultural, economic, historical, geographic, and other contexts.

Achieving and sustaining UHC requires a range of reforms in health service delivery, health stewardship, and health financing. In particular, health financing reforms are needed to determine: (1) how resources or funds for health are raised; (2) the extent of pooling of funds that will ensure social solidarity; (3) how to strengthen the purchasing power and capacity of the purchaser; and (4) the strategies to modify behaviors of patients and health care providers (see Chapter 5).

17.2 Concept of Prepayment, Pooling, and Purchasing

Universal health coverage requires increased reliance on *prepayments* in financing health services, which are funds or resources raised ex-ante (in advance) to pay for or purchase health services on behalf of the users. Prepayments can be in the form of taxation, health insurance contributions/premiums, or individual/household health saving accounts. All these prepayments are different from payments at the point of delivery, which are usually paid by households out of their pocket.

Prepayment through taxation or insurance usually results in the *pooling of funds*, which is usually managed by government institutions or insurance organizations which purchase health services on behalf of designated or assigned populations. Pooling enables risk sharing among people of different socioeconomic levels, health risk, employment status, age, and other characteristics. While they aim to share financial risk over time, individual/household health saving accounts do not contribute to the pooling of funds because of their individual nature.

The holders of pooled prepaid funds have the ability to negotiate with health care providers and demand higher-quality care for lower tariffs, rates, or fee schedules. This purchasing and negotiating power is strengthened when funds include prepayments from a large number of people. It is, therefore, best to have the prepayments pooled into as few funded pools as possible.

The nature of the pooled funds generally influences their respective *provider payment arrangements* (see Chapter 18). If the funds are pooled as *government revenues*, provider payments are usually done as budgetary allocations for the salaries of health care providers, and line-item budgets for health goods including medicines, operating expenses of health facilities and hospitals, and capital expenditures. If the funds are pooled into *health insurance funds* that pay for health services, payments for health care providers are usually based on fee-for-service, case rates, per capita, or combinations of these payment methods.

17.3 Health Care Models from a Financing Perspective

Given the wide range of health care system designs that have evolved in countries striving toward UHC, different types of financing options need consideration. One approach is to present them as either the Beveridge, Semashko, or Bismarck models [2]. This approach has particular relevance from the perspective of health financing and the evolution of health insurance arrangements.

The *Beveridge model* [3] is named after Lord William Beveridge who, in the 1942 Beveridge Report, proposed that the National Health Service, financed by the government through income tax payments, would ensure provision of health care services for all people in the United Kingdom. The *Semashko model* [4], named after Nikolai Semashko, who was People's Commissar of Public Health of the former Soviet Union from 1918 to 1930, proposed a centralized government-run health system where government-financed health services are provided to all people by doctors and other health providers employed by the government, in hospitals and health facilities owned and run by the government. The *Bismarck model* [5] is named after Chancellor Otto von Bismarck of Germany. In this model, health services are jointly financed by employers and employees through payroll deductions, also known as social health insurance (SHI). Table 17.1 presents the key features of the three models.

Table 17.1 Comparative analysis of the health care models from a financing perspective

	Beveridge model	Semashko model	Bismarck model
Year and country of introduction	Lord William Beveridge proposed the National Health Service in the United Kingdom in 1942	Nikolai Semashko, People's Commissar of Public Health, Soviet Union (1918–1930), proposed a totally government-run centralized health system	Chancellor Otto von Bismarck of Germany created in 1883 an SHI model financed jointly by employers and employees through payroll deductions
Governance/ regulation	Hospitals and ambulatory health facilities are owned, regulated, and managed by the government. Health care providers are mainly government employees but also include private providers paid by the government	Totally government-owned and -run centralized health system	Multiple health insurance funds that are tightly regulated by the government in terms of costs, provider fees, quality, and type of health services
Financing	Financed by government through taxes	The health care system is entirely financed by the government	Financed by payroll deductions from employers and employees. Funds pooled into single or several insurance funds
Eligibility	Usually based on citizenship, although long-term noncitizen residents are also covered	All citizens	Formal sector employees working in the public or private sector
Payer/ purchaser	Government/public sector	Government/public sector	Insurance funds (called "sickness funds")
Provider	Government provider but this has expanded to include contracts with private general practitioners (GPs)	Government-employed health care providers	Mostly private providers
Purchaser–provider split	Limited scope initially, which has progressed to become the predominant mode	None	Contracts with private providers for provision of care to the covered population

17.4 Social Health Insurance

17.4.1 Evolution of SHI in HICs

Social health insurance, or the Bismarckian model, started in Germany with the introduction of the Sickness Insurance Law of 1883. This approach was later adopted by other European countries, such as Belgium, Austria, the Netherlands, Switzerland, and France, and eventually by Japan and Korea. Initially, entitlements were based on one's employment status, but SHI arrangements were eventually expected to cover everybody, with payment into health insurance funds made mandatory for formal sector employees and government subsidies provided for the poor and other vulnerable populations who could not comply with the mandatory health insurance payments. People who are unable to pay the full health insurance contributions, and those from whom it would be difficult to collect contributions, are provided partial or full subsidy by the government based on "means test" estimations. SHI systems usually allow the coexistence of multiple funds or purchasers (Box 17.1).

Today, 87% of Germany's population is covered by SHI or *Gesetzliche Krankenversicherung* (GKV) [7]. Health insurance payments are paid by employers and employees into around 130 public nonprofit "sickness funds." The employer pays half and the employee pays the other half. Self-employed workers and those who are unemployed without benefits must pay the entire health insurance payments themselves. Social welfare beneficiaries (the poor) are enrolled and paid for by municipalities. Benefits are essentially similar across all health insurance funds, but payment rates differ based on complex negotiations that involve social bargaining between specified self-governing bodies (e.g., physicians' associations) and sickness funds at the level of the Länder or federal states. It is noteworthy that most civil servants benefit from a tax-funded government employee benefit scheme covering a percentage of the costs, and they usually get private health insurance coverage to cover the remaining costs (referred to as "complementary health insurance coverage"). Civil servants also get supplementary private health insurance coverage for non-SHI-covered health services, such as prescription glasses and additional dental care (referred to as "supplementary health insurance coverage") [8].

In France, the SHI scheme requires all employed people to pay part of their income to one of the nonprofit health insurance funds [9]. In addition to the payments by employers and employees, the funds are financed by a "*Contribution Sociale Généralisée*" (CSG) [10] from the general population. France's three main funds are: the General Scheme (*Régime général*) [11], which covers employees in commerce and industry and their families (about

---

Box 17.1 What Is a Means Test?

A **means test** assesses the financial status of a person or household to determine eligibility for public assistance. In health insurance, means testing is used to identify and register the poor who have no means to access health services and to make essential health services available to those enrolled in programs.

A **proxy means test** measures income and poverty in many L&MICs with a large informal sector. The concept of proxy means testing is usually understood as using observable characteristics of the household or its members to estimate their income or consumption when other income data (salary slips, tax returns) are unavailable or unreliable [6].

84% of the population); the Agricultural Scheme (*Mutualité sociale agricole*) [12], which covers farmers and agricultural employees and their families (about 7.2% of the population); and the fund for nonagricultural self-employed people (*Caisse national d'assurance maladie* [CNAM], formerly known as *Caisse nationale d'assurance maladie des travailleurs non-salariés* [CNAMTS]) [13], which covers craftsmen and self-employed people (about 5% of the population). Other major funds are those for students. The government also implements the Universal Medical Insurance (*Couverture Maladie Universelle* [CMU])[14], which provides means-tested government-financed health insurance for those who cannot pay for their insurance. In order to ensure that the benefits are harmonized across the different funds, the government sets the payment rate for medical services through yearly negotiations with doctors' representative organizations, while the Ministry of Health directly negotiates prices of medicines with the manufacturers. Almost 85% of the French population also benefits from complementary private health insurance [15] that pays for non-SHI-covered health services, which are provided mostly by nonprofit health funds and are often subsidized by employers.

In Asia, Japan's SHI system is funded primarily by taxes and individual contributions, and is either employment-based or residence-based [16]. The employment-based plans cover about 59% of the population, while the residence-based insurance plans include citizen health insurance plans for nonemployed individuals aged 74 and under, and health insurance for the elderly plans which automatically cover all adults aged 75 and older. There are more than 1,400 employment-based health insurance funds, while each of Japan's 47 prefectures, or regions, has its own residence-based health insurance fund. In order to harmonize benefits across the different health funds, the national government sets the fee schedule for health care providers and gives subsidies to local governments (municipalities and prefectures), insurers, and providers. It also establishes and enforces detailed regulations for insurers and providers. In addition, many Japanese get supplementary or complementary voluntary private health insurance that provides additional income in the case of sickness or hospitalization (usually as a lump sum or in daily payments over a defined period of time), and/or coverage of noncovered health services such as orthodontics. A separate public social assistance program for impoverished people covers the remaining 2% who are uninsured.

17.4.2 SHI Programs in L&MICs

Many developing countries, including Egypt, Indonesia, Iran, Morocco, the Philippines, Thailand, Tunisia, and several Latin American countries, have adopted SHI programs. The adoption of SHI was seen as the initial step to providing health coverage to everyone, with informal sector workers expected to be covered when they become part of the formal sector; otherwise they self-pay their health insurance payments.

However, these countries did not see their formal sector employment expand to the same scale as in Europe and Japan, which has resulted in plateauing of their SHI population coverage. In addition, other key elements for implementing and expanding SHI systems – such as increased wages and salaries and resulting payroll deductions, improved health care provider management capacities, and strengthened government regulatory capabilities – never reached the same level as for Europe and Japan. Beginning in the 1990s, the difficulty in achieving universal population coverage using SHI eventually drove these countries to hybrid models incorporating elements of the Beveridge and Bismarck models, called

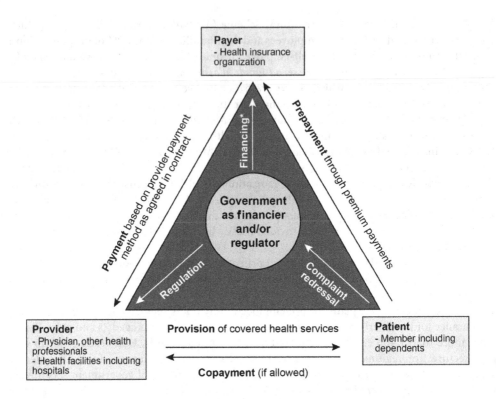

Figure 17.1 Illustrative model of an NHI scheme.

national health insurance (NHI) schemes, universal health insurance, or SHI for UHC. Figure 17.1 illustrates a simple model of the NHI scheme.

17.5 National Health Insurance Schemes

17.5.1 Financing NHI: Taxes, General Revenues, and Payroll Deductions

National health insurance schemes collect from both taxes and general revenues, besides compulsory payroll deduction. Together with their employers, formal sector workers contribute from their payroll into a health insurance fund. Informal sector workers and the rest of the population are partially or fully subsidized into health insurance funds with tax or general government revenues. Workers do not lose their coverage when they lose their formal sector jobs, as they are then deemed entitled to the partial and full subsidies that the informal sector workers and the rest of the population get. Similar to tax-based funding mechanisms, entitlements are based on one's citizenship or place of residence, not on employment status.

17.5.2 Single National Fund: The Desirable Goal

National health insurance usually attempts to pool everyone into a single fund, but not all countries have been able to successfully pool the funds from formal sector employees with those for the rest of the population. Indonesia, the Philippines, and Turkey have been among the few middle-income countries (MICs) that have established single funds or purchasers. Other countries typically have separate funds for the formal sector and for those subsidized by the government. India, Iran, Mexico, Pakistan, and Thailand are among the countries that have kept a few separate funds as part of their NHI schemes.

17.5.3 Independent Health Purchaser

Despite being financed by tax or general government revenues, NHI funds are independent and separate from the general government budget, which continues to directly finance public health services and some population-based interventions. The independence of NHI funds allows an easier split between purchasing and provision functions and allows the purchase of health services from both private and government providers. Table 17.2 provides some examples of NHI programs recently established by L&MICs.

17.5.4 Management Autonomy

National health insurance can take different legal forms. NHI institutions can have various degrees of autonomy, ranging from being departments of Ministries of Health or related ministries, semi-autonomous agencies, or independent corporations. In Asia and the Pacific, countries that have established NHI *corporations*, such as Korea and the Philippines, have been successful at moving toward UHC more quickly. Other countries are progressively providing greater autonomy to their NHI funds, such as the

Table 17.2 National health insurance organizations in selected low- and middle-income countries

Country	National health insurance program	Link
India	National Health Authority, which runs *Pradhan Mantri Jan Arogaya Yojana* (PMJAY)	https://pmjay.gov.in/about/nha
Indonesia	Social Insurance Administration Organization – Health (Badan *Penyelenggara Jaminan Sosial-Kesehatan* – BPJS-K)	https://bpjs-kesehatan.go.id/bpjs
Morocco	National Health Insurance Agency, which runs *Régime d'Assistance Médicale* (RAMED)	www.ramed.ma
Pakistan	Ministry of National Health Services, Regulations and Coordination, which runs the *Sehat Sahulat Programme* (SSP)	www.pmhealthprogram.gov.pk
Philippines	Philippine Health Insurance Corporation	www.philhealth.gov.ph
Tunisia	National Health Insurance Fund (CNAM)	www.cnam.nat.tn/lacaisse.jsp

National Health Insurance Fund in Lao PDR. Examples from other continents demonstrate that alternative legal setups can also be considered – the Bahamas recently introduced an autonomous NHI authority similar to the National Health Insurance Scheme in Ghana.

Government corporations are the most autonomous form of NHI bodies and present a number of advantages [17]: (1) they are owned by the government; (2) they do not have to follow the restrictions of public sector agencies; (3) they can borrow and lend, as well as pay providers freely; (4) they are "off-budget," which frees them from dependency on the Ministry of Finance; (5) they receive government subsidies as tax-based transfers; and (6) they are free from typical personnel, procurement, and budget restrictions, allowing them to put in place incentives and innovative human resource management strategies.

17.5.5 Social Solidarity and Risk Pooling

Similar to SHI and schemes that pool funds, NHI facilitates wealth transfers. Risk pooling transfers wealth from the healthy to the sick. The high-income population is expected to pay more than the low-income population in contributions as well as through their tax payments that fund NHI. Premium differentials transfer wealth from the young and relatively healthy to the old who need greater health care. Subsidies to rural hospitals transfer wealth out of cities and suburbs.

National health insurance facilitates larger pooling of funds and risk sharing between all members and ultimately enhances equitable access to health care. Increasing the scale of operation is recommended in the public economics literature [18] as well as in the health financing field under the motto "bigger is better." The high level of risk and financial pooling increases equity, and the larger health fund increases purchasing power.

17.5.6 Improving Financial Protection

Health insurance protects individuals from unpredictable and potentially financially catastrophic events. The larger health funds and the increased purchasing and market powers allow NHI schemes to provide more comprehensive cover for catastrophic health events. The larger funds also enable NHI schemes to leverage their market power to obtain price concessions from hospitals, physicians, and other health professionals. Covered or insured patients can also benefit from these discounts when making copayments. Settling the level and type of payments to providers a priori is usually essential for securing pre-admission authorizations from the pooled funds before an elective hospital admission will be considered for coverage and be paid for or purchased. The same might be required for a mandatory consultation with primary care providers before a specialist outpatient consultation or an elective hospital admission.

17.5.7 Enhanced Transparency and Accountability

National health insurance facilitates grievance-redressal mechanisms (or channels of complaints), and patient satisfaction surveys ensure that providers receive feedback on their performance and quality of care [19]. NHI schemes can be a perfect means to improve patients' access to information and implement feedback independent of the government. This contributes to members feeling a sense of ownership and acceptability. However, factors such as population literacy are important for beneficiaries to become fully empowered.

National health insurance also creates a climate of social acceptability to generate more financial resources for UHC and can be a catalyst in mobilizing earmarked taxes for health and UHC, as experienced in the Philippines [20]. The presence of a visible single NHI fund offers the capacity to absorb and manage the additional revenues for UHC.

17.5.8 Increased Use of Information Technologies

The need for data to manage NHI schemes has led to increased investment in information technologies (IT), and the harmonization of standards and interoperability of related systems to help improve the processing of claims submission and payment. This has led to innovative approaches in expanding the use of IT, including the accreditation of health IT providers.

17.5.9 Protected Health Funds

In a typical government setup, savings from the health budget are returned to the national treasury at the end of the budgetary cycle. This potentially diverts unspent resources to other sectors. Annual budgets do not provide the incentive for the Ministry of Health and its institutions to improve their performance as these are not linked to outcomes. NHI schemes can carry over funds to the next year even if they remain unutilized.

17.5.10 Contracting and Payment Arrangements with Public and Private Providers

A contract specifies the type and quality of services to be provided, which reflects the purchaser's health objectives based on the health needs of the population, by stating which services to provide and under what terms. Contracting fosters competition among public and private providers and results in cost-containment, as well as improved utilization, as can be seen in the value-based payment mechanisms used in the case of Turkey (Box 17.2).

Box 17.2 Value-Based Payments for Improved Access to Primary Care Services in Turkey [21]

Beginning in 2008, the existing health insurance schemes in Turkey were merged into general health insurance with a unified risk pool and harmonized benefits package. The Social Security Institution was the implementer of the Health Transformation Program (HTP), aiming at improving access and utilization of services and moving toward universal population coverage.

With the HTP, primary care service delivery was reorganized in 2005 under a new system of family medicine. Family health centers were new health care facilities operated by one or more family physicians and family health personnel. They provided primary care services which were free at the point of care, including: immunization; follow-up for pregnant, recently delivered, and childbearing age women; infants and children health care; and school health and similar services. In order to benefit from the system, patients had to register with a family physician and were not allowed to change physician for six months. For every patient registered, the physician received a capitation fee from the insurer, up to a maximum of 4,000 patients. The insurer could penalize physicians up to US$220 for any misbehavior or for failing to offer, for example, breastfeeding and contraceptive advice, growth and development monitoring, or immunization for children up to two years old.

These efforts led to increased utilization of primary care services by 3.3 times between 2002 and 2011 (from 74.8 million primary care visits to 244.3 million). This was partly due to a system of incentives for both physicians (to register more patients) and patients in terms of their improved health-seeking behavior due to minimal or no out-of-pocket expenditure.

> **Box 17.3** PhilHealth in the Philippines: Expanding Service Delivery through Private Sector Accreditation [22]
>
> The Philippine Health Insurance Corporation (PhilHealth) has been mandated by the Filipino government to manage the National Health Insurance Program since 1995. It guarantees access to quality health services for all, while pooling revenues from the government, premium contributions, and excise taxes. The Sin Tax Law and later reforms (2004 and 2012) introduced the obligation to allocate incremental revenues from excise taxes to health services (85% of incremental revenues).
>
> *To fulfill its mandate of ensuring access to quality services for all, PhilHealth uses accreditation as a quality assurance mechanism.* Accreditation means verifying the qualifications and capabilities of health care providers in accordance with the guidelines, standards, and procedures set by PhilHealth. This obliges public and private providers to fulfill minimum standards of quality and effectiveness. In particular, the case-based payments implemented by PhilHealth induce private providers to participate in the scheme.

17.5.11 Improved Quality of Care

The strategic payment mechanisms and nonfinancial incentives used by NHI schemes facilitate the implementation of quality assurance mechanisms, which in turn foster appropriate design and management and adequate equipping and staffing of facilities as a necessary requirement for private providers wishing to engage with the NHI schemes (Box 17.3). This contributes to improving quality on the path to UHC.

17.5.12 Comparison of NHI with Other Schemes

Another way to appreciate NHI is to compare it with other prepayment arrangements, as presented in Table 17.3.

17.6 Designing and Implementing NHI Schemes

17.6.1 Effective Governance of NHI Schemes

The effective governance of NHI schemes requires the development and implementation of explicit policies that clearly describe the roles and expected actions of Ministries of Health, the NHI agencies, health care providers, and beneficiary members. It requires robust information systems to detect and correct fraud, inappropriate behavior, and other undesirable trends in a timely manner. It needs data analytics to ensure transparency and accountability mechanisms and to help promote behavioral change. It requires information management systems that will enable and facilitate reporting of health care providers and institutionalize monitoring and evaluation (Box 17.4).

17.6.2 Membership and Fund Management

With NHI schemes designed to cover everyone, the challenge for countries has been how to bring in and cover the informal sector, the poor, and other vulnerable groups of the population. In nearly all developing countries that are implementing NHI, they have done this by building on the formal sector scheme financed by payroll taxes and using tax

Table 17.3 Comparison of different types of insurance schemes

Attributes	National health insurance	Social health insurance	Private health insurance	Community health insurance
Funding	Payroll deductions paid by employers and employees for formal sector workers Tax and general revenues for poor and also nonpoor informal sector	Payroll deductions paid by employers and employees	Usually, employee benefit scheme for formal sector with some employees paying a share of the premium Self-payments for voluntary members	Self-payments for members Maybe partly financed by development partners or other external financing
Membership	Based on citizenship Sometimes long-term residency	Linked to employment and usually mandatory	Linked to employment but usually voluntary for the employers	Community-based and voluntary
Pooling	Single national pool, as much as possible	Multiple pools are usually based on employer type	Pooled according to an agreement with private health insurance providers	Pooled per defined community
Health care providers	Government or private	Government or private	Usually private	Government or private
Management	Usually autonomous NHI organization	Maybe a government agency or an autonomous government insurance organization	Private health insurance companies	Community organizations
Examples	UC scheme in Thailand	SHI in Germany	BUPA in the UK	Community-based health insurance in Ghana

Box 17.4 Government of Thailand's National Health Insurance Schemes [23]

Formal sector schemes. In 1963, the Thai government started a Civil Service Medical Benefit Scheme (CSMBS) to pay for health services for about 2 million civil servants and their 3.2 million dependents. The CSMBS is financed by taxes and overseen by the Comptroller's General Department of the Ministry of Finance.

In 1990, Thailand enacted the Social Security Act, which introduced SHI in Thailand. The following year, the Social Security Organization (SSO), which is under the Ministry of Labor, started providing health insurance coverage to formal sector workers financed by health insurance payments by employers, employees, and the government. The insurance scheme did not cover workers' dependents, informal sector workers, or unemployed and other vulnerable populations. It covered 12.6 million formal sector employees, or 19% of Thailand's population.

Universal coverage. In 2002, the Universal Coverage Scheme (UCS) was introduced to cover all noninsured people, which currently covers 49 million people, or 73% of the total population. The UCS is financed by tax and other government revenues, and provides health insurance to all Thais not covered by the CSMBS and SSO. UCS is managed by the National Health Security Office.

National Health Security Office (NHSO). The NHSO is supervised by the National Health Security Board, which is chaired by the minister of public health (see Chapter 30). Among others, the NHSO prescribes the covered health services and payment levels, provides advice on the appointment of officials, encourages cooperation with local government organizations, advises on how to improve the quality and standard of services, and prescribes rules on penalties and revocation of enrollment. In addition, a Standard and Quality Control Board was established to oversee and monitor the standard and quality of health services.

NHSO and the Ministry of Public Health. NHSO's governance of the NHI scheme is complemented by the Ministry of Public Health's regulation of public hospitals and community health clinics through ministerial decrees and regulations, budgetary processes, and administrative oversight, and by its key institutions. The Department of Health Service Support gives licenses and regulates private hospitals. The Food and Drugs Administration regulates medicines. The National Drug System Development Committee approves the National List of Essential Medicines. Finally, the Health Accreditation Institute ensures quality assurance of health care services offered at an international level.

revenues to cover the informal sector and the poor. Several countries, including Indonesia (Box 17.5), the Philippines, and Turkey, have successfully consolidated the formal and informal sectors and the rest of the population into a single pool. Other countries, including Iran, Morocco, Thailand, and Tunisia, have maintained separate funds for the formal sector, mostly financed by payroll taxes, and the informal sector and other population groups, who are financed by tax and other government revenues.

A similar situation existed in Turkey, where four health insurance schemes were consolidated into a single NHI. These schemes covered: (1) public sector, private sector, and blue-collar workers; (2) retired civil servants; (3) craftsmen, businessmen, professionals, agriculture workers, and others; and (4) those earning less than the minimum level of income as defined by the law. With the implementation of legislation establishing a universal (national) health insurance scheme in 2008, all individuals living in Turkey became members of the NHI scheme, especially those who were unable to pay the health insurance premium, as assessed by a means test, who were fully subsidized by the

Box 17.5 National Health Insurance Scheme, Indonesia

Prior to 2014, Indonesia had three separate funds: the Askes health insurance, Jamsostek health insurance, and the tax-financed Jamkesmas as shown in Table 17.4.

Table 17.4 Health insurance funds in Indonesia

	Jamkesmas*	Askes	Jamsostek
Started in	2005	1960	1992
Members	Poor and near-poor, including dependents	Current and retired civil servants Retired military personnel Includes spouse and two unmarried nonworking children under 21 years	Employees of private employers with >10 employees Employees paid more than one million Rupiah per month by private employers with ≤10 employees Includes spouse and three unmarried nonworking children under 21 years
Financed by	Taxes	Employees 66%; employers 34%	Employers 100%

Jaminan Kesehatan Masyaraka (managed by the Ministry of Health).

In 2014 Indonesia implemented the national health insurance scheme *Jaminan Kesehatan Nasional* (JKN), managed by the Social Security Organizing Agency – Health (*Badan Penyelenggara Jaminan Sosial-Kesahatan*, or BPJS-K) which was the former PT Askes. This led to the merger of the three schemes. Members of Askes and Jamsostek were enrolled into JKN and the poor and near-poor were subsidized with tax financing. Initial membership in 2014 was 121.6 million, with 96.4 million poor and near-poor members. In 2018 almost 80% of the population was covered by JKN, *which makes it the largest single-payer system in the world, covering 203 million members.*

government. These were those who were determined to have domestic average monthly income per capita less than one-third of the gross minimum wage.

17.6.3 Benefits Design and Provider Management

Traditionally, designing benefits and provider payment methods would simply require deciding on what health services to cover and selecting from a range of provider payment methods (see Chapter 15 for designing benefit packages). The benefits design of NHI schemes would usually include: (1) ambulatory patient services (outpatient care which one gets without being admitted to a hospital); (2) emergency services; (3) hospitalization (such as surgery and overnight stays); and (4) pregnancy, maternity, and newborn care. Other health services that are eventually covered include outpatient prescription medicines and laboratory services, and rehabilitative services and devices. NHI in many developing countries has yet to pay for mental health services, including counseling and psychotherapy, or dental and vision care coverage.

> **Box 17.6** Options and Means for Strategic Purchasing
>
> - Protect funding for primary care services and pay relatively high amounts to reflect their priority
> - Disincentivize by limiting the provision of high-cost services, including by paying providers relatively low prices for high-cost but low-priority services
> - Implement payments methods such as diagnosis-related groups and/or capitation, together with a global budget to control overall levels of spending
> - Introduce performance-based payments
> - Enforce copayments for patients who bypass primary care
> - Negotiate prices of medicines
> - Use hospital accreditation as a tool to benchmark safety and quality to established standards

In recent years, designing the benefits and provider payment mechanisms of NHI essentially means moving from passive to strategic health purchasing (Chapter 18), which means active, evidence-based engagement in defining the service mix and volume, and selecting the provider mix in order to maximize societal objectives. It is therefore important that the following questions be asked: (1) Which health services need to be covered as a priority? (2) How cost-effective are the available interventions for these priority services? (3) Which staff and facilities are needed to deliver these services? (4) How well are interventions currently being delivered by providers? (5) What are the projections of available resources? (6) How much money does the purchaser expect to have in the next 2–3 years? NHI schemes also have several options to become strategic purchasers of health services, as shown in Box 17.6.

17.7 NHI Schemes: Prerequisites for Success

National health insurance schemes are too precious to fail and require certain capacities and a commitment to function efficiently. For instance, having a culture of cost-effective management and adoption of appropriate public financial management rules demonstrate this commitment. The key success factors include the following:

- Enhanced institutional and individual capacity by having experts skilled and competent in, for instance, system management, health financing, procurement, billing, information systems, and information technology. These are critical for NHI schemes to become strategic purchasers.
- Government's support to the NHI approach through continued financial commitment and degree of autonomy in its operations (e.g., by encouraging purchaser–provider split) is a precondition for success. At the same time, strong oversight by NHI of its subunits and entities is essential to harmonize practices and resources at the local level.
- Responsiveness of health service providers to ensure translation of incentives into effective quality of care and efficiency gains. One of the implications of NHI is to guarantee a level playing field that ensures fair competition among providers.
- Robust communication strategy and awareness-raising mechanisms toward beneficiaries are crucial to achieving the goal of equitable use of services. Alternatively, it can lead to misinformation about NHI benefits, resulting in frivolous or underutilization of services.

References

1. World Health Organization. *Health Systems Financing: The Path to Universal Coverage.* Geneva, World Health Organization, 2010. https://apps.who.int/iris/bitstream/handle/10665/44371/9789241564021_eng.pdf?sequence=1&isAllowed=y (accessed November 19, 2021).

2. T. R. Reid. *The Healing of America: A Global Quest for Better, Cheaper, and Fairer Health Care.* New York, Penguin, 2010.

3. W. Beveridge. Social insurance and allied services. 1942. http://pombo.free.fr/beveridge42.pdf (accessed November 20, 2021).

4. C. Davis. The organization and performance of the contemporary Soviet health system. In G. Lapidus, G. Swanson, eds., *State and Welfare, USA/USSR: Contemporary Policy and Practice.* Berkeley, University of California Press, 1988, pp. 114–130.

5. Physicians for a National Health Program. Health care systems: four basic models. 2010. www.pnhp.org/single_payer_resources/health_care_systems_four_basic_models.php (accessed December 5, 2021).

6. World Bank Group. Measuring income and poverty using proxy means tests. https://olc.worldbank.org/sites/default/files/1.pdf (accessed January 15, 2022).

7. Institute for Quality and Efficiency in Health Care. Health care in Germany: health insurance in Germany. 2018. www.ncbi.nlm.nih.gov/books/NBK298832 (accessed December 5, 2021).

8. Encyclopedia of Health Economics. Health insurance systems in developed countries. 2014. www.sciencedirect.com/referencework/9780123756794/encyclopedia-of-health-economics (accessed February 7, 2022).

9. European Observatory of Health Systems and Policies. France. 2021. https://eurohealthobservatory.who.int/countries/france (accessed December 5, 2021).

10. Republique Francaise. What is the CSG? 2021. www-vie–publique-fr.translate.goog/fiches/21973-quest-ce-que-la-csg-contribution-sociale-generalisee?_x_tr_sl=fr&_x_tr_tl=en&_x_tr_hl=en&_x_tr_pto=sc (accessed December 5, 2021).

11. Previssima. General scheme. 2021. www-previssima-fr.translate.goog/lexique/regime-general.html?_x_tr_sl=fr&_x_tr_tl=en&_x_tr_hl=en&_x_tr_pto=sc (accessed December 5, 2021).

12. Ministere de Lagriculture et de Lalimentation. Agricultural social mutuality, social security for farmers. 2017. https://agriculture-gouv-fr.translate.goog/mutualite-sociale-agricole-la-securite-sociale-des-agriculteurs?_x_tr_sl=fr&_x_tr_tl=en&_x_tr_hl=en&_x_tr_pto=sc (accessed December 5, 2021).

13. OECD. *The Future of Social Protection: What Works for Non-standard Workers?* Paris, OECD, 2018. https://doi.org/10.1787/9789264306943-en (accessed December 5, 2021).

14. Republique Francaise. Does universal health coverage (CMU) still exist? 2020. www-service–public-fr.translate.goog/particuliers/vosdroits/F34306?_x_tr_sl=fr&_x_tr_tl=en&_x_tr_hl=en&_x_tr_pto=sc (accessed December 5, 2021).

15. J. Ambler. *The French Welfare State: Surviving Social and Ideological Change.* New York, NYU Press, 1993.

16. Commonwealth Fund. International health care system profiles: Japan. 2020. www.commonwealthfund.org/international-health-policy-center/countries/japan (accessed December 5, 2021).

17. J. E. Stiglitz, J. K. Rosengard. *Economics of the Public Sector: Fourth International Student Edition.* New York, W.W. Norton, 2015.

18. I. Joumard, Z. Lonti, T. Curristine. Improving public sector efficiency. *OECD J Budgeting* 2007; 7(1): 1–41.

19. D. Cotlear, S. Nagpal, O. Smith, et al. Going universal: how 24 developing countries are implementing universal health coverage from the bottom up. 2015. https://openknowledge.worldbank.org/bitstream/

handle/10986/22011/9781464806100.pdf (accessed October 19, 2020).

20. A. Madore, J. Rosenberg, R. Weintraub. Sin taxes and health financing in the Philippines. Module Note for Cases in Global Health. 2015. www.globalhealth delivery.org/case-collection/case-studies/ asia-and-middle-east/sin-taxes-and-health-financing-in-the-philippines (accessed October 19, 2020).

21. H. H. Yildrim, H. O. Ari, M. K. Uslu. Value-based healthcare: the Turkish case.

J Presid Turkish Health Instit 2021; 4(1): 33–48.

22. Asian Development Bank. Overcoming public sector inefficiencies towards universal health coverage: the case for national insurance systems in Asia and the Pacific. 2018. www.adb.org/publications/ overcoming-public-sector-inefficiencies-universal-health (accessed October 18, 2020).

23. T. Puttasuwan. Governance risk assessment on Thailand's health sector (unpublished). 2020.

18

From Passive to Strategic Purchasing in Low and Middle Income Countries

The What and How of Getting the Most from Limited Resources

John C. Langenbrunner, Cheryl Cashin, Michelle Wen, and Mariam Zameer

Key Messages
• Countries want more funding for health and health care, but resources are always limited.
• Over the last 50 years, countries focused on ways to spend better to improve health sector performance, enhance financial protection and (over time) achieve better health outcomes.
• For this, countries have utilized what has come to be known as strategic purchasing (SP).
• SP is understood as the allocation of financial resources to providers that moves from passive line-item budgeting reflecting last year's inputs plus inflation, to more demand-driven (or service-driven) approaches that encourage activities and outputs to improve equity of access, efficiency of delivery, quality, financial protection, and (ultimately) health outcomes and population gains.
• To move toward SP, purchasers should focus on core subfunctions called "policy levers." These include: (1) understanding population coverage ("for whom to buy"); (2) supply or benefits package ("what to buy"); (3) contracting ("from whom to buy"); (4) prices and incentives or provider payment systems (how to pay and at what price); and (5) accountability and measurement of achieving performance (what impact?).
• SP requires a complex network of interventions and institutions, so transition to SP is not straightforward nor easily accomplished.

18.1 Introduction

Strategic purchasing in health is not new. It started in Western Europe in the 1960s as an approach to improve health system responsiveness, and better match supply with demand to improve efficiency. Western Europe in the 1960s suffered from empty beds in some facilities and overcrowding in others; doctors not showing up for work and establishing dual practices; patient queues; and complaints that providers were "inhuman." In response, purchasers in high-income countries (HICs), such as those in the Organisation for Economic Co-operation and Development (OECD), moved from paying for inputs to paying for outputs and now outcomes, with the aim to improve health system efficiency and equity, and ensure better responsiveness. Non-OECD countries face similar challenges today. This chapter discusses the concept, design, and implementation of SP in low- and lower-middle income countries (LICs and LMICs, respectively), where successful models are emerging, with lessons for all low- and middle-income countries (L&MICs).

18.2 Purchasing and Health Financing

Health care financing is the "function of a health system concerned with the mobilization, accumulation and allocation of money to cover the health needs of people, individually and collectively" [1] – see Chapter 5 for a description of the three health financing functions of revenue raising, pooling, and purchasing.

Providers respond differently to how they are paid, and at the same time data on true diagnosis and optimal interventions may not be available. The *purchasing function* is concerned with the allocation and use of funds in the health system to ensure "more" value for the existing money for health – that is, greater equity, efficiency, and quality. It does so by setting the right financial incentives to providers to ensure that all individuals have effective access to the "right" set of their needed health services [1]. This is the focus of this chapter. For a discussion on the *revenue raising* and *pooling* functions, refer to Chapters 5, 16, and 17. Figure 18.1 describes how the purchasing function fits within the overall health financing system [2].

One strategy to enhance the value for money is to use SP (Box 18.1). SP achieves this through different approaches, including by focusing on more cost-effective interventions that address high-burden diseases at the primary care level; redirecting existing allocations toward services that improve access to the poor; and changing the way providers are paid in a manner to influence their behaviors.

18.3 Passive Purchasing versus Strategic Purchasing

All countries, regardless of income, are constantly searching for ways to improve the performance of their health systems, to provide "more health for money." There is a marked difference across countries in terms of how they purchase health care. All allocations for health are different forms of purchasing. Historically, countries with public sector delivery systems received line-item budgets from the Ministries of Finance for inputs such as salaries, infrastructure, utilities, pharmaceuticals, food, and so on. These line-item budgets typically cannot be moved across lines flexibly to respond to demand or needs. Budgets are released late to the service-level implementers, and often too late to be fully spent, hence ultimately being returned to the Ministry of Finance. This is termed "passive purchasing." This still occurs today in parts of Asia (India, Bangladesh, and Pakistan) and in many countries in sub-Saharan Africa (e.g., Liberia, Nigeria, and Mozambique). This is in contrast to SP, which involves a continuous search for the best ways to maximize health system performance by deciding which interventions should be purchased, how, and from whom.

Line-item budgeting, however, does offer strong administrative controls which are valued by the Ministries of Finance. It assumes that governments understand how the right allocation of funds under different line-items are expected to achieve the desired outputs and can track progress of the intended results. In reality, they cannot for lack of a good monitoring process and information, which impairs their ability to identify and address demand for health care in a timely way. Further, annual budgets from the Ministries of Finance are often subjected to political and stakeholder pressures. The latter

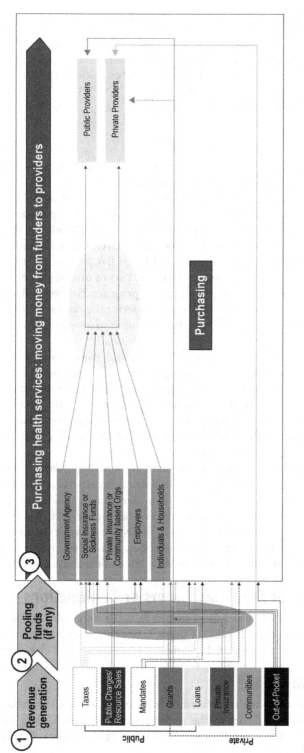

Figure 18.1 Three functions of the health financing system with a focus on the purchasing function.

> **Box 18.1** Strategic Purchasing
>
> Strategic purchasing is understood as the allocation of financial resources to providers that moves from passive line-item budgeting exercises reflecting last year's inputs plus inflation, to more demand-driven (or service-driven) approaches that encourage activities and outputs to improve equity of access, efficiency of delivery, quality, financial protection, and (ultimately) health outcomes and population gains.

results in focusing fund allocations to urban and tertiary facilities, away from rural and primary care. This has both efficiency and equity implications.

In the *World Health Report 2000*, SP was seen as a policy tool that should be embraced by all countries, including L&MICs [1]. Today, SP is increasingly being utilized by countries across every income level, whether it is Germany or Ghana, Estonia, or the Democratic Republic of Congo; several Gulf Cooperation Council (GCC) countries have similarly revamped their systems over the last decade; and Egypt has proposed a similar structural reform for the coming decade. Countries utilize it as part of overall system reforms (as in Kosovo, Bahrain, and Nigeria), or as part of special programs for population groups (e.g., the HIV/AIDS program in Indonesia), or parts of the sector (i.e., at state or region levels). In moving toward SP, some countries decide to fully abandon passive purchasing, as in Eastern Europe and several GCC countries, or partly, as in Thailand.

International organizations such as WHO, the World Bank, and the IMF, as well as research universities, have reported the growing evidence of SP to improve efficiency (both technical and allocative), equity across population groups, and financial protection [2]. The World Bank has funded efforts for SP in every region of the world through its lending programs. The Joint Learning Network (JLN) that has members and associate members comprising 34 countries, mostly middle- and low-income, shows how consistently countries are progressively moving toward SP (Table 18.1) [3].

Since it requires a complex network of interventions and institutions, transition to SP is not straightforward nor easily accomplished. Countries can experience unintended consequences if SP is not implemented correctly or in harmony across actors. For example, unnecessary hospital admissions could increase, or the wrong mix of services could be reimbursed. Nevertheless, countries need to stop passive purchasing (line-item budgeting) and increasingly funding urban and tertiary services, and move toward SP of pro-poor primary care and other priority services in both urban and rural areas.

18.4 The "How" of SP: Policy Levers or Subfunctions

In order to move toward SP, purchasers should focus on core subfunctions (sometimes termed "policy levers") at their disposal to improve health system performance. Five main subfunctions are outlined in Table 18.2 and described in more detail elsewhere [4].

18.4.1 For Whom to Buy?

Many countries are now moving to universal health coverage (UHC). Purchasers, whether providing coverage to all or part of the population, must have a clear picture of the individuals and families for whom they will be purchasing health care. This can start with

Table 18.1 Summary of Joint Learning Network (JLN) country experiences in health care financing in selected L&MICs

Country	Purchaser–provider split	Population coverage and share of funds of insurance/purchasing agency	Benefit package (HTA capacity)	Contracting	Purchaser and payment models	Scale of new model implementation	Comments
Low-income countries							
Ethiopia	✓	Community-based health insurance and formal sector insurance schemes	✓	✓	Fee-for-service	SS	
Tanzania	✓	20% coverage (2015): • Community health fund (CHF) (7.2%) and • National health insurance fund (NHIF) (12.8%)	✓	✓	MOH: PBF CHF/NHIF: fee-for-service since start; capitation proposed	SS	Single national health insurance fund planned
Lower middle-income							
Egypt	✓	National insurance agency (NIA): 55% population coverage; 22% of government health expenditure	✓		Budget; salaries		NIA (55% coverage) but no purchaser–provider split
India	✓	Multiple government-sponsored insurance schemes (e.g., Aarogysori; RSBY; others): 45% population coverage	✓	✓ (P)	Fee-for-service; case-based ("package rates")	LS	

Table 18.1 (cont.)

Country	Purchaser–provider split	Population coverage and share of funds of insurance/purchasing agency	Benefit package (HTA capacity)	Contracting	Purchaser and payment models	Scale of new model implementation	Comments
Upper middle-income countries							
Colombia	✓	96% population coverage by three public insurance schemes (EPS; EPC; IPS) 83% of government health expenditure	✓	✓ (P)	Capitation (PHC); fee-for-service (outpatient specialty); case-based (inpatient)	LS SS SS	The public insurers contract further with entities (EPS) that are selected by individuals, and carry out the contracting and purchasing with health providers
Mexico	✓	Three public insurance schemes: social health insurance for formal sector employed; civil servant scheme; and subsidized Segura Popular for the poor and informal sector – together nearly 100% population coverage and 56% of government health spending	✓ (HTA)		All purchasers: budget and salaries		100% public insurance coverage but no purchaser–provider split

- **Purchaser–provider split** means that there is a separate public insurance or purchasing agency that manages at least a portion of government health funding.
- **Population coverage and share of funds of insurance/purchasing agency**: percentage of the population covered and percentage of total government health expenditure and/or premiums being channeled through public insurance or purchasing agency.
- **Benefit package (health technology assessment (HTA) capacity)**: entitlement to services defined either as benefits package or essential services package.
- **HTA** means there is a process in the country for explicit decision-making and priority-setting for adding new tools, services, or benefits.
- **Contracting** means that there is some explicit contracting mechanism through a public purchaser (Ministry of Health or insurance agency).
- **P** means the public purchaser also contracts with private health care providers.
- **Purchaser and payment models:** The payment models used by public purchasers are: input-based payment model: budget/salaries – the purchaser uses traditional input-based line-item budgets and salaries to pay health care providers; and output-based payment models: case-based, capitation, fee-for-service (FFS); performance-based financing (PBF).
- **Scale of new payment model implementation:** SS = new approaches being piloted or implemented on a small scale; LS = new approaches being implemented nationally or paid through the purchasing agency.
- **Comments:** Additional context about the health system or SP approaches.

Table 18.2 Policy levers or subfunctions related to the use of financing and SP

1. Demand or "population coverage" (**for whom** to buy)
2. Supply or "benefits package" (**what** to buy, in which form, and what to exclude)
3. Contracting (**from whom** to buy, **who** the providers to buy from are, and **how much** to buy)
4. Prices and incentives or "provider payment systems" (**how to pay** and at **what price**)[a]
5. Accountability and the measurement of achieving performance (**what impact**)

[a] Arguably, price for services and payment method can be thought of as separate levers, with overall incentives embedded in these levers.
Source: [4].

a simple analysis of demographics and disease burden, as well as a mechanism to verify eligibility and record the services encounters. Over time, information about the population can help to better customize services to match population needs and demands.

18.4.2 What to Buy?

While all countries would like to offer a comprehensive benefits package to all citizens, budget constraints impose restrictions on what services can be bought. Defining the benefits package involves making decisions about who will benefit from publicly financed services (breadth of coverage), the types of services to be financed (depth of coverage), and the levels of out-of-pocket (OOP) contributions beneficiaries will need to make – see Chapter 15. These decisions are influenced by economic, social, and political factors specific to each country. Difficult trade-offs have to be made while protecting the poor and near-poor. Some countries must choose between covering fewer poor and near-poor individuals with a comprehensive package (deep coverage) or covering more of them with a less comprehensive package (broad coverage) [5]. In L&MICs, low levels of health expenditure per capita result in measures to limit utilization (i.e., rationing) through user fees, limit the volume of services provided, or limit the service quality.

In Pakistan, the principal criteria considered in defining its nationally endorsed UHC benefit package included: the burden of disease/risk factors, the cost-effectiveness of interventions, the budgetary impact, and the feasibility of implementation. Additional criteria that were also considered included the impact on equity and financial risk protection [6]. In some countries packages have omitted certain benefits, resulting in delayed progress in some areas, such as maternal and neonatal health in Indonesia and tuberculosis (TB) care in India. Globally, health promotion and disease prevention, immunizations and vaccinations, infectious disease control, and essential primary health care (PHC) services are typically part of national benefit packages funded by the government.

18.4.3 From Whom to Buy?

A purchaser could buy services from all providers or from a selected group of providers based on predefined criteria. Through contracting, purchasers can establish minimum standards in terms of the necessary staff qualifications and infrastructure to be awarded a contract with the scheme (see Chapter 28). Purchasers can also establish service-specific standards, whereby providers are reimbursed for particular services only if they are performed by staff with adequate qualifications and in a manner consistent with established practice protocols and prescription guidelines. Contracting could also be utilized to develop benchmarks and performance standards with an organization such as a hospital or clinic. This could be used as part of the civil service code or outside of it in the case of private and nongovernmental organizations.

Progress with contracting both public and private providers can be seen in Indonesia, Thailand, Malaysia, and Mongolia, as well as in HICs such as Germany, Japan, South Korea, and Taiwan, where private providers dominate the sector. Based on global experience, however, contracting out requires some caution and adherence to "pre-conditions," such as: a competitive environment; well-defined services; coordination with public and private sector activities; assessment of quality; specification of service standards; and close monitoring of contract performance [7]. When contracting is limited to an *exclusive* or *preferred* network of providers, with additional conditions or criteria, it is referred to as "selective contracting" [8].

18.4.4 How to Pay and at What Price?

There are many payment systems that have emerged globally in the last few decades which move from payment for inputs to payment for outputs and outcomes. New payment models should be put in place in response to an explicit hierarchy of policy priorities as well as practical considerations. Purchasers first have to decide on the policy objectives of the payment system; e.g., increased revenues, equity, efficiency, cost-containment, access, quality, administrative simplicity, or some combination of these. The payment system chosen, and the associated incentives, have to address one or more health sector policy objectives at that particular time. Related incentives must be chosen in tandem with other factors, such as improved knowledge about clinical outcomes, cultural factors, and providers' professional ethics. In addition, when purchasers begin to consider new incentives, decisions are typically based on factors such as readily available information, technical capacity, and time available to design, implement, and monitor the payment systems.

No one model is perfect. The world is moving to blended payment models. An example from Estonia

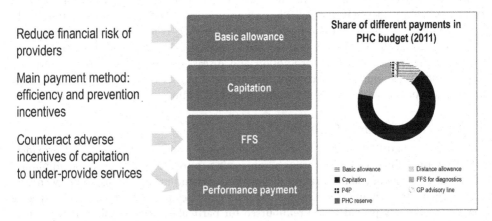

Figure 18.2 Provider payment methods and health policy objectives: an example from Estonia [9].

More recently, *performance-related pay*, sometimes called *pay-for-performance* (P4P), has been employed to directly link payment to the performance of the health care provider. Ideally, the link is based on achieving an outcome, though because of measurement challenges it is more often based on some ideal process of care delivery. P4P can be used to pay either an individual provider or a facility (e.g., a primary care facility). "Performance" is measured by how well a specified task is implemented against the set target (e.g., all immunizations provided to the child), or some established threshold (e.g., 90% of children immunized). P4P programs can and should be used as an integral part of the new incentive structures within the health sector. The P4P models are emergent in countries like Indonesia, the Philippines, and India, and are becoming well established in Africa in countries such as Rwanda [10].

18.4.5 Recent Developments: Moving to "Blended" Payment Methods

Which payment system works best? Unfortunately, there is no one best payment method. No single set of incentives is able to address the multiple objectives of purchasers, providers, and patients. Table 18.3 shows the relative advantages and disadvantages of each of the payment methods.

In response, "blended payments" are increasingly being utilized in OECD countries and some middle-income countries (MICs). "Blended payments" mix more than one method to discourage negative incentives and encourage optimal allocations and performance. For example, in primary care, blended payments can include capitation plus FFS for immunizations and preventive care, plus P4P for containing referrals. As a component of the overall "blend," P4P may have greater impact. On the hospital side, a blend of case mix and global budgets is used in several European countries, Taiwan, and Thailand [12]. Figure 18.2 illustrates the use of blended payment methods in Estonia.

Sophisticated payment systems may lead to higher transaction costs and may require expanded capacity to use information and management systems. This is true both for purchasers and providers, as the unit of payment increases, and the risk necessarily shifts relative to providers. Management information systems cannot always be designed and implemented quickly.

18.5 "Enablers" and "Choke Points" for Successful Implementation of Payment Systems to Providers

The best planned and implemented payment systems may fail due to a variety of factors, which if not properly addressed can dilute or neutralize their benefits. In addition, a set of "enablers" could help advance the implementation of SP. Technicians and policymakers need to address these potential "chokepoints" and leverage the various "enablers" to ensure progress. Table 18.4 summarizes both chokepoints and enablers of the payment systems [13].

18.6 How to Hold the Purchaser and Providers Accountable?

Lack of proper accountability systems and culture is one of the key areas for improvement in health systems of many L&MICs. For the health system to deliver good-quality care in an efficient manner it is essential to establish systems and processes for tight monitoring of performance, as well as possible administrative mechanisms to address poor performance. Public and private providers should be subject to minimal standards and requirements in terms of reporting, mostly limited to basic accounting and monitoring of quality/outcomes.

Table 18.3 Different output-based options to pay providers: each creates certain risks and incentives

Payment mechanism	Risk borne by		Provider incentive to			
	Payer	Provider	Increase number of patients/ users	Decrease number of services per unit	Increase reported illness severity	Select healthy patients
Fee-for-service	All risks borne by payer	No risk borne by provider	✓	✗	✓	✗
Case mix adjusted per admission (e.g., DRG)	Risk of number of cases and risk severity classification	Risk of cost of treatment for a given case	✓	✓	✓	✓
Per admission	Risk of number of admissions	Risk of number of services per admission	✓	✓	✗	✓
Per diem	Risk of number of days to stay	Risk of cost of services within a given day	✓	✓	✗	✗
Capitation	Amount above "Stop loss ceiling"	All risk borne by provider up to a given ceiling (stop loss)	✓	✓	NA	✓
Global budget	No risk borne by payer	All risk borne by provider	✗	NA	NA	✓

DRG, diagnosis related group.
Source: [11].

Table 18.4 "Enablers" and "choke points" of provider payment systems, with country examples

"Chokepoints"	"Enablers"
• *Fragmented pooling and purchasing*: In Indonesia, while it succeeded in enhancing coverage to a large segment of the population, still less than 25% of all funding is streamlined under the insurance fund. Providers have other sources of revenues, e.g., OOP payment, fiscal transfers, Ministry of Health vertical funds – each with its own set of rules and constraints.	• *Operational autonomy of providers* [14]: New incentives require flexibility to respond regarding the use of resources, both financial and human, as well as the needed and timely inputs such as equipment, labs, and medicines.
• *Poor complementarity of design across service settings* (e.g., inpatient and outpatient): In Croatia, primary care providers when paid by capitation referred patients to save funds. Higher levels of care used FFS, per visit and per admission, thereby creating unnecessary volumes of care.	• *Timely information and routine management and information systems*: Minimum but critical information on each encounter in both public and private provider settings allow purchasers to track utilization, quality, and appropriateness of referrals up the levels of care. It further allows performance comparisons across providers.
• *Institutional or governance impediments*: Countries may face governance issues with Ministry of Health taking most decisions and insurance fund too few, or vice versa. Thailand is a good model of balanced governance and SP.	• *Quality assurance systems*: This is needed to identify and offset unintended consequences created by new incentives. (See Section 18.6)
• *Lack of technical capacity and management skills*: This is seen when purchasers have limited understanding of the benefits and risks of various provider payment methods.	• *Good monitoring and evaluation systems*: This is needed to create dynamics of improvement over time. (See Section 18.6)

These processes include, among others:

- tracking inappropriate admissions treatable at lower levels of care;
- measurement of volume (and type) of services delivered;
- measurement of outcome – from basic indicators (e.g., hospital mortality and infection rates) to more complex measures (e.g., 30-/60-/90-day readmission rates, especially for major procedures). These would need to be risk-adjusted using the case mix index and other mechanisms;
- tracking of financial performance against budgets; and
- prevention, detection, and deterrence of fraud.

A progressive escalation process in case of lack of performance could include, for example: initial warning, auditing, publication of relative performance, commissioning interventions, stopping new agreement plans, and even closure or interruption of services provision. Once in place, these mechanisms foster the creation of a widespread culture of performance in the health system.

It is worth noting that purchasers can often collect many of these performance indicators through routine claims payment systems. South Korea reviews 36 indicators – an increase from

24 indicators initially used – for every provider through its routine claims data processing system. The new Modi-care program in India is now instituting a series of accountability measures, as well as publicizing bad performers and using instruments to jail repeatedly offending providers [10]. The accreditation status may further offer a tool to publish facility performance through online "scorecards" for users shopping for quality care, and as a motivator for providers to continually improve quality.

Low- and middle-income countries sometimes lack minimal but essential data, something which undermines proper monitoring. This is largely due to: lack of standards; underdeveloped information technology systems; lack of contractual requirements related to reporting back; and inadequate regulations. Such measures, once implemented, need to be also synchronized across all levels of allocation for services – district, province, and central.

In the end, sophisticated payment models will not work without performance contracting and accountability measures. Synchronization across all five subfunctions/levers (Table 18.2) is key for purchasers to realize the full potential of SP as intended. Overall, these levers and subfunctions create a type of network of institutions and interventions. It is critical that countries put together a full network of cohesive and coordinating interventions to avoid the "unintended consequences" mentioned above. This tends to occur across all countries to some degree, but more often in L&MICs.

18.7 Best Practices: Strategic Purchasing Experiences from L&MICs

All HICs have been engaging in SP to some degree since the 1960s. The United States progressed in the 1970s and 1980s when health care costs began to get out of control, though due to the multiplicity of purchasers there was limited success. The following subsections shed light on successful experiences with SP in L&MICs.

18.7.1 Middle-Income Countries

Strategic purchasing has been successful in a number of MICs, including Thailand [15], Estonia [16], Turkey [1], and Argentina. The "Plan Nacer," Argentina's health coverage program for pregnant women and children under six years, utilized performance contracting and payment to improve health outcomes for the poor. Over a five-year period, prenatal visits and well-baby check-ups increased, quality of care improved, and probability of low birth weight and in-hospital neonatal death reduced by 23% and 74%, respectively [16]. Countries such as India, Egypt, and Ukraine are now engaged in the design and implementation of similar reforms. An expanding number of MICs have also initiated SP over the last three decades. Three MIC countries that are typically pointed to as best-practice models are Thailand, Turkey, and Estonia (Table 18.5). These countries have worked to ensure the following:

- purchaser–provider splits with new purchaser-based social insurance funds have been created;
- increased levels of pooling: in Thailand, 70% of the population is covered by one pool of funds (the Universal Coverage Scheme); in Estonia and Turkey, multiple funds were merged to form a single-payer model;
- benefits packages are based on explicit criteria related to cost-effectiveness, equity, patient preference, and other factors;

Table 18.5 SP policy levers in three best-practice MICs

	Thailand	Turkey	Estonia
For whom to purchase (*agency, population groups*)	Social Security Scheme: formal sector employees and families; civil servants and families Universal Coverage Scheme: covers 70% of the population	Three insurance organizations merged to form a single-payer model (see Chapter 17)	Transition from line-item MOH-driven model to new insurance model (single-payer) with universal coverage The insurance fund is autonomous relative to the MOH
	Overall coverage: 98%	90–97% coverage	100% coverage for citizens
What to buy (*benefit package*)	Inpatient and outpatient care; preventive and promotive care; family planning; essential medicines; renal therapy and dialysis; antiretroviral treatment for HIV/AIDS; cancer care	Inpatient and outpatient care; emergency care; preventive care; essential medicines; organ, tissue, and stem-cell transplantation; renal dialysis; cancer care; cardiovascular surgery	Extensive package of primary, secondary, and tertiary care, updated with sophisticated technology assessment process
Copayment	None	20% for medicines/medical devices, capped for procedures in the private sector	OOP for home and outpatient visits, hospital stays and medicines Pensioners and children below 16 have lower OOP payment
Institutional arrangements	National Health Security Board Health Intervention and Technology Assessment Program Expert stakeholder group	Reimbursement Commission; Social Security System (SSI) Medical and Economic Evaluation Commission	Insurance fund identifies changes in medicines, procedures, and technologies MOH reviews safety, efficacy, and cost-effectiveness Health insurance sets tariffs for new procedures/services

Table 18.5 (cont.)

	Thailand	Turkey	Estonia
From whom to buy (*provider type*)	Mostly public providers Private providers primarily in urban areas Overall, 79% public and 21% private	Primarily public providers at the hospital level Autonomous or private PHC providers In 2010: public beds 86%, private beds 14%	In the 1990s, over 90% of providers became autonomous or private Hospitals were merged from 120 hospitals to 19 networks with financial autonomy
How to pay (*payment methods*)	Capitation for outpatients Per admission, DRGs with capped budgets and fixed fee for inpatients Global budgets in rural districts	Capitation for GPs and PHC and P4P for outpatients Case-based payment for inpatients. Developing DRG system FFS for specialists and diagnostics	Blended payment models Hospitals: DRGs and global budgets Line-item and capitation for infrastructure and outpatient FFS for specialists Pay-for-performance
Accountability	Accreditation system with payment tied to level of accreditation Indicators of volume, efficiency, and quality	Accreditation system Purchaser in UHC scheme developed various indicators related to volume, efficiency, and quality	Accreditation system Purchaser (insurance fund) developed various indicators related to volume, efficiency, equity, and quality
Other subfunctions	Sophisticated IT system Autonomy of public providers	Full autonomy has not yet been reached at hospital level	Sophisticated IT systems E-services

Source: [17, 18].

- contracting is done with both the public and private providers;
- person-level management information systems for payment and quality assurance have been established;
- new provider payment models for PHC, hospitals, and performance-based bonus pools for priority services (e.g., immunizations, family planning, preventive care) have been put in place;
- SP focuses on resources and management attention for primary care and family health; and
- accreditation mechanisms and quality assurance systems are functioning.

18.7.2 Low-Income Countries

Low income countries face formidable challenges, including low public allocations for health, large OOP payments, and reliance on donor support, which is often provided in fragmented streams of funding. Donor support is waning in several countries, creating pressure for LICs to spend wisely, and making domestic financing and SP more important. Nevertheless, there are some notable successes with LIC experience in SP:

1. **Kyrgyzstan** is a small country in central Asia with a population of five million, and is mostly rural. It underwent economic freefall following the break-up of the Soviet Union and GDP fell to levels less than US$300 per capita. Kyrgyzstan responded to the fiscal crisis by catalyzing health systems transformation, with wide-ranging structural and SP reforms that included an expanded benefits package and delivery of primary care services, PHC capitation payments, and hospital DRG payment reforms, which has driven significant health improvements over 10 years [15].

2. **Ghana** is one of very few African countries to take significant, large-scale steps toward SP for health. The country has focused on expanding enrolment of vulnerable groups (increasing by 10% in the last five years), increasing access and utilization through new payment models.

3. **Guatemala** established its *Programa de Extension de Cobertura* (PEC) as a large-scale contracting-out program to NGOs with the aim of scaling up primary care in poor, rural, underserved areas. The PEC serves 4.3 million people; it is managed by the Ministry of Health and is 75% funded by the government. Contract renewal was conditional on NGOs meeting 28 targets related to prenatal health, family planning, and vaccinations. A difference-in-differences study[1] showed increase vaccination coverage and woman and child care [5, 16].

Although many LICs have embarked on SP reforms, they continue to face capacity and political economy challenges in attaining the full network of institutions and interventions necessary to achieve successful SP.

18.8 Going Forward

The recent COVID-19 pandemic has shown the need to respond quickly and build more resilient and effective health systems (Chapter 34). Countries also face increasing fiscal shocks: higher debt and deficit and interest rates pushing health sectors to perform efficiently. SP is an important tool to help countries achieve greater resilience. The interest of L&MICs in SP is expected to grow over time. It is important to manage the risk and potential harm that could result from purchasing being "captured" by elites and tertiary care, or being oversimplified into a one-size-fits-all approach. This calls for:

1. **Building technical capacity and the evidence base** to design and implement provider payment systems and other SP levers, especially the availability of – and skills to analyze – data for purchasing decisions. Part of this is a larger IT and health management information system issue (Chapter 22).

---

[1] A difference-in-differences study is a statistical technique used in econometrics and quantitative research that attempts to mimic an experimental research design using observational study data, by studying the differential effect of a treatment on a "treatment group" versus a "control group" in a natural experiment.

2. **Creating greater "policy coherence"**: Case studies show that many LICs are taking steps on individual elements of purchasing (e.g., changing provider payment mechanisms, introducing HTA, or establishing facility accreditation programs). It would be productive to link these initiatives into a more coherent overall purchasing function so that pooled funds are used to purchase a benefit package that is based on evidence of cost-effectiveness, using a provider payment mechanism that sends clearer incentives to providers, and that links with measures to improve quality (e.g., clinical guidelines or accreditation) and equity (e.g., no extra billing permitted).

3. Building **institutional relationships between Ministries of Health and the purchasers**, such as an insurance fund, which are often frayed and sometimes in conflict, both of which can stall the implementation of SP. The relationship must extend to Ministries of Finance and higher levels of governance. This can help ensure that purchasing is not "captured" by tertiary care, but is targeted toward PHC, prevention, and promotion.

4. **Building a step-by-step strategy**: As every country starts at a different point, it needs to prioritize which reforms are most required to start with. As a general rule, countries with traditional public systems will need to establish a good information system as a first step, codify a clear benefits package, followed by new payment incentives and autonomy of public providers – best done in parallel. In the process, countries would be wise to integrate public and private providers through contracting.

References

1. World Health Organization. *The World Health Report 2000: Health Systems Improving Performance*. Geneva, World Health Organization, 2000. www.who.int/whr/2000/en/whr00_en.pdf (accessed November 12, 2020).

2. P. Gottret, G. Schieber, H. R. Waters. Good practices in health financing: lessons from reforms in low and middle-income countries. 2008. https://openknowledge.worldbank.org/handle/10986/6442 (accessed November 12, 2020).

3. Joint Learning Network. Webinar: coordinating multisectoral, multi-level pandemic responses. 2021. www.jointlearning network.org/events/webinar-coordinating-multi-sectoral-multi-level-pandemic-responses-2/ (accessed February 8, 2022).

4. A. S. Preker, J. C. Langenbrunner. Spending wisely: buying health services for the poor. 2005. https://openknowledge.worldbank.org/handle/10986/7449 (accessed November 16, 2020).

5. World Bank Group. Social health insurance for developing nations. 2007. https://openknowledge.worldbank.org/handle/10986/6860 (accessed November 14, 2020).

6. DCP3 Economic evaluation for health: translation – Pakistan. 2021. http://dcp-3.org/translation/pakistan (accessed February 8, 2022).

7. S. Siddiqi, T. I. Masud, B. Sabri. Contracting but not without caution: experience with outsourcing of health services in countries of the Eastern Mediterranean Region. *Bull World Health Organ* 2006; **84**(11): 867–875.

8. R. E. Bes, E. C. Curfs, P. P. Groenewegen, et al. Selective contracting and channelling patients to preferred providers: a scoping review. *Health Policy* 2017; **121**(5): 504–514.

9. Eesti Haigekassa. Estonian health insurance fund yearbook 2016. 2017. https://haigekassa.ee/sites/default/files/2017-11/haigekassa_eng_loplik.pdf (accessed February 11, 2022).

10. A. Agarwal, A. Kumar, C. Baeza, et al. Health system for a New India: building blocks. Ministry of Finance, Government of India. 2019. https://niti.gov.in/sites/default/files/2019-11/NitiAayogBook_compressed.pdf (accessed January 14, 2022).

11. W. C. Hsiao, D. L. Dunn, D. K. Verrilli. Assessing the implementation of physician-payment reform. *N Engl J Med* 1993; **328**(13): 928–933.

12. J. C. Langenbrunner, A. Somanathan. Financing health care in East Asia and the Pacific: best practices and remaining challenges. 2011. https://openknowledge .worldbank.org/handle/10986/2321 (accessed November 18, 2020).

13. C. Avila, R. Bright, J. C. Gutierrez, et al. Guatemala health system assessment. 2015. www.hfgproject.org/guatemala-health-system-assessment-2015/ (accessed November 1, 2020).

14. A. Harding, A. S. Preker. *Introduction to Private Participation in Health Services.* Washington, DC, World Bank, 2003.

15. A. Dixon, J. Langenbrunner, E. Masiolis. Ten years of experience: health financing in Eastern Europe and the former Soviet Union. In *Ten Years of Health Reform Conference* 2002.

16. R. Cortez, D. Romero. Argentina: increasing utilization of health care services among the uninsured population – the Plan Nacer program. 2013. https://openknowledge.worldbank .org/handle/10986/13289 (accessed November 11, 2020).

17. K. Xu, A. Chu, R. Eng, et al. Experiences on benefit package design: Turkey, Mexico and Thailand. In *WHO Western Pacific Region Conference* 2015.

18. Eesti Haigekassa. Estonia health insurance fund yearbook. 2018. www.haigekassa.ee/ en/infomaterjalid (accessed November 17, 2020).

Chapter 19

Good Governance and Leadership for Better Health Systems

Fadi El-Jardali and Nour Ataya

Key Messages

- Participatory governance is effective for strengthening participation and achieving a common strategic vision as a key principle of good governance.
- Building policy capacity and institutionalizing procedures to incorporate evidence in policymaking and its implementation across the health system are critical for strengthening transparency and accountability.
- Effective regulatory capacity depends on the regulator's political autonomy and reputation for possessing expertise and moral authority.
- There is a variety of strategies that health system managers can adapt to improve governance of health systems at the policy, institutional, and health care professional levels.
- Policy-level strategies include effective decentralization in low- and middle-income countries (L&MICs), which requires local technical capacity, political leadership, and support from the central level.
- Health care and related institutional strategies include:
  - linking accreditation status to incentives, such as public funding, preferential reimbursement, or contractual agreements, which is a potential regulatory strategy in L&MICs; and
  - multifaceted interventions that include training of inspectors, public–private collaboration, and legal actions against counterfeiters, which may be effective in medicine regulation.
- Health care professional strategies include professionally led self-regulation, which combines regulation through professional associations or unions with co-regulation by the government or external bodies, and is seen as enabling transparency and accountability of health care professionals to external authorities.
- Effective control of corruption requires political reforms to enhance participation, transparency, and accountability, and to enforce the rule of law with a focus on (1) open exchange of information, (2) channels for participation of citizens in policymaking, and (3) penalties for the misuse of power.

19.1 Introduction

This chapter provides health policymakers, managers, and care providers with an overview of strategies that can potentially improve the governance of health systems in L&MICs, and of key success elements that they can build on to help ensure effective implementation of these strategies. It builds on the principles of health system governance presented in Chapter 4 and proposes illustrative examples on how to enhance participation, rule of law, transparency, and accountability as key governance principles.

The chapter first explores participatory governance as potentially effective for achieving a common vision and enhancing participation and accountability. It then discusses the importance of strengthening policy capacity for making evidence-informed policies and regulatory capacity for potentially strengthening transparency and accountability and enforcing the rule of law. It then presents an overview of strategies at the policy, institutional, and health care professional levels that can potentially strengthen the governance of health systems in L&MICs. It is important to note that the evidence on governance in L&MICs remains elusive. As such, a variety of information sources, including local contextual evidence and deliberations with stakeholders, should be used when adapting the strategies to local settings.

19.2 Participatory Governance for Effective Leadership of the Health System

Participatory governance, which empowers diverse groups and enables them to contribute to the functioning of a health system in a harmonized and coordinated manner, emerges as potentially effective for achieving a common vision – a key principle of good governance [1, 2]. Experiences from L&MICs, including from Bangladesh, Brazil, Kenya, Thailand, and Turkey, demonstrate how participatory governance that involves multiple providers, civil society organizations, other government sectors, and the media, along with support from global health partners, such as the World Health Organization (WHO), was instrumental in driving successful multisectoral action for a public health priority such as tobacco control [3].

Strengthening participatory governance in health requires an ecosystem that fosters engagement and collaborative learning, and builds new competencies such as collective problem-solving and teamwork, including for those in nonconventional leadership positions [4]. Institutionalizing participatory governance can help make the system less vulnerable to change of individual leaders. It can actively engage multiple actors in participation and consensus orientation to set priorities and monitor implementation, which can also act to keep individual leaders in check and enhance accountability (see Chapter 29) [1].

19.3 Policy Capacity and Evidence-Informed Policymaking

This section focuses on strengthening policy capacity of health systems and incorporating evidence in policymaking as key components for successful leadership and governance [5].

19.3.1 Enhancing Policy Capacity

Policy capacity is defined as the competencies, financial and human resources, and experiences that governments use to identify, formulate, implement, and evaluate solutions to public problems [6]. It includes having the technical and political skills and resources to gather and understand data – for example, on the performance of interventions and the context that shapes policymaking. This capacity is critical for making evidence-informed policies that can potentially strengthen transparency, accountability, and performance of health systems [7].

Capacity-building in L&MICs has largely focused on strengthening technical capacity, such as delivery of health care services, with much less attention to enhancing system-wide capacities such as participatory governance, political advocacy, and navigating complexity [4]. Health system managers can build the policy capacity of local organizations by establishing policies and norms that help foster a conducive environment for organizational exchange and learning, as well as strengthening procedures to incorporate evidence in policymaking, as discussed below.

19.3.2 Incorporating Evidence into Policymaking

In L&MICs, the use of evidence in policymaking is complicated by the lack of high-quality and relevant research, poor access to research (due to lack of a national research database), and lack of policymakers' capacity to access, interpret, and use research evidence [8, 9]. To effectively support policymakers in using evidence, governmental bodies should adopt processes that institutionalize engagement with experts in relevant fields, ensuring that their participation in informing policymaking becomes an integral and sustainable part of the organization [10]. Such institutionalization, including the location of platforms that foster this engagement, funding sources, and governing bodies, should be strategic, such that it provides access to support and opportunities to influence policies [11, 12]. For example, EVIPNet Ethiopia, a platform that brings health system stakeholders together to facilitate use of evidence into policy, was established as a permanent structure within the Ministry of Health, which helped sustain funding and forged direct links with policymakers [11]. Such initiatives can build policy capacity by bringing policymakers, experts, and stakeholders, including citizens and civil society organizations, together for knowledge sharing and exchange. Box 19.1 provides lessons learned from the experience of the Knowledge to Policy (K2P) Centre in Lebanon, which has empowered various health systems actors and helped strengthen government stewardship in addressing health policy

---

Box 19.1 Knowledge to Policy Centre: Lessons Learned

The K2P Centre, a WHO Collaborating Centre for Evidence-Informed Policymaking and Practice, was established within a university setting in Lebanon. It seeks to bridge the gap between science, policy, and politics by making evidence accessible to diverse stakeholders, and to build capacities for evidence-informed policymaking. The Centre's experience provides important lessons for strengthening evidence-informed policymaking in L&MICs [13, 14].

1. **Invest in raising awareness** of policymakers, stakeholders, civil society organizations, and media on the importance of using evidence in policymaking, developing capacities in accessing and using evidence, raising demand for evidence, and building trust.

2. **Adopt a holistic knowledge-to-policy approach** that covers priority-setting, systematic review production, and knowledge uptake. This also includes proactively shaping the policy agenda by seizing opportunities to advocate and influence the policy cycle.

3. **Tailor products, services, and dissemination channels** to the policymaking context, type of priority, and stakeholders involved. For example, in responding to the COVID-19 pandemic, the Centre operationalized its rapid response services, activated the "K2People" initiative to educate citizens, and diversified its search of evidence to include nonconventional sources such as media websites and social media platforms.

priorities, such as the Syrian refugee crisis and the COVID-19 pandemic [13]. Incorporating evidence into policymaking also requires information systems that track a wide range of data; however, in L&MICs information systems often do not meet the needs of regulatory and policymaking bodies.

19.4 Strengthening Regulatory Capacity

Regulatory capacity refers to the capacity for oversight of safety, efficacy, and quality of health services and pharmaceuticals; enforcement capacity for guidelines, standards, and regulations; and perception of the burden imposed by excessive regulation [15]. In L&MICs, governments often lack context-specific policy and regulatory instruments and the human, technical, and financial resources needed to implement these instruments and enforce regulations [15–17]. This is an essential condition for enhancing accountability and enforcing the rule of law (see Chapter 4).

The ability of a regulator to effectively implement regulatory strategies depends on the regulator's political autonomy and reputation for possessing expertise and moral authority [7, 18]. However, it may be challenging to establish a positive reputation when the public has a low level of trust in governments, as is prevalent in several L&MICs. A number of strategies can help the regulator establish a positive reputation, such as hiring skilled individuals, publicly reporting information about the performance of the regulator, and establishing clear conflict-of-interest policies and codes of conduct [7, 18].

19.5 Governance Strategies at the Policy, Institutional, and Health Care Professional Levels: Illustrative Examples

This section provides an overview of strategies that health system managers can use to improve accountability, transparency, and participation. These strategies are targeted at different levels in health systems: the policy (e.g., Ministry of Health), institutional (e.g., hospitals and pharmaceutical industry), and health care professional (e.g., physicians, nurses) levels.

It is important to note that much of the evidence on governance strategies comes from high-income countries (HICs), which differ significantly from L&MICs in the availability of resources and access to advanced technology and specialized skills [19]. When making decisions about governance strategies, health system managers need context-specific information to make judgments about their applicability [7, 19].

19.5.1 Governance Strategies at the Policy Level: Enhancing the Effectiveness of Decentralization

Decentralization is a strategy that transfers authority from central to regional or local levels, to potentially improve participation, responsiveness, equity, and accountability (see Chapter 9) [19, 20].

Despite widespread adoption of decentralization in L&MICs, empirical evidence on its impact on the health system remains limited [20, 21]. A review of case studies from L&MICs found that the use of decentralization to improve the management of human resources for health enhanced community trust in the government and increased ownership and flexibility in planning, and had a likely positive influence on retention of health workers. However,

---

Box 19.2 Conditions for Effective Decentralization

Different forms of decentralization in governance have been implemented in the Philippines since the 1950s, providing key insights on the conditions for effective decentralization [23]:

- utilize a multistakeholder approach for planning;
- build capacity to raise revenues for health services at local levels and make evidence-informed funding decisions;
- use central-level capacity to provide resource needs locally through bulk procurement and deploying human resources to areas in need;
- use central-level capacity to ensure alignment of local authorities with national objectives and promote cooperation among local health facilities; and
- use central-level capacity to ensure timely and accurate local data collection for monitoring.

---

decentralization was generally associated with mismatches between transfer of roles and responsibilities and transfer of resources and lack of accountability and transparency [22].

Lessons learned from L&MICs suggest that adequate technical skills at the local level to perform decentralized tasks, effective decentralization of decision-making to the periphery, and political leadership are key for successful decentralization [21]. Box 19.2 summarizes key insights based on the Philippines' 25 years of experience with decentralization.

19.5.2 Governance Strategies at the Health Care and Related Institutions Level

Health Care Accreditation

Recent years have seen a shift away from voluntary self-regulation of health institutions, whereby organized groups (e.g., medical or hospital associations) regulate the behavior of their members – for example, by establishing a code of practice [24]. Instead, mandatory external inspection of adherence to standards through an external national body, such as the Punjab Health Care Commission in Pakistan, or international accreditation bodies has become increasingly common. If the standards are not adhered to, the external inspection body can take action to reinforce them, such as withdrawing designation as accredited. As such, accreditation is increasingly being used by governments as a tool for regulation, transparency, and public accountability [25]. However, it is uncertain whether external inspection of standards improves adherence with these standards and quality of care in hospital settings [26].

While several reviews have found benefits of health care accreditation (see Chapter 26) [27–29], there is uncertainty about whether health care accreditation improves the quality of care and health-related outcomes [19, 27, 30]. Many countries are encouraging participation in voluntary accreditation through linking accreditation status to incentives such as access to public funding, preferential reimbursement, health insurance benefits, contractual agreements, or designation as a medical travel destination. For example, in India, Brazil, and Costa Rica, insurers and employers are increasingly relying on accreditation award as a prerequisite for provider participation in their health care reimbursement programs [31]. In Lebanon, there are no legislative mandates for implementing quality improvement strategies and a patient safety system. In order to regulate the behavior of health care institutions, particularly in the private sector which is the dominant health care provider, the Ministry of Public Health linked accreditation status, along with other risk adjustment factors, to contracting with private and public health care facilities as an incentive for quality improvement [32, 33].

Public Disclosure of Performance Data

There is moderate-strength evidence that public disclosure of performance data for hospitals in HICs encourages them to implement quality improvement activities, and low-strength evidence that it may lead to slight improvements in hospital clinical outcomes and little or no difference in patient selection of hospitals [34]. In Qatar, for example, the Ministry of Public Health developed mandatory contractual performance agreements with public and private health care institutions with the intention to publish performance data as a tool for driving improvements in health care quality, accountability, and transparency [35]. Although Qatar is a HIC, its educational system for training health care professionals and health system regulation is less developed compared to other HICs from Europe or North America [36]. It therefore presents important lessons to L&MICs with similar capacities in human resources and information infrastructure. A focus on feasibility in measuring performance and building on existing information infrastructures while strengthening the capacity of health care institutions for measurement are critical to implementing contractual agreements, especially with the private sector [35].

Medicine Regulation

There is uncertainty that licensing of medicines outlets reduces the prevalence of counterfeit medicines or the failure rates of medicines undergoing quality testing in L&MICs [37]. Medicine registration, in which medicine regulatory authorities assess medicine manufacturers and products to ensure they meet international standards, may decrease the prevalence of counterfeit and substandard medicines, although the evidence is of low certainty [19]. Prequalification of medicines by WHO, whereby manufacturers receive WHO-approved certificates, may lead to a decrease in the failure rates of medicines undergoing quality testing. Finally, multifaceted interventions that include a mix of regulations, training of inspectors, public–private collaborations, and legal actions against counterfeiters may be effective in decreasing the prevalence of counterfeit and substandard medicines, although the evidence is of low certainty [19, 32, 37].

19.5.3 Governance Strategies at the Health Care Professionals' Level

Professionals' self-regulation, through professional associations or unions, is the dominant approach for regulating health care professionals. It can be combined with co-regulation and enforcement by the government, particularly in countries where the government is the main financier and provider of health care, such as Iran and Turkey. It is important to note the paucity of research on governance strategies of health care professionals, particularly from L&MICs [19].

Preservice: Pre-Licensing and Licensing

Evidence on the effects of governance strategies that improve pre-licensure education and ensure supply of adequately qualified health care professionals is generally limited, particularly from L&MICs [19, 38]. Low-certainty evidence indicates that academic advising programs that target minority groups may increase the number of minority students enrolled in and graduating from health training institutions [19, 38]. Other promising strategies that require further evaluation in L&MICs include providing financial support to health care professional students or introducing mechanisms to identify and encourage potential students [19, 38].

Licensing is commonly used by governments in L&MICs to regulate health care professionals and hold them accountable upon their entry into the workforce. Its implementation varies across countries and health care professional categories. For example, Angola does not require licensing of allied health professionals, physiotherapists, and opticians [39].

A recent comparative analysis among seven countries – of which four were L&MICs – of mandatory regulations and voluntary guidelines to control standards for medical education, clinical training, licensing, and relicensing of physicians revealed that there is no gold standard model for medical education and practice regulation. Combination of controls used in different countries enables identification of innovations and regulatory approaches to address specific contextual challenges, such as decentralization of regulations to subnational bodies or privatization of medical education [40].

In-service: Training and Revalidation

Health care professionals' self-regulation through professional associations or unions is a dominant strategy for regulating in-service training and revalidation [41]. It can be combined with regulation by government or external bodies. Professionally led self-regulation is seen as enabling transparency and accountability of health care professionals to external authorities [41].

In-service training programs of district health system managers that focus on developing managers' competencies, including knowledge, job performance, coordination, and communication skills, may increase knowledge of planning processes and monitoring and evaluation skills compared with no training, although the evidence is of low certainty [19, 42].

19.6 Means of Controlling Corruption

Corruption can be broadly defined as the abuse of entrusted power for private gain [43]. The health sector is particularly susceptible to corruption as: (1) it involves various actors, including patients who are considered vulnerable and often unaware of their rights; (2) private providers are entrusted with important public roles; and (3) large amounts of public money are allocated to health spending [44]. The cost of corruption in the health sector is substantial: the amount of health care funds wasted each year could achieve universal health coverage (UHC) [45]. Corruption has a significant adverse impact on access to and quality of health care services and health outcomes. It is estimated that annually more than 140,000 child deaths could indirectly be attributed to corruption, which exceeds the total of cholera, rabies, Ebola, and combat-related deaths [46]. Corruption can undermine a country's efforts toward equity, reform, and achieving all goals of the Sustainable Development Agenda. Its effects are likely to be debilitating in L&MICs, where the Corruption Perceptions Index (CPI), a measure of public sector corruption as perceived by business people and country analysts, is persistently high [47].

Jain [48] provides a theoretical overview of how corruption influences the provision of publicly provided health care services: (1) corruption can drive up the price and lower the level of government output and services; (2) it can reduce investment in human capital; and (3) it can reduce government revenue, which can lower the quality of publicly provided services and create incentives for seeking privately provided services. In countries where private markets for health care are limited, this can lead to congestion and delays in obtaining public services. Similarly, in countries where private markets are extensive, the poor may lack the ability to pay for private services, further deepening inequities [48].

19.6.1 Political Reform for Corruption Control

Corruption likely results when those in positions of power misuse their authority for their own rather than the public's interest and are not held accountable by the political system. It also likely depends on the extent of inclusivity of various interest groups in decision-making. For example, if the political system does not serve the interests of a specific group, this group may then explore weak points, such as through corrupt policymakers, to serve its own interests [48]. As such, effective control of corruption requires political reform with a focus on three main areas [48, 49]:

1. Open exchange of information, particularly with regards to how decisions are made by those in power, likely contributes to strengthening transparency and accountability. In Kyrgyzstan, for example, the government carried out several strategies, including providing the public with information about how much they should be paying providers, as well as increasing health care workers' salaries. These strategies may have led to reductions in informal payments, although the evidence is of low certainty.
2. Establishing legitimate channels for citizens and interest groups to participate in policymaking, express their interests, and exert influence. This may reduce corruption and increase participation, transparency, and accountability.
3. Mechanisms for controlling misuse of power, including penalties, must be strengthened in order to enforce the rule of law. A recent systematic review reported that combining improved detection and punishment of corruption with establishing an independent agency to coordinate anti-corruption activities can potentially detect and reduce corruption [49]. For example, in the United States there is high-certainty evidence that establishing a national independent agency to coordinate efforts to investigate and punish corruption in the health sector led to convictions and recovery of large amounts of money [49]. India's experience with an ombudsman for detecting corruption shows that reducing corruption depends on continued political support and is limited by a dysfunctional judicial system (Box 19.3) [49, 50]. Another promising intervention is establishing guidelines that prohibit doctors from accepting benefits from the pharmaceutical industry. Low-certainty evidence from Germany suggests that such guidelines may improve doctors' attitudes about the influence of pharmaceutical companies on their choice of medicines [49].

Importantly, health policymakers, managers, and providers working on addressing corruption in L&MICs should implement robust situation analyses to enable tailoring interventions to specific country needs [51], taking into account the availability of human and technical resources to combat fraud, the acceptability and costs of the interventions, and the increased vulnerability to fraud and its consequences [19].

> **Box 19.3** Lessons Learned from Controlling Corruption in India
>
> In Karnataka state in India, the Karnataka Lokayukta (KLA), a public complaints agency with the authority to investigate citizen complaints and initiate prosecution, had been criticized for failing to hold governments accountable. Upon the election of a new government, a new economically independent ombudsman with technical expertise in jurisdiction and health care was selected. Following this change in leadership, improvements to governance were seen within the KLA and to some extent in the wider health system.
>
> **Mobilizing the Media and Citizens**
>
> The KLA collaborated with the media to inform and mobilize citizens about corruption scandals. The approach was particularly successful in areas where citizens were better educated and of high economic status, but failed at the state level, mainly due to lack of political support.
>
> **Lack of Political Support Hindered Sustainable Change**
>
> Complaints increased after the first year of new leadership. Convictions increased only during the fourth year, as the initial aim was public education rather than legal action. Some junior officials were prosecuted for corruption, but political and judicial barriers limited convictions at senior levels.
>
> **Factors Influencing Governance and Corruption**
>
> Committed, powerful, and skilled leadership and a participatory citizenship movement were key positive factors for effective governance, while a shortage of financial resources, perception of weak sanctions, and poor education and representation of citizens hindered sustainable change.
>
> *Source:* [50].

19.7 Conclusion

The evidence is unclear about how different health system governance strategies work in different contexts, particularly in L&MICs. Health policymakers, managers, and providers need to cautiously assess and adapt strategies to their own contexts. A lot more research is needed to discover innovative ways of measuring, monitoring, and improving governance of the health system in L&MICs.

References

1. World Health Organization. Open mindsets: participatory leadership for health. 2016. www.who.int/alliance-hpsr/resources/publications/participatory-leadership/en/ (accessed June 15, 2021).

2. S. Chunharas, D. S. C. Davies. Leadership in health systems: a new agenda for interactive leadership. *Health Syst Reform* 2016; 2(3): 176–178.

3. S. Bennett, D. Glandon, K. Rasanathan. Governing multisectoral action for health in low-income and middle-income countries: unpacking the problem and rising to the challenge. *BMJ Glob Health* 2018; 3 (Suppl. 4): e000880.

4. R. C. Swanson, R. Atun, A. Best, et al. Strengthening health systems in low-income countries by enhancing organizational capacities and improving institutions. *Global Health* 2015; **11**: 5.

5. P. C. Smith, A. Anell, R. Busse, et al. Leadership and governance in seven developed health systems. *Health Policy* 2012; **106**(1): 37–49.

6. P. G. Forest, J. L. Denis, L. D. Brown, et al. Health reform requires policy capacity. *Int J Health Policy Manag* 2015; **4**(5): 265–266.

7. World Health Organization. Strengthening health system governance: better policies, stronger performance. 2016. www .euro.who.int/__data/assets/pdf_file/0004/ 307939/Strengthening-health-system-governance-better-policies-stronger-performance.pdf (accessed June 14, 2020).

8. V. I. Murunga, R. N. Oronje, I. Bates, et al. Review of published evidence on knowledge translation capacity, practice and support among researchers and research institutions in low- and middle-income countries. *Health Res Policy Syst* 2020; **18**(1): 16.

9. F. El-Jardali, J. N. Lavis, N. Ataya, et al. Use of health systems evidence by policymakers in eastern Mediterranean countries: views, practices, and contextual influences. *BMC Health Serv Res* 2012; **12**: 200.

10. A. Zida, J. N. Lavis, N K. Sewankambo, et al. The factors affecting the institutionalisation of two policy units in Burkina Faso's health system: a case study. *Health Res Policy Syst* 2017; **15**(1): 62.

11. F. El-Jardali, J. Lavis, K. Moat, et al. Capturing lessons learned from evidence-to-policy initiatives through structured reflection. *Health Res Policy Syst* 2014; **12**: 2.

12. J. M. Kasonde, S. Campbell. Creating a knowledge translation platform: nine lessons from the Zambia Forum for Health Research. *Health Res Policy Syst* 2012; **10**: 31.

13. F. El-Jardali, L. Bou-Karroum, R. Fadlallah. Amplifying the role of knowledge translation platforms in the COVID-19 pandemic response. *Health Res Policy Syst* 2020; **18**(1): 58.

14. F. El-Jardali, E. Akl, L. Bou Karroum, et al. Impact story: policy-responsive systematic reviews: the case of Syrian refugees in Lebanon. 2018. www.ncbi.nlm.nih.gov/ books/NBK569575/ (accessed June 17, 2020).

15. USAID. *Health Systems Assessment Approach: A How-To Manual.* 2007. http:// conflict.lshtm.ac.uk/media/USAID_health_ systems_assessment_approach_2007.pdf (accessed August 16, 2022).

16. D. Clarke, S. Doerr, M. Hunter, et al. The private sector and universal health coverage. *Bull World Health Organ* 2019; **97**(6): 434–435.

17. L. Roth, D. Bempong, J. B. Babigumira, et al. Expanding global access to essential medicines: investment priorities for sustainably strengthening medical product regulatory systems. *Global Health* 2018; **14**(1): 102.

18. D. P. Carpenter. *The Forging of Bureaucratic Autonomy.* Princeton, NJ: Princeton University Press, 2001.

19. C. A. Herrera, S. Lewin, E. Paulsen, et al. Governance arrangements for health systems in low-income countries: an overview of systematic reviews. *Cochrane Database Syst Rev* 2017; **9**(9): CD011085.

20. R. S. Saltman, V. Bankauskaite, K. Vrangbaek. Decentralization in health care, strategies and outcomes. 2007. www .euro.who.int/en/publications/abstracts/dece ntralization-in-health-care.-strategies-and-outcomes-2007 (accessed June 12, 2021).

21. D. Cobos Muñoz, P. Merino Amador, L. Monzon Llamas, et al. Decentralization of health systems in low and middle income countries: a systematic review. *Int J Public Health* 2017; **62**(2): 219–229.

22. M. Dieleman, D. M. Shaw, P. Zwanikken. Improving the implementation of health workforce policies through governance: a review of case studies. *Hum Resour Health* 2011; **9**: 10.

23. H. J. Liwanag, K. Wyss. What conditions enable decentralization to improve the health system? Qualitative analysis of perspectives on decision space after 25 years of devolution in the Philippines. *PLoS One* 2018; **13**(11): e0206809.

24. J. Healy, J. Braithwaite. Designing safer health care through responsive regulation. *Med J Aust* 2006; **184**(S10): S56–S59.

25. World Health Organization. Quality and accreditation in health care services: a global review. 2003. https://apps.who.int/iris/handle/10665/68410 (accessed June 11, 2020).

26. G. Flodgren, M. P. Pomey, S. A. Taber, et al. Effectiveness of external inspection of compliance with standards in improving healthcare organisation behaviour, healthcare professional behaviour or patient outcomes. *Cochrane Database Syst Rev* 2011; **11**: CD008992.

27. D. Greenfield, J. Braithwaite. Health sector accreditation research: a systematic review. *Int J Qual Health Care* 2008; **20**(3): 172–183.

28. G. K. Ng, G. K. Leung, J. M. Johnston, et al. Factors affecting implementation of accreditation programmes and the impact of the accreditation process on quality improvement in hospitals: a SWOT analysis. *Hong Kong Med J* 2013; **19**(5): 434–446.

29. D. Greenfield, M. Pawsey, R. Hinchcliff, et al. The standard of healthcare accreditation standards: a review of empirical research underpinning their development and impact. *BMC Health Serv Res* 2012; **12**: 329.

30. E. Patouillard, C. A. Goodman, K. G. Hanson, et al. Can working with the private for-profit sector improve utilization of quality health services by the poor? A systematic review of the literature. *Int J Equity Health* 2007; **6**: 17.

31. K. S. Mate, A. L. Rooney, A. Supachutikul, et al. Accreditation as a path to achieving universal quality health coverage. *Global Health* 2014; **10**: 68.

32. F. El-Jardali, R. Fadlallah. A review of national policies and strategies to improve quality of health care and patient safety: a case study from Lebanon and Jordan. *BMC Health Serv Res* 2017; **17**(1): 568.

33. W. Ammar, J. Khalife, F. El-Jardali, et al. Hospital accreditation, reimbursement and case mix: links and insights for contractual systems. *BMC Health Serv Res* 2013; **13**: 505.

34. C. H. Fung, Y. W. Lim, S. Mattke, et al. Systematic review: the evidence that publishing patient care performance data improves quality of care. *Ann Intern Med* 2008; **148**(2): 111–123.

35. H. Al-Katheeri, F. El-Jardali, N. Ataya, et al. Contractual health services performance agreements for responsive health systems: from conception to implementation in the case of Qatar. *Int J Qual Health Care* 2018; **30**(3): 219–226.

36. J. I. Sheikh, S. Cheema, K. Chaabna, et al. Capacity building in health care professions within the Gulf Cooperation Council countries: paving the way forward. *BMC Med Educ* 2019; **19**(1): 83.

37. F. El-Jardali, E. A. Akl, R. Fadlallah, et al. Interventions to combat or prevent drug counterfeiting: a systematic review. *BMJ Open* 2015; **5**(3): e006290.

38. G. W. Pariyo, S. N. Kiwanuka, E. Rutebemberwa, et al. Effects of changes in the pre-licensure education of health workers on health-worker supply. *Cochrane Database Syst Rev* 2009; **2**: CD007018.

39. A. D. Kaplan, S. Dominis, J. G. Palen, et al. Human resource governance: what does governance mean for the health workforce in low- and middle-income countries? *Hum Resour Health* 2013; **11**: 6.

40. W. Aftab, M. Khan, S. Rego, et al. Variations in regulations to control standards for training and licensing of physicians: a multi-country comparison. *Hum Resour Health* 2021; **19**(1): 91.

41. S. Merkur, P. Mladovsky, E. Mossialos, et al. Do lifelong learning and revalidation ensure that physicians are fit to practise?

2008. www.euro.who.int/__data/assets/pdf_file/0005/75434/E93412.pdf (accessed June 10, 2020).

42. P. C. Rockers, T. Bärnighausen. Interventions for hiring, retaining and training district health systems managers in low- and middle-income countries. *Cochrane Database Syst Rev* 2013; **4**: CD009035.

43. Transparency International. What is corruption? 2020. www.transparency.org/en/what-is-corruption (accessed August 25, 2020).

44. W. D. Savedoff. *The Causes of Corruption in the Health Sector: Corruption and Health*. London, Pluto Press, 2006.

45. Transparency International. Health. 2021. www.transparency.org/en/our-priorities/health-and-corruption (accessed August 28, 2020).

46. M. Hanf, A. Van-Melle, F. Fraisse, et al. Corruption kills: estimating the global impact of corruption on children deaths. *PLoS One* 2011; **6**(11): e26990.

47. Transparency International. Persistently high corruption in low-income countries amounts to an "ongoing humanitarian disaster." 2008. www.transparency.org/en/press/20080930-persistently-high-corruption-in-low-income-countries (accessed August 25, 2021).

48. A. K. Jain, ed., *Power, Politics, and Corruption: The Political Economy of Corruption*. London, Routledge, 2001.

49. R. Gaitonde, A. D. Oxman, P. O. Okebukola, et al. Interventions to reduce corruption in the health sector. *Cochrane Database Syst Rev* 2016; **8**: CD008856.

50. R. Huss, A. Green, H. Sudarshan, et al. Good governance and corruption in the health sector: lessons from the Karnataka experience. *Health Policy Plan* 2011; **26**(6): 471–484.

51. World Health Organization. Reinforcing the focus on anti-corruption, transparency and accountability in national health policies, strategies and plans. 2019. www.who.int/publications/i/item/reinforcing-the-focus-on-anti-corruption-transparency-and-accountability-in-national-health-policies-strategies-and-plans (accessed January 16, 2021).

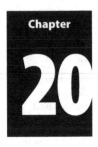

Developing a Balanced Health Workforce
Understanding the Health Labor Market Dynamics

F. Gulin Gedik and Mario Dal Poz

Key Messages

- The development of health workforce strategies and implementation plans requires significant technical skills and competence, but it does not offer a blueprint for countries to replicate.
- The development of health workforce strategies and implementation plans is a technical as well as a political exercise as it involves many actors, often with diverging interests; hence, engaging stakeholders is a necessity, not merely an option.
- It will rarely be possible to meet the objectives of all stakeholders, but their engagement, including health care providers and communities, public and private sector representatives, and of course planners and policymakers, reduces avoidable misunderstandings and resistance.
- The traditional planning methods will fail if the preferences and behaviors of the supply and demand sides and health labor market dynamics are overlooked.
- Each country has its own unique circumstances. Although expert planners can use the experience of comparable countries as a source of lessons and good practice, each country must find its own way of addressing its health workforce challenges.

20.1 Introduction

The health workforce is well recognized as a critical component of any health system. Challenges with health workforce development have persisted for decades and are more prominent in low- and middle-income countries (L&MICs). The shortage of health workers and the limited absorptive capacity[1] of the health system have delayed implementation of related strategies and interventions even when sufficient funds are available. The *World Health Report 2006* identified a threshold of 2.3 doctors, nurses, and midwives per 1,000 population as essential to deliver basic services to achieve the Millennium Development Goals, and signaled critical shortages of health workers in 57 countries [1]. The Agenda for Sustainable Development further recognized the importance of the health workforce and set in its Goal of Health and Wellbeing (SDG 3) an ambitious target (3c): "substantially increase health financing, and the recruitment, development, training and retention of the health workforce in developing countries" [2].

---

[1] The ability to recruit people within the system.

The WHO Global Strategy on Human Resources for Health: Workforce 2030 examined the contemporary evidence and provided recommendations and policy options for transformative actions to tackle incipient health workforce challenges, toward attaining universal health coverage (UHC). The health workforce has a fundamental role in enabling progress toward UHC and Sustainable Development Goals (SDGs), and WHO estimates an indicative threshold of aggregate density of around 4.45 health workers, comprising doctors, nurses, and midwives, per 1,000 population that corresponds to the median score of SDG tracer indicator attainment (25%) [3].

There is a growing recognition that the demand for health services generated by population growth, aging, and economic development is placing an increased emphasis on how countries train, recruit, deploy, retain, and manage their health workforces. This has led to an unprecedented and much-needed focus on health workforce policy, planning, production, deployment, and continued professional development, while giving due consideration to labor market factors [4]. To address their health workforce challenges, L&MICs need to develop effective strategies to optimize the supply of the health workforce, as well as support their recruitment, deployment, retention, and performance [3]. The challenge ahead is to determine what to do and, more importantly, how to do it.

Every country has its unique demographic, epidemiological, cultural, economic, and health system milieu. Planners can use the experience of comparable countries as a source of lessons and good practices, but attempting to replicate the experience of other countries is unlikely to be successful. Each country must find its own path to address health workforce challenges [5], with an understanding of the labor market dynamics. Chapter 6 highlighted some of the conceptual underpinnings and associated frameworks that can help identify health workforce challenges and the factors that influence them. This chapter focuses on the application of those concepts and frameworks in framing policies and strategies that can help address the prevailing workforce challenges in L&MICs.

20.2 Understanding the Health Labor Market

Traditionally, health workforce policy development has largely been oblivious to health labor market dynamics, which is one of the reasons that health workforce policies in the past have failed to achieve their objectives [6–8]. The analyses of health workforces have been framed as a supply crisis, to be answered with *training more*, with the demand-side factors receiving little attention. The use of a labor market analysis permits greater insight into key factors that affect need for and demand and supply of health workers in a dynamic system. In many countries there is a misalignment between:

- **need:** the number of health workers required to provide health care to everyone;
- **demand:** the number of jobs a country's public and private sectors can create with the budget and funds it has; and
- **supply:** the number of trained health workers in the country that can potentially be recruited and are willing to work.

There is often a mismatch between the financial resources available – and therefore the ability to recruit health workers – and the number of workers required to address the health needs of the population. Beyond the numbers, the imbalances in the skill mix and the distribution of health workers across levels of the health system and geographical areas amplify the problem. This is affected by the capacities, behaviors, and preferences of actors on both the supply (health workers) and the demand (employers) sides [9]. It is hence necessary to understand and take into account the diverse and dynamic aspects of the health labor market to be able to develop effective health workforce policies and strategies.

Sousa et al. [10] developed a comprehensive framework to analyze and understand the health labor market, addressing not only the supply and demand for health workers, but also key areas for policy interventions (Figure 20.1). Building on the framework, the supply of and demand for health workers will be discussed next, with the aim of contributing to a better understanding of policies to address health workforce challenges through a labor market approach, particularly in relation to key issues such as production, maldistribution and retention, attrition and mobility of health workers, and regulation of health workers' education and practice.

20.2.1 Supply of and Demand for Health Workers

The supply of health workers is determined by the number of qualified health workers who are willing to work in the health sector under given conditions, including prevailing wages in health institutions such as hospitals, clinics, pharmacies, diagnostic centers, and training centers. The supply of health workers is shaped by labor market demands, the health workforce production capacities, and the education market – that is, the availability, capacity, and quality of health professional education institutions.

Conversely, the demand for health workers is determined by what employers (the government, the private sector, and different actors) are willing and able to pay to hire the health workers. "Willingness to pay" makes a distinction between demand and need. The demand for health workers, which is linked to – or derived from – the demand for health care, depends on the capacity and willingness of public and private institutions to hire health workers. The "willingness to pay" of employers depends on the availability of financial resources. Hence, there is often a mismatch between the demand, as a measure of the absorptive capacity, and the actual need for health workers in a health system. The demand and supply of workers in the health sector are influenced by many factors, as shown in Box 20.1; it is thus useful to identify **enabling** labor market and public policies.

Financial considerations are increasingly becoming a significant determinant of the demand for health workers and their recruitment. Health workers respond to economic incentives that are unrelated to the health care needs of the population. Employers also respond to economic, social, and political incentives, and the demands of consumers in addition to the health care needs of the population. A better understanding of the health labor market helps to identify challenges in a more rational manner and allows the development of policies tailored to address the identified problems, as shown in Figure 20.1.

20.3 Policies to Address Health Workforce Challenges Using a Labor Market Approach

20.3.1 Policies on Production of Health Workers

As the overall global shortages of health workers continue, more attention is being paid to training more health professionals. The production of health professionals is influenced by the availability of resources, the rate of return to education, educational approaches,

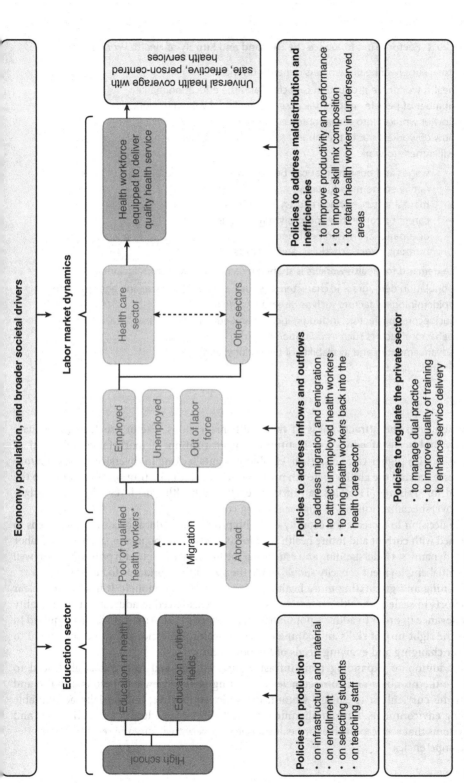

Figure 20.1 Health labor market framework for UHC [10].

The labeled content within the figure:

Economy, population, and broader societal drivers

Education sector | **Labor market dynamics**

Universal health coverage with safe, effective, person-centred health services

High school

Education in health

Education in other fields

Pool of qualified health workers*

Migration

Abroad

Employed

Unemployed

Out of labor force

Health care sector

Other sectors

Health workforce equipped to deliver quality health service

Policies on production
- on infrastructure and material
- on enrollment
- on selecting students
- on teaching staff

Policies to address inflows and outflows
- to address migration and emigration
- to attract unemployed health workers
- to bring health workers back into the health care sector

Policies to address maldistribution and inefficiencies
- to improve productivity and performance
- to improve skill mix composition
- to retain health workers in underserved areas

Policies to regulate the private sector
- to manage dual practice
- to improve quality of training
- to enhance service delivery

Box 20.1 Factors That Influence the Demand and Supply of Health Workers

The total supply of health workers depends on the:

- health workforce production capacities and the education market;
- number of people educated/licensed to work and willing to work;
- flow of workers into the labor force (graduations);
- flow of workers out of the labor force (retirements); and
- willingness to work:
  - wages and benefits that can be earned;
  - family economic situation;
  - marital status, having children and other dependents;
  - career opportunities and growth trajectories;
  - occupational environment; and
  - burnout, stress, schedules, and interests.

The demand for health workers is shaped by a number of factors, including:

- population demographic characteristics such as population size and age structure;
- epidemiological factors such as disease patterns;
- socioeconomic factors, including income and education levels;
- behavioral factors such as utilization patterns;
- advancement in and availability of technology; and
- financial resources.

regulation, and the attractiveness of the health professions. Factors such as inadequate capacity and scale of education institutions, prioritization of marketable skills and of specialties with higher rates of return, eligible students lacking in diversity, and regulatory weaknesses curtail the ability of health professional education institutions to respond to the demand for training [11]. This can further result in a health workforce with skills imbalances, overspecialization, and a higher training cost.

The decision to increase the capacity of health professional education institutions needs to be aligned with current and future health workforce needs of the population, considering labor market dynamics. Understanding and estimating the future need for health professionals as well as potential employment capacity should guide the size of the workforce to be trained.

Training and graduating more health professionals is not enough. It has become clear that efforts to scale up health professionals' education also need to address issues of quality and relevance in order to address population health needs [12]. Attention is also required to attain the right mix of skills and competencies of health professionals who can respond to the ever changing and evolving needs of the population.

In addition to expanding their infrastructure, educational institutions also need to improve the numbers and competencies of existing staff, review admissions criteria, and adjust the curriculum to ensure vibrant, dynamic, supportive, and socially accountable learning environments. Greater alignment is needed between educational institutions and the systems that are responsible for health service delivery to ensure the required quantities and competencies.

20.3.2 Policies to Address Maldistribution and Retention

The demand side introduces the challenges of recruitment and retention. The health labor market model outlined above offers a structure for evaluating the role of incentives in recruiting and retaining health workers. A health worker will accept a job if the benefits of doing so outweigh the opportunity cost. Improving recruitment and retention requires providing the type and level of compensation that reduces the appeal of alternative employment, such as reducing external (international) pressure to recruit health workers in certain countries [13].

Financial incentives, career development, and management issues are key factors that affect health workers' motivation to remain. Recognition is obviously highly influential in incentivizing health workers. Moreover, adequate supplies and facilities are factors that can dramatically increase morale [14]. To enhance staff motivation [15, 16], work incentives such as salary increments and payment of extra duty hours allowance are often implemented. While these incentives are effective, relying on them without adequate complementary nonfinancial incentives has proven to be insufficient to sustain staff motivation and performance [14, 17, 18].

Limited health budgets in L&MICs make financial rewards unsustainable and impractical as the sole or main strategy to incentivize health workers. Although a significant proportion of domestic health expenditures goes toward the wage bill (staff salaries) in low-income countries [19], staff productivity and quality of health care service delivery remain a major challenge. Considering that staff motivation can be determined by factors beyond material and financial rewards, there is the need to explore the possible nonfinancial incentives that could be potentially cost-effective and sustainable in the long term [20].

Studies have shown that besides financial incentives, a good working relationship between staff and clients promotes staff motivation and quality of health care delivery, especially at the primary care level [21]. Health workers who perceive a sense of duty to the community they serve are more likely to be intrinsically motivated and have better working experience with clients [22, 23].

The WHO's global recommendations on increasing access to health workers in remote and rural areas through improved retention were updated and revised in 2021 [24]. These can be classified into four categories of interventions related to education, regulation, financing, and external environment (Table 20.1) [25].

Different interventions can be applied in different contexts and for different types of health workers. Despite the lack of rigorous evaluations, it is proposed that: (1) interventions need to be implemented in packages, addressing different but interrelated issues; and (2) health workers' preferences need to be considered in the design of interventions. The latter is especially important as employment decisions are a function of those preferences and the success of any recruitment and retention strategy depends on making work in rural and remote jobs more attractive to health workers [26]. A recent review of effective strategies to develop the rural health workforce in L&MICs proposes, among others, that rural pathways only work if rural workers are supported once they have been trained [27].

The process for designing and implementing strategic and effective recruitment and retention plans should include a comprehensive situation analysis, including a systematic health labor market analysis. Such an analysis provides accurate information on key aspects

Table 20.1 Interventions that enhance retention of health workers in rural and remote areas [25]

Category of intervention	Examples
Education	• Students from rural backgrounds • Health professional schools outside of major cities • Clinical rotations in rural areas during studies • Curricula that reflect rural health issues • Continuous professional development for rural health workers
Regulatory	• Enhanced scope of practice • Different types of health workers • Compulsory service • Subsidized education for return of service
Incentives	• A package of fiscally sustainable financial and nonfinancial incentives, including all benefits (i.e., remuneration, allowances, housing, transportation, etc.)
Professional and personal support	• Decent living conditions • Safe, secure, and supportive working environment • Decent work • Outreach support and support networks • Career development programs • Professional networks • Social recognition measures

of the health workforce in the country (e.g., current number and distribution of health workers by skills, gender, geographical region, distribution across public and private sectors, the existence of dual practice, and the level of unemployment) and identifies the main factors leading to a mismatch between demand and supply of health workers in rural and remote areas (i.e., the push and pull factors).

Quantitative analysis and planning. It is critical to have information on the number and distribution of various cadres of health workers. However, many countries are challenged in ensuring the availability of comprehensive, accurate, and reliable data. Different data sources and mechanisms to strengthen health workforce data and information are elaborated in Section 20.4.

Qualitative work to identify employment decision contexts. This step is essential for reaching an understanding of the context in which health workers make employment decisions, as well as specific characteristics of health workers' preferences and expectations. Carefully designed qualitative research may help to identify critical job attributes most valued by health workers, and their relative importance and intensity of preferences.

Scale-up interventions. After a package of recruitment and retention interventions is developed based on the analyses and other considerations, policy effectiveness needs to be monitored and evaluated as the interventions are implemented in a phased manner.

Therefore, the recruitment and retention of health workers in remote and rural areas depend both on the factors influencing the preferences of health workers for rural or remote areas and the health system's ability to meet such preferences. In other words, the interventions must respond to the factors that health workers value when choosing to work in these areas [25, 28].

20.3.3 Policies to Address Attrition and Mobility of Health Workers

With globalization, the international mobility of people, services, and goods has increased. Thus, health workforce mobility has also increased. Historically, international workforce mobility has been seen as "brain drain" from L&MICs, which oftentimes exacerbates health workforce shortages. The migration of skilled health workers has become more complex, more global, and of growing concern to the countries that lose much-needed health workers. The migration of skilled health workers occurs for a variety of reasons, many of which are common across different countries. They include income, job satisfaction, career opportunity, management and governance, and social and family motivations. Some countries suffer disproportionately from the effects of migration. If a country has a fragile health system, the loss of part of its trained workforce adds further strain on the health systems and on the remaining health workers, especially in rural and underserved areas. The impact of aging populations, innovations in technology, and changing consumer demands will most certainly affect the demand for health care and accelerate the movement of health workers [29].

There are concerns around the severe shortage of health workers in many countries as a major threat to the performance of health systems. Even more alarming is the increasing migration of highly educated and trained health personnel from countries in conflicts and crises that further weakens the fragile health systems of these countries. As a response, the World Health Assembly adopted the WHO Global Code of Practice on International Recruitment of Health Personnel in 2010 [30]. This Code outlines some principles for managing health workforce mobility and ethical international recruitment, emphasizing that countries should strengthen their health systems and ensure self-sustainability in ensuring retention of health workers. It also highlights a rationale for improved collaboration and information exchange among countries, including multilateral and bilateral agreements to manage the mobility of health workers. The voluntary and nonbinding nature of this Code does not oblige countries to implement its guidelines, with little impact on transnational workforce mobility. The WHO developed the Health Workforce Support and Safeguard List in February 2021, which has identified 47 priority countries for health personnel development and health system-related support. These countries are to be provided with safeguards that discourage active international recruitment of health personnel [31].

Although it is challenging to be even-handed, policies and interventions related to health workforce mobility should consider balancing the relationship between the rights of health personnel, including the right to leave their countries and to migrate, and the right to the highest attainable standard of health of the populations of countries.

20.3.4 Policies to Regulate Health Workers' Education and Practice

The regulation of health workforce education and practice is getting greater attention with rising concerns about the quality of training, especially with the increasing involvement of the private sector in both education and employment of health workers. Regulation of the health workforce aims to improve the quality of education and services provided to protect the users.

The core elements of many regulatory systems include: the standards set for entry into a profession (i.e., the minimum criteria to be admitted to a school of medicine or nursing); the standards required to become registered or licensed (i.e., prescribed educational pathways and qualifications); the standards required to maintain registration (including continuing professional development); and the mechanisms for dealing with people who breach the standards [32]. Consequently, new oversight and appraisal systems and mechanisms need to be put in place, such as school self-assessment, external evaluation, institution and program accreditation, and the like [33–35]. The institutional arrangements, approaches, and processes that are established to implement these systems may vary among countries, according to the legislation and the purpose of the regulation itself.

Another significant challenge for health systems in advancing toward UHC is to tackle dual practice. Having individual providers simultaneously holding multiple positions in the public and private sectors is becoming increasingly prevalent among health workers in many L&MICs. Internationally, there is wide cross-country heterogeneity in government responses to dual practice in the health sector. Countries consider three broad sets of interventions to address this recalcitrant problem – banning dual practice, offering rewarding contracts to public physicians, and limiting dual practice (including both limits to private earnings of dual providers and limits to involvement in private activities). In theory, there is support for different regulations in different economic environments; however, it is a challenge to implement these in practice in most countries [36]. An assessment of the impacts of dual practice and its causes may allow policymakers to offer appropriate solutions. Where needed, countries could implement optimal regulatory policies on dual practice and ensure progress toward UHC (see Chapter 27) [35–37].

20.4 Data Needs for Health Workforce Planning, Production, Deployment, and Performance

While there is no single source of data that captures the various health workforce dynamics, there are a number of data sources that can potentially be used to collect information on the health workforce in most countries (see Box 20.2). These include population censuses, labor force and employment surveys, health facility assessments, and administrative databases for human resource management and planning (such as health information systems, payroll data, and databases of regulatory bodies). However, none of these sources are primarily designed for the purpose of supporting health workforce policy and planning. Consequently, the evidence on the impact of various health workforce strategies on health system performance and health outcomes remains largely fragmented and incomplete, in part due to the lack of institutional capacity in many countries to collect, analyze, and use this data to support health workforce management decisions [37].

It is essential that health workforce data goes beyond simply counting the number of health workers, but also includes their basic characteristics to help understand the determinants of and solutions to labor market imbalances. In this way, better data can be used to

Box 20.2 National Health Workforce Accounts

As part of the Global Strategy on Human Resources for Health for 2030 [3], approved by the World Health Assembly in 2016, WHO defined as relevant the improvement of data and information on the health workforce. The goal is for all countries to make progress in their records to monitor stock, education, distribution, flow, demand, capacity, and compensation of the health workforce. To this end, WHO proposes to organize data and information into a National Health Workforce Account (NHWA) to standardize information architecture and interoperability, as well as to monitor health workforce policy performance. The NHWA contains a set of 78 core indicators distributed in 10 modules, aiming at supporting health workforce policies at the national level. The indicators and the modules are structured in three crucial components of the health labor market: education, labor market participation, and the relationship with the health of the population.

Source: [42].

generate information to develop evidence-informed health workforce policies built on comprehensive health workforce analysis [38].

In order to adequately outline the characteristics and dynamics of the health workforce, the multiple sources identified above, as well as data on employers and health services and on training, registration, and licensing can be consulted [39, 40]. It is not always possible to have all the information; however, a minimum amount of information about the available workforce is always required. The availability of more data increases the likelihood of more comprehensive planning and projections [41].

Assuming that L&MICs have less data, they can begin by using simple approaches such as the worker–population ratio or service-based benchmarks for planning to address their current imbalances. Once more data becomes available, as is the case in many middle and higher income countries, other L&MICs can work toward improving their models, adding less tangible and still relevant dimensions such as productivity or skill mix.

20.5 Governance Arrangements for Policy and Planning of the Health Workforce

Strategic planning is not reducible to the production of a plan. It is important to have a plan, but the real challenge is the implementation of change. It is critical to see planning as a process that is flexible enough to consider contextual factors. Planners and policymakers need to be continuously attentive and be flexible in adapting their strategies [5]. For example, one study showed that the extent and eventual success of health workforce planning varies considerably between European countries, depending on two key aspects [43]: (1) identification, development, and use of models and tools to balance and obtain forecasts on the demand and supply of the health workforce; and (2) development of an integrated system of health workforce planning, involving multiple institutions and stakeholders and influencing cross-cutting policies (health care, education, labor market, and others).

Therefore, undertaking strategic planning and implementation processes requires well-established health workforce governance capacities and mechanisms. Strengthening governance capacities among all stakeholders is important, and the capacity of the Ministry of Health is critical, as it should take the leadership and coordination functions in the development, implementation, and monitoring of health workforce strategic plans. The units in the Ministry of Health in charge of the health workforce need to have the technical capacity, adequate mandate, responsibilities, resources, and accountability for a standard set of core functions of health workforce governance, policy, planning, information, reporting, and other functions.

Similarly, mechanisms for multistakeholder coordination, partnership, and policy dialog for the health workforce, such as human resources for health committees or stakeholder boards, are key for successful monitoring and evaluation of health workforce policies, strategies, and plans.

20.6 Conclusion

This chapter has focused on the use of labor market dynamics concepts and frameworks in developing policies and strategies to address the current workforce challenges in L&MICs. There is a growing recognition that the increased demand for health services brought about by population growth, aging, and economic development is putting greater emphasis on how countries train, recruit, deploy, retain, and manage their health workforces. This has resulted in an unprecedented and much-needed focus on health workforce policy, planning, production, deployment, and ongoing professional development, while taking labor market factors into account. L&MICs must develop effective strategies to optimize health workforce supply while also supporting recruitment, deployment, retention, and performance in order to address their health workforce challenges. The challenge ahead is to decide on what to do and, more importantly, how to do it.

References

1. World Health Organization. *Working Together for Health: The World Health Report 2006*. Geneva, World Health Organization, 2006. www.who.int/whr/2006/whr06_en.pdf (accessed May 11, 2021).

2. United Nations. SDG indicators, metadata repository. 2022. https://unstats.un.org/sdgs/metadata/?Text=&Goal=3&Target=3.c (accessed March 7, 2022).

3. World Health Organization. *Global Strategy on Human Resources for Health: Workforce 2030*. Geneva, World Health Organization, 2016. https://apps.who.int/iris/bitstream/handle/10665/250368/9789241511131-eng.pdf;jsessionid=1BF3D138816BD89DEDEA7F726FB6DCAF?sequence=1 (accessed March 12, 2021).

4. F. G. Gedik, J. Buchan, Z. Mirza, et al. The need for research evidence to meet health workforce challenges in the Eastern Mediterranean Region (Editorial). *East Mediterr Health J* 2018; **24**(9): 811–812.

5. N. Arya, J. S. Barbara. *Peace through Health: How Health Professionals Can Work for a Less Violent World*. West Hartford, Kumarian Press, 2008.

6. S. Birch, G. Kephart, G. T. Murphy, et al. Health human resources planning and the production of health: development of an extended analytical framework for needs-based health human resources planning. *J Public Health Manag Pract* 2009; **15**(6 Suppl.): S56–S61.

7. M. Vujicic, P. Zurn. The dynamics of the health labour market. *Int J Health Plann Manage* 2006; **21**(2): 101–115.

8. B. McPake, A. Maeda, E. C. Araújo, et al. Why do health labour market forces matter? *Bull World Health Organ* 2013; **91**: 841–846.

9. R. M. Scheffler, C. H. Herbst, C. Lemiere, et al. *Health Labor Market Analyses in Low- and Middle-Income Countries: An Evidence-Based Approach.* Washington, DC, World Bank, 2016.

10. A. Sousa, R. M. Scheffler, J. Nyoni, et al. A comprehensive health labour market framework for universal health coverage. *Bull World Health Organ* 2013; **91**: 892–894.

11. T. Evans, E. C. Araujo, C. H. Herbst, et al. Addressing the challenges of health professional education: opportunities to accelerate progress towards universal health coverage. 2016. www.researchgate.net/ profile/Christopher-Herbst/publication/ 317689924_Addressing_the_challenges_ of_health_professional_education_ Opportunities_to_accelerate_progress_ towards_universal_health_coverage/links/ 59493395aca272f02e0f3799/Addressing-the- challenges-of-health-professional-education -Opportunities-to-accelerate-progress- towards-universal-health-coverage.pdf (accessed May 12, 2021).

12. World Health Organization. Transforming and scaling up health professionals' education and training. 2013. www.who.int/ publications/i/item/transforming-and- scaling-up-health-professionals%E2%80% 99-education-and-training (accessed March 11, 2021).

13. C. Hongoro, C. Normand. Health workers: building and motivating the workforce. In D. T. Jamison, R. Nugent, H. Gelband, et al., eds., *Disease Control Priorities 2015– 2018*, 3rd ed. Washington, DC, World Bank, 2019, pp. 1309–1322.

14. M. Willis-Shattuck, P. Bidwell, S. Thomas, et al. Motivation and retention of health workers in developing countries: a systematic review. *BMC Health Serv Res* 2008; **8**: 247.

15. J. Antwi, D. C. Phillips. Wages and health worker retention: evidence from public sector wage reforms in Ghana. *J Dev Econ* 2013; **102**: 101–115.

16. S. D. Ndima, M. Sidat, H. Ormel, et al. Supervision of community health workers in Mozambique: a qualitative study of factors influencing motivation and programme implementation. *Hum Resour Health* 2015; **13**(1): 63.

17. I. A. Agyepong, P. Anafi, E. Asiamah, et al. Health worker (internal customer) satisfaction and motivation in the public sector in Ghana. *Int J Health Plann Manage* 2004; **19**(4): 319–336.

18. I. Mathauer, I. Imhoff. Health worker motivation in Africa: the role of non-financial incentives and human resource management tools. *Hum Resour Health* 2006; **4**: 24.

19. P. Hernandez, S. Dräger, D. B. Evans, et al. Measuring expenditure for the health workforce: evidence and challenges. 2006. www.who.int/hrh/documents/measuring_ expenditure.pdf (accessed April 13, 2021).

20. V. Hicks, O. Adams. Pay and non-pay incentives, performance and motivation: towards a global health workforce strategy. 2003. http://193.190.239.98/bitstream/ handle/10390/2554/2003shso0257.pdf? sequence=2 (accessed May 10, 2021).

21. T. Frank, K. Källander. Developing intervention strategies to improve community health worker motivation and performance. 2012. www .malariaconsortium.org/upscale/local/ downloads/1234-inscale-learning-paper- developing-intervention-strategies- english.pdf (accessed May 12, 2021).

22. D. L. Strachan, K. Källander, M. Nakirunda, et al. Using theory and formative research to design interventions to improve community health worker motivation, retention and performance in Mozambique and Uganda. *Hum Resour Health* 2015; **13**(1): 1–3.

23. J. A. Greenspan, S. A. McMahon, J. J. Chebet, et al. Sources of community health worker motivation: a qualitative study in Morogoro Region, Tanzania. *Hum Resour Health* 2013; **11**: 52.

24. World Health Organization. *WHO Guideline on Health Workforce Development, Attraction, Recruitment and Retention in Rural and Remote Areas.* Geneva, World Health Organization, 2021.

www.who.int/publications/i/item/9789240024229 (accessed January 31, 2022).

25. World Health Organization. *Increasing Access to Health Workers in Remote and Rural Areas through Improved Retention: Global Policy Recommendations.* Geneva, World Health Organization,2010. www.ncbi.nlm.nih.gov/books/NBK138618/ (accessed March 12, 2021).

26. E. Araujo, A. Maeda. How to recruit and retain health workers in rural and remote areas in developing countries: a guidance note. 2013. https://openknowledge.worldbank.org/bitstream/handle/10986/16104/78506.pdf (accessed March 2021).

27. B. G. O'Sullivan, I. Couper, P. Kumar, et al. Editorial: effective strategies to develop rural health workforce in low and middle-income countries (LMICs). *Front Public Health* 2021. doi: 10.3389/fpubh.2021.702362.

28. C. Dolea, L. Stormont, J. M. Braichet. Evaluated strategies to increase attraction and retention of health workers in remote and rural areas. *Bull World Health Organ* 2010; 88(5): 379–385.

29. World Health Organization. International migration of health personnel: a challenge for health systems in developing countries. Resolution WHA57. 2004. www.who.int/workforcealliance/who04.pdf?ua=1 (accessed January 11, 2021).

30. World Health Organization. International recruitment of health personnel: draft global code of practice. 2010. https://apps.who.int/gb/ebwha/pdf_files/WHA63/A63_8-en.pdf (accessed February 11, 2021).

31. World Health Organization. Health workforce support and safeguards list, 2020. 2020. https://cdn.who.int/media/docs/default-source/health-workforce/hwf-support-and-safeguards-list8jan.pdf?sfvrsn=1a16bc6f_10 (accessed January 31, 2022).

32. World Health Organization. Health workforce regulation in the Western Pacific Region. 2016. www.who.int/publications/i/item/health-workforce-regulation-in-the-western-pacific-region (accessed May 12, 2021).

33. M. C. Scheffer, M. R. Dal Poz. The privatization of medical education in Brazil: trends and challenges. *Hum Resour Health* 2015; 13(1): 96.

34. A. Mitchell, T. J. Bossert, Politics and governance in human resources for health. In A. Soucat, R. Scheffler, eds., *The Labor Market for Health Workers in Africa: New Look at the Crisis.* Washington, DC, World Bank, 2013.

35. V. R. Keshri, V. Sriram, R. Baru. Reforming the regulation of medical education, professionals and practice in India. *BMJ Glob Health* 2020; 5(8): e002765.

36. P. González, I. Macho-Stadler. A theoretical approach to dual practice regulations in the health sector. *J Health Econ* 2013; 32(1): 66–87.

37. P. L. Riley, A. Zuber, S. M. Vindigni, et al. Information systems on human resources for health: a global review. *Hum Resour Health* 2012; 10(1): 1–2.

38. F. Pozo-Martin, A. Nove, S. C. Lopes, et al. Health workforce metrics pre- and post-2015: a stimulus to public policy and planning. *Hum Resour Health* 2017; 15 (1): 1–6.

39. K. A. Grépin, W. D. Savedoff. 10 best resources on health workers in developing countries. *Health Policy Plan* 2009; 24(6): 479–482.

40. A. Siyam, P. Zurn, G. Gedik, et al. Monitoring the implementation of the WHO Global Code of Practice on the International Recruitment of Health Personnel. *Bull World Health Organ* 2013; 91: 816–823.

41. M. A. Lopes, A. S. Almeida, B. Almada-Lobo. Handling healthcare workforce planning with care: where do we stand? *Hum Resour Health* 2015; 13: 38.

42. World Health Organization. *National Health Workforce Accounts: A Handbook.* Geneva, World Health Organization,2017. https://apps.who.int/iris/handle/10665/259360 (accessed February 10, 2022).

43. Matrix Insight. EU level collaboration on forecasting health workforce needs, workforce planning and health workforce trends – a feasibility study. 2012. www.yumpu.com/en/document/view/4915 0015/eu-level-collaboration-on-forecasting-health-workforce-geko (accessed May 12, 2021).

Chapter 21

Enhancing Equitable Access to Essential Medicines and Health Technologies

Veronika J. Wirtz and Raffaella Ravinetto

Key Messages

- Pharmaceutical systems are a core part of health systems, and their failure to work adequately severely undermines the performance of the entire health system.
- The view that medicines are mere commodities managed for technical aspects by the national regulatory authority disregards the need for and role and complexity of a system to ensure access to essential medicines. This has serious consequences as it leaves key functions underfunded and underrepresented in national and international platforms where decisions related to health care systems and for achievement of universal health coverage (UHC) are made.
- Key strategies to strengthen pharmaceutical systems are well documented. Their effective implementation requires political commitment, institutional oversight and adequate financial allocation.
- Good governance of pharmaceutical systems promotes transparency and accountability to prevent corruption and inefficiencies.
- Assessing pharmaceutical systems is often neglected but essential to improving their performance. This chapter presents a series of key performance measures that countries should routinely use to measure and report on.

21.1 Introduction

Within the framework of UHC [1], the concepts of health technologies as a component of the health system, the regulation and supply of health products, and the major challenges faced by pharmaceutical systems in low- and middle-income countries (L&MICs) were presented in Chapter 7. This chapter focuses on enhancing equitable access to essential medicines and health technologies as a key contributor to health system performance. We consider in turn key strategies to improve the performance of pharmaceutical systems, ways in which pharmaceutical systems and policies contribute to achieving the overarching goals of equity in health, financial protection, and responsiveness to the needs of all, and the performance indicators for activities and functions related to finance, procurement, supply, quality assurance, and use of medicines and vaccines.

The term *pharmaceutical system refers here to all structures, people, resources, processes, and their interactions within the broader health system that aim to ensure equitable and timely access to safe, effective, quality pharmaceutical products and related services that promote their appropriate and cost-effective use to improve health outcomes* [2]. A pharmaceutical system includes, but is not limited to, the national regulatory authority (NRA) or equivalent body, the central medical store or equivalent purchasing unit(s), the quality control laboratory, the pharmacovigilance program, and all agencies or units responsible for financing health products and their appropriate use, including the training of prescribers.

To achieve its goals, a pharmaceutical system needs to have functional or collaborative links with other bodies that influence its performance, such as professional orders or associations, the social insurance system, and patent offices. Those in charge of each component of the pharmaceutical system, or related functions (e.g., selection, financing, regulation, quality assurance, appropriate use, services planning and monitoring, and others) are collectively responsible for the performance of the system in ensuring access to medicines. All stakeholders need to implement routine measures, such as frequency and characteristics of stock-outs, number of batch recalls and quality incidents, compliance of prescriptions with guidelines, and household and facility surveys on medicines access and utilization, in order to assess the system's performance. Similar to a functioning fuel gauge in a car, which monitors when to fill the tank and safely reach a given place at a given time, appropriate indicators of the pharmaceutical system guide policy decisions and determine progress toward universal, equitable, and sustainable access to medicines.

While the focus here is on medicines, including vaccines, similar principles apply to diagnostics, medical devices, and nutritional supplements. Integration of traditional medicines into pharmaceutical systems is important and requires a contextualized approach that goes beyond the scope of the chapter.

21.2 Strategies and Performance Indicators to Ensure Access to Medicines within UHC

Pharmaceutical systems strengthening is the process of identifying and implementing strategies and actions that achieve coordinated and sustainable improvements in the critical components of a pharmaceutical system, to make it more responsive and resilient, and to enhance its performance [2]. Different assessment frameworks have been proposed to that end [2–5]. This chapter is informed by the Lancet Commission on essential medicines [6] and proposes the following five strategic areas for pharmaceutical system strengthening in L&MICs:

1. paying for a basket of essential medicines;
2. making essential medicines affordable;
3. ensuring equitable distribution and continuous supply;
4. assuring the quality and safety; and
5. promoting quality use.

In addition to the framework proposed by the Lancet Commission, we consider the area of "supply," as it is critical for the performance of national systems. The development of essential medicines that do not currently exist (or that have suboptimal efficacy or safety profiles, or are otherwise not adapted to a population's needs) is an important public health-oriented strategy for pharmaceutical research and development, but requires reform of the global innovation ecosystem that goes beyond the capacities of individual systems [7]. Table 21.1 presents an overview of the five areas, core strategies, and key performance measurements.

Table 21.1 Overview of core strategies and performance measurements of pharmaceutical systems

Area	Examples of key strategies	Some key performance measures
Financing essential medicines	Defining and regularly updating the benefit package Financing of the benefit package	Publication and regular updates of the national essential medicines list Management of conflict of interest in the selection committee Publication and regular updates of pharmaceutical benefit packages[a] Pharmaceutical expenditure as a percentage of total expenditure on health Per capita expenditure on pharmaceuticals[b] Percentage of out-of-pocket expenditure out of total pharmaceutical expenditure[b]
Making essential medicines affordable	Price policies and regulations Generic medicines policies Use of TRIPS (Trade-Related Aspects of Intellectual Property Rights) flexibilities (for new medicines) Transparency on price information	TRIPS flexibilities are included in national legislation Median price ratio paid for a set of tracer medicines that was part of the last regular Ministry of Health (public sector) procurement Median price ratio paid for a set of tracer medicines in the private and public sectors Medicine price per daily defined dose + subsistence/salary of lowest government worker
Ensuring equitable distribution and continuous supply	Ongoing monitoring of consumption and need Matching needs and procurement Integrating public, private for-profit, and private not-for-profit sectors	Number of registered products per essential medicine Availability of standardized data on consumption at all levels/in all sectors Number and duration of stock-outs in the public and private sector Consumption versus needs for a set of tracer medicines Transparent procurement process (e.g., tenders)
Assuring quality and safety of medicines	Stringent regulation (e.g., good manufacturing practice, good distribution practice) Stringent regulatory oversight Functional pharmacovigilance Functional postmarketing surveillance (PMS)	NRA institutional development plan, based on Global Benchmarking Tool (GBT), within the last three years Availability of information on licenses to pharmaceutical facilities (issued, renewed, withdrawn) Number of notifications to WHO Alert systems Number of batch recalls

Table 21.1 (cont.)

Area	Examples of key strategies	Some key performance measures
Promoting the quality use of medicines	Standard treatment guidelines Surveillance of utilization Payment for performance	Percentage of medicines prescribed according to standard treatment guidelines Percentage of generic medicines out of total pharmaceutical sale volume

[a] Depending on the historic development of the health systems, not every country has a national essential medicines list, but each insurance scheme should have a defined benefit package to enable effective entitlement and accountability.
[b] Many countries do not routinely report data on pharmaceutical per capita expenditure or out-of-pocket expenditure on pharmaceuticals.

21.2.1   Paying for a Basket of Essential Medicines

Medicines represent one of the largest proportions of health expenditures [8], accounting for about US$1 in US$4 of health expenditures globally and up to 70% in some low-income countries (LICs) [9]. The percentage of pharmaceutical expenditures from public sources is a sensitive measure of whether governments provide adequate financial protection for medicine use. While roughly 60% of total pharmaceutical expenditures are covered by public funds in high-income countries, that proportion is less than 40% in L&MICs (Table 21.2). Thus, pharmaceutical expenditure in L&MICs is overwhelmingly financed by households via out-of-pocket financing. This contradicts the principles of pooling and risk sharing, and is the most inequitable way of financing health expenses as poorer households spend proportionally more on medicines than richer households [10], and either incur catastrophic expenditure or simply forgo the medicines because they cannot afford them [11].

There is evidence that public financial protection arrangements, funded by taxes and mandatory insurance contributions, are critical to prevent catastrophic expenditure [12]. Traditionally, social health insurance was tied to employment, but many L&MICs are now moving toward an essential package of "health care for all," for which costs should be covered by the public sector regardless of the ability to pay [13]. Unfortunately, such packages are often limited. For instance, they may reimburse the hospital stays and outpatient visits but exclude the costs of auxiliary services (e.g., laboratory tests) and essential medicines [14]. Furthermore, policies that cover only a percentage of total cost (coinsurance) instead of fixed copayment have been shown to decrease adherence to treatment and can result in catastrophic household expenditure (see Chapters 16 and 17) [15].

It is critical that countries measure their progress toward provision of an essential package of "health care for all." The costs of a standardized basket of essential medicines can be a good indicator of this, as indicated in Table 21.1. Other, more general indicators include: the percentage of out-of-pocket expenditure on pharmaceuticals relative to total pharmaceutical expenditure; the percentage of pharmaceutical expenditure relative to total health expenditure; and per capita expenditure on pharmaceuticals. Unfortunately, even when countries track health expenditure (e.g., using national health accounts), data is seldom disaggregated so as to provide information about medicines versus other expenditure; and when it is, it is

Table 21.2 Mean per capita total pharmaceutical expenditure (TPE) and total health expenditure (THE) in countries by income group in 2010

	Mean per capita TPE* (US$)			Mean per capita THE (US$)			
	Public expenditure	Private expenditure	Total	Public expenditure	Private expenditure	Total	%TPE of THE
High-income (n = 49)	279.2 (60.9%)	179.2 (39.1%)	458.4	2203.0 (73.1%)	811.7 (26.9%)	3,014.7	15.2%
Upper middle-income (n = 53)	39.6 (37.2%)	66.7 (62.8%)	106.3	334.4 (63.9%)	189.0 (36.1%)	523.4	20.3%
Lower middle-income (n = 48)	11 to 9 (32 to 4%)	24.8 (67.6%)	36.7	88.9 (60.1%)	59.1(39.9%)	148.0	24.8%
Low-income (n = 32)	2.0 (22.7%)	6.8 (77.3%)	8.8	13 to 9 (40.1%)	20.8 (59.9%)	34.7	25.4%
Total (n = 182)	90.2 (54.3%)	75.8 (45.7%)	166.0	716 to 4 (71.0%)	292.8 (29.0%)	1,009.2	16.4%

Source: [6].

typically not disaggregated by source, such as differentiating between public and private (see Chapter 13) [10]. Improving data reporting, particularly for data on household out-of-pocket expenditures versus public spending, is essential for guiding governments and insurance arrangements to allocate resources and increase equity and efficiency in spending.

21.2.2 Making Essential Medicines Affordable

Affordability by Governments

The cost of medicines presents a challenge for the financial sustainability of all health systems. Apart from direct price regulation, the affordability of medicines is shaped by multiple functions of pharmaceutical systems, such as financing, selection, procurement, and distribution; and by their ability to coordinate these functions. To improve access to all essential medicines, governments need to measure the performance of these functions individually and collectively, and enact policy adjustments accordingly.

Table 21.1 summarizes key indicators of affordability, and Table 21.3 outlines key policies to make medicines affordable. Transparent price regulation is only one of the many policy measures that governments need to put in place to promote affordable medicines. Policies and strategies should differentiate between single- and multi-source medicines. Single-source medicines are produced by only one supplier, either due to a monopoly in the case of patented medicines or due to market structure, such as for generic medicines for which there is little commercial incentive for multiple competing formulations. If there is only one (or few) suppliers, the de facto monopoly always pushes toward high prices: for instance, the price of generic pyrimethamine for toxoplasmosis famously increased by 5,000 times, taking advantage of the de facto monopoly for an essential and potentially lifesaving product [16]. When generics are available from multiple suppliers, conversely, prices generally decrease as a result of competition [17].

Making single-source patented medicines affordable requires consideration of intellectual property (IP). Health policymakers may be unfamiliar with international rules, and particularly with the areas of flexibility in the World Trade Organization (WTO). Agreements on Trade-Related Intellectual Property Rights (TRIPS) [17], such as applying stringent criteria for patentability, allowing compulsory licensing and particularly government use, encouraging voluntary patent pooling, or – at WTO level – implementing temporary IP waivers under extraordinary circumstances, and other measures. Or, they can be pressured not to implement them by interest groups or other governments. This results in inadequate legislation and practices, such as granting patents on noninnovative products, extending the patent protection ("evergreening"), and other consequences that directly impact on access to innovative essential medicines [18]. A detailed discussion on TRIPS and its flexibilities is beyond the scope of this chapter and can be found elsewhere [6]. Direct price negotiations are also used to lower prices of single-source medicines, but they have limited effectiveness and often come with the unfair requirement to keep prices confidential [19]. Advanced market commitments, or bulk procurement, have also been used by groups of countries, such as in Latin America, particularly for vaccines [20], as well as patent pools [21].

Affordability by Users

Affordability for users depends on whether the cost of given medicines is covered by health insurance or national health service; on the amount of out-of-pocket cost charged to the user;

Table 21.3 Policies affecting medicines prices

Area of intervention	Policy	The policy mainly directed at	
		SSM	MSM
IP rights	Delayed deadlines for enforcing medicines patents and test data protection in least developed countries (TRIPS agreement, now valid until 2033)	x	
	Application of strict (and TRIPS-compliant) patentability criteria	x	
	Government use of licensing	x	
	Compulsory licensing	x	
	Voluntary licensing	x	
	(Supporting) temporary IP waivers under exceptional circumstances	x	
	Patent pooling	x	
Market authorization	Incentivizing market entry of quality-assured essential medicines to increase healthy market competition		x
Pricing	External reference pricing	x	
	Internal reference pricing		x
	Value-based pricing	x	
	Removal or reduction of import taxes or sales taxes	x	x
	Regulation of distribution chain mark-ups	x	x
	Regulation of dispensing fees	x	x
Procurement	Price negotiation based on the volume procured	x	x
	Competitive tenders across prequalified suppliers		x
	Parallel importation	x	
Prescription	Mandatory use of the international nonproprietary name (INN)	x	x
Dispensing	Mandatory or voluntary substitution of originator for lower-priced generic product		x

SSM, single-sourced medicines; MSM, multi-source medicines.

and on individual purchasing power. In settings with higher purchasing power more people will be able to afford medicines (excluding vulnerable groups) compared to settings with (very) low purchasing power. Purchasing medication in the long term to treat chronic conditions poses a high financial burden on many households and can result in treatment interruption or nonadherence. Financing health care and medicines through taxes and mandatory insurance is a core strategy to improve access. Among the methods to measure affordability, the proposed *affordability indicator* in SDG 3, the goal of Health and Wellbeing, is *the sum of the medicine price per daily defined dose (DDD) treatment and the minimum cost of daily subsistence (defined as the national poverty line [NPL]), divided by the minimum daily wage of the lowest-paid unskilled government sector worker (LPGW)* (Box 21.1) [22].

Box 21.1 Medicine Affordability

Extra daily wages (EDW) = (NPL + price per DDD)/daily wage of the LPGW

If EDW ≤ 1, then affordability = 1; otherwise affordability = 0
For example, where NPL = US$2; price per DDD = US$1; daily wage of LPGW = US$6:

EDW = US$2 + US$1/US$6 = 3/6 = 0.5

Since EDW = 0.5, which is ≤1, the price is affordable.

21.2.3 Ensuring Equitable Procurement, Distribution, and Continuous Supply

Procurement, distribution, and supply encompass all activities needed to ensure that quality-assured medicines are available at the best prices, to satisfy all needs, in line with essential medicines lists and prescribing guidelines. In L&MICs barriers to achieving this aim include: scarce resources, limited purchasing power, complex global and national supply chains, variable regulatory capacities, poor coordination among pharmaceutical sector and national/international stakeholders, and in some cases the poorly planned withdrawal of donor support [23, 24].

The strategic objectives of *procurement* include:

- accurate quantification of the need;
- adequate prequalification and continuous requalification, including licensing, marketing authorization, postmarketing surveillance, pharmacovigilance, and others;
- adequate purchasing methods, such as restricted tenders, competitive negotiation, and direct procurement (open tender is never appropriate for health products because it precludes the limiting options to quality-assured products) [25];
- maintaining a constant, secured supply of medicines, as well as their integrity and quality; and
- fair and transparent setting of prices and mark-ups along the supply chain, guided by appropriate policies such as external or internal reference pricing, value-based pricing, mark-up regulation, tax exemptions or reductions for pharmaceutical products, and others [26].

Distribution should minimize stock-outs and losses, assure good storage and distribution practices, and rationalize storage points and transport resources. It can follow a pull or push system, or a combination of the two. In *push systems*, a given quantity of a limited list of products is pushed from the central level of the supply system during a defined timeframe [27]. In *pull systems*, conversely, orders are sent from decentralized (local, district, regional) levels based on actual consumption and need. Pull systems are preferred in stable settings. They require well-trained staff, accurate and comprehensive data on actual *needs* and *consumption*, and harmonized stock management tools.

The Lancet Commission recommends information systems for monitoring countrywide data on availability, affordability, and price. To be able to detect early signals of problems, data and key indicators from different sources should be triangulated within and beyond national systems, as illustrated in Table 21.4. All stakeholders must promote transparency and information-sharing about quality, availability, and price-setting mechanisms [28]. Table 21.5 illustrates some cases of access problems related to inadequate procurement strategies.

Table 21.4 Institutional stakeholders involved in the evaluation of needs and consumption

Institutional stakeholder	Examples of data that can be provided
NRA	Manufacturers', wholesalers', and importers' licenses Marketing authorizations Quality incidents and batch recall (For multi-source medicines) How many products are registered, for each item on the national essential medicines list or the insurance benefit package
Disease control and vaccination programs	National coverage by disease (e.g., TB, malaria, HIV) National coverage by-products (e.g., opioids, condoms)
Departments of procurement, supply, and distribution	All-levels data on consumption (consumption can be lower than need) All-levels data on overstocks All-levels data on number and duration of stock-outs All-levels data on pharmaceutical wastes (expired products)
Social security schemes	Health insurance population coverage
Academic and public health institutions	Comparisons of payment for a given treatment course vs. households' resources (surrogate indicator of gaps between consumption and need) [29] Monitoring of needs vs. availability/affordability of a group of "tracer" products

Table 21.5 Examples of challenges in medicines procurement

Case	Key issues	Reference
Benzathine penicillin: global shortages	"Sole sourcing" (no ready alternative supplier) Inadequate forecasting and monitoring of needs Lack of economic interest: manufacturers abandon production	[30]
Insulin in L&MICs	Purchase of (costly) analog insulin, instead of human insulin No effective (joint) price negotiations Market is dominated by the three companies (quasi-monopoly)	[31]
Controlled medicines [33, 34]	Complexities due to needs for medical use vs. potential for illicit use Measures to improve access should address the contents of drug control, drug control legislation and policy; role of authorities; policy planning; health care professionals' training; estimates and statistics; procurement; etc.	[32]

21.2.4 Assuring the Quality and Safety of Medicines

Pharmaceutical quality assurance (QA) is a prerequisite for attaining UHC [35]. It is states' obligation to protect public health by assuring the quality and safety of medicines, and effective regulatory systems are an essential component of national health systems [36]. Unfortunately, medicine quality is variable on the global market. The risk of poor-quality medicines is particularly high in countries with weak regulatory authorities [37–39]. Poor-quality medicines include "falsified medicines" that stem from illegal activities, and "substandard medicines" that fail to meet adequate standards due to undetected poor practices [40]. Both falsified and substandard medicines cause therapeutic failure, toxicity, and resistance [41], harm confidence in medicines and in health care systems, and inflate health expenditures for households and governments. Table 21.6 presents indicators that can be used to evaluate the adequacy of national pharmaceutical quality systems [5, 42].

These indicators reflect NRAs' capacities. To reach an adequate maturity level as defined by WHO, an NRA needs: a clear mission statement; adequate legislation, regulations, and organizational structure; and human and financial resources. Harmonizing standards and reliance on assessments done by WHO-listed (stringent) authorities improves regulatory efficiency. Positive examples include the harmonization initiative of the East African Community [45]; the Common Technical Dossier and Technical Requirements of the Association of Southeast Asian Nations; and WHO's collaborative registration procedure [46]. Importantly, the WHO GBT for Evaluation of National Regulatory System of Medical Products allows NRAs to identify strengths and weaknesses, and to formulate institutional strengthening plans [33].

21.2.5 Promoting the Appropriate Use of Medicines

While sometimes underappreciated, the appropriate use of medicines (traditionally called "rational use") has a strong impact on the performance of the pharmaceutical and health systems and, in turn, on health outcomes. Inappropriate use can harm patients (e.g., clinical deterioration if insulin doses are skipped), increase mortality (e.g., opioid illicit use), and create public health challenges (e.g., suboptimal doses leading to antimalarial and antibiotic resistance). Inappropriate use also wastes system resources, making it inefficient and expensive.

Key strategies to ensure appropriate use include the adoption of evidence-based standard treatment guidelines; stringent regulatory oversight of medicines promotion; prescribers' (re)training; awareness-raising at patient and community levels; and making essential medicines available and affordable to all.

The NRA should have a function dedicated to control promotion materials [47], as unregulated marketing practices foster inadequate prescribing patterns and influence patients' expectations. The appropriate use of medicine is influenced by a number of stakeholders, including patients, prescribers, dispensers, professional boards, consumer organizations, pharmaceutical manufacturers and associations, third-party payers, scientists, and traditional and social media. For instance, nudges for medicine users through social marketing strategies can enhance appropriate but also (severely) inappropriate use [48]. Furthermore, apart from poor prescribing or poor compliance, the lack of availability and affordability is a determinant of inappropriate underuse of medicines.

Unfortunately, many countries lack a dedicated function that coordinates activities and strategies to promote appropriate use of medicines. As a result, performance is low, jeopardizing quality of care and creating inefficiencies. Table 21.7 outlines examples of

Table 21.6 Some indicators of pharmaceutical quality standards

Activity	Proposed outcome indicators	Conditions
Licensing and inspecting (manufacturers, importers, wholesalers, outlets)	Number of inspections by the NRA Number of inspection reports published by the NRA Compliance with good practices as assessed by the NRA Frequency of violations, and how these are addressed by the NRA Renewal of licenses by the NRA Number of national manufacturers approved by the WHO PQ or licensed by a stringent regulatory authority	Availability of an established list of all facilities Availability of legal provisions, regulations, and guidelines to ensure that inspecting and licensing are based on stringent assessments The NRA is empowered to issue, suspend, or revoke licenses
Marketing authorization	Number of product application dossiers and assessment reports published Time to review/approve innovator and generic medicines Proportion of products with valid authorization Number of market authorizations granted based on a mutual recognition program, or WHO prequalification collaborative program	Only products authorized by the NRA are manufactured, imported, distributed, sold, or supplied to end-users
Pharmacovigilance (PV) and postmarketing surveillance (PMS)	Is there a PV program? Is there a risk-based PMS system? Is there a (functional) national quality control laboratory? Number of batch recalls Number of confiscations of poor-quality batches Number of samples tested, and analysis reports published Membership of WHO Programme for International Drug Monitoring Number of reports to VigiBase [43] Focal point(s) for the WHO Alert system [44]	
Transparency	Availability of a public regulatory website, updated with information on legislation, registered products, and public assessment reports	

Table 21.7 Examples of indicators of appropriate use of medicines

Appropriate use	Example indicator	Level of care
Quality of prescription	Availability of standard treatment protocols (and compliance with it)	General
	Availability of a (facility) essential medicines list	General
	Percentage of encounters with antibiotic prescribed	Primary level of care
	Percentage of encounters with an injectable formulation prescribed	Primary level of care
	Percentage of prescriptions with >3 medicines	Primary level of care
	Average time for dispensing	Primary level of care
	Percentage of medicines prescribed by generic name	General
	Volume of psychotropic medicines in one area exceeds average by factor of 2 or more	General
Patients' adherence	Percentage of medicines prescribed but not purchased out of total medicines prescribed	Primary level of care
Characteristics of the medicines	Availability of clear instructions (leaflet, packaging); availability of an easy-to-use dosing tool; etc.	Primary level of care
Characteristics of the health system	Percentage outlets dispensing medicines without prescriptions even when they should	Retail sector

indicators to be considered when measuring the performance of the pharmaceutical system related to appropriate use of medicines.

21.3 Regulation and Governance Challenges Related to Essential Medicines and Technologies

Measuring pharmaceutical systems performance is a multidisciplinary task that requires continuous monitoring of a complex set of services, policies, laws, regulations, financing, and information. The pharmaceutical system, like any other system that manages substantial budgets, is particularly prone to lack of transparency and corruption.

Corruption, in any of the critical decision points and at any level in the pharmaceutical system, is harmful to a country's ability to improve the health of its population [49]. Corrupt practices potentially have a threefold impact: *health impact*, as waste of public resources reduces the capacity to provide and finance quality-assured essential medicines; *economic impact*, as large amounts of public funds are wasted; and *image and trust impact*, as inefficiency and lack of transparency reduce the credibility of public institutions, decrease donors' trust, and discourage in-country investments [50]. Such deleterious effects result from illegal practices, but also from borderline practices, such as nonevidence-based selection of essential medicines and/or promotion of inappropriate use of medicines for financial gain (e.g., inappropriate antibiotic combinations which fuel antimicrobial resistance) [51].

Strengthening the performance of the pharmaceutical system should start by raising awareness about the importance of good governance. WHO recommends *increasing transparency and accountability in medicine regulatory and supply management systems; promoting individual and institutional integrity in the pharmaceutical sector; and institutionalizing good governance by building national capacity and leadership* [52]. These general principles have practical implications. For instance, at each level of the pharmaceutical system, the technical and commercial components need to be kept separated. Hence, the QA department of a manufacturer or a wholesaler should be totally independent from commercial and financial functions.

The WHO Pharmaceutical System Transparency Assessment is meant to assist countries with the assessment of key documentation, to facilitate transparency and accountability of the pharmaceutical system [50]. It guides policymakers through the detailed assessment of five cross-cutting areas: (1) access to information; (2) public participation; (3) medicines policy; (4) code of conduct and anti-corruption measures; and (5) management of conflicts of interest. It also explains how the five "areas" are applicable in the different regulatory and supply functions, as well as in medicine selection and reimbursement. Even though governance activities require adequate funding, they provide an important return on investments by boosting systems protection from inefficiencies, harm, and erosion of trust.

21.3.1 Access to Medicines in Public Health Emergencies

The COVID-19 pandemic that started in 2019–2020 has reinforced the lessons learned in the past for HIV/AIDS, hepatitis C, cancer, and other diseases by highlighting that essential medicines and vaccines are global goods, and that equitable access is essential for global development. The first 18 months of the pandemic also cruelly illustrated the lack of global solidarity when it comes to equitably sharing innovative health products, including vaccines and therapeutics, among all those in need [53]. There is a need for a new approach to innovation and access, for stronger global coordination, for stronger supply systems, and for strengthening national pharmaceutical systems as a whole, so as to ensure that production meets global needs, that the distribution of quality-assured medical products is timely and equitable, and that appropriate use is promoted for all in need [54].

21.4 Conclusion

Enhancing equitable access to essential medicines and health technologies is a key contributor to health system performance. Five strategic areas for pharmaceutical system strengthening in L&MICs include: (1) paying for a basket of essential medicines; (2) making essential medicines affordable; (3) ensuring equitable distribution and continuous supply; (4) assuring quality and safety; and (5) promoting quality use. Assessing pharmaceutical systems is often neglected but essential to improving their performance. Well-performing pharmaceutical systems require increasing transparency and accountability; promotion of individual and institutional integrity; and institutionalization of good governance by building national capacity and leadership.

References

1. S. K. Perehudoff, N. V. Alexandrov, H. V. Hogerzeil. The right to health as the basis for universal health coverage: a cross-national analysis of national medicines policies of 71 countries. *PLoS One* 2019; **14**(6): e0215577.

2. T. Hafner, H. Walkowiak, D. Lee, et al. Defining pharmaceutical systems strengthening: concepts to enable measurement. *Health Policy Plan* 2017; **32** (4): 572–584.

3. M. Bigdeli, D. H. Peters, A. K. Wagner. Medicines in health systems: advancing access, affordability and appropriate use. 2014. www.who.int/alliance-hpsr/resources/publications/9789241507622/en/ (accessed December 15, 2020).

4. E. Pisani, A. L. Nistor, A. Hasnida, et al. Identifying market risk for substandard and falsified medicines: an analytic framework based on qualitative research in China, Indonesia, Turkey and Romania. *Wellcome Open Res* 2019; **4**: 70.

5. World Health Organization. Monitoring the components and predictors of access to medicines. 2019. www.who.int/medicines/areas/policy/monitoring/monitoring-the-components-of-access-to-medicines.pdf (accessed December 19, 2020).

6. V. J. Wirtz, H. V. Hogerzeil, A. L. Gray, et al. Essential medicines for universal health coverage. *Lancet* 2017; **389**(10067): 403–476.

7. E. Torreele. Business-as-usual will not deliver the COVID-19 vaccines we need. *Development (Rome)* 2020; **63**: 191–199.

8. World Health Organization. *The World Health Report: Health Systems Financing – the Path to Universal Coverage.* Geneva, World Health Organization, 2010. https://apps.who.int/iris/handle/10665/44371 (accessed December 19, 2020).

9. Y. Lu, P. Hernandez, D. Abegunde, et al. The world medicines situation 2011: medicine expenditures. 2011. http://digicollection.org/hss/documents/s18767en/s18767en.pdf (accessed December 19, 2020).

10. World Health Organization, International Bank for Reconstruction and Development, World Bank. *Global Monitoring Report on Financial Protection in Health 2019.* Washington, DC, World Bank, 2019. www.who.int/healthinfo/universal_health_coverage/report/fp_gmr_2019.pdf?ua=1 (accessed December 19, 2020).

11. World Health Organization. Public spending on health: a closer look at global trends. 2018. www.who.int/publications/i/item/WHO-HIS-HGF-HFWorkingPaper-18.3 (accessed December 18, 2020).

12. A. Wagstaff, G. Flores, J. Hsu, et al. Progress on catastrophic health spending in 133 countries: a retrospective observational study. *Lancet Glob Health* 2018; **6**(2): e169–e179.

13. D. A. Watkins, D. T. Jamison, A. Mills, et al. Universal health coverage and essential packages of care. 2018. www.ncbi.nlm.nih.gov/books/NBK525285/ (accessed December 19, 2020).

14. G. Sum, T. Hone, R. Atun, et al. Multimorbidity and out-of-pocket expenditure on medicines: a systematic review. *BMJ Glob Health* 2018; **3**(1): e000505.

15. S. Thomson, J. Cylus, T. Evetovits. Can people afford to pay for health care? New evidence on financial protection in Europe. *Eurohealth* 2019; **25**(3): 41–46.

16. S. Luthra. "Pharma bro" Shkreli is in prison, but Daraprim's price is still high. 2018. https://khn.org/news/for-shame-pharma-bro-shkreli-is-in-prison-but-daraprims-price-is-still-high/ (accessed December 13, 2020).

17. World Health Organization. Multisource (Generic) pharmaceutical products: guidelines on registration requirements to establish interchangeability, revision. 2014. www.who.int/medicines/areas/quality_safety/quality_assurance/guideline-be-revision_qas14-583rev1_15072014.pdf (accessed December 18, 2020).

18. Y. A. Vawda, B. Shozi. Eighteen years after Doha: an analysis of the use of public health TRIPS flexibilities in Africa. 2020. https://papers.ssrn.com/sol3/papers.cfm?abstract_id=3559478 (accessed December 17, 2020).

19. S. G. Morgan, S. Vogler, A. K. Wagner. Payers' experiences with confidential pharmaceutical price discounts: a survey of public and statutory health systems in North America, Europe, and Australasia. *Health Policy* 2017; **121**(4): 354–362.

20. S. Vogler, V. Paris, D. Panteli. Ensuring access to medicines: how to redesign pricing, reimbursement and procurement? 2018. www.euro.who.int/__data/assets/pdf_file/0009/379710/PolicyBrief_AUSTRIA_PB30_web_13082018.pdf (accessed December 11, 2020).

21. S. Juneja, A. Gupta, S. Moon, et al. Projected savings through public health voluntary licences of HIV drugs negotiated by the Medicines Patent Pool (MPP). *PLoS One* 2017; **12**(5): e0177770.

22. United Nations. Sustainable Development Goals 3.b.3. 2020. https://unstats.un.org/sdgs/metadata/?Text=&Goal=3&Target=3.b (accessed December 11, 2020).

23. M. Tatay, E. Torreele. Ensuring access to life-saving medicines as countries shift from Global Fund support. *Bull World Health Organ* 2019; **97**(5): 311–311A.

24. World Health Organization. How pharmaceutical systems are organized in Asia and the Pacific. 2018. www.oecd-ilibrary.org/docserver/9789264291706-en.pdf?expires=1627889008&id=id&accname=guest&checksum=681DA63B02A99996497E034891549E24 (accessed December 18, 2020).

25. World Health Organization. Forty-eighth report of the WHO Expert Committee on specifications for pharmaceutical preparations. 2014. https://apps.who.int/iris/handle/10665/112733 (accessed December 19, 2020).

26. World Health Organization. *WHO Guideline on Country Pharmaceutical Pricing Policies.* Geneva, World Health Organization, 2020. www.who.int/publications/i/item/9789240011878 (accessed September 15, 2021).

27. World Health Organization. Interagency reproductive health kits for crisis situations. 2011. www.who.int/publications/i/item/inter-agency-reproductive-health-kits-for-crisis-situations (accessed December 12, 2020).

28. E. R. Fletcher, Health Policy Watch. World Health Assembly approves milestone resolution on price transparency. 2019. https://healthpolicy-watch.news/world-health-assembly-approves-milestone-resolution-on-price-transparency (accessed December 16, 2020).

29. S. Vogler, ed. *Medicine Price Surveys, Analyses and Comparisons: Evidence and Methodology Guidance.* New York, Academic Press, 2018.

30. S. Nurse-Findlay, M. Taylor, M. Savage, et al. Shortages of benzathine penicillin for prevention of mother-to-child transmission of syphilis: an evaluation from multi-country surveys and stakeholder interviews. *PLoS Med* 2017; **14** (12): e1002473.

31. M. Ewen, H.-J. Joosse, D. Beran, et al. Insulin prices, availability and affordability in 13 low-income and middle-income countries. *BMJ Glob Health* 2019; **4**: e001410.

32. S. Berterame, J. Erthal, J. Thomas, et al. Use of and barriers to access to opioid analgesics: a worldwide, regional, and national study. *Lancet* 2016; **387**: 1644–1656.

33. International Narcotics Control Board. The yellow list of narcotic drugs under international control. 2019. www.incb.org/incb/en/narcotic-drugs/Yellowlist_Forms/yellow-list.html (accessed September 20, 2020).

34. International Narcotics Control Board. The green list of psychotropic substances under international control. 2020. www.incb.org/incb/en/psychotropics/green-list.html (accessed December 18, 2020).

35. S. Ozawa, C. R. Higgins, T. T. Yemeke, et al. Importance of medicine quality in

achieving universal health coverage. *PLoS One* 2020; **15**(7): e0232966.

36. World Health Organization. Good regulatory practices: guidelines for national regulatory authorities for medical products. 2016. www.who.int/medicines/areas/quality_safety/quality_assurance/GoodRegulatory_PracticesPublicConsult.pdf (accessed December 17, 2020).

37. P. N. Newton, A. A. Amin, C. Bird, et al. The primacy of public health considerations in defining poor quality medicines. *PLoS Med* 2011; **8**(12): e1001139.

38. A. Johnston, D. W. Holt. Substandard drugs: a potential crisis for public health. *Br J Clin Pharmacol* 2014; **78**(2): 218–243.

39. P. N. Newton, K. C. Bond; Oxford Statement signatories. Global access to quality-assured medical products: the Oxford Statement and call to action. *Lancet Glob Health* 2019; **7**(12): e1609–e1611.

40. World Health Organization. Substandard and falsified medical products. 2022. www.who.int/news-room/fact-sheets/detail/substandard-and-falsified-medical-products (accessed February 15, 2022).

41. P. N. Newton, C. Caillet, P. J. Guerin. A link between poor quality antimalarials and malaria drug resistance? *Expert Rev Anti Infect Ther* 2016; **14**(6): 531–533.

42. WHO. WHO expert committee on specifications for pharmaceutical preparations. 2016. www.who.int/medicines/publications/pharmprep/WHO_TRS_996_web.pdf (accessed December 19, 2020).

43. Uppsala Monitoring Centre. Making medicines safer for patients. 2020. www.who-umc.org (accessed December 10, 2020).

44. World Health Organization. WHO Global Surveillance and Monitoring System for Substandard and Falsified Medical Products. 2017. www.who.int/medicines/regulation/ssffc/publications/GSMSreport_EN.pdf?ua=1 (accessed December 18, 2020).

45. M. Ndomondo-Sigonda, G. Mahlangu, M. Agama-Anyetei, et al. A new approach to an old problem: overview of the East African Community's Medicines Regulatory Harmonization initiative. *PLoS Med* 2020; **17**(8): e1003099.

46. World Health Organization. World Health Organization prequalification. 2021. https://extranet.who.int/prequal/content/collaborative-registration-faster-registration (accessed January 20, 2021).

47. R. Laing, H. Hogerzeil, D. Ross-Degnan. Ten recommendations to improve use of medicines in developing countries. *Health Policy Plan* 2001; **16**(1): 13–20.

48. E. Gabarron, S. O. Oyeyemi, R. Wynn. COVID-19-related misinformation on social media: a systematic review. *Bull World Health Organ* 2021; **99**(6): 455–463A.

49. World Health Organization. Good governance for medicines: model framework, updated version 2014. 2014. https://apps.who.int/iris/handle/10665/129495 (accessed December 19, 2020).

50. D. Dimancesco. Pharmaceutical system transparency and accountability assessment tool. 2018. https://apps.who.int/iris/bitstream/handle/10665/275370/WHO-EMP-2018.04-eng.pdf?ua=1 (accessed December 19, 2020).

51. V. J. Wirtz, P. G. Mol, J. Verdijk, et al. Use of antibacterial fixed-dose combinations in the private sector in eight Latin American countries between 1999 and 2009. *Trop Med Int Health* 2013; **18**(4): 416–425.

52. World Health Organization. Good governance for medicines (GGM) overview. 2021. www.who.int/medicines/areas/policy/goodgovernance/en/ (accessed January 20, 2021).

53. A. Herlitz, Z. Lederman, J. Miller, et al. Just allocation of COVID-19 vaccines. *BMJ Glob Health* 2021; **6**(2): e004812.

54. K. Perehudoff, E. 't Hoen, P. Boulet. Overriding drug and medical technology patents for pandemic recovery: a legitimate move for high-income countries, too. *BMJ Glob Health* 2021; **6**(4): e005518.

Health Information and Information Technology

The Path from Data to Decision

Jeremy C. Wyatt and Hamish Fraser

Key Messages

- The collection and analysis of relevant, high-quality data form the foundation of quality improvement and high-performing health systems.
- It is important to agree on the aims of each health program before defining the minimum set of data for collection and what level of data quality is good enough to support analysis and decision-making based on this data.
- The WHO has developed a wide range of useful indicators covering most aspects of health system activity, so it is wise to start with these. However, each indicator may require several items of data from different sources.
- The collection of accurate personal identifiers is important to allow linkage of data from different sources, but these identifiers should be substituted with a number once linkage is complete, to preserve individual privacy.
- Ensuring regular audits of data quality will usually help information systems to deliver on their promise.
- Data analysts should always consider the users of each report they write and choose graph and table formats that make sense to these users and support their decisions.
- Developing a self-service dashboard rather than numerous reports makes it easier for decision-makers to explore data and draw new inferences from it.
- There are already a large number of high-quality, open source, free-to-use data capture, analysis, and information sharing tools that communicate well with one another and can support health systems in improving their data processing, so it is rarely necessary to develop your own.
- While big data analytics, AI, and machine learning capture many headlines, much can be achieved using simple tools to capture relevant, high-quality data and turn it into actionable knowledge to support health system decision-makers.

22.1 Introduction

This chapter is about information and how it is used in health systems as a core function for health and system improvement, while Chapter 7 focused on the sources of information. Since information is an abstract concept, this chapter is organized according to how information is used to support health improvement in low- and middle-income countries (L&MICs). Figure 22.1 shows how information can be used to help a health system reach its

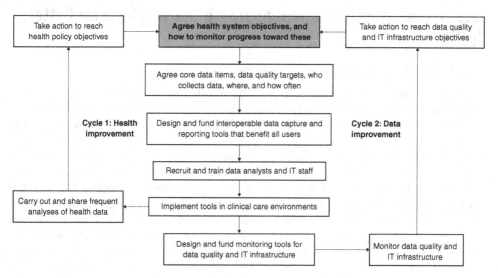

Figure 22.1 A whole-systems approach to health improvement using data.

objectives. In the description that follows, each concept highlighted in bold is further addressed in subsequent sections.

For "Cycle 1: Health improvement," having agreed with a project board and its leadership on health system objectives and how these are to be defined and monitored, the project staff need to develop a shortlist of core data items and data quality targets to support the monitoring process. Negotiation with health and other professionals helps to determine who collects these data items, and how often, as well as what tools are available for data capture – either on paper or digitally. A sufficient number of trained data analysts need to be available to produce timely reports based on the data collected.

The next stages are to develop or purchase appropriate data capture tools, which are usually easy to use, and to seamlessly share the data collected using appropriate technical standards and internet-based infrastructure. The development of data analysis reports and online dashboards to produce timely, appealing reports tailored to specific purposes for local, regional, and national decision-makers allows staff involved in data handling to see the benefits of their work from day one. In-depth analyses can be carried out periodically by trained analysts, who produce and share visually accessible summaries as infographics or short reports designed to show the current state of the health system and what proportion of patients or health facilities reach the agreed system objectives. The final stage in the process of using data to manage and improve health status is for relevant staff and organizations to act based on the reports to move population health status closer to the agreed objectives. This is covered in Chapter 23 as well as multiple other chapters in this book.

In addition to the measurement and improvement of population and individual health described as Cycle 1, a second cycle is required. "Cycle 2: Data improvement" is related to measuring and improving the quality of the collected data. This in turn requires the development of monitoring tools to assess the quality of data being captured and information technology (IT) infrastructure, followed by informed action to continually improve data quality.

22.2 A Quality Improvement Approach to Using Data for Better Health

22.2.1 Developing a Shortlist of Core Data Items

In 1990, Shortliffe, one of the founders of the medical informatics discipline, defined information as "organised data and knowledge used to inform decisions" [1]. This means that data or knowledge is only useful if they inform someone – for example, a patient, clinician, support worker, lab manager, or regional medical director in the case of health-related data. If a specific item of data is not actually used by anyone, either directly or to generate a derived variable, then it is not information by this definition, and is not worth collecting. Every item of data collected has a cost – in the time of people collecting and analyzing it, in the effort taken to process it, and in the risk it poses for generating errors of various kinds. Therefore, the data collector and data manager need to know the purpose of each data item, and need to limit the number of items collected to the minimum necessary. There is a wide range of data items that can serve to measure and improve health status (Box 22.1).

To support health systems in deciding which indicators are relevant at the local, regional, and national levels, WHO developed a Global Reference List of 100 Core Health Indicators (plus health-related Sustainable Development Goals) for national use. These cover four domains: health status, risk factors, service coverage, and health systems (Table 22.1) [2].

Typically, the more people are involved in deciding which data items to collect, the more data items are added. However, it is possible to limit the number of data items to be measured and avoid "dataset creep" if the project board decides early on how many data items will be collected and processed, at least in the first phase. Then, project workers have to prioritize suggested data items and select the top 100 items, for example, for the first phase of data collection. The list of data items selected, their definitions, and how each is coded is called a *data dictionary*. A related approach by Puttkammer and colleagues used a qualitative Delphi process, with the stakeholders identifying the types of information

---

Box 22.1 Some of the Kinds of Data That May be Relevant to Measuring and Improving Health Status

Individual patient data: demographics, education level, ethnic group and other risk factors, nutrition, and performance status; number and severity of long-term conditions, past medical history, mental health status, acute conditions, current and previous treatments, family history, and support at home; ability to travel to health facilities; ability to self-care; level of digital literacy.

Population data: local disease prevalence, usage of alcohol, tobacco, or recreational drugs; nutrition levels, prevalence and location of air or water pollution; local education and employment rates, proximity of health care facilities.

Data about health care facilities: location, range of services offered, size, staff number and skills, availability of supplies, medicine/vaccine cold chain, facilities to contain epidemic spread, local transport links, geography, timing of seasonal weather, electricity supply, internet access quality.

Table 22.1 Examples of the four indicator categories from the WHO Global Reference List of 100 Core Health Indicators

Domain: Health status

Mortality by age and sex: Life expectancy at birth, under-five mortality rate (SDG 3.2.1)

Mortality by cause: Maternal mortality ratio (SDG 3.1.1), TB, AIDS-related and malaria mortality rate, premature NCD mortality (SDG 3.4.1), suicide rate (SDG 3.4.2), the death rate due to road traffic injuries (SDG 3.6.1)

Fertility: Adolescent birth rate (SDG 3.7.2), total fertility rate

Morbidity: New cases of vaccine-preventable, IHR-notifiable diseases and other notifiable diseases, HIV prevalence and incidence rates (SDG 3.3.1), sexually transmitted infections incidence rate, TB incidence (SDG 3.3.2) and notification rates

Domain: Risk factors

Nutrition: Exclusive breastfeeding rate 0–5 months of age, incidence of low birth weight among newborns, children under five years who are stunted (SDG 2.2.1), wasted (SDG 2.2.2), or overweight (SDG 2.2.2)

Infections: Prevention of HIV in key populations

Environmental risk factors: Population using safely managed drinking water services (SDG 6.1.1) or safely managed sanitation services (SDG 6.2.1a/6.2.1b), air pollution level in cities (SDG 11.6.2)

Noncommunicable diseases: Total alcohol per capita (age 15+ years) consumption (SDG 3.5.2), tobacco use among persons aged 15+ years (SDG 3.a.1), raised blood pressure among adults, raised blood glucose/diabetes among adults

Injuries/harmful traditional practices: Intimate partner violence prevalence (SDG 5.2.1), nonpartner sexual violence prevalence (SDG 5.2.2), prevalence of female genital mutilation (SDG 5.3.2), sexual violence against children (SDG 16.2.3)

Domain: Service coverage

Reproductive, maternal, newborn, child, and adolescent: Demand for family planning satisfied with modern methods (SDG 3.7.1), antenatal care coverage, births attended by skilled health personnel (SDG 3.1.2), postpartum care coverage – women and newborn, vitamin A supplementation coverage

Immunization: Immunization coverage rate by vaccine for each vaccine in the national schedule (SDG 3.b.1)

HIV: People living with HIV who know their status, prevention of mother-to-child transmission, antiretroviral therapy (ART) coverage

Tuberculosis: TB treatment coverage, treatment coverage for drug-resistant TB

Malaria: Intermittent preventive therapy for malaria during pregnancy, use of insecticide-treated nets, indoor residual spraying coverage

Neglected tropical diseases (NTDs): Number of people requiring interventions against NTDs (SDG 3.3.5), coverage of preventive chemotherapy for selected NTDs

Screening and preventive care: Cervical cancer screening

Mental health: Coverage of services for severe mental health disorders

Substance abuse: Treatment coverage for alcohol/drug dependence (SDG 3.5.1)

Essential health services: Coverage of essential health services (SDG 3.8.1)

Domain: Health systems

Quality and safety of care: Perioperative mortality rate, obstetric and gynecological admissions owing to abortion, institutional maternal mortality ratio, ART retention rate, TB treatment success rate

Table 22.1 (cont.)

Utilization and access: Outpatient service utilization, inpatient admissions and surgical volume, health facility density and distribution, access to a core set of relevant essential medicines (SDG 3.b.3)

Health workforce: Health worker density and distribution (SDG 3.c.1), output training institutions

Health information: Birth registration (SDG 16.9.1), death registration (SDG 17.19.2), completeness and timeliness of reporting by facilities for notifiable diseases

Health financing: Total current expenditure on health as percentage of GDP, proportion of population with impoverishing health expenditure, total net official development assistance to medical research and basic health sectors (SDG 3.b.2)

Health security: International Health Regulations (IHR) core capacity index (SDG 3.d.1)

Governance: Existence of national health sector policy/strategy/plan

Source: [4].

crucial for competent clinical care and public health reporting [3], and focused data quality procedures and evaluation studies on those variables.

22.2.2 From Data to Indicators: An Example of Maternal Mortality Ratio

It is important to distinguish person-level data (i.e., data about individuals – such as a specific woman's pregnancy and its outcome) from the kind of information that is needed to run and improve health systems. In this case, the number of women who are receiving prenatal care, who are developing complications, the rate of resolving these complications, delivery rates, measures of perinatal morbidity and mortality, and maternal mortality are key variables for managing a maternity service at local, regional, and national levels. However, maternity units may not use standard definitions and may not have access to the relevant data to calculate the indicator. For example, maternal death is defined by WHO as: "the death of a woman while pregnant or within 42 days of termination of pregnancy, irrespective of the duration and site of the pregnancy, from any cause related to or aggravated by the pregnancy or its management but not from accidental or incidental causes" [5]. Maternal mortality ratio is defined as: "the annual number of female deaths per 100,000 live births from any cause related to or aggravated by pregnancy or its management (excluding accidental or incidental causes)." Three separate information systems and six different data items are needed to calculate this important indicator (Figure 22.2). This diagram also demonstrates how generating an accurate indicator centrally requires the data collected at the point of maternity care, in death certificates, and in vital statistics to be accurate. We consider data quality issues and point-of-care data capture next.

22.2.3 Agreeing Data Quality Targets

Data is only worth collecting, sharing, and analyzing if it is of high quality, which is defined by the International Organization for Standardization (ISO) as "fit for purpose" [6]. This perspective is useful to help limit the number of data items collected. The main dimensions of data quality based on the work of Wyatt and Sullivan are listed in Box 22.2 [7].

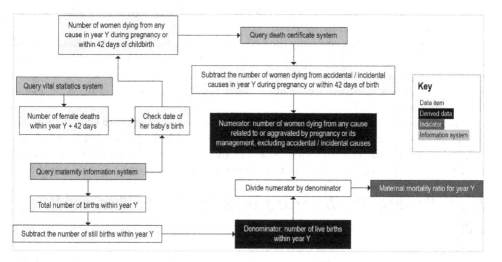

Figure 22.2 From data items to indicators: an algorithm showing one way to calculate the indicator maternal mortality ratio from data items obtained from local information systems.

Box 22.2 Dimensions of Data Quality

1. **Accuracy:** Does the data item correspond to the true state of that variable for the person observed and at the time of data recording? For example, was the systolic BP recorded close enough to the true BP to make no clinically relevant difference?
2. **Completeness and timeliness:** Is enough data available for analysis when it is needed for decisions to be made?
3. **Analysis-ready:** What proportion of the data is ready for analysis without needing further work? For example, is it collected in coded format rather than free text?
4. **Standards-based:** Does the structure and coding of the data correspond to widely used clinical data standards such as ICD11, SNOMED-CT, HL-7 FHIR, CDISC, or OpenEHR?
5. **Context:** This is a free text description of the data and is often essential to make sense of data items. For example, was a BP taken lying down or standing, or before or after medication? What kind of BP measuring device was used? When was it last calibrated?
6. **Structural and statistical metadata:** This ensures the data is well documented so that analysts can understand the meaning of each data item and carry out their analysis with confidence. This often requires information about the source of the data, how each item has been coded or processed, the method of data collection or the intended uses of the data (e.g., billing, clinical care, or research), and potentially other information.

One important issue associated with data quality is the coding of the data. While free text is useful when working with patients or trying to understand local circumstances, in order to be analyzed meaningfully data needs to be converted to a coded format. This means that all the terms and expressions that describe the same problem, including abbreviations and synonyms, are represented by a single code that data analysis software can analyze. For example, the following words or phrases would all be coded as asthma in the ICD-10 CM classification: *I think this patient probably has asthma*; *Asthma?*; *Diagnosis: asthma*; *Bronchial asthma*; and *Asthme* (French for asthma).

There are a number of commonly used coding systems, including two commonly used internationally: SNOMED-CT and ICD-11. SNOMED is used within clinical information systems to represent the details of a person's clinical findings, while ICD is used for diagnosis, including aggregate information about populations to give an overview of the rates of disease [8].

It is common for data that is of sufficient quality for some purposes to be of insufficient quality for other purposes. Therefore, it is important to decide the primary purposes of data collection upfront and ensure it is of sufficient quality to support that purpose. The concept of "data readiness level," analogous to technology readiness level, can be useful here [9].

22.2.4 Deciding Who Will Collect These Data Items, When, and How Often

The four principles of good data capture are:

1. **Capture data once**, from the most reliable source, and reuse it elsewhere. If a clinical sign is needed, then ask the clinician to observe the patient and record the data. When capturing lab data, do not copy the data from the patient's record but instead link directly to the laboratory information system or analysis device. Similarly, capture the patient's medication data from the outpatient prescription, or the prescription chart for inpatients. Increasingly, patients are invited to enter their symptoms directly using a simple questionnaire on a tablet or a computer in the waiting room, or a symptom checker app on their smartphone at home [10].

2. **Define your data.** The operational definition of a data item is crucial to how it is interpreted, so ensure people know how you are defining the data item. For example, when collecting data on COVID-19 symptoms from a patient, give them advice on how each symptom is defined and how to grade its severity. Provide clinicians with advice on how to define and measure a clinical sign (e.g., which instrument to use to measure blood pressure, should the patient be sitting, lying or standing?).

3. **Minimize over-collection.** For time-varying data, only collect the data after a suitable interval, meaning when the data value is likely to have changed. Often, only the latest value needs to be analyzed, but sometimes the rate of change over a period is also important.

4. **Check data quality at the point of capture** rather than later, so that missing or incorrect data can be corrected. Some data capture tools such as a tablet, computer, or smartphone make it easy to check that each data item on a page is of the allowed data type (number, text, multiple choice, etc.), is within the normal range, and has not changed more than expected from a previous value. The device can then issue a reminder to correct invalid data items before the data moves elsewhere for further processing. This also increases the value of the data for immediate use.

The methods for capturing data depend on the kind of data needed. For example, all patient-level data such as clinical, educational, occupational, or housing data needs to be linked and anonymized before it leaves each health care organization, to protect patient identity. The broad approach is shown in Figure 22.3.

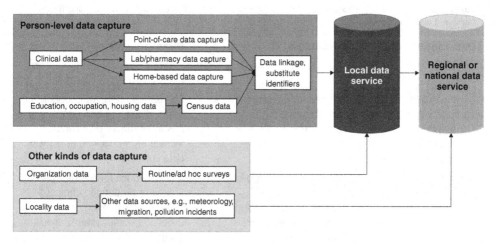

Figure 22.3 Simplified view of how data is captured and identifiers are removed in a health system.

Figure 22.3 shows how clinical person-level data is first linked with person-level data from other sources using identifiers such as name, date of birth, health service number, or postcode, then all these identifiers are removed to reduce the chances of identifying any person, and a numerical pseudo-identifier is substituted. Any free text data that might provide clues to a person's identity is also removed or converted to coded data. The unique pseudonymized identifier is used if there is a need to reidentify the person – for example to obtain further data or for contact-tracing purposes. The database matching the substitute identifier to personal identifiers is encrypted and the key is kept securely by a local trusted organization. The person-level dataset can then be safely shared with local, regional, or national data services for further analysis in a safe haven or trusted research environment. Additional data needed, such as results of routine or ad hoc surveys of local organizations, or data about localities, such as climate, migration, quality of water supplies, or pollution incidents, are included in the local, regional, or national data pipeline.

22.2.5 Deciding What Support Will be Available for Data Capture

Capturing patient data to derive population indicators is demanding. Before computers, most health care professionals used either paper and pen or a dictating machine, which was later transcribed into a typed or word-processed encounter note or clinic letter. A range of alternative data capture methods are now available. Those overseeing clinical data collection need to decide which data capture methods to use, based on consultation with the health professionals who will be collecting data, those funding the project, local technology suppliers, and the characteristics of the main data capture methods. Table 22.2 lists the major data collection methods and their main advantages and disadvantages.

22.2.6 Developing or Purchasing Appropriate Data Capture and Processing Tools

Creating good user interfaces and workflow patterns and support for open data standards requires good information system architecture, software development, and extensive cycles

Table 22.2 The main data capture methods for face-to-face or point-of-care data collection, and their advantages and disadvantages

Data capture method	Advantages	Disadvantages
Preprinted forms used in health facilities with transcription at the district level	No equipment or network needed in local facility; centralizes the transcription process	Labor intensive; delays in transport and transcription; transcription errors; difficult to find people with missing information; cannot include error checking at point of data collection
Preprinted paper forms with optical mark recognition	Cheaper than point-of-care technology but requires dedicated form reader; provides users with a checklist they keep in record; newer software and low-cost document cameras are improving this approach for low income settings	Inflexible once form is designed; limited to predefined choices – cannot collect patient name or other text; some systems need a supply of custom forms; others can use any structured paper form; cannot give immediate feedback based on data
Preprinted paper forms with optical character recognition	Widens range of data collected to text and numbers, written in boxes	May require a form reader that gets dirty over time; not 100% accurate, needs operator supervision
Web-based forms on a laptop or PC, e.g., DHIS2 [11]	Flexible, can check errors, give feedback, issue alerts and carry out calculations e.g., BMI	Expensive to deliver to all locations – requires computers at point of care; maybe security risk to hardware or data collected
Tablet computer or smartphone app, e.g., DHIS2 Mobile	Flexible, can give feedback, issue alerts, and carry out calculations, e.g., BMI Less expensive to deliver, especially if staff have own devices; can work in sites with unreliable power and connectivity	Potential risk of theft for tablets in particular
Machine translation for speech	Quick, intuitive, can be combined with form filling	Higher-performance hardware may be needed; may only work in quiet surroundings and with certain speakers; may not exist for certain languages or cover limited vocabulary; not 100% accurate but can be better than handwritten notes
	Captures risk factors, health-related behaviors,	People may not use the same language as clinicians, may delay

Table 22.2 (cont.)

Data capture method	Advantages	Disadvantages
Data capture by individuals using an online app	treatment compliance, etc.; symptom checker apps now widely used in middle- and high-income countries	data capture until just before a clinic appointment or sometimes may even fabricate data; limited to symptoms, cannot capture clinical examination results, etc.; symptom checkers have limited evidence base and rarely connect to electronic health records (EHRs) or other health information systems (HIS)
Data capture by community health workers in home settings using tablet computers/smartphone apps + cellular network links	Capture demographics, symptoms, some examination data and vital signs, treatment compliance; rapidly growing approach	Requires good user interfaces, training, and supervision; apps may not connect to EHRs or other HIS but this is improving (e.g., DHIS2, CommCare, OpenSRP)
Direct data capture from medical devices via wired or Bluetooth network	Immediate frequent objective data capture form, e.g., bedside monitors, blood glucose meters, ultrasound fetal heart rate monitoring, audiometry data for screening infants	Devices need to be calibrated and maintained; currently limited range of data that can be collected but growing; successful use in remote areas such as rural Guatemala [12]

of monitoring, evaluation, and improvement. For health systems looking to improve data collection, reporting, and utilization, adapting well-designed and tested systems is usually the best approach, unless the application is very specialized. As health management information systems (HMISs) become more widely used in L&MICs, it is increasingly important to identify those that will function in the specific clinical or public health setting and with the available infrastructure. After two decades of rapid innovation in HMIS worldwide there is increasing consolidation on a limited number of systems that address the main requirements.

In many L&MICs, open source HMIS has become widely used. These systems have been developed collaboratively with health systems and software development experts in many locations, fostering local innovation and ownership. They have been recognized by a group of funding and development organizations such as Digital Square [13] as Global Public Goods and increasingly share standards for data coding and exchange (Box 22.3).

Combined with health information exchange systems (e.g., *OpenHIM*, *OpenHIE*), whose purpose is to facilitate data communication between data management systems

Box 22.3 Leading Examples of Open Source Systems

Mobile Health Applications

CommCare and MedicMobile CHT. Both are designed primarily to support community health care workers in L&MICs, and are also used for case finding and contact tracing for Ebola and COVID-19 [14].

OpenSRP has similar functionality and uses, with a focus on maternal child care. *OpenDataKit* is used widely for data collection and management for community health care and other uses, such as agriculture.

Electronic Health Records

OpenMRS is used clinically in 44+ countries for a wide range of diseases and clinical settings, with a strong focus on HIV. It has strong support for open standards and interoperability, including FHIR [15, 16].

OpenClinics is used clinically in larger clinics and hospitals in many West African countries such as Rwanda [17].

National Reporting Systems

SORMAS is a disease surveillance system developed during the West African Ebola outbreak. It supports case finding surveillance and contact tracing [18].

Laboratory Information Systems

OpenELIS [19] is an open source laboratory information system inituially developed by US public health organizations and now supported by the University of Washington. It has been adapted for use in LMICs such as Vietnam and as a component of the Bahmni EHR system combined with OpenMRS and other applications.

Pharmacy and Supply Chain Management

OpenLMIS [20] is an open source, electronic logistics management information system (LMIS) built to manage health commodity supply chains in LMICs. It is used in nine African countries, covering a wide range of commodities in more than 10,000 health facilities.

iDart [21] is an open source medication dispensing system for HIV care in LMICs such as South Africa. It includes tools to track patient collection of medications.

OpenBoxes [22] is an open source supply chain management system for warehouses and pharmacies developed by the health care NGO Partners in Health. It is deployed in Haiti, Sierra Leone, Liberia, Cameroon, Rwanda, and Kazakhstan, and in pharmacy warehouses in the United States.

that serve different users or purposes, these systems can be rapidly linked to address new challenges. An example is the *mHero* two-way communication platform used to support dialog between Ministries of Health and health workers during the Ebola outbreak in West Africa [23].

Many of these systems have been adapted and deployed to support case finding, contact tracing, and clinical management for the COVID-19 pandemic [24]. In addition, there are vibrant local software development communities in a number of L&MICs such as Kenya [25] and in the Philippines. This has resulted in many high-quality commercial health information systems in those countries, although extensive use is made of open source systems such as *OpenMRS* in both countries [26].

22.2.7 Seamlessly Sharing Data

With the move to support open data standards for data storage and transmission, there is an increasing ability to share person-level data: (1) between different components of HIS in a health facility; and (2) between other systems at the district or national level. Figure 22.4 shows examples of such systems used in L&MICs settings, and the types of standards used to share data.

While there are examples of such links between information systems, there is still a long way to go to ensure seamless access to all important data when and where it is required. For example, the immunization data needed to optimize immunization levels in a community may be recorded in a community or school health system, primary or pediatric services, or pharmacies, in the public or private sectors. The new data exchange standard HL7 FHIR (*Fast Health care Interoperability Resources*)[27, 28] is increasingly being used as the common connector for different types of HIS. For example, the link between *OpenMRS* and the *OpenELIS* laboratory information system in some Ministry of Health-run clinics in Haiti was upgraded to use FHIR in 2020 and started a nationwide roll-out in 2021 to speed

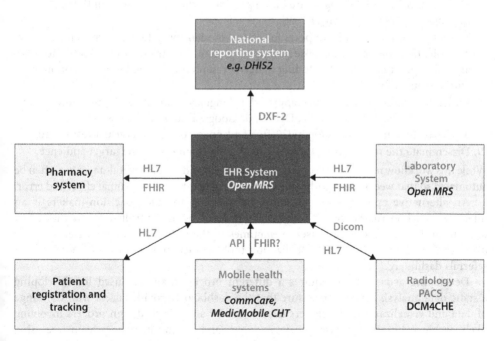

Figure 22.4 How different information systems within and outside a health facility can exchange data with an OpenMRS electronic health record using interoperability standards. Example systems (italics) are from the Digital Square Global Goods list.

the updates to national statistics requiring lab results [16]. M-health applications are also being adapted to use FHIR. Data export for analysis, reporting, and research in data warehouses is also possible using FHIR. Interoperability standards work best when used with information systems with strong support for standards-based data dictionaries, such as OpenMRS. Careful testing with real data and networking environments is essential to ensure reliability and accuracy of data exchange. Any changes to data dictionaries in systems exchanging data must be shared to ensure that the terms mean the same in both systems.

22.2.8 Developing Data Analysis Reports and Online Dashboards

To generate useful insights about health using pooled person-level data, the following steps are needed:

1. Agree on the main audience for the report and the questions to be answered using data.
2. Check the quality – especially the completeness – of the relevant data and where necessary contact health care provider organizations to fill in missing data items.
3. Use appropriate methods to infer or impute missing data items (see www .missingdata.org).
4. Calculate derived variables as required (e.g., age at diagnosis, socioeconomic class, distance from nearest health care facility) using variables that will later be removed as part of the anonymization process.
5. Anonymize the data as much as possible, removing patient identifiers and potentially health care provider and provider organization identifiers.
6. Carry out the data analysis using statistical analysis tools such as SPSS, Excel, R, SAS, Stata, or others, while being aware of the possibility that these tools can themselves introduce errors to the analysis [29].
7. Submit preliminary results to peers for review to identify systematic errors introduced by earlier data manipulation, false assumptions (about the origin or purpose of the data), and other potential biases (including underrepresentation of gender, socioeconomic, or ethnic groups) [30].
8. Present the findings in audience-appropriate language using data visualization tools such as Candela, Tableau Public, DHIS2, or Google Data tools (see www .hackerearth.com/blog/developers/20-free-and-open-source-data-visualization-tools).
9. Disseminate the report using the most acceptable channels for the target audience.

While this workflow may seem complex, once it is set up and tested, several stages can often be automated so that weekly or monthly reports can be generated with minimal effort and error.

An alternative approach to presenting information to guide decision-makers is an interactive dashboard. These are web-based platforms with controlled access that allow users to drill down into a database – sometimes to the individual (anonymized) records using various data analysis and visualization tools. An example is the UK online urgent referrals dashboard [31].

Developing a dashboard requires a different process than that used for developing a static data analysis report. To ensure that the dashboard provides users with the range of data and visualizations, developers need to follow an agile co-design process involving likely dashboard users. Increasingly, data analysts and health intelligence teams are using dashboards to empower users to carry out their own analyses. This frees up analysts' time to carry out more in-depth analyses as required. DHIS2 includes some of this functionality.

22.2.9 Monitoring Tools to Assess the Quality of Data and IT Infrastructure

When HIS are deployed in settings with limited infrastructure and technical expertise, particularly in remote sites, it is essential to monitor system and user performance. Too often information systems stop functioning due to easily correctable issues such as power supply problems. Mobile health applications can integrate data for monitoring users and locations in their design. For electronic health records (EHRs), additional software is typically required for monitoring users or locations. An example is a server monitoring tool developed for the *OpenMRS* EHR, which tracks uptime and episodes of downtime, data entry per day, and completeness of key variables. This allows early intervention to correct problems and maintain momentum in system use and data entry – which typically translates into better-quality data. A survey of OpenMRS EHR users in 54 health centers in Rwanda [32] showed generally high levels of user satisfaction, although clinical users were less likely to use certain functionalities such as updating records and running reports than technical staff. In intervention sites with added decision support tools, users were significantly more likely to use key functionality, and agree that the EHR provides useful alerts and reminders. In 25% of the sites, users reported reduced EHR availability, and 7% said it was rarely available.

The WHO now publishes a Data Quality Review (DQR) Toolkit [33], which can be used at regional and national levels to monitor the quality of key variables (see www.who.int/healthinfo/tools_data_analysis/en/).

22.3 Emerging Areas of Importance in Data-Driven Health Care

Artificial intelligence (AI) is an umbrella term referring to the substitution of human reasoning with software for machine translation, machine learning, machine vision, robotics, or decision support, using rules or algorithms derived from human experts or from data. *Machine learning* (ML) is a subtype of AI in which the automated analysis of large datasets is used to predict outcomes with increasing levels of precision [38]. We discuss them together here as AI and ML are often used interchangeably. Most ML uses a neural network "deep learning," such that resulting algorithms are unable to explain findings – a black box that has been known for decades to be unsuitable in medicine for ethical and legal liability reasons [39, 40]. An example is a video-streaming service suggesting films to a viewer based on the viewing patterns and ratings of a large database of people with similar viewing and rating histories. Accuracy does not matter much here as viewers can easily stop watching a boring film. In the medical context, however, such as in the choice of a medication to treat a particular patient, accuracy is essential and requires rigorous validation, which is expensive to carry out. Most studies of medical AI are retrospective. For example, 72 (88%) of 82 studies in a 2019 *Lancet* review comparing AI with doctors were retrospective, and only 25 (36%) of the subgroup of 69 studies that could be checked provided sufficient detail to allow validation of the algorithm's results based on calculations on an external sample [41].

The detection of melanoma from skin photographs provides another useful example. A Stanford team developed a very accurate diagnostic algorithm that exceeded the performance of a specialist team [42]. However, it later emerged that the algorithm was based on images of melanoma that had been confirmed by biopsy [43]. The algorithm had "learned" from data that was different from that available to providers *prior* to referral when it is

---

Box 22.4 An Example of Data Science

Targeting and **predictive analytics** are often used together to focus limited services on patients who need them the most [34]. For example, detecting alcohol-related liver disease using routine lab investigations can help target community-based alcohol-reduction measures to people who are most likely to benefit [35]. **Cluster analysis** uses a variety of analytical techniques to detect novel clusters of patients that have not been previously identified. For example, it is now known from cluster analysis of facial images that vitiligo includes three distinct subtypes [36]. **Causal inference** is a speculative branch of data analytics that attempts to estimate the effectiveness of a public health intervention from routine datasets, and is fraught with difficulty because of a number of well-known biases such as confounding by indication [30, 37].

---

needed to make a management decision and was therefore of limited use. A well-designed study of the convolutional neural networks processing of optical coherence tomography retinal images with prospective validation provides a more positive example. The technology's performance was comparable to that of leading ophthalmologists [44] and further guided management by highlighting areas of concern on retinal images.

Much has been written about the exciting potential of data science, ML, and AI to improve health in L&MICs, but before adopting these approaches a thoughtful consideration of positive as well as negative accounts of performance on the ground and concerns about bias is warranted [45, 46]. Simpler statistical ML techniques such as logistic regression have a long history of success in creating reliable clinical prediction models, such as the well-known Framingham cardiac risk index [47]. The use of ML algorithms to assist clinicians in the diagnosis of patients with an unusual and/or serious disease based on risk factors or laboratory data is useful and can be further improved as experts contribute further information to optimize the algorithm's accuracy.

The most important determinant of AI success is the use of high-quality unbiased data collected from populations with a representative range by gender, age, ethnicity, location, and socioeconomic status. These datasets must be large enough for deriving models and testing validity, with additional testing with new datasets before algorithms are released for wider use. Thus, the principles of high-quality data collection, cleaning, and coding discussed above are also essential for applying AI or ML to health care.

22.4 Conclusion

Health information is a core function for *health and system improvement* that requires developing a shortlist of core data items and data quality targets, determining who collects data, making available data capture tools, sharing data collected, and developing analytical reports and online dashboards. A parallel stream focuses on *data improvement* to assess the quality of data being captured and IT infrastructure, followed by informed action to improve data quality.

Equally important for L&MICs is to develop understanding of the various high-quality, open source data capture, analysis, and sharing tools for improved data processing. While it is important to know the potential of big data analytics, AI, and ML, much can be achieved using simple tools to capture data and turn it into actionable knowledge for informed decisions.

References

1. E. H. Shortliffe, L. E. Perreault, G. Wiederhold, et al. *Medical Informatics: Computer Applications in Health Care.* Reading, MA, Addison-Wesley, 1990.

2. World Health Organization. Toolkit on Monitoring Health Systems Strengthening: health information systems. 2008. www.who.int/healthinfo/statistics/toolkit_hss/EN_PDF_Toolkit_HSS_Information Systems.pdf (accessed January 11, 2021).

3. N. Puttkammer, J. G. Baseman, E. B. Devine, et al. An assessment of data quality in a multi-site electronic medical record system in Haiti. *Int J Med Inform* 2016; **86**: 104–116.

4. World Health Organization. 2018 Global reference list of 100 core health indicators (plus health-related SDGs). 2018. https://apps.who.int/iris/handle/10665/259951 (accessed November 22, 2021).

5. World Health Organization. Maternal mortality ratio (per 100 000 live births). 2021. www.who.int/data/gho/indicator-metadata-registry/imr-details/26 (accessed November 22, 2021).

6. ISO 9000. Glossary of words used in the ISO9000 family of standards. 2019. www.iso.org/files/live/sites/isoorg/files/standards/docs/en/terminology-ISO9000-family.pdf (accessed August 20, 2022).

7. J. C. Wyatt, F. Sullivan. What is health information? *BMJ* 2005; **331**(7516): 566–568.

8. World Health Organization. International statistical classification of diseases and related health problems (ICD). 2021. www.who.int/standards/classifications/classification-of-diseases (accessed November 22, 2021).

9. N. D. Lawrence. Data readiness levels. 2017. https://arxiv.org/abs/1705.02245 (accessed August 20, 2022).

10. H. Fraser, E. Coiera, D. Wong. Safety of patient-facing digital symptom checkers. *Lancet* 2018; **392**(10161): 2263–2264.

11. Open Health News. District Health Information System 2 (DHIS2). 2020. www.openhealthnews.com/resources/district-health-information-system-2-dhis2 (accessed November 22, 2021).

12. L. Stroux, B. Martinez, I. E. Coyote, et al. An mHealth monitoring system for traditional birth attendant-led antenatal risk assessment in rural Guatemala. *J Med Eng Technol* 2016; **40**(7–8): 356–371.

13. Digital Square. Addressing the need for a thriving marketplace for digital health. 2021. https://digitalsquare.org (accessed November 22, 2021).

14. S. Kaphle, S. Chaturvedi, I. Chaudhuri, et al. Adoption and usage of mHealth technology on quality and experience of care provided by frontline workers: observations from rural India. *JMIR Mhealth Uhealth* 2015; **3**(2): e61.

15. B. W. Mamlin, P. G. Biondich, B. A. Wolfe, et al. Cooking up an open source EMR for developing countries: OpenMRS – a recipe for successful collaboration. *AMIA Annu Symp Proc* 2006; **2006**: 529–533.

16. I. Bacher, P. Mankowski, C. White, et al. A new FHIR-based API for OpenMRS. Poster presented at AMIA Clinical Informatics Conference, May 2021.

17. Medfloss. OpenClinic GA. 2020. www.medfloss.org/node/722 (accessed August 20, 2022).

18. D. Tom-Aba, B. C. Silenou, J. Doerrbecker, et al. The Surveillance Outbreak Response Management and Analysis System (SORMAS): digital health global goods maturity assessment. *JMIR Public Health Surveill* 2020; **6**(2): e15860.

19. OpenELIS global. Homepage. 2020. https://openelis-global.org (accessed August 20, 2022).

20. Open Logistics Management Information System. Homepage. https://openlmis.org (accessed May 29, 2022).

21. iDart. iDart pharmacy dispensing system. www.cell-life.org/idart (accessed May 28, 2022).

22. OpenBoxes. Homepage. https://openboxes.com (accessed May 28, 2022).

23. E. Tambo, A. Kazienga, M. Talla, et al. Digital technology and mobile applications

impact on Zika and Ebola epidemics data sharing and emergency response. *J Health Med Inform* 2017; **8**: 254.

24. S. Agarwal. Digital solutions for COVID-19 response: an assessment of digital tools for rapid scale-up for case management and contact tracing. 2020. www.comminit .com/covid/content/digital-solutions-covid-19-response-assessment-digital-tools-rapid-scale-case-management (accessed March 19, 2020).

25. N. Muinga, S. Magare, J. Monda, et al. Digital health systems in Kenyan public hospitals: a mixed-methods survey. *BMC Med Inform Decis Mak* 2020; **20**(1): 2.

26. V. Muthee, A. F. Bochner, A. Osterman, et al. The impact of routine data quality assessments on electronic medical record data quality in Kenya. *PLoS One* 2018; **13**(4): e0195362.

27. R. Saripalle, C. Runyan, M. Russell. Using HL7 FHIR to achieve interoperability in patient health record. *J Biomed Inform* 2019; **94**: 103188.

28. M. Baskaya, M. Yuksel, G. B. L. Erturkmen, et al. Health4Afrika: implementing HL7 FHIR based interoperability. *Stud Health Technol Inform* 2019; **264**: 20–24.

29. B. R. Zeeberg, J. Riss, D. W. Kane, et al. Mistaken identifiers: gene name errors can be introduced inadvertently when using Excel in bioinformatics. *BMC Bioinformat* 2004; **5**: 80.

30. M. Porta. A dictionary of epidemiology. *Revista española de salud pública* 2008; **82**(4): 433.

31. NHS e-Referral Service Open Data Dashboard. UK online referrals dashboard. 2021. https://digital.nhs.uk/dashboards/ers-open-data (accessed March 19, 2020).

32. H. S. Fraser, M. Mugisha, E. Remera, et al. User perceptions and use of an enhanced electronic health record in Rwanda with and without clinical alerts: cross-sectional survey. *JMIR Med Informat* 2022; **10**(5): e32305.

33. World Health Organization. Data collection and analysis tools. 2021. www .who.int/healthinfo/tools_data_analysis/ en/ (accessed March 15, 2020).

34. C. O'Neil. *Weapons of Math Destruction: How Big Data Increases Inequality and Threatens Democracy*. London, Penguin Books, 2017.

35. N. Sheron, N. Moore, W. O'Brien, et al. Feasibility of detection and intervention for alcohol-related liver disease in the community: the Alcohol and Liver Disease Detection study (ALDDeS). *Br J Gen Pract* 2013; **63**(615): e698–e705.

36. J. M. Bae, Y. S. Jung, H. M. Jung, et al. Classification of facial vitiligo: a cluster analysis of 473 patients. *Pigment Cell Melanoma Res* 2018; **31**(5): 585–591.

37. E. Gray, J. Marti, J. C. Wyatt, et al. Chemotherapy effectiveness in trial-underrepresented groups with early breast cancer: a retrospective cohort study. *PLoS Med* 2019; **16**(12): e1003006.

38. E. J. Topol. High-performance medicine: the convergence of human and artificial intelligence. *Nat Med* 2019; **25**(1): 44–56.

39. A. Hart, J. Wyatt. Evaluating black-boxes as medical decision aids: issues arising from a study of neural networks. *Med Inform (Lond)* 1990; **15**(3): 229–236.

40. J. Wyatt. Nervous about artificial neural networks? *Lancet* 1995; **346**(8984): 1175–1177.

41. X. Liu, L. Faes, A. U. Kale, et al. A comparison of deep learning performance against health-care professionals in detecting diseases from medical imaging: a systematic review and meta-analysis. *Lancet Digit Health* 2019; **1**(6): e271–e297.

42. A. Esteva, B. Kuprel, R. A. Novoa, et al. Dermatologist-level classification of skin cancer with deep neural networks. *Nature* 2017; **542**(7639): 115–118.

43. A. Narla, B. Kuprel, K. Sarin, et al. Automated classification of skin lesions: from pixels to practice. *J Invest Dermatol* 2018; **138**(10): 2108–2110.

44. J. De Fauw, J. R. Ledsam, B. Romera-Paredes, et al. Clinically applicable deep learning for diagnosis and referral in retinal disease. *Nat Med* 2018; **24**(9): 1342–1350.

45. A. Rajkomar, J. Dean, I. Kohane. Machine learning in medicine. *N Engl J Med* 2019; **380**(14): 1347–1358.

46. D. A. Vyas, L. G. Eisenstein, D. S. Jones. Hidden in plain sight: reconsidering the use of race correction in clinical algorithms. *N Engl J Med* 2020; **383**(9): 874–882.

47. W. B. Kannel, T. R. Dawber, A. Kagan, et al. Factors of risk in the development of coronary heart disease: six year follow-up experience – the Framingham study. *Ann Intern Med* 1961; **55**: 33–50.

Using Health Research for Evidence-Informed Decisions in Health Systems in L&MICs

23

Kabir Sheikh, Aku Kwamie, and Abdul Ghaffar

Key Messages

- Research evidence is one of the many diverse influences on decisions by different stakeholders at all levels of the health system.
- Decisions by stakeholders in health systems benefit from the use of different forms of evidence, drawn from heterogeneous research fields and disciplines – including epidemiology, clinical and basic biomedical research, and health policy and systems research.
- Out of these diverse forms of evidence, health policy and systems research (HPSR) is relatively underused and underfunded. Challenges associated with the use of HPSR in health systems in low- and middle-income countries (L&MICs) include lack of opportunities and resources, the need for greater capacity for the generation and use of evidence, and fundamental problems around how the research agenda is framed.
- As such, evidence-informed decision-making in L&MICs can be improved by better alignment of research with health system needs, institutionalizing the use of such evidence, and strengthening individual capacities to generate and use evidence.
- Several global, national, and local initiatives have helped take strides in these areas, but more work and investment is needed to strengthen the use of appropriate evidence, especially HPSR evidence, in health systems.

23.1 Background

23.1.1 Who Are the Decision-Makers in Health Systems?

Health systems have been described as the sum of all organizations, institutions, and resources that produce actions whose primary purpose is to improve health [1]. Health systems function as a result of decisions taken by stakeholders at different levels of the system. For instance, policymakers at the helm of health systems take decisions that might involve introducing or changing policies, undertaking reforms, setting up new schemes, allocating funds, and interpreting the change and impact that results from these actions. Similarly, program and health facility managers make decisions regarding a range of topics – from financing to human resources to general management – for their program or facility to function. And finally, frontline practitioners (e.g., community health workers, nurses, and physicians) make decisions about how best to serve users and treat patients, as well as how to implement policy and manage organizational imperatives [2].

23.1.2 What Types of Evidence-Informed Decisions Are Taken in Health Systems?

Decisions can be major – when they concern choices around large-scale or high-impact policies and finances – or minor, such as adjustments in policy and practice with the intention of improving implementation on a day-to-day basis. Decisions taken by various stakeholders at different levels of the health system have a potential impact on the performance of the health system. Therefore, it is important for them to be well informed by relevant, timely, and good-quality research and evidence. Figure 23.1 provides a broad framework of the types of decisions taken by health system decision-makers, and the corresponding types of evidence needed.

23.1.3 What Type of Evidence Is Needed to Inform Decisions in the Health System?

The evidence needed to inform each of these decisions varies and can be drawn from a heterogeneous range of research fields and disciplines, including epidemiology, clinical and basic biomedical research, and a suite of research subfields that can be clustered under the broad umbrella of HPSR. Table 23.1 presents a map of these different fields of research. These fields produce different types of knowledge; the research conducted within them, as well as how resulting evidence is assessed and used, can follow different (but overlapping) rules and principles. This can cause confusion and conflict when using evidence to inform decisions. Nonetheless, the choice of research design and methodology should vary according to the nature of the research question or the problem to be resolved (see Chapter 14).

23.1.4 How Does Evidence Inform Decision-Making?

Health system problems are often complex and multifaceted, and so is decision-making in health systems. The policy theorist Vickers postulated that public policy decisions are driven

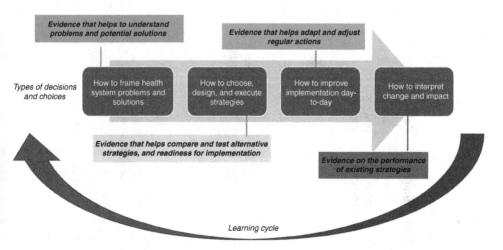

Figure 23.1 Diverse evidence needs of health system decision-makers.

Table 23.1 Fields of research that contribute to evidence needs of health systems

Contributing research field	Types of evidence	Purpose of evidence	Types of decisions informed
Epidemiology, demography, social behavioral research, clinical and biomedical research	Evidence on the population, on the nature and scale of health concerns, and potential therapies and public health measures		
	Evidence on the nature and scale of health system and policy problems, and on potential measures to address them	Helping decision-makers understand health system problems and their potential solutions	Framing health system problems and solutions
Health systems research, health economics, health policy analysis	Evidence on the nature and scale of health system and policy problems, and on potential measures to address them		
	Evidence on the effectiveness of policies, programs, and other health system interventions and their viability	Helping decision-makers compare and test alternative health systems strategies, and readiness for implementation	Choosing, designing, and executing strategies
Implementation research	Context-specific evidence on policy/program implementation gaps and how to resolve them	Helping decision-makers adapt and adjust regular actions	Improving implementation day-to-day
Evaluation research	Context-specific evidence on the processes and outcomes of health system interventions, reforms, and policies	Helping decision-makers assess the performance of existing strategies	Interpreting change and impact

Health policy and systems research

by a combination of judgments about the facts (What is?) and value judgments (What ought?) to arrive at action judgments (What to do? How to do it?) [3]. As such, evidence is only one of the multitude of influences informing decisions in the health system. Political and pragmatic factors and value judgments play a significant, and often greater, part.

Evidence can inform decisions in the health system in two distinct ways. First, evidence can contribute to making adjustments and corrections to regular actions – helping to adapt routines and practices within the system – without examining the underlying root causes of problems or contributing to reframing strategies and policies. This is known as single-loop learning [4]. Implementation research initiatives, for example, have helped program managers around the world to overcome implementation bottlenecks and improve the delivery of programs to prevent noncommunicable diseases (NCDs) [5].

Second, evidence can serve a deeper purpose by helping decision-makers question fundamental frameworks, models, and assumptions that underpin problems and their solutions, which may require changes at the level of policies or objectives. This is known as double-loop learning. For example, in Nigeria, economic recession led the government to fundamentally rethink existing social protection and health financing policy, instigating a policy reform process that led to the establishment of the National Health Insurance Scheme [6]. Single and double learning loops are both mechanisms of evidence-informed decision-making that have an important role in health systems [7].

23.2 Key Challenges

There are several challenges associated with the use of research evidence to inform decisions in health systems in L&MICs. While some of these challenges relate to the need to develop more capacity for the generation and use of evidence and the lack of opportunities and platforms for evidence use, there are also fundamental problems related to how the research agenda is framed.

23.2.1 The "Framing" Challenge

Much of the research generated worldwide about health systems in L&MICs does not adequately consider the needs and priorities of decision-makers, and is instead driven by the interests of research funders and researchers, often situated in high-income countries (HICs) [8, 9]. It is important that research agendas be closely aligned with the needs of health system decision-makers who are the ultimate end-users of research on health systems (Figure 23.1). There are several reasons why such alignment is needed, the foremost of which are that this,

- improves the likelihood that research findings will be utilized and hence the quality of decisions; and
- improves the efficiency of research funding, ensuring that resources are directed toward knowledge products that will not be wasted.

Another critical challenge in framing the research agenda for evidence use is the persistent dominance of the biomedical research model. As demonstrated in Table 23.1, biomedical research addresses only one of the multiple types of evidence needs of decision-makers within health systems. Yet, biomedical research continues to be dominant over applied social sciences and HPSR due to better research capacity, greater funding, and a higher volume of publications, including in L&MICs [8].

An unfortunate consequence of this imbalance is that traditional standards for biomedical research are often applied to HPSR, favoring designs based on hypothesis testing and randomization over more context-sensitive methods and study designs, even when less appropriate. These unhelpful knowledge hierarchies have constrained the contribution of diverse research disciplines and fields to address the different evidence needs of health systems (see Figure 23.1 and Table 23.1).

23.2.2 The "Opportunity" Challenge

A more tangible challenge to the effective use of evidence to inform decision-making is limited opportunity. Decision-makers in L&MICs often lack ready and rapid access to the evidence they need. This "opportunity" challenge has multiple facets, including:

- the lack of institutional mechanisms to promptly analyze, synthesize, and present relevant evidence to decision-makers [10];
- inadequate funding for research, contributing to a low critical mass of useful evidence – notably, many L&MICs do not have a national health research budget [8]; and
- limited opportunities for researchers in L&MICs to meaningfully engage and collaborate with decision-makers [8].

23.2.3 The "Capacity" Challenge

Underpinning and worsening the other two challenges is the inadequate capacity that prevails in L&MICs to generate and use evidence relevant to health systems. HPSR is still a nascent discipline and has not yet found a foothold as an area of specialization in higher education institutions in L&MICs, compounding the more generic problem of the low numbers of skilled researchers engaging in the generation of all forms of health research.

Coupled with the capacity problem in the generation of research is the problem of capacity to engage, interpret, and use diverse forms of research, especially HPSR, among health system decision-makers. These capacity gaps underpin the low demand for HPSR from decision-makers, which in turn also impedes the generation of more relevant evidence, completing a vicious cycle of obstacles to evidence use in L&MIC health systems [8].

23.3 Options and Opportunities

What can be done to address these challenges and strengthen evidence-informed decision-making in L&MICs? The key opportunities that correspond to each of the aforementioned challenges include: (1) aligning research with health system needs; (2) institutionalizing knowledge use; and (3) strengthening individual capacities to generate and use evidence for health systems.

23.3.1 Aligning Research with Health System Needs

It is important that the objectives and processes of research on health systems align closely with the evidence needs of decision-makers, so as to increase the likelihood of uptake and reduce research waste. The WHO 2012 Strategy on HPSR advocated a six-point agenda for action to facilitate evidence-informed decision-making and the strengthening of health systems [11]:

1. embedding research within decision-making processes;
2. supporting demand-driven research;

3. strengthening capacity for research and use of evidence;
4. establishing repositories of knowledge;
5. improving the efficiency of investments in research; and
6. increasing accountability for actions.

Nearly a decade later, the agenda remains as relevant as ever, yet progress, while steady, remains limited and difficult to track. For instance, improvements in research investments are unclear. In fact, lack of data on health research budgets in several L&MICs (and almost no disaggregated data on allocations for HPSR) makes this virtually impossible to assess and reinforces the need for greater advocacy for increased domestic financing for health research. This is similarly the case with increasing accountability for actions. Some progress has been made on establishing knowledge repositories at the global (e.g., the WHO Observatory on R&D) and regional (e.g., the Asia Pacific Observatory on Health Systems and Policies and the African Health Observatory) levels, which are a significant resource for L&MICs. Yet, greater investments are needed to support national and subnational knowledge repositories that can more effectively serve local needs.

Notable progress has been made on embedding research within decision-making processes, supporting demand-driven research, and strengthening research capacity for research and use of evidence. We address these below.

Embedding Research within Decision-Making Processes

Ghaffar and colleagues [12] have argued that embedding research into decision-making processes within health systems is a critical step to improve the use of evidence. Embedded research brings together researchers and decision-makers to design, produce, and interpret research findings. It empowers health system decision-makers by prioritizing their needs and questions in defining the research agenda; engages and equips them to own and participate in research; and potentially increases the utilization of research findings for system improvements. A multi-site study in Latin America demonstrated that embedded implementation research fostered stakeholder "buy-in" early on in the research process, increased research focus, and resulted in fewer hindrances in translating research findings [13].

Supporting Demand-Driven Research

Demand-driven research is a related approach that specifically responds to the needs and priorities of health system decision-makers. Demand-driven research is useful in enhancing the legitimacy and ownership of research findings, but can also, crucially, orient policy-makers and practitioners to the value and promise of research on health systems. In Ghana, an analysis of demand-driven research questions revealed that there was a disconnect between the research needs of local decision-makers – which were mostly related to strengthening health systems – and the interests of international researchers and donors – mostly related to biomedical and disease-specific issues [14]. Demand-driven research calls for a balance between generating universally applicable findings and ensuring well-contextualized locally relevant research.

A corollary to supporting demand-driven research is promoting research thinking and capacity so that decision-makers can be much more strategic and directive in scoping, commissioning, and using research. Currently, the bulk of efforts in this domain are "demand-responsive supply," and not truly "demand-led" [15]. Experience from South

Africa's establishment of a national evaluation system demonstrates that stimulating demand for evidence yields more promising results when it is accompanied by institutionalizing support systems that can foster demand for evidence. These include introducing change management processes to support the organizational changes that arise as a result of increased demand for evidence, establishing coalitions and technical working groups to routinize demand for evidence, and increasing learning-by-doing and short-course opportunities that strengthen capacities for demanding evidence [16].

23.3.2 Institutionalizing Knowledge Use

A second critical step in strengthening evidence-based decision-making is institutionalization, which refers to the mainstreaming or routinization of the generation and use of relevant knowledge within the health system. Two mechanisms for institutionalization of evidence use are described below.

Building Knowledge Platforms for Evidence Synthesis

Policymakers frequently need reliable evidence that can support time-sensitive decisions in relation to health systems. Rapid reviews and evidence synthesis approaches are important means of accelerating informed decision-making. They can help policymakers to make decisions by providing evidence that is relevant and actionable at various stages of the policymaking process. This is particularly important in the context of emergencies, as was observed during the early onset of the COVID-19 pandemic (see Box 23.1).

Embedding Implementation Research into Large-Scale Global Health Funds

Implementation research has been widely used to improve and course-correct the implementation of health system interventions and health programs. In this chapter we refer to embedded implementation research (eIR) as an action-oriented approach that brings

---

Box 23.1 Embedding Rapid Reviews in Health Systems Decision-Making

In 2018, the Alliance for Health Policy and Systems Research launched a program in several countries to establish rapid review platforms directly within health decision-making institutions. The platforms aimed to respond to decision-makers' requests in real time, while strengthening capacities to develop and disseminate timely and relevant knowledge products such as rapid evidence syntheses and policy briefs.

In Georgia, the platform was established as a partnership between the Committee on Health and Social Affairs of the Parliament of Georgia and Curatio Foundation. In India, the platform was a partnership between the National Health Systems Resource Centre, Ministry of Health and Family Welfare, and the George Institute for Global Health. The credibility attributed to these evidence platforms made them readily available to generate new evidence synthesis in record time.

During the ongoing COVID-19 pandemic, in Georgia the platform published a rapid response for policy options to respond to the emergency that included modeling to support the government working group. In India, the platform responded to the government's need to develop guidelines for personal protection for frontline health workers.

Source: [17].

together researchers and decision-makers to design, produce, and interpret research findings. eIR is useful to spotlight the role of decision-makers throughout the research process in order to deepen the impact of implementation research (IR) by embedding it into "real-world" contexts of implementation. In general, while eIR shares similarities to IR, operations research (OR), implementation science (IS), and delivery science (DS), universally agreed-upon definitions of these evidence approaches do not exist as yet.

Increasingly, large-scale global health initiatives are embedding IR into their programs. For example, the US President's Emergency Plan for AIDS Relief uses IR alongside its monitoring and evaluation and impact evaluations to build evidence on how global clinical trial findings translate into local health settings [18]. The Global Fund to Fight AIDS, Tuberculosis and Malaria also promotes IR as part of its support to disease control programs. Since 2015, Gavi the Vaccine Alliance, UNICEF, and the Alliance for Health Policy and Systems Research have partnered in several countries to test and refine embedded implementation approaches to scaling up immunization coverage in underimmunized populations [19].

23.3.3 Strengthening Individual Capacities to Generate Evidence for Health Systems

A third critical step is the development of human capacities to generate and use relevant evidence for health systems. As outlined in Table 23.1, the types of evidence relevant for health systems range from epidemiological, clinical, and biomedical research to different forms of HPSR.

Epidemiological, Clinical, and Biomedical Research Capacities

Epidemiological, clinical, and biomedical research capacities are still inadequate in many L&MICs, yet several opportunities exist to redress these challenges. At the individual level, formalized and incentivized career paths for young researchers offer one way to attract and motivate researchers into viable research careers within their countries, while reducing the push to seek international training opportunities [20]. This can be assisted by better integrating research training into undergraduate, medical, nursing, and other health professional educational programs. L&MICs can further seek to elevate research career paths by introducing national recognition or awards for scientists.

At the institutional level, incentives that reward network exchange, institutional mentorship, and processes for developing research leaders [21] are much-needed to further support the development of individual capacities. Appropriate legal and governance frameworks for research are also needed to provide an overarching enabling environment to nurture in-country research capacities.

Health Policy and Systems Research Capacities

The need to enhance capacity to generate and use HPSR is urgent, especially in many L&MICs [22]. Most frequently, capacity strengthening examples have demonstrated partnerships (mostly North–South, but increasingly South–South) that combine individual- and institutional-level capacity inputs. For instance, Thailand demonstrates a long-term case of nurturing HPSR capacities through the establishment of national and international collaborations for graduate-level training, followed by posting of trainees to government institutions. In time, trainees became mentors for junior researchers within the institutions, and enabling environments were fostered by expanding a critical mass [23]. More recently, options to strengthen both national and subnational HPSR capacities through local centers of excellence are increasingly observed. One such example is eHealthLab Ethiopia, a health informatics partnership between the Federal Ministry of Health and the University of Gondar. eHealthLab exists to conduct embedded research into the country's health information agenda, while offering postgraduate degrees to train new cohorts of researchers and health planners.

23.4 Global Efforts and Movements

It is useful to situate the options and opportunities for strengthening evidence-informed decision-making in L&MICs within the broader canvas of global efforts in this area. A selection of pertinent global movements is outlined in this section.

23.4.1 Evidence-Based Medicine and Evidence-Based Health Policy

The past few decades have seen the development of a movement of evidence-based medicine – formalized in developments such as the International Cochrane Collaboration, and other global mechanisms for updating clinical guidelines. During the 1990s, concepts associated with evidence-based medicine began to be applied in relation to health policy. This approach has, however, faced a number of challenges. Health decision-makers have diverse backgrounds and, unlike colleagues with expertise in a common specific subclinical domain, may not share norms and language [24]. Furthermore, while clinicians commonly make decisions within the scope of their expertise and authority, health policymakers often take fewer, larger-scale decisions over a longer time horizon, influenced by unique externalities, which do not lend themselves to standard solutions [25]. Over the years, more sophisticated and practical approaches to strengthening the relationship between evidence and policy have begun to emerge (Box 23.2).

23.4.2 Establishment of the Alliance for Health Policy and Systems Research

The Alliance for Health Policy and Systems Research was established in 1999 as a response to the findings of the 1996 WHO Ad Hoc Committee on Health Research. In particular, that

---

Box 23.2 Terminology

Evidence-based medicine (EBM): the integration of clinical expertise, patient values, and the best research evidence into the decision-making process for patient care [26].

Evidence-based policymaking (EBPM): the continuum of three domains, encompassing policy process (i.e., approaches to enhance the likelihood of policy adoption), policy content (i.e., specific elements likely to be effective), and policy outcome (i.e., potential impact) [27].

Evidence-based management (EBMgt): the systematic application of the best available evidence to management decision-making, aimed at improving the performance of health care organizations [28].

Evidence-informed decision-making (EIDM): the process of distilling and disseminating the best available evidence from research, context, and experience, and using that evidence to inform and improve public health practice and policy [29].

report made clear that some knowledge gaps related to health systems could not be addressed by the existing approaches to research, and that investment was needed to develop the field of HPSR in terms of capacities, methods, guidelines, and approaches. Since that time, the Alliance has provided thought-leadership on strengthening capacities for evidence-informed health policy [30], pioneered the embedded research approach [14], developed guides on conducting evidence synthesis [10] and rapid reviews [31], and established the production of rapid review and evidence synthesis platforms directly into health decision-making institutions (see Box 23.1).

The *World Report on Health Policy and Systems Research* [8] identified that international funding committed to HPSR from 2000 to 2014 had steadily increased. In 2000, annual HPSR funding from international donors was less than US$100 million; it peaked at US$540 million in 2010 and averaged US$400 million in 2011–2014 (Figure 23.2).

23.4.3 Other Initiatives

At the global level, clinical guidelines and public health policy recommendations are developed by WHO as part of its normative and standard-setting work when the Member States or other stakeholders request guidance. When guidelines are available, countries may still need guidance on selecting and implementing the guidelines most appropriate to them.

Within countries, a refocus on strengthening health information systems is growing, especially to achieve universal health coverage (UHC). Strengthened health information systems – and the myriad data initiatives that support them – are important for decision-makers at all levels of the system to make informed decisions in real time (see Chapters 8 and 22). A coordinated and well-functioning health information system enables data from households, facilities, and districts to be communicated up to the national level, enabling responsive decisions on policy and practice to be communicated back. Countries can take action to strengthen health information systems by improving their interoperability (i.e., the ability for subdomains to speak across others), investing in digital systems and harnessing emerging technologies, and investing in capacities for use, dissemination, and accountability.

Bringing the global and country-based evidence considerations together, the 2004 Mexico Summit on Health Research advocated the need for countries to strengthen mechanisms to use health research in policymaking and health systems strengthening. This resulted in the adoption of key resolutions by the 58th World Health Assembly, which in turn led WHO to launch the Evidence-Informed Policy Network (EVIPNet) in June 2005. EVIPNet supports networks in many countries of the world to strengthen capacities and information exchange among researchers and policymakers to develop policy briefs, host policy dialogs, support priority-setting mechanisms, and establish evidence clearinghouses and observatories [32].

The Way Forward

As we consider future global efforts to strengthen evidence-based decision-making, the final two points of WHO's six-point agenda for HPSR bear close attention – improving the efficiency of investments in research and increasing accountability for actions [11].

For *investments in research* to be more effective, it is crucial that they increasingly align with system priorities and be contextually relevant and locally generated – domestic research funding is key to making this happen. There are increasing calls globally to raise domestic financing for HPSR in L&MICs. Many L&MICs do not have a national health

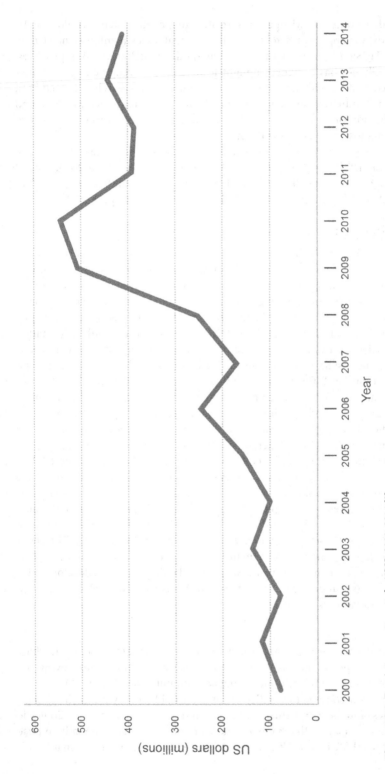

Figure 23.2 Trends in commitments for HPSR, 2000–2014 [8].

research budget. Where they do, these budgets are rarely disaggregated. Frequently, HPSR budgets are embedded within disease programs [33].

Ultimately, as policy theorists have recognized for a long time, evidence is one of a multitude of influences on decisions taken by stakeholders in the health system [3]. However, it is possible to increase the use of evidence by holding stakeholders more accountable. Public transparency laws, publishing the evidence behind policy decisions and the results of reviews and evaluations, and different forms of deliberative health policymaking (such as health assemblies, facility committees, and health councils) are key mechanisms that help to increase accountability and build stakeholders' trust in health systems [34].

Genuine progress in evidence use will occur when decision-makers improve funding for contextually relevant, locally owned research, complemented with rules and procedures to ensure that evidence is taken into account when decisions are made regarding health systems. One notable example of this is Thailand's experience of preparing for UHC reforms in the 1970s, through investments in domestic health systems research capacity, and by linking trained researchers in collaborative arrangements with policymakers. This allowed the reforms to be continuously adapted and improved through the application of evidence on their implementation over three to five decades, with a salutary impact on levels of financial protection across the country [22].

Decisions in relation to health systems influence the health and wellbeing of innumerable people, and the improved use of evidence in making those decisions should be a matter of the highest priority for governments across the world.

References

1. World Health Organization. *The World Health Report 2000: Health Systems – Improving Performance*. Geneva, World Health Organization, 2000. www.who.int/whr/2000/en/whr00_en.pdf (accessed July 11, 2021).

2. M. Lipsky. Street-level bureaucracy and the analysis of urban reform. *Urban Aff Q* 1971; **6**(4): 391–409.

3. G. Vickers. *The Art of Judgment: A Study of Policy Making*. London, Chapman & Hall, 1965.

4. C. Argyris. *Organizational Learning II. Theory, Method, and Practice*. London, FT Press, 1996.

5. N. Gibbs, J. Kwon, J. Balen, et al. Operational research to support equitable non-communicable disease policy in low-income and middle-income countries in the sustainable development era: a scoping review. *BMJ Glob Health* 2020; **5**(6): e002259.

6. C. A. Onoka, K. Hanson, J. Hanefeld. Towards universal coverage: a policy analysis of the development of the National Health Insurance Scheme in Nigeria. *Health Policy Plan* 2015; **30**(9): 1105–1117.

7. World Health Organization. Learning health systems: pathways to progress: flagship report of the Alliance for Health Policy and Systems Research. Geneva, World Health Organization, 2021. https://apps.who.int/iris/handle/10665/344891 (accessed February 16, 2022).

8. World Health Organization. *World Report on Health Policy and Systems Research*. Geneva, World Health Organization, 2017. https://apps.who.int/iris/bitstream/handle/10665/255051/9789241512268-eng.pdf (accessed July 18, 2021).

9. S. Abimbola. The foreign gaze: authorship in academic global health. *BMJ Glob Health* 2019; **4**(5): e002068.

10. E. V. Langlois, K. Daniels, E. A. Akl. Evidence synthesis for health policy and systems: a methods guide. 2018. www.who.int/alliance-hpsr/resources/publications/hsr-synthesis/en/ (accessed July 10, 2021).

11. World Health Organization. Changing mindsets: strategy on health policy and systems research. 2012. www.who.int/ alliance-hpsr/alliancehpsr_changing mindsets_strategyhpsr.pdf (accessed July 11, 2021).

12. A. Ghaffar, E. V. Langlois, K. Rasanathan, et al. Strengthening health systems through embedded research. *Bull World Health Organ* 2017; **95**(2): 87.

13. N. Tran, E. V. Langlois, L. Reveiz, et al. Embedding research to improve program implementation in Latin America and the Caribbean. *Rev Panam Salud Publica* 2017; **41**: e75.

14. M. O. Kok, J. O. Gyapong, I. Wolffers, et al. Towards fair and effective North–South collaboration: realising a programme for demand-driven and locally led research. *Health Res Policy Syst* 2017; **15**(1): 96.

15. S. Witter, K. Andrew, S. Molly, et al. Generating demand for and use of evaluation evidence in government health ministries: lessons from a pilot programme in Uganda and Zambia. *Health Res Policy Syst* 2017; **15**: 86.

16. I. Goldman, J. E. Mathe, C. Jacob, et al. Developing South Africa's national evaluation policy and system: first lessons learned. *AEJ* 2015; **3**(1): 9.

17. Alliance for Health Policy and Systems Research. Rapid research responders: the life-saving power of embedded research. 2021. www.ahpsr.org/stories/rapid-research-responders-the-life-saving-power-of-embedded-research (accessed July 11, 2021).

18. D. Kerrigan, C. E. Kennedy, A. S. Cheng, et al. Advancing the strategic use of HIV operations research to strengthen local policies and programmes: the Research to Prevention Project. *J Int AIDS Soc* 2015; **18**(1): 20029.

19. Z. Shroff, B. Aulakh, L. Gilson, et al. Incorporating research evidence into decision-making processes: researcher and decision-maker perceptions from five low- and middle-income countries. *Health Res Policy Syst* 2015; **13**: 70.

20. Academy of Medical Sciences. Strengthening clinical research capacity in low- and middle-income countries. 2017. https://acmedsci .ac.uk/policy/policy-projects/strengthening-clinical-research-capacity-in-low-and-middle-income-countries (accessed July 14, 2021).

21. S. R. Franzen, C. Chandler, T. Lang. Health research capacity development in low and middle income countries: reality or rhetoric? A systematic meta-narrative review of the qualitative literature. *BMJ Open* 2017; **7**(1):e012332.

22. L. Gilson. *Health Policy and Systems Research: A Methodology Reader*. Geneva, Alliance for Health Policy and Systems Research, 2012.

23. S. Pitayarangsarit, V. Tangcharoensathien. Sustaining capacity in health policy and systems research in Thailand. *Bull World Health Organ* 2009; **87**(1): 72–74.

24. K. Walshe, T. G. Rundall. Evidence-based management: from theory to practice in health care. *Milbank Q* 2001; **79**(3): 429–457, iv–v.

25. K. Oliver, T. Lorenc, S. Innvær. New directions in evidence-based policy research: a critical analysis of the literature. *Health Res Policy Syst* 2014; **12**: 34.

26. D. L. Sackett, W.M. Rosenberg, J. A. Gray, et al. Evidence based medicine: what it is and what it isn't. *BMJ* 1996; **312**: 70–72.

27. R. C. Brownson, J. F. Chriqui, K. A. Stamatakis. Understanding evidence-based public health policy. *Am J Public Health* 2009; **99**: 1576–1583.

28. A. Janati, E. Hasanpoor, S. Hajebrahimi, et al. An evidence-based framework for evidence-based management in healthcare organizations: a Delphi study. *Ethip J Health Sci* 2018; **28**(3): 305–314.

29. H. Husson, C. Howarth, S. N. Sztramko, et al. The National Collaborating Centre for Methods and Tools (NCCMT): supporting evidence-informed

decision-making in public health in Canada. 2021. www.canada.ca/en/public-health/services/reports-publications/canada-communicable-disease-report-ccdr/monthly-issue/2021-47/issue-5-6-may-june-2021/evidence-informed-decision-making-national-collaborating-centre-methods-tools.html (accessed July 12, 2021).

30. A. Green, S. Bennett. *Sound Choices: Enhancing Capacity for Evidence-Informed Health Policy*. Geneva, Alliance for Health Policy and Systems Research, 2007.

31. A. C. Tricco, E. V. Langlois, S. E. Straus. *Rapid Reviews to Strengthen Health Policy*

and Systems: A Practical Guide. Geneva, World Health Organization, 2017.

32. M. Hamid, T. Bustamante-Manaog, V. D. Truong, et al. EVIPNet: translating the spirit of Mexico. *Lancet* 2005; **366** (9499): 1758–1760.

33. World Health Organization. Partners' health policy and systems research report – 2021. 2021. www.ahpsr.org/partners-hpsr-report/ (accessed February 16, 2022).

34. G. Argyrous. Evidence based policy: principles of transparency and accountability. *AJPA* 2012; **71**(4): 457–468.

Integrated People-Centered Health Care
What It Is and How It's Done!

Katherine Rouleau, Shatha Albeik, Sayed Masoom Shah,
Kenneth Yakubu, and Akihiro Seita

Key Messages

- The evolution of people's health needs from mainly acute infectious and perinatal conditions requiring punctual treatment, to multiple chronic comorbidities underpinned by multifactorial risk factors and requiring complex and prolonged management demands a different approach to the delivery of health services.
- The integration of services through funding, administrative, organizational, and clinical service delivery mechanisms aims to respond to health needs in a way that optimizes coordination, minimizes care gaps, improves outcomes, and enhances patient satisfaction.
- People-centered services include a collective dimension, centered on the needs of a defined population, as well as an individual dimension, responsive to the unique needs and circumstances of the person.
- Family practice (also called family medicine) is a medical discipline that addresses most of the health and medical needs of individuals and their family, at all ages, throughout the life course. While its scope, organization, and role within health systems varies across settings and jurisdictions, it is practiced according to specific principles and a clinical approach centered on the whole person.
- Where it is most contributory to health systems, family practice is community-based and community-oriented, anchored in lasting relationships between the user and providers, is accountable to a defined population, sometimes includes empanelment, and is delivered by highly skilled clinicians. It is increasingly delivered through multidisciplinary teams that ideally include trained family physicians. Family practice purposefully delivers integrated person-centered care.
- Transformation toward integrated people-centered health systems is enabled through leadership (clear vision), organizational strategies (governance and accountability, and funding and allocation), patient-engagement strategies, and health worker-oriented strategies.
- The reform of primary care services by the United Nations Relief and Works Agency for Palestine Refugees in the Near East (UNRWA) in 2011 provides important lessons about the reorientation of services into an integrated and people-centered model.

24.1 Introduction and Objectives

The delivery of integrated and people-centered services is key to improving health systems' performance. Both integration and people-centeredness feature prominently in the renewed global commitment to primary health care (PHC) for universal health coverage as expressed in the 2018 Declaration of Astana [1]. While intuitively inviting, the concepts of integrated health services and people-centeredness are subject to a wide range of interpretations. Moreover, whereas consensus exists on the merits of health services integration, its expected outcomes are diverse and "how" to achieve them often remains unclear.

In this chapter, we explore why and how health systems deliver integrated and people-centered health services. To do so, we outline the rationale for integrated care; review key concepts, definitions, and models of integrated health services; describe the unique role of family practice in delivering integrated and people-centered health services; list strategies for integration; highlight common barriers, enablers, and promising approaches for the delivery of integrated and people-centered health services; and illustrate the reorientation from a vertical to a more comprehensively integrated service delivery model through a case study of the adoption of a family health team approach by UNRWA in 2011.

24.2 Rationale and Definitions

24.2.1 Rationale

As noted throughout this book, despite medical advances, more than half of the world's population does not have access to the health services they need, particularly in many resource-constrained settings [2]. When care is available, lack of accessibility and acceptability, and poor quality, result in the underutilization of services [3, 4]. Health systems historically organized to respond to episodic and acute issues are not adapted to meeting the diverse and increasingly complex health needs of the population in the twenty-first century. In low- and middle-income countries (L&MICs) efforts to move beyond vertically organized services focused on single diseases or targeted populations have often been limited to the combination or simple colocation of services for infectious diseases, child and maternal health (e.g., integrated management of childhood diseases), and TB and HIV, [5] excluding care for other health needs (e.g., care for noncommunicable diseases and palliative care) [6, 7] and failing to achieve true integration.

Yet the need for integration has never been greater. The aging of the population and the double burden of disease that prevails in L&MICs call for new models of care [8]. An integrated approach to care and fit-for-purpose competencies, ideally rooted in a continuous therapeutic relation over the life course, are particularly indicated to address multiple concurrent chronic conditions and their overlapping risk factors, as well as to provide self-management support and enable long-term adherence to complex therapeutic regimens [9]. These require the combination of medical, social, and multidisciplinary approaches to care [10].

Growing consumerism and increasing access to health information have also raised the expectations of users regarding quality of care as patients everywhere increasingly demand health services that are effective, easy to access and navigate, and responsive to their values, preferences, and unique environments, including in L&MICs [11].

The reorientation of health systems to deliver integrated people-centered care is proposed as a solution to address multiple and sometimes conflicting objectives, including: improvements in access, efficiency, care continuity, clinical outcomes, provider satisfaction, patient satisfaction, and cost reduction, to name only a few [12]. Striving to achieve some of the objectives may steer away from others. For example, efforts to increase access can result in increased cost. In high-income countries, new models of integrated care are sometimes linked to enhanced patient satisfaction, improved quality, and increased access, but the impact on other outcomes, including reduced cost and cost-effectiveness, is less clear [13].

There is also weak evidence that organizational integration alone, without patient-centered integrated care, results in improved outcomes [14].

24.2.2 Definitions

The concepts of integrated health services and of people-centeredness are subject to diverse and sometimes conflicting interpretations.

Integration and integrated care: Integration has been defined as "a coherent set of methods and models on the funding, administrative, organisational, service delivery and clinical levels designed to create connectivity, alignment and collaboration within and between the cure and care sectors" for the purpose of improving patient care and experience. When such processes achieve improved patient care and experience, the result is termed integrated care [15].

People-centered care: This includes a collective and an individual dimension. Health services centered on *people-as-community* are responsive to the prevalent needs of a given population, and sociocultural diversities and preferences are recognized and addressed [16]. The notion of people-centered care is not new. In many resource-constrained settings, a people-centered approach to health services prevailed well before their exposure to allopathic medicine. At the micro level of delivery (i.e., during clinical consultations or service provision), services centered on *people-as-individuals* are *person-centered* and engage each person's entire reality, unique needs, and personal experience of health or illness [16]. This is distinct from the more limited concept of *patient-centeredness* associated with a medical model that assumes a single, more passive, and "sickness informed" role for the person. Some consider integrated services to be inherently people- and person-centered.

In short, an integrated people-centered health system is one that plans, funds, manages, and delivers health services in a way that acknowledges the perspectives, comprehensive needs, and social preferences of the people it serves, as individuals and populations. Integrated services enable seamless access to the full continuum of care (including promotion, prevention, treatment, rehabilitation, and palliation), coordinated between health and social services, within and across different levels and sites in the health system to address all health needs throughout the life course.

24.3 Frameworks for Integrated Care and the Contribution of Family Practice

A number of frameworks and guidance documents have been published to inform the implementation of integrated care. They include the Chronic Care Model [17], the Rainbow Model [18], the WHO framework on Integrated People-Centered Health Services [19], and the Innovative Care for Chronic Conditions Framework [20]. While not a model of care *per se*, family practice (also called family medicine or general practice) espouses the features of integrated and people-centered care especially where it constitutes the foundation of health services.

24.3.1 Family Practice and Its Relevance to Integrated and People-Centered Care

Globally, health systems are best able to deliver integrated and people-centered health services when anchored in high-quality multidisciplinary family practice because the discipline itself is fundamentally and inherently people-centered and integrative.

Family medicine has historically referred to a medical specialty practiced by physicians with postgraduate training and having achieved a set of defined competencies (which may vary from one country to another), rooted in a generalist philosophy [21, 22] and applied according to specific principles and clinical approaches central to that discipline. While its unique competencies and training requirements make family medicine a specialty, its breadth and scope, including its key role in diagnosing and addressing undifferentiated presentations, requires a generalist approach. In other words, the family physician is a specialist in generalism who addresses the majority of health and medical needs of people at all ages. By contrast, in many parts of the world, a general practitioner (GP) is a physician who enters practice without having completed postgraduate training in a specialty, often immediately after graduating from medical school. In the UK, however, the term general practitioner is used instead of (and is equivalent to) *family doctor* to refer to generalist physicians who have undergone postgraduate training to deliver expert, comprehensive, person-centered primary care medicine.

While the discipline of family medicine is often practiced by solo physicians, it is increasingly recognized as being best delivered through multidisciplinary teams that include a range of allied health professionals with unique and essential competencies, such as pharmacists, nutritionists, and rehabilitation experts. The term *family practice* is used in some contexts to underscore the central role of nonphysicians in delivering services according to the principles and clinical approach of the discipline of family medicine. There is persistent debate as to whether a minimum number of family physicians (and if so, how many and in what specific role) are required for family practice to deliver the desired and expected outcomes. This debate is part of a broader and crucial discussion of how a limited number of health workers in L&MICs and elsewhere can best be trained and organized to deliver high-quality primary care, including in a family practice model that is increasingly recognized as the preferred model.

Family medicine, then, is "the medical specialty which provides continuing, comprehensive and responsive health services to individuals and families, integrating the biological, clinical and behavioural sciences to deliver care to people of all ages, all genders, and to address every disease entity across the life course" [23]. While organized differently in different countries, the practice of family medicine around the world expresses a number of common defining principles. We present them here as adapted from the Canadian principles of family medicine, which are only one of multiple formulations of these principles [24, 25].

Family practice is a "community-based discipline" delivered in, through, and in alignment with the values and priorities of the community in which it is rooted [26]. The term "community-oriented primary care" has been defined as "a continuous process by which primary health care is provided to a defined community on the basis of its assessed health needs, by the planned integration of primary care practice and public health" [27]. While some argue that they are distinct, they have common roots and principles, and both acknowledge the central role of the community in the planning and delivery of primary care. While in some L&MICs family physicians are "pushed" to practice mainly in hospitals due to a variety of labor market and other pressures, in its optimal model, family practice is the first entry point into the health system and the bridge to the community. Traditionally, and still in many settings, family practice includes home visits carried out by various members of the team, such as community health workers, nurses, or physicians. The community-based nature of family practice and its anchor in the provider–patient relationship as described below also means that family practice is instrumental in engaging with families as carers and at supporting self-care.

The family practice team is equipped to identify and address the health needs of a *"defined population."* This principle captures the mutual accountability of providers and users and is sometimes operationalized through empanelment, a process that explicitly links individual patients to individual or teams of primary care providers.[1] This principle also means that family practice delivers a comprehensive scope of services informed by the specific needs of the people served, as individuals and as collectives. Accountability to a defined patient population includes responsibility for coordinating services both within primary care and beyond as required.

The *patient–provider relationship* is central to family practice and distinguishes it from other specialties which are organized primarily around a disease (infectious diseases, oncology, or others) or a body system (cardiology, urology, or others). The relationship at the core of family practice results in and from accountability, continuity, and person-centeredness. It makes family practice the natural clinical model for the delivery of integrated and people-centered health services.

Last but not least, family practice is delivered by *"skilled clinicians,"* including physicians and allied health professionals, purposively trained in a family practice model as highly competent "specialized generalists" to deliver high-quality, evidence-informed care.

Family practice is "conceptually designed" to deliver integrated services, enhance equity, and improve cost-effectiveness. The key characteristics that link primary care to better outcomes are often referred to as "the 5Cs"; these are (first) contact, continuity, comprehensiveness, coordination, and care centered on the patient, as described in Chapter 10.

In most settings, family practice shares the primary care space with a range of providers that may or may not be fully integrated into the family practice team, including: other physicians (general internists, pediatricians, and obstetricians), allied health professionals (nurse practitioners, physician assistants, pharmacists, rehabilitation experts, and midwives) and lay health workers (community health workers). In some settings, family physicians deliver services beyond the narrow description of primary care (e.g., surgery and anesthesia) and may strengthen the delivery of comprehensive care through enhanced competencies beyond those identified as core to family practice, in areas such as palliative care, sports medicine, care of the elderly, emergency medicine, and others.

The way in which family medicine is integrated in any given health system, including the scope of practice of family practice teams, varies greatly globally and neither guarantees nor is sufficient in and of itself to ensure the delivery of integrated and people-centered services. Nonetheless, health systems anchored in high-quality family practice have been repeatedly shown to gravitate toward integrated care and to contribute to better health outcomes, more equity, and improved cost-effectiveness [28–31].

24.3.2 Translating Principles into Integrative Models of Care

In addition to the blueprint for the delivery of integrated and people-centered services provided by the principles of family medicine, indicators of the WHO PHC Monitoring and Indicators Framework [32] offer concrete guidance on how to structure health systems to

---

[1] For empanelment in health insurance, see Chapter 17.

Table 24.1 Principles of family medicine and related PHC M&E model of care indicators

Principles of family medicine	PHC M&E framework: elements of models of care
Community-based	• System to promote first contact through regular provider(s) • Linkages to community-based and social services • Community engagement in services organization and management • Self-management and health literacy in primary care • Proactive population outreach
Resource to a defined population	• Empanelment • Service package meeting criteria • Care pathways for tracer conditions
Relationship-based	• Self-management and health literacy • System to promote first contact through regular provider
Clinical expert	• Care pathways for tracer conditions • Multidisciplinary team • Management capability and leadership • Supportive supervision in place • Information system in place • Protocols for patient transfer, referral, and counter-referral

Source: [32].

effectively deliver such services. Table 24.1 presents some of the WHO PHC framework indicators alongside the related principles of family practice to illustrate their relationships.

24.3.3 Additional Strategies for Integrated Care

In addition to health systems anchored in family medicine, three broad strategies are commonly used to integrate care, often in combination with one another. We describe these briefly here [12]:

1. **Case management** is "a collaborative process that assesses, plans, implements, coordinates, monitors and evaluates the options and services required to meet the user's health and human service needs" [33]. It is focused on, and primarily benefits individuals with complex health needs such as multiple chronic conditions, severe illness in the context of highly precarious social circumstances or the combination of physical and severe mental illness.

2. **Multidisciplinary teams (MDTs)** refer to two separate but often combined strategies, namely: (1) the deliberate engagement of health workers representing a range of health disciplines; and (2) working as a team. This second strategy highlights the fact that engaging various providers does not *per se* constitute a team. Obtaining the full benefits of MDTs requires the investment of time, leadership, and expertise to transform a group of providers into an optimally functioning team. MDTs are often used in combination with other strategies and can bridge care across a range of functions (from promotion to palliation), scopes, across primary and secondary care, and between health and social services

3. **Networking of organizations** to drive integration includes at least three broad approaches: (1) the development of evidence-based *clinical care pathways* (e.g., assessment and management of low back pain, stroke care from acute presentation to long-term care and rehabilitation, or the management of breast cancer); (2) *partnerships* that enable multiagency collaboration through strategic alliances and shared governance (e.g., partnership between health and social agencies to support long-term care for older people, as in the UK) [12]; and (3) *collective accountability (financial and clinical)*, which aims for best value care and provides payment and incentives that drive toward prevention and primary care to avoid more expense downstream (e.g., capitated or bundled payments that include key preventive maneuvers and quality measures).

24.4 Transforming Health Systems to Deliver Integrated and People-Centered Health Services: Challenges and Enablers

A number of barriers and enablers commonly impact the reorientation of health systems to deliver integrated and people-centered health services. We outline some of them here according to five broad categories of "influencing factors" adapted from Baxter et al. [13], namely those related to: (1) leadership and management, (2) organization and systems, (3) patients, (4) the workforce, and (5) equipment or facilities. Some of these same enablers also apply to the implementation of effective family practice as summarized in Table 24.2.

24.4.1 Leadership and Management

Effective leadership and a "compelling vision" are essential to transform systems for the delivery of integrated people-centered health services. A clear rationale and explicit goals avoid confusion and concentrate collective efforts [34]. Highlighting the benefit to patients or users in the vision can be particularly effective.

At the macro level, leadership is needed to develop the required policy frameworks and engage a broad range of stakeholders and actors; at the meso level it enables networking and collaboration; and at the micro level leadership is required to support effective multidisciplinary services.

"Top-down" leadership alone is unlikely to lead to successful integration of services where it requires the transformation of pre-existing structures and processes. "Bottom-up" input and direction from the community and other stakeholders, and the involvement of "champions," can advance engagement and buy-in [13].

24.4.2 Organization and Systems

Some barriers and enablers of a reorientation toward integrated and people-centered services, including the implementation of family medicine, relate to organizations and systems.

Governance and Accountability

The optimal integration of services across organizations or programs often requires a reform of governance structures and processes at the macro, meso, or micro levels to achieve the right balance of engagement and mutual accountability [35]. Integration is best implemented initially in a "workable geographic and political space," meaning on a smaller scale. The urge to "boil the ocean" and integrate all services, across all settings and for all

Table 24.2 Examples of enablers of effective family medicine/practice and related strategies and mechanisms

Enablers	Mechanisms and strategies
Strategy and policy	
Policy that enshrines clear, distinct, and valued role for family practice in the health system	• System organization that values family practice • Partnership with professional associations • Family medicine as first contact • Empanelment • Strategies that promote trust through high-quality care
Engagement of key stakeholders	
Patients	• Clear communication regarding the nature and role of family medicine in the health system • Mechanism for input by patients at macro, meso, and micro levels. • Engaged champions • Deliberate process to engage those most difficult to reach
Providers	• Clear role in the health system including how to collaborate and coordinate with other providers/levels • Engaged champions and professional associations • Support and enablers of interprofessional learning and service delivery • Adequate and commensurate remuneration (amount and model)
Communities	• Active process to identify community priorities • Mechanisms for ongoing input and engagement by community
Operational considerations	
Skilled clinicians	• Robust competency-based postgraduate training • Certification • Accredited training programs • Accredited continuing professional development • Family practice-focused training for allied health • Training on team process • Practice tools/academic detailing • Training anchored in universities/academic institutions • Foster/fund family medicine research
Relationship-focused	• Training curriculum and environment • Continuity of care • Appointment system • Provider/team/clinic continuity • Reliability of access and care
Community-based	• Located in the community • Partnerships with communities and community organizations, institutions (school, agencies, others)

Table 24.2 (cont.)

Enablers	Mechanisms and strategies
Resource to a defined population	• Empanelment • Population-based data • Explicit collaboration with public health • Incentives • Quality improvement processes

users at once must be resisted. Instead, focusing on a modest but achievable integration goal and a careful process for evaluation and improvement before scaling up is much more likely to be successful [35].

Decentralization potentially brings the planning and service delivery, as well as governance and decision-making, closer to the users and can also enable people-centeredness (see Chapter 9). At the local level, shifts in governance within the team should enable optimal team function, collaboration, and mutual accountability. This requires all professional groups but especially physicians to be able to relinquish unnecessary control to allow the whole team to function in the best interest of the patient.

The implementation of effective integrated health services also requires appropriate accountability mechanisms. Policies that foster professional and clinical accountability, quality improvement, performance-enabling incentives, empanelment, and the integration of people's perspectives in the planning and delivery of services are among the many strategies to enhance accountability in the delivery of integrated health services.

Funding and Allocation

While the integration of health services is presumed to result in improved efficiency and cost reduction, this is not always the case and it is important for the primary goal(s) of integration to be explicitly identified to ensure that efforts meant to improve care outcome and experience, for example, are not solely and mistakenly evaluated based on an assumption of cost reduction. The transformation process and the sustainable delivery of integrated services require adequate resources. Integration is most successful when it builds on existing knowledge and a pre-existing level of capacity [36]. A lack of resources, either as salaries and incentives, and the unavailability of equipment and medication, even if modest, constitute a barrier to effective integration [34, 36]. Where integration is interpreted as a covert strategy to reduce services, it is likely to fail (see the UNRWA case study below). Furthermore, the development of the processes and relationships needed for successful integration require time.

Equally important to effective integration is the reallocation of resources toward primary care, community, and social services. Funding and allocation should ultimately support the "wrapping of services" around the user. Capitation-based funding and remuneration (see Chapter 18) can help integration, especially when combined with empanelment [34].

24.4.3 Patient-Related

The implementation of integrated and people-centered health services should obviously engage patients. At the micro or individual level, as discussed, the adoption of family practice supports integration. At the meso and macro levels, the perspectives of patients can be integrated in health services planning through structures such as "*assemblées sanitaires*" or "*états généraux*" (*health assemblies* common in some countries, such as Thailand or Iran), village health committees, and patient advisory panels, and through direct solicitation, such as questionnaires and surveys.

Achieving authentic and full representation including the voice of those most marginalized is challenging. Moreover, even when dissatisfied with the existing level of care, patients often resist change when they feel they risk losing whatever unsatisfactory services they have [13]. A clear outline of the gaps and overlaps in services for specific hard-to-reach populations and the implementation of acceptable integrative solutions requires deliberate and sustained efforts, innovative solutions, and, frequently, additional resources [37]. Engaging users, especially highly regarded and trusted community or patient representatives, can help transition toward integration. The examples of participatory governance in Thailand (see Chapter 29) and more recently the "*dialogue societal*" in Tunisia provide lessons on how this can be implemented in practice [38]. Supporting the development of new sustainable relations with providers and consistently centering the provision of services on the users help both providers and users during transition toward integration.

24.4.4 Workforce-Related

While the people at the center of integrated services are primarily the users, the successful, sustainable, and effective delivery of care that is both integrated and people-centered ultimately relies on the performance of providers, as providers are the ones who "care."

The literature points to a few provider-focused enablers of service integration. First, providers need to be *willing* to deliver integrated and people-centered care. This can be cultivated through recruitment, selection, and training, including through family practice programs, which have been shown to enhance continuity and coordination [39]. It can also be nurtured by leadership that creates a sense of common purpose and clearly expressed values. Adequate resources and incentives can also help providers adapt and deliver integrated care in a way that enables them to fulfill their clinical responsibilities safely and effectively while also feeling valued and supported [36].

Building on existing knowledge at the individual and organizational levels helps effective integration as it validates and recruits existing expertise. It can be further bolstered by continuing professional development activities such as training, retraining, and coaching.

Also key to effective integration are measures that enhance providers' ability to work effectively as a team. Bringing providers together is not sufficient to generate the benefits of teamwork. Clearly defined roles with some flexibility and overlap in scope of expertise allows team members to fulfill part of each other's responsibilities when needed, and promotes a common focus. Additionally, nurturing the development of effective relationships among team members is needed to deliver effective team-based care. This might involve regularly working with the same individuals, hosting care coordination meetings, and constructively addressing tensions when they arise. The organization of the workflow and support by managers is also important for effective teamwork.

24.4.5 Rational Use of Technology for Quality Services

Lastly, the availability of technology, equipment, and medicines required to deliver quality services, and access to facilities that support the delivery of effective, comfortable, and confidential care can enable a transition to integrated services [36]. Conversely, their unavailability undermines trust in the health system and may result in people bypassing services close to their home in order to go directly to hospitals where the cost of care for managing the same problem can be much higher.

While not essential to the delivery of quality health services *per se*, digital technology is increasingly acknowledged as a key enabler of integration (see Chapter 22). It allows rapid access to information that can support clinical decision-making and allows for seamless communication among providers (and increasingly patients). Digital tools and technology can support effective task shifting. Digital technology also facilitates the collection and analyses of data, including in the form of metrics and performance indicators, and improves data visualization. Without thoughtful implementation, digital technology can hinder rather than support service delivery.

24.5 A Case Study of Integrated People-Centered PHC Based on Family Medicine: UNRWA's Experience

We conclude by presenting an example that illustrates a pivot toward a family care model as implemented by UNRWA [40]. In the Middle East, UNRWA provides primary care for more than 5.7 million Palestine refugees residing in Jordan, Lebanon, Syria, the Gaza Strip, and the West Bank including East Jerusalem through 141 PHC clinics with 3,000 staff. Historically, UNRWA's health clinics have provided primary care services in three main areas: maternal and child health care (MCH) including immunization; noncommunicable diseases (NCDs) care, particularly for diabetes and hypertension; and general outpatient services.

In 2012, UNRWA engaged in a reform of its health service delivery model and introduced a family practice approach, called Family Health Team (FHT). The following sections describe UNRWA's experience, highlight key challenges, and describe enablers encountered while transitioning to integrated care.

24.5.1 A Clearly Defined Problem or Gap, Supported by Data

UNRWA's health reform started with clear recognition of the demographic and epidemiological transitions taking place in the Palestine refugee population, including the extremely high burden of NCDs, with diabetes and hypertension affecting more than 300,000 individuals and together with cancer accounting for 70–80% of all morbidity and mortality. This information prompted a reform of UNRWA's primary care services and the adoption of a person-centered FHT approach in 2011.

Health services provided by UNRWA had not evolved in pace with the needs of the population and continued to be delivered in fragmented and siloed disease- or condition-specific clinics dedicated to MCH, NCDs, and general walk-in clinics. Clinics were extremely crowded, and each doctor routinely consulted 100 patients per day – too many to provide quality services.

24.5.2 Clear Vision and Rationale

UNRWA undertook a reform in 2011 to address NCDs, particularly diabetes and hypertension, with a goal to improve efficiency and reduce the high costs of treatment. Accordingly, a family medicine approach was introduced based on an FHT model. The FHT model consisted of a treating team comprising at least a physician, a nurse, and a midwife who provided care not only for the individual patient but also all family members.

24.5.3 Engagement of Stakeholders

Prior to implementing the planned changes, UNRWA engaged in extensive discussions with four distinct groups of stakeholders: Palestine refugees (beneficiaries), UNRWA staff, host governments, and donors to overcome the skepticism and the concern that "reform" implied a distinct improvement rather than a reduction of services. In the past, refugees had been dissatisfied with the prevailing reduction of services due to financial constraints and were skeptical about reforms. UNRWA staff shared the many concerns of the refugee populations – the majority being refugees themselves. Host governments, aware of the dissatisfaction of both patients and staff, shared the concern that the health reform may do more harm than good. Donors, for their part, were concerned that UNRWA had not yet made decisive reforms despite the urgent need to do so. In response, UNRWA adopted two strategies:

1. A *compelling common focus*, by putting the refugees at the center of the reform. It was expected that if the refugees were "happy," the staff would be as well, and their satisfaction would in turn alleviate the concerns of host governments and compel donors to provide additional support. This served to facilitate stakeholders' buy-in while also avoiding strong opposition.

2. *Engaging champions by identifying agents of change*, specifically among the Chief Field Health Programme who head UNRWA health services, and who are themselves from the refugee communities and have a strong influence on the staff in the field while also being highly respected and listened to by refugees.

24.5.4 Delineation of a Clear Goal and Indicators

The stated goal of the FHT approach was to improve the quality of UNRWA's primary care services in the context of highly prevalent NCDs. Clear, meaningful, and achievable initial target indicators included: the number of daily consultations per doctor; the rate of antibiotics prescription for general outpatients; and rates of diabetes control. Introducing electronic health records was a central pillar in the integration of health services for UNRWA and in monitoring target indicators.

24.5.5 Piloting and Initial Evaluation

UNRWA piloted the FHT approach in two health clinics: one each in Gaza and Lebanon starting in 2011. Patients expressed high overall rates of satisfaction. One patient in Lebanon said: "This new system is excellent. The time that nurses and doctors devote to me, and my family is much more than before." Doctors also responded positively to the new model. The average number of daily medical consultations decreased from roughly 80 per doctor per day to 50 in Lebanon, and from roughly 100 to 90 in Gaza.

In July 2012, a joint assessment of the FHT approach was conducted by UNRWA and the Mailman School of Public Health at Columbia University, New York in three health centers in Jordan, Lebanon, and the West Bank [41]. The assessment concluded that, thanks to the FHT approach, most patients had their needs met in a single visit by a single provider, thus decreasing repeat visits and leading to an overall decline in the number of daily doctor consultations and waiting times. In the West Bank, for example, waiting time decreased from 24 minutes to 6 minutes per patient on average. Duration of doctor–patient encounter, however, did not show an increase and remained a major concern.

24.5.6 Scale-up, Health Promotion, Continuity, and Intensified Patient Support

UNRWA expanded the FHT approach to all clinics by the end of 2017. Services included health promotion activities and education for patients with diabetes through a network of small peer support groups (known as a "Microclinic approach" [42]), healthy eating advice, oral health screening, anemia screening for school children, and preconception counseling. Continuity of care was assured using the same team for each visit.

24.5.7 Intermediate Evaluation

Output indicators remained favorable throughout the scale-up of FHT approach. The number of daily medical consultations decreased in all five fields from around 100 to 80 per doctor per day. Antibiotics prescription rates also decreased from around 30% to 25%. The average number of pregnant women's visits to antenatal care remained between six and seven. The proportion of controlled diabetics measured by HbA1c did not improve and remained high for 30–35% of patients. This clearly indicated that medical treatment alone was not sufficient and underscored the need for community outreach with a more preventable approach, which was introduced using the above-mentioned "Microclinic approach."

24.5.8 Electronic Health Records and Data

Electronic medical records, or e-health, is a core component of the FHT approach [43]. E-health is a web-based electronic medical record, developed by UNRWA to support all clinical transactions within the FHT approach, including the registrations of patients at reception, the recording of clinical encounters with doctors, nurses, midwives, and dentists, laboratory examinations, and the prescription and delivery of medicines at pharmacies. E-health includes a built-in appointment system and is now installed in almost all health clinics, except for a few clinics in Syria where access to the Internet is limited. Clinics using e-health are entirely digitalized, foregoing the use of paper records and registrations. E-health can produce a set of 22 reports, from daily statistics to monthly and annual reports, as needed, and helps in monitoring and evaluation of health services at each health clinic. At present, the e-health program has a total of 3.2 million records of patients in the central server.

The e-health program uses the International Classification for Diseases (ICD) for the recording of morbidities and mortalities. The most up-to-date ICD-11 version has been introduced since 2020 with the support of WHO. All morbidities and mortalities are now coded and recorded using ICD-11.

24.5.9 Training and Continuing Professional Development

Continued training of health staff, particularly doctors, is an important component of the reform. During the introduction of the FHT approach, it became evident that up-skilling of doctors in the discipline of family medicine would be required. Formal training opportunities in family medicine in the region are few, and where available it is a four-year specialized fulltime postgraduate degree. UNRWA's limited resources precluded access to such training for most providers, as well as financing the recruitment of replacement doctors during such extended training.

Instead, UNRWA developed a one-year on-the-job training program in family medicine and, with support from the Rila Institute of Health Science (UK), established a formal, structured training program leading to a family medicine diploma [44]. The Imperial College London's WHO Collaborating Center for Public Health Education and Training also supported the training.

The diploma curriculum was aligned with the core curriculum of the Royal College of General Practitioners and was delivered through a blended training and work-based format, with a dedicated e-learning platform, direct face-to-face contact, interactive webinars, online core reading, formative assessments, self-assessed clinical case studies, and a practical skills module using video clips and clinical videos. There was a formal final summative examination [45].

The first training started in Gaza from July 2015 with 15 selected doctors. The assessment of these doctors after the training indicated that all those who participated found the training extremely beneficial. They acquired a better understanding of the psychosocial elements affecting patient health; felt more inclined toward team-working and collaborative approaches to health care; and gained more insight into nonverbal communication such as active listening and tactile gestures. Encouraged by the assessment, UNRWA continues the family medicine diploma course every year. To date, around 150 doctors have completed the training course. UNRWA is seeking continued donor support to enroll its roughly 500 physicians in the bespoke family medicine diploma program.

The aging of the population, the increasing prevalence of concurrent complex chronic conditions, the changing expectations of populations worldwide, and mounting evidence about models of care that offer optimized outcomes all supported the transition of the UNWRA health system toward the delivery of integrated and people-centered services. Doing so effectively requires a good understanding of the pre-existing gaps, a clear vision of the desired outcome, and the careful orchestration of a number of processes at the macro, meso, and micro levels. The establishment of family practice as the core of health systems can help achieve integrated and people-centered care.

24.6 Conclusion

The reorientation of health systems to deliver integrated and people-centered services is essential to effectively address the complex, concurrent, and chronic health issues of individuals, families, and populations across the life course. Driven by a clear vision, various funding, administrative, organizational, and clinical service mechanisms can be used to integrate services and achieve the expected improvements in effectiveness, clinical outcomes, and patient experience. Family practice is inherently integrated and people-centered, and health systems anchored in clinically robust and well-resourced family practice naturally drive toward the delivery of integrated people-centered care.

References

1. World Health Organization, United Nations Children's Fund (UNICEF). Declaration of Astana 2018. 2018. www.who.int/docs/default-source/primary-health/declaration/gcphc-declaration.pdf (accessed December 12, 2021).

2. World Health Organization, World Bank. *Tracking Universal Health Coverage 2017 Global Monitoring Report.* Geneva, World Health Organization, 2017. https://apps.who.int/iris/bitstream/handle/10665/259817/9789241513555-eng.pdf (accessed January 24, 2022).

3. S. K. Bakeera, S. P. Wamala, S. Galea, et al. Community perceptions and factors influencing utilization of health services in Uganda. *Int J Equity Health* 2009; 8: 25.

4. S. Sermsri. *The Triumph of Practicality: Tradition and Modernity in Health Care Utilization in Selected Asian Countries.* Singapore, Institute of Southeast Asian Studies, 1990. https://bookshop.iseas.edu.sg/search?type_code=book&subject=21 (accessed July 13, 2021).

5. S. Mounier-Jack, S. H. Mayhew, N. Mays. Integrated care: learning between high-income, and low- and middle-income country health systems. *Health Policy Plan* 2017; 32(Suppl. 4): iv6–iv12.

6. L. Court, J. Olivier. Approaches to integrating palliative care into African health systems: a qualitative systematic review. *Health Policy Plan* 2020; 35(8): 1053–1069.

7. A. Garrib, J. Birungi, S. Lesikari, et al. Integrated care for human immunodeficiency virus, diabetes and hypertension in Africa. *Trans R Soc Trop Med Hyg* 2019; 113(12): 809–812.

8. M. A. Bautista, M. Nurjono, Y. W. Lim, et al. Instruments measuring integrated care: a systematic review of measurement properties. *Milbank Q* 2016; 94(4): 862–917.

9. L. Borgermans, Y. Marchal, L. Busetto, et al. How to improve integrated care for people with chronic conditions: key findings from EU FP-7 project INTEGRATE and beyond. *Int J Integr Care* 2017; 17(4): 7.

10. Y. Mahendradhata, A. Souares, R. Phalkey, et al. Optimizing patient-centeredness in the transitions of healthcare systems in low- and middle-income countries. *BMC Health Serv Res* 2014; 14: 386.

11. A. K. Niazi, S. Kalra. Patient centred care in diabetology: an Islamic perspective from South Asia. *J Diabetes Metab Disord* 2012; 11(1): 30.

12. G. Hughes, S. E. Shaw, T. Greenhalgh. Rethinking integrated care: a systematic hermeneutic review of the literature on integrated care strategies and concepts. *Milbank Q* 2020; 98(2): 446–492.

13. S. Baxter, M. Johnson, D. Chambers, et al. Understanding new models of integrated care in developed countries: a systematic review. *Health Soc Care Deliv Res* 2018; 6(29).

14. R. Q. Lewis, R. Rosen, N. Goodwin, et al. Where next for integrated care organisations in the English NHS? 2010. www.nuffieldtrust.org.uk/files/2017-01/where-next-integrated-care-english-nhs-web-final.pdf (accessed December 14, 2021).

15. S. Shaw, R. Rosen, B. Rumbold. What is integrated care? 2011. www.nuffieldtrust.org.uk/files/2017-01/what-is-integrated-care-report-web-final.pdf (accessed December 11, 2021).

16. J. D. Maeseneer, C. V. Wee, L. Daeren, et al. From "patient" to "person" to "people": the need for integrated, people centered health care. *IJPCM* 2012; 2: 601–614.

17. E. H. Wagner, C. Davis, J. Schaefer, et al. A survey of leading chronic disease management programs: are they consistent with the literature? *Manag Care Q* 1999; 7(3): 56–66.

18. P. P. Valentijn, S. M. Schepman, W. Opheij, et al. Understanding integrated care: a comprehensive conceptual framework based on the integrative functions of primary care. *Int J Integr Care* 2013; 13: e010.

19. World Health Organization. WHO global strategy on people-centered and integrated health services. 2015. www.who.int/teams/

integrated-health-services/clinical-services-and-systems/service-organizations-and-integration (accessed July 11, 2021).

20. J. E. Epping-Jordan, S. D. Pruitt, R. Bengoa, et al. Improving the quality of health care for chronic conditions. *Qual Saf Health Care* 2004; **13**(4): 299–305.

21. C. Handford, B. Hennen. The gentle radical: ten reflections on Ian McWhinney, generalism, and family medicine today. *Can Fam Physician* 2014; **60**(1): 20–23.

22. M. Nutik, N. N. Woods, A. Moaveni, et al. Assessing undergraduate medical education through a generalist lens. *Can Fam Physician* 2021; **67**(5): 357–363.

23. American Academy of Family Physicians. Definition of family medicine. 2019. www.aafp.org/about/policies/all/family-medicine-definition.html (accessed July 15, 2021).

24. N. Arya, C. Gibson, D. Ponka, et al. Family medicine around the world: overview by region. *Canadian Family Physician* 2017; **63**(6): 436–441.

25. College of Family Physicians of Canada. Vision, mission, values, and goals. 2021. www.cfpc.ca/en/about-us/vision-mission-principles (accessed July 19, 2021).

26. College of Family Physicians of Canada. Vision, mission, values and goals. 2022. www.cfpc.ca/en/about-us/vision-mission-principles (accessed January 24, 2022).

27. B. Mash, S. Ray, A. Essuman, et al. Community-orientated primary care: a scoping review of different models, and their effectiveness and feasibility in sub-Saharan Africa. *BMJ Glob Health* 2019; **4**(Suppl. 8): e001489.

28. B. Starfield, L. Shi, J. Macinko. Contribution of primary care to health systems and health. *Milbank Q* 2005; **83**(3): 457–502.

29. B. Starfield. Is US health really the best in the world? *JAMA* 2000; **284**(4): 483–484.

30. B. Starfield. Global health, equity, and primary care. *J Am Board Fam Med* 2007; **20**(6): 511–513.

31. B. Starfield. Family medicine should shape reform, not vice versa. *Fam Pract Manag* 2009; **16**(4): 6–7.

32. World Health Organization, United Nations Children's Fund (UNICEF). Primary health care monitoring framework and indicators. 2022.

33. Commission for Case Manager Certification. Definition and philosophy of case management. 2021. https://ccmcertification.org/about-ccmc/about-case-management/definition-and-philosophy-case-management (accessed July 17, 2021).

34. L. Spigel, M. Pesec, O. Villegas Del Carpio, et al. Implementing sustainable primary healthcare reforms: strategies from Costa Rica. *BMJ Glob Health* 2020; **5**(8): e002674.

35. M. M. N. Minkman. Suitable scales: rethinking scale for innovative integrated care governance. *Int J Integr Care* 2020; **20**(1): 1.

36. S. M. Topp, S. Abimbola, R. Joshi, et al. How to assess and prepare health systems in low- and middle-income countries for integration of services: a systematic review. *Health Policy Plan* 2018; **33**(2): 298–312.

37. G. Bloch, L. Rozmovits. Implementing social interventions in primary care. *CMAJ* 2021; **193**(44): E1696–E1701.

38. H. Ben Mesmia, R. Chtioui, M. Ben Rejeb. The Tunisian societal dialogue for health reform (a qualitative study). *Eur J Public Health* 2020; **30**(Suppl. 5): ckaa166-1393.

39. A. G. Jantsch, B. Burström, G. H. Nilsson, et al. Residency training in family medicine and its impact on coordination and continuity of care: an analysis of referrals to secondary care in Rio de Janeiro. *BMJ Open* 2022; **12**(2): e051515.

40. UNRWA. Homepage. 2022. www.unrwa.org (accessed January 24, 2022).

41. UNRWA. Update on health reform. 2012. www.unrwa.org/userfiles/file/AdCom_en/2012/october/2012%20Oct%20SubAdCom%20Health%20Reform%20FINAL.pdf (accessed July 17, 2021).

42. Y. M. Shahin, N. A. Kishk, Y. Turki, et al. Evaluation of the Microclinic social network model for Palestine refugees with

diabetes at UNRWA health centers. *J Diabetes* 2018; **8**(4): 99.

43. G. Ballout, N. Al-Shorbaji, N. Abu-Kishk, et al. UNRWA's innovative e-health for 5 million Palestine refugees in the Near East. *BMJ Innov* 2018. http://dx.doi.org/10.1136/bmjinnov-2017-000262.

44. B. Lovell, R. Dhillon, A. Khader, et al. Delivering and evaluating a scalable training model for strengthening family medicine in resource-limited environments: the Gaza experience. A mixed-methods evaluation. *BJGP Open* 2019; **3**(2): bjgpopen 19X101647.

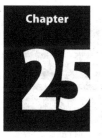

Chapter

25

Strengthening Hospital Governance and Management to Become High-Performing Organizations

Ann-Lise Guisset and Eric de Roodenbeke

Key Messages

- Hospitals play a key role in health systems and can enable or hinder their effective reorientation toward primary health care (PHC).
- A new paradigm is required for hospitals to drive toward universal health coverage (UHC), including in the positioning of hospitals as key contributors and enablers in the overall health system, accountable to the communities they serve, and as high-performing organizations.
- Well-performing hospitals require highly competent executives, purposely trained to lead complex organizations.
- Robust governance and operational frameworks are essential to optimize hospital performance, including in the context of leadership turnover.
- Hospital performance ultimately requires the full investment and the optimal contribution of health workers. Appropriate and constructive monitoring and recognition mechanisms can foster such contribution.

25.1 Introduction: Vision for a High-Performing Hospital

Hospitals and their performance are central to health system strengthening efforts in all countries. Despite being critical assets, hospitals often fail to meet the needs of the communities they serve. Globally, 40% of countries have fewer than 18 hospital beds for every 10,000 people – the estimated minimum number needed to achieve the Sustainable Development Goals [1]. It is also estimated that more than one-third of hospitals offering surgical care in low- and middle-income countries (L&MICs) lack a reliable source of water supply, continuous electricity, or a functioning generator. Furthermore, people's hospital experience is often bewildering and depersonalized – a maze of congested corridors and waiting rooms, beeping machines, and hectic staff. Reports of staff absenteeism, high out-of-pocket payment, and lack of respect for privacy and dignity are common and undermine community trust and effective use of hospital services. In emergencies, hospitals are often unable to maintain their usual activities, depriving affected communities of services when they are most needed.

Hospitals not only play a vital role as a service delivery platform, they are also essential settings for training and research, and are major employers and important consumers of goods and services with a significant impact on social cohesion and local economies. Hospitals receive an important share of health spending. They impact public perception on reliability of

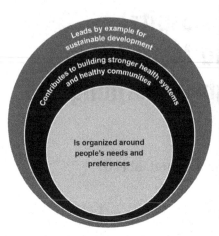

- Embraces social responsibility principles, and aims at reducing impact of its activities on the environment

- Engages with the community to set hospital's strategic direction
- Goes one step further to "leave no one behind" (understands who is missed and reaches out to them)
- Distributes knowledge and resources with other health and social care providers, and in particular supports primary health care
- Contributes to reorient models of care toward more ambulatory, home- and community-based care

- Is organized around people's needs, smoothens process of care and administration and logistics both within hospital walls and with community for increased continuity and coordination of patient care
- Systematically strives for long-term functional outcomes and improved user experiences
- Engages and empowers patient/user to take an active role in their health, informs patient/users about their rights and gives them a voice
- Is internally efficient and constantly strives for improved quality

Leads by example for sustainable development

Contributes to building stronger healthy communities and healthy communities

Is organized around people's needs and preferences

Figure 25.1 A vision for high-performing hospitals actively contributing to universal health coverage and building strong PHC-oriented health systems.

health services and are commonly considered representative of the performance of a country's health system. Hence, optimizing their performance is critical. In a PHC-oriented health system, high-performing hospitals [2, 3] are expected to deliver high-quality people-centered services, and contribute to improving population health outcomes and sustainable development (Figure 25.1) [4]. Achieving these objectives requires a shift in paradigm from hospitals operating in isolation, or even in competition with primary care providers, to hospitals fully embedded in, and contributing to their local health systems (Table 25.1) [5, 6].

Beyond efforts to address the insufficient number of hospitals, priority should be given to improving how hospitals operate internally and how they contribute to the health system. This requires two simultaneous approaches:

- **External:** (re)defining the position, role, and functions of hospitals, and setting clear objectives to foster a new health and social care model with an appropriate role for hospitals.
- **Internal:** (re)organizing hospitals and optimizing the production process to strengthen their institutional delivery of patient-centered care.

The two approaches are closely interrelated. A hospital's internal organization and how production processes are defined across service delivery platforms (e.g., community-based services, primary care, rehabilitation, and longer-term facilities) are shaped by forces such as its position, role, and function in the broader health system. Conversely, a hospital that is poorly governed or chaotically managed, that does not collect, analyze, or present performance data, that focuses on volume and profits or provides low-quality and high-risk care with poor infection control, will be unable to take on and sustain new roles.

25.2 National and Subnational Levers to Improve the Performance of the Hospitals in L&MICs?

National and subnational authorities can create the conditions to drive, enable, and sustain hospital integration in the local service delivery architecture and its community. As system

Table 25.1 The changing paradigm for hospitals

Element	Hospitals operating in isolation	Hospitals contributing to a PHC-oriented health system
Mission, role	Seek to save lives and increase patient satisfaction for distinct episodes of care Focus on patient outcomes at discharge; set clinical objectives for individual users	Seek to save or improve lives through timely intervention, restore functionality, and improve quality of life throughout patients' health pathways by working with care providers at different tiers of the health system Embrace public health objectives and act as a resource for the community
Key functions	Directly deliver clinical and support services	Directly deliver clinical services for patients requiring high-intensity, multispeciality or multidisciplinary complex care or complex technologies Increasingly support other health and social care providers when needed to ensure people can be cared for closer to their homes and in their communities
Interaction with other health care providers and the environment	Compete to increase volume of services (with other health care providers, including PHC providers) Passively react to patient demands or adopt marketing techniques to increase volume (or profit) for targeted patient categories Retain patients to return to hospital-based specialists for post-acute outpatient treatment	Collaborate within network of care to increase relevance of services and develop solid ties with primary care (PC) providers by sharing: (1) resources and knowledge to support other care providers, (2) patient information for continuity of care, (3) epidemiological data to inform public health services Proactively influence demand to ensure adequate use of hospital services by: (1) understanding those being missed and identifying ways to overcome organizational, cultural, and financial bottlenecks to access; (2) actively promoting PHC or alternative care for people who do not need inpatient care; (3) engaging with other care providers for smooth return to home or to less intensive care settings
Planning and strategy definition	Are defined as physical entities in a bureaucratic system; resources and scope of work are defined according to strict norms based on a hierarchical delineation, not taking into account health needs of local population and map of other care providers in the area	Are defined as functional entities; engage with the local communities to define strategic orientation of hospitals based on their health needs and analysis of supply of local health and social services Central or regional planning ensures that high-cost, specialized care is centralized in regional and tertiary care centers in

Table 25.1 (cont.)

Element	Hospitals operating in isolation	Hospitals contributing to a PHC-oriented health system
	In the private sector, define strategic orientations based on market analysis, profit opportunities, or owners' interests	a coordinated and complementary manner
Care processes	Consider patients as passive recipients of care, adopting a paternalist perspective	Empower patients, families, and communities to take an active role in their health and health care
	Services are delivered in silos around diseases: the more complex the patients' needs, the more the patients are moved around wards	Team jointly deliver services around people's complex needs: the more complex the patients' needs, the more effective the navigation system and integration of services (which might reduce the number of persons the patient would interface with)
Organizational culture	Hierarchical and bureaucratic organizational culture	Collaborative culture where teamwork and innovation are promoted through participatory and transformative leadership style

Source: World Health Organization, forthcoming.

architects who oversee health system reforms, authorities can ensure that policies and incentives are coherent and drive hospital engagement toward UHC while supporting continued improvement of the institutional performance of hospitals. Implementing a national vision of the role of hospitals and of their contribution to UHC requires a set of policy and operational levers that [5]:

1. strengthen *system design* (degree of vertical and/or horizontal integration, public–private mix, hospital typologies and role delineation across providers), autonomy, accountability, regulation, and people's participation; and
2. design and implement provider *payment systems and monitoring and feedback mechanisms* to encourage, recognize, or reward hospitals that demonstrate desired roles and functions; and
3. ensure *adequate resources* (infrastructure, technologies, human resources, and information systems) as preconditions to deliver on hospitals' roles and functions.

Table 25.2 identifies a limited number of illustrative interventions most relevant for L&MICs. It also touches on how these interventions have been implemented in countries.

Table 25.2 Key policy orientations and illustrative interventions to strengthen hospital sector performance in L&MICs

Dimension	Key policy orientations and interventions
System design	1. Establish governance structures with clear population-based responsibilities and with a role to ensure comprehensive planning and coordination of services, including private facilities. 2. Strengthen accountability of hospitals toward the public and ensure effective functioning of governance boards (with community representatives). 3. Adopt a rights-based approach to make explicit providers' and patients' rights and responsibilities; facilitate establishment of patients' organizations and associations and strengthen their roles. 4. Extend beyond command and control to include a full range of regulatory mechanisms, including incentives and self-regulatory instruments to ensure quality and safety.

Performance drivers: payment systems and monitoring and feedback mechanisms	1. Develop comprehensive performance assessment frameworks and publicly report on performance indicators.
	2. Move away from historical budgets or payments strictly based on volume of activity:
	  • simultaneously use a variety of payment modalities adapted to the various functions or types of services that hospitals offer;
	  • link hospital remuneration to performance, including achievement of public policy objectives measured by smart indicators.
	3. Consider opportunities for joint contracting of health and social care, e.g., through regional or local health authorities.

Performance enablers: adequate resources	1. When minimum requirements to ensure access to essential hospital care are not met, rally all stakeholders for the development of a comprehensive health sector development plan, with a component on hospitals:
	  • adopt a population health approach and inform local plans by community health needs assessment;
	  • ensure all hospitals have acceptable environmental conditions, available essential commodities, and adequate deployment of health care workers;
	  • implement comprehensive health facility assessments to provide an overview of service availability, readiness, and quality;
	  • make hospitals safe from disasters;
	  • identify opportunities to leapfrog: expand on opportunities offered by e-health to enhance outreach to patients and collaboration with other providers (e.g., m-health, telemedicine, home monitoring); and
	  • beyond initial investments, ensure their sustainability by systematically allocating sufficient maintenance budgets and integrating flexibility in hospital design.
	2. In health workforce policies, promote teamwork and collaboration across care settings by integrating opportunities for educational outreach and staff rotation between care levels; empower the nursing profession to

Table 25.2 (cont.)

Dimension	Key policy orientations and interventions
	make hospitals more people-centered and strengthen nursing management.
	3. Establish the enabling conditions for professionalization of management and sound clinical governance.
	4. Establish information systems to gather data on resources and activities as a prerequisite for sound management and strategic purchasing of hospital services; ensure interoperability to enable sharing of information between hospitals and other parts of the systems.

Source: World Health Organization, forthcoming.

While governments can align incentives and create an enabling environment to improve performance of hospitals (see Chapter 12), it is the role of managers and clinicians to optimize the performance of the organization in the context of prevailing constraints and opportunities. Hospital managers can consider several initiatives to improve the performance of their hospitals.

1. Hospital managers can *build credibility, trust, and shared ownership* with both staff and community by ensuring that the foundations for safe delivery of essential services are met, such as continued access to water and energy, infection prevention processes and equipment, maintenance of infrastructure, availability of essential medicines, payment of salaries on time, and others, while taking decisive steps to tackle the most pressing performance issues. The improved relations will facilitate the next steps on the path to transformation.

2. Hospital managers can simultaneously *improve patient-centeredness, quality, safety, and efficiency* by strengthening and streamlining monitoring and analysis of care flows, new ways of working in teams and sharing knowledge, standardized clinical pathways and operational procedures, and patient management approaches.

3. On their path to transformation, hospitals will also need to *develop new roles to help staff develop new skills and ways of working* [7]. Cultural barriers may present challenges, often requiring a widespread shift in professional attitudes. This requires a high level of strategic leadership and clinical ownership. Fit-for-purpose hospitals require a high level of empowerment of frontline staff, including clinicians and allied health care providers. They also require hospital managers with a wide skill set and demonstrated achievement of core competencies.

25.3 Control Knobs Approach for Strengthening Hospital Governance and Management

Strengthening a hospital's internal management and its relationship with external stakeholders requires acting simultaneously and coherently on three "control knobs," namely: (1) increase the competencies of individual managers; (2) institutionalize essential leadership and management functions through adequate structures and processes; and (3) monitor

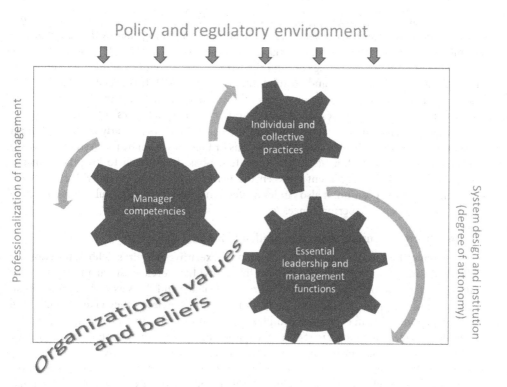

Figure 25.2 Control knobs for hospital performance management.

and reward constructive individual and collective practices (Figure 25.2). We provide below more details on how to strengthen the three control knobs.

25.3.1 Control Knob #1: Ensuring Hospital Managers Have the Required Competencies

What Leadership and Management Competencies Are Important for Hospital Managers?

Hospitals are very complex organizations and their managers should have the required knowledge and skills to carry out their responsibilities [8, 9]. Ensuring that hospital managers are competent is an essential first step to ensure that internal operations run smoothly. Investing in professional development to ensure that managers have achieved the expected level of competencies, including leadership proficiencies, should precede or at least go hand in hand with investments in infrastructure and equipment as it enhances the likelihood that the latter will be effectively and efficiently used. Ensuring that hospitals are led by capable managers is critical and works in tandem with effective organizational framework and governance rules (see Figure 25.2).

The knowledge and skills required to effectively manage hospitals are different than those required for clinical and public health activities. They are derived from business and administration practices, with a specific focus on health services. Competency in hospital management is required to achieve optimal hospital performance regardless of previous training, including (and some would argue especially) for those trained as physicians.

Building on the work done by the Healthcare Leadership Alliance [10], a global consortium of prominent health service leaders' associations brought together by the International Hospital Federation has developed a global competency directory [11] for health care managers operating in all settings around the world. This directory includes 80 competencies classified into 5 domains and 26 subdomains (Table 25.3). It is expected that hospital managers demonstrate competency across all domains. The relative importance of each competency depends on responsibilities and expected activities of each manager (Figure 25.3). Hence, in both the public and the private sectors a clearly outlined skill set is recommended for all health care organizations or facilities, local health systems (district) and/or national/state authorities. This competency-based approach to hospital management allows for better alignment between the personal capacities of individuals and the requirements of the position. It also guides professional development, resulting in a positive impact on the hospital's performance.

How to Support and Sustain Professionalization of Hospital Management?

Strengthening the capacity and quality of hospital executives requires deliberate action on individual and organizational drivers. At the individual level, hospital managers need training and education to acquire the required knowledge and skills as well as professional opportunities to apply, develop, and deepen these competencies as they take on increasing levels of responsibility in ever more complex organizations. Health services management is generally not suited to being a part-time occupation and competency cannot be achieved by relying exclusively on short and episodic training activities. Expertise is cultivated by engaging with the work and is supported by a range of clear and deliberate professional development measures. These can include self-assessment using existing tools [12], regular individual performance management reviews that ensure that executives fulfill their roles and drive performance in the organization they lead [13], and the development of formalized individual continuous plans for professional development.

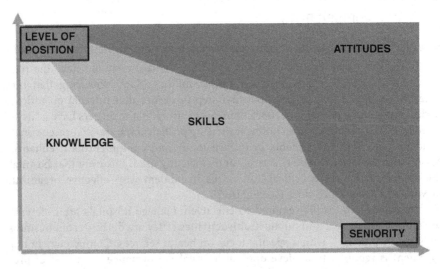

Figure 25.3 Priorities for growing competencies during the professional life course.

Table 25.3 Core competencies for health leaders

Domains	Leadership	Communication and relation management	Professional and social responsibility	Health and health care environment	Business and operations
Subdomains	• Leadership skills and behavior • Engaging culture and environment • Leading change • Driving innovation	• Relationship management • Communication skills and engagement • Facilitation and negotiation	• Personal and professional accountability • Professional development and learning • Contribution to the profession • Self-awareness • Ethical conduct and social consciousness	• Health systems and organizations • Health workforce • Person-centered care • Public health	• General management • Laws and regulations • Financial management • Human resource management • Strategic planning and thinking • Information management • Risk management • Quality improvement • System thinking • Supply chain management

Source: [11].

At the organizational level, hospitals can strengthen their capacity through a competency-based approach to recruitment and hiring, and by supporting career pathways that allow for professional growth. Talent management strategies and recruitment processes that are merit-based, competitive, and transparent are increasingly used to attract and retain competent and desirable executives. Already well established in most private organizations, these are equally relevant for public hospitals where management and leadership positions with the possibility of attractive career development and outcome-based compensation can support the recruitment and retention of talented executives. Well-written role descriptions related to clear time-bound organizational objectives can also enable effective recruitment and retention.

Furthermore, career paths that support or even encourage "horizontal/diagonal professional mobility" between hospitals, primary care facilities, and district-level positions can foster a more comprehensive understanding of how health systems work and ensure hospitals are fit for purpose in their environments.

25.3.2 Control Knob #2: Governance and Operational Framework for Improving Hospital Performance

Having well-trained and competent managers is necessary but not sufficient to achieve optimal hospital performance. In addition, the establishment of clear governance and organizational structures, policies, and procedures that do not rely on any single or small group of individuals are required to ensure sustainability and continuity when there is a turnover of managers. Thus, optimal performance requires the combination of competent managers and appropriate organizational processes (Figure 25.4).

Stewardship through Sound Governance Structures: The Role of Hospital Boards

In all systems and types of organizations, including public and private hospitals, it is important that the leadership, including the chief executive officer or "head" of the organization, be accountable to a governing body, usually named a "board of directors" or simply "board." A board is a collective body of directors who share a commitment to

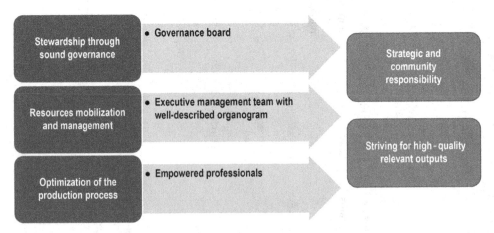

Figure 25.4 Essential leadership and management functions supported by governance and organizational frameworks.

the mission of the institution and ideally represent the interests of a range of stakeholders. The board is responsible for setting the strategic direction, framing policies, and overseeing performance of the organization. It enjoys a degree of autonomy, buffers against the interests of individual stakeholders, and seeks accountability from the managers. Boards are common in private hospitals but are not consistently present in publicly funded hospitals [14, 15]. Without a board, institutions are at risk of being governed by a single or small group of decision-makers without clear accountability for performance nor responsiveness to local needs and capacities. Optimal performance, in private and public hospitals, requires a clear mission and vision, well-aligned policies, and effective oversight, all of which are enabled by the autonomy of a board of directors. Autonomy in public hospitals is often confused with independence. Rather, it should be understood to reflect a degree of authority for making choices toward agreed goals, translated into locally adapted strategic objectives. The high-level goals are set by national policymakers, negotiated with state or local health authorities, and then translated into the mission of the organization. The board is accountable, on behalf of the organization, for contributing to the implementation of national and local public health priorities.

For a board to be effective, its role and responsibilities need to be well described. This can be achieved through a legal act or regulations that give clear terms of reference. A board can – in addition – set its own rules and mechanisms for their implementation. In the absence of clear "rules of engagement," accountability cannot be established, opening the possibility for boards to favor the interests of board members at the expense of the mission of the organization.

Board models vary according to countries' legal environments. Board models for public and not-for-profit hospitals are often similar to those of other public autonomous organizations, while boards of private for-profit hospitals are often under the same regulations as commercial companies. A board's nomination process should be transparent and should ensure that key stakeholders are represented. The stakeholders vary from country to country; in general they represent the health authorities and payers, clinical staff, community, and patients. The term of office for board members should be time-limited and members should be selected based on merit.

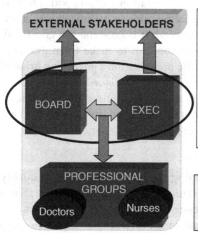

Board: generic definition for the body in charge of strategic decisions, policies, and procedures, and overseeing the organization's performance.

Executive team: generic definition for the body in charge of running the hospital day to day but also implementing board decisions and inspiring the strategy. The executive team can vary in components and levels.

Extensive versus restricted power of the board: the right balance is critical for operational autonomy of the executive team.

Figure 25.5 Respective roles of board and executive team. *Source:* Author from unpublished training material used with WHO-EMRO.

A board should focus on strategic and tactical decisions and should not be involved in operational decisions such as day-to-day management (Figure 25.5).

Respective Role of the Board and the Executive Team

Boards are expected to take decisions regarding service planning (e.g., activities to be developed or downsized) and capital asset investments (e.g., infrastructure, equipment, and information systems). These decisions are based on a thorough assessment of the revenue and cost implications (including considerations regarding maintenance and staff mobilization) and are aligned with long-term goals negotiated with national and local authorities (their "mandate").

Sound governance requires the right balance of power between the board chair (or president) and the hospital's chief executive. The hospital leadership can be organized as a team with a chain of command that may vary from one organization to another. It is important that the hospital's leadership and management structure be clearly outlined in an organizational chart. A series of organizational charts can be used to convey increasing levels of detail about the lines of command, including the decision-making hierarchy, reporting structure, and the flow of information [16].

Delegation is necessary to avoid counterproductive micromanagement. Micromanagement results from the absence of trust and, in complex organizations like hospitals, can cause major bottlenecks in the flow of activities. Delegation protocols should be established to empower managers to make the decisions required for them to manage effectively. Establishing clear delegation regulations allows high levels of accountability while mobilizing people's talents and competencies. It requires clear measurable objectives and regular monitoring and evaluation of achievements. Effective delegation also requires prior assessment of the competencies of the delegate. Delegation is effective when delegates have a clear knowledge of their responsibilities and have the authority to mobilize and use the resources required to carry out the activities under their responsibility. Delegation can be temporary, typically when related to a specific task, or permanent when related to a function. When responsibilities are delegated to a unit rather than to an individual it can be advisable to resort to contracts [17] that outline explicit and mutually agreed rules, results, and outputs, and a review process to assess achievements.

In many countries, hospitals have *standard* organizational charts with predetermined roles and reporting structures. This is unfortunate because an organizational chart should reflect the unique vision and needs of a given hospital. It is important to give the development of the organizational chart(s) careful attention and to make them available to the public. The organizational chart should reflect the organization's governing principles that have been validated by the board; and it should reflect and be aligned with the organization's leadership and management style and culture. It should also reflect the modalities adopted for managing the hospital. Hospitals that are more people- and project-oriented will adopt different organizational charts than those focusing on processes and structures.

Resources Mobilization and Management

Hospital executives are in charge of implementing the information system, quality assurance, and financial management. These three critical components of management require a strong combination of well-established processes and technical competencies.

The hospital management team is responsible for overseeing the whole production function and should therefore ensure that core processes are in place. Each process can be organized as a department headed by qualified managers responsible for the

---

Box 25.1 Core Processes of Effective Hospital Management

Hospital workforce planning and management covers all aspects of workforce planning in terms of norms and standards, and appropriate staff and skill mix. In addition, it covers developing job descriptions and adhering to standard processes of recruitment, selection, deployment, continuing professional development, and performance appraisal of staff. Special attention is needed to create a cadre of well-trained hospital executives and develop strategies for team building, staff motivation, and conflict resolution.

Financial management serves to manage funds and minimize risks to achieve the financial goals of the hospital while providing efficient health care to all patients. Hospital executives need to understand the different types of hospital costs. They should be knowledgeable in the areas of resource allocation, expenditure, and utilization that help achieve the goals of the hospital. Importantly, they should be conversant with the process of budgeting as an important tool for financial management and monitoring.

Supply chain management in hospitals oversees the flow of goods and services and includes processes that ensure efficient resource use, prompt operations, and better health outcomes. Hospital executives need to understand basic concepts, terminologies, and components of supply chain management. An important component is procurement, which is a process of purchasing the services, equipment, and supplies in sufficient quantities and at cost-effective prices to fulfill hospital requirements. Procurement requires a high level of transparency and accountability to mitigate the risks of corruption.

Hospital information and use of digital technology is critical for monitoring and improving all aspects of hospital performance. It entails documenting information related to patient care as well as hospital management systems. For patient care, transitioning to electronic medical records is essential for efficient and timely retrieval of information. Executives also need to ensure adherence to the Family of International Classifications, such as the International Classification of Diseases (ICD) (see Chapter 8) and its application in cataloging diseases based on this internationally accepted method.

Delivery of safe and quality health care in the hospital setting is essential under routine circumstances, as well as in emergencies. Hospital executives should be conversant with the six domains of quality and the strategies, approaches, and tools available for providing quality and safe care (see Chapter 26). These relate to externally driven programs such as hospital accreditation, as well as internal quality assurance programs. Executives should strive to inculcate a culture conducive to providing safe and quality-assured care to patients.

Disaster preparedness and hospital resilience are essential elements to prepare a hospital in the event of an emergency or disaster. Hospital executives should know the core components and the tools to develop a hospital emergency preparedness plan and comprehend core features of the hospital's response in terms of its surge capacity in the event of a disaster.

---

implementation and oversight of that process. Box 25.1 provides a brief description of some of the core processes, which are discussed in greater detail in the relevant chapters of the book.

Hospital Productivity Optimization

Hospital productivity can be measured by a set of indicators that can serve as a benchmark. Productivity indicators can be divided into measures for inputs, processes, outputs, and outcomes (Table 12.2, Chapter 12) [18, 19]. The productivity of hospitals can be monitored using a dashboard that provides live information on selected key performance indicators.

Indicators used to monitor the level of activity of hospitals, especially at the inpatient level, include the average length of stay, bed occupancy, rates for bed turnover, unit cost per bed day, as well as the number of diagnostic and therapeutic procedures conducted. In the outpatient setting, measures of service utilization and consultation time are used to measure performance. See Chapter 12 for an in-depth discussion of the measures of hospital performance (Table 12.2).

25.3.3 Control Knob #3: Monitor and Reward Individual and Collective Practices

Having managerial competencies and appropriate governance structures and mechanisms is essential, but not sufficient to ensure the highest level of performance. The limitations of "management by orders" call for a better recognition of the human dimension of health services management and provision, from both users and staff perspectives. Hence, the third control knob calls for monitoring and rewarding individual and collective practices by nurturing the organizational culture, developing feedback mechanisms on staff and user experiences, establishing staff performance evaluation and rewarding systems, and supporting staff to strengthen their skills, develop new competencies, and adopt new ways of working.

High-performing hospitals adopt and nurture collaborative cultures where teamwork and innovation are encouraged. They also place value on "people's voice" and ensure collective practices are monitored through the perspectives of their key stakeholders: community/users (patient and relatives) and staff. A variety of mechanisms can be used to capture "people's voices," such as organizational climate surveys, patient experience surveys, patient interviews, hotlines, ombudsman to monitor complaints, suggestion boxes, and others.

The performance monitoring and reward system [20] must simultaneously deal with two targets: (1) making sure that each individual staff member is held accountable and gives their best for the work accomplished; while (2) also nurturing a team dynamic that rewards collective effort. The leadership of the organization plays a major role in ensuring a results-driven mindset and in setting an example through its own behavior. It is challenging to develop a performance-driven incentive system in hospitals lacking transparency and assessment of individual performance. A contracting approach [21] is a powerful tool to align achievement of objectives in terms of internal operation and in terms of contribution to the local health system and population health. Even in the context of civil service employment in public budgetary hospitals, incentive systems can be set up, for instance by mobilizing community support to provide financial or material incentives. According to the local culture and legal possibilities, a variety of incentive mechanisms can be set up, from personal or team financial benefit to public recognition awards.

While monitoring staff performance, it is also critical to create "protected spaces" for staff to dare to innovate and to foster a culture of safety and continuous quality improvement. A performance monitoring and reward system [22] is only one element to drive staff's contribution to align with the hospital's vision. Hence, human resource management cannot entirely rely on such an incentive system. This control knob is intrinsically embedded in human resource management and must be built on a shared set of organizational values and staff skills development (i.e., by aligning staff performance assessment with staff development mechanisms).

25.4 Conclusion: Fostering Innovation in People-Centered Hospitals

The key to dealing with today's public health challenges, such as COVID-19 and the expected consequences of climate change, is not to change strategic direction – PHC is the path to universal health coverage and health system resilience – but to transform the way health and social services are delivered and funded. Health care and coverage that are truly universal require a shift from systems organized around diseases and health institutions toward systems organized around people's needs, and hospitals are an integral part of this agenda [23].

Hospital leaders need to be empowered to tailor hospital operations to better respond to community health needs and local conditions, to facilitate achieving a shared goal, and to ensure adequate organizational resources and support. A range of approaches is available toward that end, including effective communication, efficient resource mobilization, and engagement of all stakeholders based on their roles and abilities.

A high level of strategic leadership and clinical ownership is a critical enabler, with a shift from overreliance on top-heavy, bureaucratic processes to value bottom-up initiatives that resonate with frontline care providers and appeal to their intrinsic motivation to care for people and communities. Achieving this requires hospital leadership to create an enabling environment for frontline initiatives to flourish. Supportive elements for people-centered hospitals include developing care pathways to support transition across care settings, putting in place communication tools and e-health applications, finding new ways to deliver patient and family education, and reorienting hospital outreach programs to serve the disadvantaged and marginalized. Shared decision-making in patient care requires not only a shift in the relationship between practitioners and patients, but also a change in the organizational culture to give a place to patients, families, and the community [24]. In summary, giving greater visibility and support to the development, scale-up, and adoption of frontline innovations in hospitals is vital to the shared vision of integrated and people-centered services in a PHC-oriented health system.

References

1. World Health Organization. World Health Statistics 2022: Monitoring Health for the SDGs, Sustainable Development Goals. 2022. www.who.int/publications/i/item/9789240051157 (accessed August 26, 2022).

2. N. Taylor, R. Clay-Williams, E. Hogden, et al. High performing hospitals: a qualitative systematic review of associated factors and practical strategies for improvement. *BMC Health Serv Res* 2015; **15**: 244.

3. S. R. Adhikari, V. P. Sapkota, S. Supakankunti. A new approach of measuring hospital performance for low- and middle-income countries. *J Korean Med Sci* 2015; **30**(Suppl. 2): S143–S148.

4. World Health Organization. The transformative role of hospitals in the future of primary health care. 2018. https://apps.who.int/iris/bitstream/handle/10665/326296/WHO-HIS-SDS-2018.45-eng.pdf?sequence=1&isAllowed=y (accessed February 10, 2022).

5. World Health Organization. Introducing the framework for action for the hospital sector in the Eastern Mediterranean Region. 2019. https://applications.emro.who.int/docs/RC_Technical_Papers_2019_5_en.pdf?ua=1 (accessed February 10, 2022).

6. World Health Organization. Interview with the WHO inter-regional taskforce on hospitals. 2018. https://apps.who.int/iris/

handle/10665/324845 (accessed February 12, 2022).

7. L. Doshmangir, A. Takian. Capacity building to improve hospital managers' performance in West Asia. *Int J Health Policy Manag* 2019; **8**(5): 319–320.

8. L. Gilson, I. A. Agyepong. Strengthening health system leadership for better governance: what does it take? *Health Policy Plan* 2018; **33**(Suppl. 2): ii1–ii4.

9. M. Kitchener. The "bureaucratization" of professional roles: the case of clinical directors in UK hospitals. *Organization* 2000; **7**(1): 129–154.

10. M. E. Stefl. Common competencies for all healthcare managers: the Healthcare Leadership Alliance model. *J Healthc Manag* 2008; **53**(6): 360–373; discussion 374.

11. International Hospital Federation. Leadership competencies for healthcare services managers. 2015. www.ache.org/-/media/ache/about-ache/leadership_competencies_healthcare_services_managers.pdf (accessed March 12, 2021).

12. International Hospital Federation. IHFSIG healthcare management. 2016. https://healthmanagementcompetency.org/base (accessed April 11, 2021).

13. M. Vainieri, F. Ferrè, G. Giacomelli, et al. Explaining performance in health care: how and when top management competencies make the difference. *Health Care Manage Rev* 2019; **44**(4): 306–317.

14. A. M. Lipunga, B. M. Tchereni, R. C. Bakuwa. Emerging structural models for governance of public hospitals. *Int J Health Gov* 2019; **24**(2).

15. P. A. Abor, G. Abekah-Nkrumah, J. Abor. An examination of hospital governance in Ghana. *Leadersh Health Serv* 2008; **21**(1).

16. USAID, CIPE. Health sector governance better governance for better health principles & guidelines for governance in hospitals Egypt 2014. 2015. https://cipe-arabia.org/wp-content/uploads/2018/08/Principles_and_Guidelines_for_Governance_in_Hospitals_EN.pdf (accessed February 12, 2022).

17. E. de Roodenbeke. *Strategic Contracting for Health Systems and Services*. London, Routledge, 2017.

18. M. Ali, R. Salehnejad, M. Mansur. Hospital productivity: the role of efficiency drivers. *Int J Health Plann Manage* 2019; **34**(2): 806–823.

19. J. Du, S. Cui, H. Gao. Assessing productivity development of public hospitals: a case study of Shanghai, China. *Int J Environ Res Public Health* 2020; **17** (18): 6763.

20. G. Kacholi, O. H. Mahomed. Perceptions of hospital staff on the performance of quality improvement teams in the regional referral hospitals in Tanzania: a cross sectional study. *PLoS One* 2021; **16**(2): e0246927.

21. World Health Organization. Performance incentives for health care providers. 2010. https://apps.who.int/iris/handle/10665/85701 (accessed June 14, 2022).

22. K. B. Walker, L. M. Dunn. Improving hospital performance and productivity with the balanced scorecard. *Acad Health Care Manag* 2006; **2**.

23. World Health Organization. Introducing the framework for action for the hospital sector in the Eastern Mediterranean Region. 2019. https://applications.emro.who.int/docs/RC_Technical_Papers_2019_5_en.pdf (accessed February 17, 2022).

24. I. Gabutti, D. Mascia, A. Cicchetti. Exploring "patient-centered" hospitals: a systematic review to understand change. *BMC Health Serv Res* 2017; **17**(1): 364.

Chapter 26

Improving the Quality and Safety of Health Care in Low and Middle Income Countries
What Works!

Salma W. Jaouni, Mondher Letaief, Samer Ellaham, and Samar Hassan

Key Messages

- Improving quality and safety of health care will require several components, including:
  - application of quality improvement (QI) and patient safety principles in all aspects of care, with a focus on patients, team involvement, accountability, and use of data;
  - adoption of multimodal approaches, with attention to the proper selection of QI models as fit to the goal and situation;
  - use of approaches that ensure the sustainability and continuity of QI and safety in health care, such as external evaluation; and
  - a focus on the rationale, purpose, objectives, and outcomes of any approach or model and how to continuously expand and improve them.

26.1 Introduction

The concept of quality in health care includes several dimensions and has evolved over time. Quality improvement (QI) is a systematic process to optimize performance, which has evolved from lessons learned outside the health sector and has led to improvement in many settings while having limited impact in others. Patient safety has emerged as a critical and core objective of QI in the health sector. While quality can be considered as an end in itself, it is increasingly recognized as an integral component of health care reforms and an essential dimension of universal health coverage (UHC).

Improved quality of care can be achieved through a multitude of approaches, including institution-specific and health system-wide strategies; patient-centric and process-centric approaches; and external and internal quality assessment. While all approaches have merit, choosing an improvement strategy appropriate for a given setting is important to achieve optimal and sustainable benefits and avoid wasteful investment. This is especially relevant in low- and middle-income countries (L&MICs).

This chapter looks at the evolution of QI in health care over time; the types of health care QI approaches and their relation to patient safety and UHC; the opportunities to improve common health care quality and safety challenges in L&MICs; and what has and has not worked and how.

26.1.1 Definition of the Problem

Poor quality of care is a leading cause of excess morbidity and mortality in many L&MICs. Improving the quality of health care is complex, and it can be challenging to identify the specific problem, devise a potential solution, make the intended improvement, and ensure it is well measured and sustained. In low-resource settings, poorly designed approaches and lack of human and financial resources add another layer of challenges to QI. L&MICs nonetheless offer many successful QI examples that highlight the requirements for success and offer rich lessons.

26.2 The Evolution of Quality and Safety in Health Care

Quality improvement emerged outside the health care industry. Specifically, many of the techniques currently used in health care QI were developed for the manufacturing sector. QI originated with the craftsmanship guilds of the Middle Ages. In the 1920s, pioneers including Shewarts [1], Deming [2], Juran [3], Crosby [4], and Donabedian [5] advocated for the use of measurement and data to judge the effectiveness of processes in achieving desired outcomes (see Box 26.1) [6].

Although the idea of QI was not heavily emphasized within the health care industry until the 1980s, efforts to improve and develop quality care for patients had in fact already been in existence. In 1910, hospital care improvement was led by Ernest Codman, who followed up on patients to ensure treatments were effective, leading to the development of a "minimum standard of care" for hospitals by the American College of Surgeons [10]. Nearly 40 years later, these efforts led to the establishment of the Joint Commission on Accreditation of Health Care Organizations, now known as The Joint Commission, and with it a more concerted effort in external assessment based on standards [6].

Table 26.1 summarizes the evolution of QI since 1910, reflecting the prevailing thinking in the health care sector throughout the years. Key milestones include the invention of the Toyota Production System in 1950, now known as "Lean Six Sigma," by Taiichi Ohno, chief engineer at Toyota [11]; the description of the three elements of the Donabedian Model by Avedis Donabedian in his 1966 article, "Evaluating the quality of medical care" [12]; the publication of a paper describing early quality failures by Dr. Mikel J. Harry in 1985 [13]; and the launch of Motorola's Six Sigma program in 1987 [14].

Box 26.1 Definitions

Health care quality: The degree to which health services for individuals and populations increase the likelihood of desired health outcomes and are consistent with current professional knowledge [7].

Health care QI: The framework used to systematically improve the ways care is delivered to patients. Processes have characteristics that can be measured, analyzed, improved, and controlled. QI entails continuous efforts to achieve stable and predictable process results; that is, to reduce process variation and improve the outcomes of these processes both for patients and the health care organization and system [8].

Patient safety: The avoidance, prevention, and amelioration of adverse outcomes or injuries stemming from the process of health care [9].

Table 26.1 The evolution of quality improvement

1910	• *Ernest Codman* led the idea of improving hospital care by following up on patients to ensure treatments were effective. Codman's ideas laid the groundwork for the American College of Surgeons to develop a "minimum standard" of care, which generally focused on improving care provided in the hospital [15].
1930	• *Walter A. Shewart* developed control charts and the principles of modern statistical process control [16].
1950–1970	• *W. Edwards Deming* taught methods for statistical analysis and control of quality to Japanese engineers and executives, and introduced principles to improve health care quality and safety without wasting available resources [2]. • *Joseph M. Juran* taught the concepts of controlling quality and managerial breakthrough [17]. • *Philip B. Crosby's* promotion of zero defects paved the way for QI in many companies [4]. • *The Joint Commission on Accreditation of Health Care Organizations*, now known as The Joint Commission was established and became responsible for implementing and advocating for quality programs not only at the organizational level but also for the entire health care system [6].
1980	• *Donabedian* was one of the first authors who focused attention on the importance of examining health care quality from different perspectives, considering inputs, processes, and outcomes. • Motorola developed *Six Sigma* to improve its business processes by minimizing defects, evolved into an organizational approach that achieved breakthroughs – and significant bottom-line results [13].
1990	• The term *TQM (total quality management)* was initially coined in 1985 by the Naval Air Systems Command to describe its Japanese-style management approach to QI. TQM is the name for the philosophy of a broad and systemic approach to managing organizational quality [18]. • *Quality standards* such as the ISO 9000 series and quality award programs such as the Deming Prize and the Malcolm Baldrige National Quality Award specify principles and processes that comprise TQM [6].
1999–2001	• The *Institute of Medicine (IOM)* published *To Err Is Human: Building a Safer Health System* (1999) which focused on patient safety and brought to the public's attention the fact that 44,000 to 98,000 deaths occur each year due to medical errors [19]. • The *IOM* published *Crossing the Quality Chasm: A New Health System for the 21st Century* (2001) built on *To Err is Human*. It called for a fundamental change in the health care delivery system through a complete redesign of patient–provider relationships and revised patient care processes, leading to improved health care outcomes [4].

Arguably, some of the defining moments in the evolution of QI in health care were the publication of two landmark documents by the Institute of Medicine (IOM) in the United States: *To Err Is Human* (1999) [19] and *Crossing the Quality Chasm* (2001) [4], which included one of the most influential frameworks for health care quality assessment and improvement based on six domains of health care quality (Figure 26. 1).

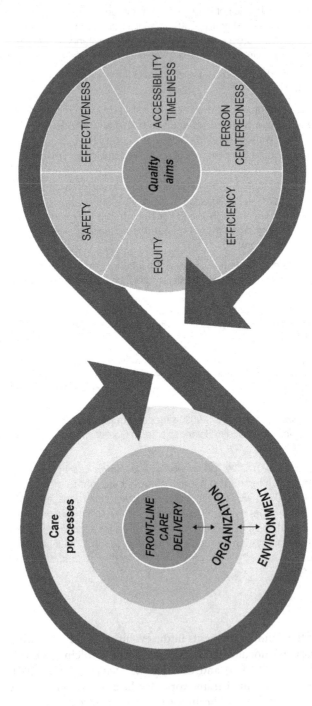

Figure 26.1 IOM crossing the quality chasm [4].

> **Box 26.2 Definitions**
>
> **Patient safety incidents:** Any unintended or unexpected incident which could have or did lead to harm for one or more patients [21].
>
> **Patient safety resolution:** The Global Action on Patient Safety resolution was adopted in 2019 by the 72nd World Health Assembly. The resolution recognizes patient safety as a global health priority and endorses the establishment of World Patient Safety Day, observed annually on September 17. In this regard, the Global Patient Safety Action Plan is a commitment from WHO, international health agencies, and Member States to organize and implement actions to reduce the overall burden of patient harm due to unsafe health care [22].

26.2.1 Patient Safety

Safety is the first domain to be considered in QI, positioning patient safety initiatives at the forefront of QI efforts. The value of patient safety can be traced back to the tenet of the Hippocratic Oath to "First do no harm" [20]. Despite this principle, there is still considerable harm being done, with 1 in 10 patients being harmed while receiving care in hospitals (Box 26.2) [21].

Patient safety encompasses more than doing no harm. It includes, but is not limited to, behavioral and structural changes in infection prevention and control, such as hand hygiene and sanitation. Patient safety remains a significant problem globally and requires systematic and individual cultural changes through leadership, commitment, transparency, learning from errors and best practices, and a judicious balance between a no-blame policy and accountability.

According to WHO, unsafe care in L&MICs results in 134 million adverse events and 2.6 million deaths annually [21]. Major patient safety challenges in L&MICs include lack of well-trained providers; inadequate infrastructure and equipment; weak monitoring practices; budget constraints; and absence of meaningful data to guide policies and programs [23]. Patient safety challenges are not unique to L&MICs, and in all settings are dependent on attitudes, expectations, perceived accountability, and resources.

We note two key approaches to improve patient safety: (1) harm prevention (mitigating adverse effects *prior to* their occurrence); and (2) changing practice *after* a critical incident occurs so that it does not happen again. One example of prevention strategy is the WHO safe surgical checklist. The checklist includes a number of procedures that are consistently carried out before, during, and at the end of surgical interventions. These include: verifying that the correct surgery is performed on the correct patient using the correct method; double-checking the doses of medicines administered; and making sure that all equipment is in working order and sterilized at the start of surgery, and all used materials are accounted for at the end of the procedure [23].

26.3 Quality of Care: An Integral Element of UHC

Universal health coverage has been endorsed by WHO and the World Bank as a means to improve access to health care without the risk of catastrophic financial burden. It is endorsed as target 3.8 of the UN Sustainable Development Goals (SDGs) – see Chapter 3 [24]. To achieve its expected benefits for health and wellbeing, UHC must not only include improved access to health care but also ensure the quality of the care provided.

Box 26.3 The Costs of Poor Quality in Numbers

- More than eight million people per year in L&MICs die from conditions that should be treatable by the health system.
- In 2015 alone these deaths resulted in US$6 trillion in economic losses.
- 60% of deaths from conditions amenable to health care are due to poor-quality care, whereas the remaining deaths result from nonutilization of the health system.
- High-quality health systems could prevent 2.5 million deaths from cardiovascular disease, 1 million newborn deaths, 900,000 deaths from tuberculosis, and half of all maternal deaths each year.

Poor quality of health care leads to poor outcomes – and wastes time and money. Therefore, ensuring that quality is an integral part of UHC is essential to achieve longer and better lives. However, quality is not inherent or automatic; it requires planning and concerted efforts, and hence should be clearly identified as a priority in any initiative that aims to advance UHC [24].

It is important to acknowledge that quality comes at a cost. Nevertheless, if applied intelligently, investments in quality will deliver better individual and population health in a cost-effective manner; that is, quality adds "value for the money." Building quality in health systems is affordable for countries at all levels of economic development. In fact, the *lack* of quality is an unaffordable cost, especially for the poorest countries (Box 26.3) [25].

26.4 Barriers to Improving Quality & Safety of Health Care in L&MICs

The barriers to delivering high-quality care are similar across all health systems. However, these barriers can be more pronounced in resource-poor settings and can have a greater impact on QI interventions. Investing resources in health systems without continuous QI is thought to be futile. Conversely, focusing on narrow QI initiatives in a resource-limited context without addressing the broader health system issues is of limited value. Hence, both must be strengthened concurrently.

While many countries, including L&MICs, recognize the need to improve quality as part of health care delivery and health systems, many lack the knowledge, skills, financial resources, and accountability systems to implement the required changes. As a result, expressed commitments to health care QI often remain unimplemented. Challenges hindering QI in L&MICs include: weak leadership, staffing shortages, scarcity of resources, lack of adherence to treatment protocols, inadequate staff training, weak performance monitoring systems, and nonempowered patients and families (see Boxes 26.4 and 26.5) [26–28].

26.5 Health Care QI Models

Developing a quality culture is key to any sustainable effort toward QI. More than just a mechanical process, QI is a culture to be nurtured, a philosophy, an approach, and a collective commitment to the common goal of patient safety and performance improvement.

Box 26.4 A Closer Look at L&MICs Health Systems

- Between 5.7 and 8.4 million deaths are attributed to poor-quality care in L&MICs, which represents up to 15% of overall deaths in these countries.
- Health providers in L&MICs often do less than half of the recommended evidence-based care actions.
- Approximately one-third of patients experience disrespectful care, short consultations, poor communication, or long waiting times.
- Inadequate integration across platforms and weak referral systems undermine the ability of health systems to care for complex and emerging conditions.
- Less than one-quarter of people in L&MICs believe that their health system works well, compared with half of the people in high-income countries.

Box 26.5 Quality and Safety of Care in Fragile, Conflict-Affected, and Vulnerable Settings

Definition: The term fragile, conflict-affected, and vulnerable settings broadly describes situations of crisis. People living in such settings include all those experiencing humanitarian crises, prolonged disruption to critical public services, significant armed conflict, extreme adversity or acute, protracted, or complex emergencies.

Currently, two billion people live in countries where development outcomes are affected by fragility, conflict, and violence; 60% of preventable maternal deaths, 53% of deaths in children younger than five years of age; and 45% of neonatal deaths are in settings of conflict, displacement, and natural disasters.

A range of constraints exist in such settings: breakdown in health systems, inadequate workforce, lack of safety and security, including attacks on health care, and scarcity of resources.

The challenge of addressing quality is compounded because fragile, conflict-affected, and vulnerable settings do not represent a homogeneous set of circumstances. Therefore, addressing quality in extreme adversity requires coordinated action at all levels of the health system.

QI initiatives in health care are frequently implemented in response to adverse events or patient complaints. Stakeholders tend to be passive or reactive rather than being proactive or adopting a systematic approach. The KAIZEN QC-7 tool (Figure 26.2) followed by a clinical value compass (Figure 26.3) can be used to prioritize, plan, identify, and implement QI initiatives [28, 29].

There are a number of well-developed QI models that are either patient-, or process- and result-centric (Table 26.2). All models involve setting the right goals; charting a structured path to achieve them; bringing attention to cost-effectiveness, timeliness and efficiency, accountability, and transparency; and engaging in repeated improvement cycles. Table 26.2 describes five models commonly used to shape quality program infrastructure and guide QI initiatives to improve patient care. The different models can be applied to the same quality challenge. Understanding their inherent strengths and weaknesses is key to selecting the right one. The plan–do–study–act model (PDSA) is cyclical, whereas the lean model seeks to eliminate waste and streamline processes to provide maximum value to patients. Six Sigma is data-driven to solve large-scale problems. Table 26.3 summarizes the characteristics of each model.

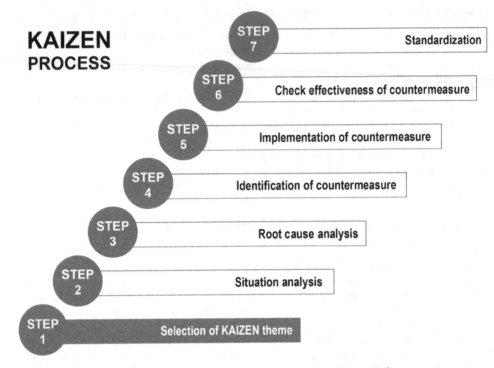

Figure 26.2 Planning, identifying, and implementing a QI project: KAIZEN QC-7 tool [28].

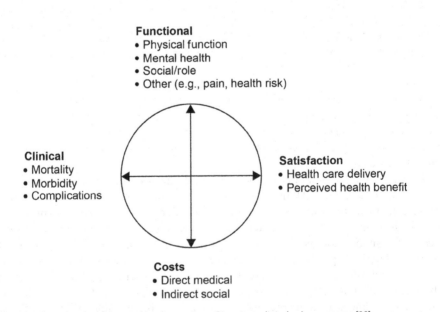

Figure 26.3 Planning, identifying, and implementing a QI project: clinical value compass [29].

Table 26.2 Quality improvement models

Focus	Framework	Types	Description
Patient-centric QI models		Plan–do–study–act (PDSA)	These are the backbone of QI in health care (Figure 26.4). QI teams study and analyze data and then design the PDSA cycles. These are repeated cycles of validity tests that help adapt and implement the QI model in the right context. At each cycle, the QI team assesses the success of the QI model/intervention. This goes on until an intervention is successfully designed and is ready to be implemented.
	Provide a framework to monitor processes and care results	IHI model	This model was developed by Associates of Process Improvement (API) and is based on the work by W. Edwards Deming (1900–1993). This model facilitates the application of QI by defining the aim of improvement, designing a specific idea/plan to bring out the improvement, and planning ways to measure improvement (Figure 26.4) [30].
		Six Sigma model	The define, measure, analyze, improve, and control model (DMAIC) is a data-driven quality strategy used to improve processes. The DMAIC approach is integral to the Six Sigma model. The model also uses the DMADV (define, measure, analyze, design, verify) approach to develop new processes [31].
Process- and results-centric QI models	Provide a framework to improve patient care	Lean model	This model is based on what a patient wants. It maps out the value of patient needs and how it flows to the patient in a cost-effective and time-sensitive manner [32].
		Care model	This model is based on fundamental aspects of care to promote high-quality disease management and focuses on disease prevention. The model involves patients in their care and facilitates active interactions between patients and health care providers (Figure 26.5) [33].

26.6 Approaches to Ensure Continuous and Sustainable QI and Safety in Health Care Institutions

Quality improvement should be considered a continuous and cyclical process, requiring a consistent review of results [33]. For all QI initiatives, proper planning, use of standards, communication of guidelines, and monitoring and evaluation are critical. Success is dependent on properly defined problems, well-trained teams, correctly assigned responsibilities, and national or institutional capabilities (see Box 26.6) [35].

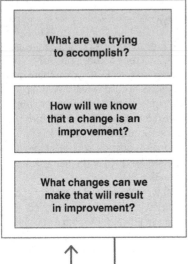

Setting aims
Improvement requires setting aims. The aim should be time-specific and measurable; it should also define the specific population of patients that will be affected.

Establishing measures
Teams use quantitative measures to determine if a specific change actually leads to an improvement.

Selecting changes
All improvement requires making changes, but not all changes result in improvement. Organizations therefore must identify the changes that are most likely to result in improvement.

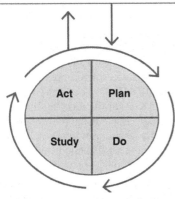

Testing changes
The Plan–Do–Study–Act (PDSA) cycle is shorthand for testing a change in the real work setting – by planning it, trying it, observing the results, and acting on what is learned. This is the scientific method used for action-oriented learning.

Figure 26.4 IHI model of improvement [34].

Quality improvement neither promises nor guarantees error-free health care. Its ultimate goal is to build trust in the quality of the health care being rendered. Trust based on high-quality care is essential to drive demand and is foundational to person-centered care.

Internal QI programs are those implemented by organizations or systems. They can be integrated into ongoing patient care and adapted to the local environment. External programs for quality evaluation serve a broader social purpose and a wider range of stakeholders. They can help maintain the improvements achieved through internal QI efforts through mechanisms such as threat of exposure, financial sanctions, or withdrawal of status. They can also identify and address outliers, assess the quality of internal QI processes and, where appropriate, offer technical assistance [36].

Approaches to ensure quality and safety of health services can be categorized into two main groups: (1) system-wide approaches based on building quality management in the whole organization; and (2) specific approaches that focus on internal assessment of quality in specific areas of care. These are reviewed in further detail below.

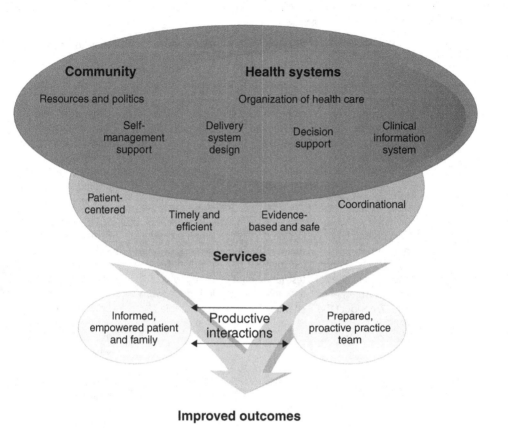

Figure 26.5 The care model [33].

26.6.1 System-Wide Approaches to Evaluate and Assure Quality in Health Care Organizations

Accreditation as an External Evaluation Approach

Accreditation falls within a group of tools known as external evaluation programs. It involves a process to assess performance in relation to established standards and to implement ways to continuously improve. The accreditation process is viewed as an external audit, serving as a QI process where organizations use it as a self-assessment tool to validate their efforts and demonstrate quality standards [36]. To optimize impact on quality, accreditation programs need to be flexible in their application and responsive to increasing variation in service delivery while ensuring that core standards of safety are embedded throughout the framework [37]. Most accreditation programs are independent, run by nonprofit, professional organizations; are instituted by medical professionals; have voluntary participation by facilities; are transparent with respect to publishing results and standards; and are funded mainly through fees charged to member facilities. However, this model is changing with more government involvement and funding as more countries make accreditation mandatory [38].

Table 26.3 Model comparative analysis

Model	Overview	Purpose	Rationale	How to use
PDSA	Cycles test change to assess impact, ensure that new ideas work, small scale before wholesale to avoid disruption	Introduce and test potential QI initiatives then refine on a small scale before expansion	When procedure, process, or system need to be introduced or changed	A procedure, process, or system is modified or newly designed, introduced in a specific timeframe, adjusted for improvements, and repeated in small cycles
IHI model [35]	Two phases: (1) pose three questions to define required changes and measurements; and (2) conduct the PDSA in live settings	Decide on measurable QI initiatives and test/refine prior to wholesale change	When procedure, process, or system needs to be changed or introduced with measurable elements	Form appropriate stakeholder team, define intended change – what is to be accomplished, how a change is actually an improvement, and what changes will result in improvement, specify its measurements, implement PDSA
Lean/Six Sigma [30]	Improve flow in a value stream and eliminate waste through statistical analysis to uncover and understand root causes and reduce them	Analyze health care systems to eliminate waste and redirect resources for improvement	When health care systems are inefficient, wasteful, and inconsistent	Use the DMAIC approach in a process-mapping form with associated stakeholders and statistical process control charts to compare current data with trends and analyze changes
Care model [31]	Consists of five core elements: health systems, delivery system, decision support, clinical information, and self-management	Promote high-quality disease and prevention management	At large scale to produce productive interactions between informed, activated patients and prepared proactive practice teams	Organized and planned approach focused on particular patient population ensuring optimal medical care by shifting from care delivered by physician to that by teams

Box 26.6 Desirable Attributes for Continuous QI Program

- Addresses overuse, underuse, and poor technical and interpersonal quality
- Deals with outlier practice and performance
- Fosters improvement throughout the health care organization and system
- Uses both positive and negative incentives for change and improvement in performance
- Provides practitioners and providers with timely information to improve performance
- Has face validity for the public and for professionals (i.e., is understandable and relevant to patient and clinical decision-making)
- Is scientifically rigorous
- Positive impact on patient outcomes can be demonstrated or inferred
- Can address both individual and population-based outcomes
- Documents improvement in quality and progress toward excellence
- Is affordable and is cost-effective
- Includes patients and the public

Box 26.7 External Evaluation Systems for Health Care

Licensure is a process by which a governmental authority grants permission to an individual practitioner or health care organization to operate or to engage in an occupation or profession.

- It exists to ensure that an organization or individual meets minimum standards to protect public health and safety.
- Organizational licensure is usually granted following an on-site inspection to determine if minimum health and safety standards have been met.
- Maintenance of licensure is an ongoing requirement for the health care organization to continue to operate and care for patients.

Accreditation is a formal process by which a recognized body, usually a nongovernmental organization (NGO), assesses and recognizes that a health care organization meets applicable predetermined and published standards. Accreditation standards are:

- optimal and achievable; and
- designed to encourage continuous improvement efforts within accredited organizations.

Accreditation is granted following a periodic on-site evaluation by a team of peer reviewers, typically conducted every 2–3 years. It is often a voluntary process in which organizations choose to participate, rather than one required by law and regulation.

Certification is a process by which an authorized body evaluates and recognizes either an individual or an organization as meeting predetermined requirements or criteria. Although the terms *accreditation* and *certification* are often used interchangeably, accreditation usually applies only to organizations, while certification may apply to individuals and organizations.

Demonstrated benefits of external evaluation programs include improved organizational efficiency and effectiveness, improved safety and quality, better risk mitigation, improved leadership, reduced liability costs, better communication and teamwork, increased satisfaction of users and staff, and better patient care (see Box 26.7) [38].

To be successful and sustainable, accreditation of health facilities needs to be an ongoing process. It also requires government support, private sector buy-in, diverse incentives to encourage participation, and well-trained teams [39]. The health care accreditation program in Jordan was launched in 2003 and is now well established (Box 26.8).

Box 26.8 Jordan's Experience in Health Care Accreditation

The Jordanian experience in driving system reform, patient safety, and quality through the design, development, and implementation of accreditation at the national level has been very successful [40]. Starting with the development of standards in 2003, Jordan now has an internationally renowned Health Care Accreditation Council (HCAC), the first and foremost entity in the Eastern Mediterranean region to achieve and maintain all three International Society for Quality in Health Care External Evaluation Association (IEEA) accreditations: standards, organizations, and surveyor training accreditation programs.

To date, HCAC has more than 11 sets of accreditation standards, around 211 accredited health care institutions (including hospitals, health care centers, breast imaging units, labs, and clinics), and around 125 surveyors.

The value of accreditation in Jordan and its positive impact on quality and patient safety have been highlighted in a number of studies, showing improved efficiency; strengthened practitioner performance, employee health and safety, and interdisciplinary team effectiveness; empowered and accountable leadership with good governance; and improved service quality (patient care practices, infection prevention, and diagnostics) [41, 42].

HCAC's multilayered accreditation strategy for success includes good governance, a collaborative approach, buy-in, evidence-based approach, and multiple services supporting health care quality and patient safety (Figure 26.6).

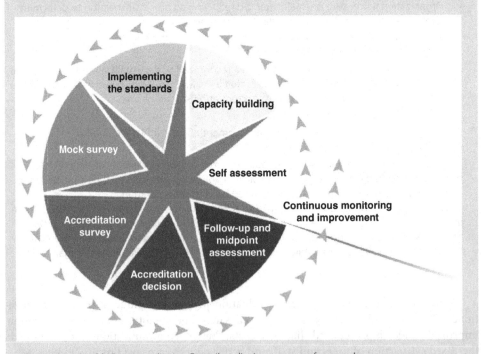

Figure 26.6 Health Care Accreditation Council quality improvement framework.

Box 26.9 Clinical Governance

"A framework through which organizations are accountable for continually improving the quality of their services and safeguarding high standards of care by creating an environment in which excellence in clinical care will flourish" [44].

Clinical Governance

Clinical governance is a general approach to QI that builds on the premise that health care professionals are the leading contributors to high-quality health care (Box 26.9) [43]. Traditionally, medical training has focused on the acquisition of knowledge and skills related to diagnostic intervention and therapeutic procedures. Clinical governance shifts the focus onto nontechnical aspects of clinical practice, including communication and teamwork.

Clinical governance is part of the corporate governance of health service organizations. It aims to ensure that everyone – from frontline clinicians to managers and members of governing bodies, such as boards – is accountable to patients and the community for the delivery of health services that are safe, effective, integrated, high quality and continuously improving (see Box 26.10) [45].

26.6.2 Specific Approaches to Evaluate and Assure Quality in Health Care Organizations

A wide range of techniques is used for assessing and ensuring the sustainability of quality and safety of defined processes in health care institutions. These include, but are not limited to, measuring the cost of quality analysis, QI teams, systematic gathering of customer data, statistical process control, clinical audit, performance benchmarking, and peer-to-peer reviews. Standards, benchmarks, and outcomes have shown good progress and impact, and include predefined criteria that support assessment and guide improvement [48, 49]. This helps guide training efforts and next steps in a QI project while using clear tools as best practices (see Table 26.4). The QI tools used during these processes include the Pareto principle, scatter plots, control charts, flow charts, cause-and-effect diagrams, histograms, and others.

26.7 Conclusion

In L&MICs, as in many other settings, improving the quality of health care is complex, requires investment, proper tools, accountability, measurable indicators, and skilled teams to design, implement, and analyze improvement interventions.

Nonetheless, addressing quality while building UHC is a huge opportunity. A health system that is maturing and becoming well established can be influenced, steered, and nurtured in the desired way. Quality can be embedded into policies, processes, and institutions as the system grows and develops.

In order to ensure successful implementation, it is important to understand the rationale for implementing QI in order to select from a number of QI models and establish approaches to continuously evaluate and sustain improvements.

Box 26.10 NHS UK Clinical Governance

The concept of clinical governance was introduced in the UK National Health Service (NHS) in 1997. It has fostered high-quality services by insisting on collaboration rather than competition, modernizing the NHS and its infrastructure, and by defining key accountabilities and responsibilities that include the quality of clinical care as well as financial performance [46].

The operation of the clinical governance framework requires (Figure 26.7) [47]:

- organizational and clinical leadership, including oversight by a designated senior clinician;
- performance review, including quality issues;
- clinical audit;
- clinical risk management;
- research and dissemination of information about the effectiveness of clinical practice;
- education, training, and continuing professional development;
- managing and learning from complaints;
- seeking and responding to user and patient views; and
- use of clinical information about patient experience.

The key benefits of effective clinical governance are:

- individual and team reflection on their practice and implementation of lessons learned;
- an open and participative climate in which education, research, and the sharing of good practice are valued;
- a commitment to quality that is shared by professionals and managers and supported by clearly identified resources, both human and financial;
- routine engagement with the public and users through an organization-wide strategy, and user representation;
- working as a multidisciplinary team; and
- strong leadership from the top.

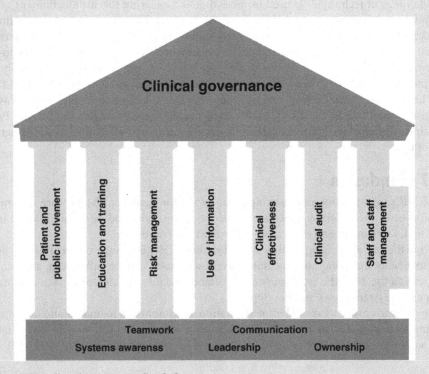

Figure 26.7 Clinical governance pillars [47].

Table 26.4 Specific approaches for quality assessment and improvement

	Purpose	Overview
1. Clinical audit [48]	To ensure that clinical care meets defined quality standards and monitor improvements to address identified shortfalls	Clinical audit can be described as a measurement of the effectiveness of health care against agreed and proven standards for high quality, followed by taking action to bring practice in line with these standards so as to assess and improve the quality of care and health outcomes. Uses a tool that requires evidence-based clinical standards drawn from best practice and audit criteria and a clearly defined population of patients (or a sample from the population) whose care will be measured using defined audit criteria.
2. Performance benchmarking [49]	To assess performance against local, national, and international performance targets, and finding and sharing best practice	Performance indicators are used as part of a benchmarking process to raise awareness of required standards and act as drivers for QI. Health care organizations and their departments strive to meet standards imposed, and those performing well demonstrate models of best practice that can be shared, becoming the benchmark against which performance is compared. Uses local, national, and international performance targets, and data collection routines for monitoring and sharing systems and processes must be in place.
3. Peer-to-peer assessment [49]	To cross-share best practices, discuss problems and actions needed in order to improve safety and quality in health care institutions	In order to create a robust and effective organizational peer-to-peer assessment process, health care systems need to: (1) establish or identify organizations, led by clinicians and supported by administrators and technical experts, to coordinate and oversee an independent, confidential, and external peer-to-peer assessment process; (2) develop and validate tools and a reliable process; (3) establish a training model and train peer evaluators; and (4) create a sustainable financial model.

References

1. Quality and Reliability Engineering International. Editorial: giants of quality – Walter Shewhart. *Qualit Reliab Eng Int* 2011. https://onlinelibrary.wiley.com/doi/epdf/10.1002/qre.1283 (accessed September 12, 2021).

2. M. Best, D. Neuhauser. W Edwards Deming: father of quality management, patient and composer. *Qual Saf Health Care* 2005; **14**(4): 310–312.

3. B. Neyestani. Principles and contributions of total quality mangement (TQM) gurus on business quality improvement. 2017. https://papers.ssrn.com/sol3/papers.cfm?abstract_id=2950981 (accessed February 16, 2022).

4. National Academies of Sciences, Engineering, and Medicine. Crossing the global quality chasm: improving health care worldwide. 2019. www.nap.edu/catalog/25152/crossing-the-global-quality-chasm-improving-health-care-worldwide (accessed September 11, 2021).

5. J. Z. Ayanian, H. Markel. Donabedian's lasting framework for health care quality. *N Engl J Med* 2016; **375**(3): 205–207.

6. J. Cantiello, P. Kitsantas, S. Moncada, et al. The evolution of quality improvement in healthcare: patient-centered care and health information technology applications. *J Hosp Admin* 2016; **5**(2): 62–68.

7. World Health Organization. Quality of care. 2022. www.who.int/health-topics/quality-of-care#tab=tab_1 (accessed February 16, 2022).

8. Agency for Healthcare Research and Quality. Practice facilitation handbook module 4. Approaches to quality improvement. 2021. www.ahrq.gov/ncepcr/tools/pf-handbook/mod4.html#:~:text=In%20health%20care%2C%20quality%20improvement,analyzed%2C%20improved%2C%20and%20controlled (accessed February 16, 2022).

9. World Health Organization. Patient safety. www.who.int/patientsafety/research/ps_online_course_session1_intro_1in1_english_2010_en.pdf (accessed February 16, 2022).

10. H. Burstin, S. Leatherman, D. Goldmann. The evolution of healthcare quality measurement in the United States. *J Intern Med* 2016; **279**(2): 154–159.

11. Toyota Production System. Lean Six Sigma definition. www.leansixsigmadefinition.com/glossary/toyota-production-system/ (accessed February 10, 2022).

12. A. Donabedian. Evaluating the quality of medical care 1966. *Milbank Q* 2005; **83**(4): 691–729.

13. M. J. Harry. Six Sigma: a breakthrough strategy for profitability. *Qual Prog* 1998; **31**(5): 60.

14. D. C. Montgomery, W. H. Woodall. An overview of six sigma. *Int Stat Rev* 2008; **76**: 329–346.

15. K. Hines. A brief history of quality improvement in health care and spinal surgery. *Global Spine J* 2020; **10**: 5S–9S.

16. M. G. Aboelmaged. Six Sigma quality: a structured review and implications for future research. *Int J Qual Reliab* 2010; **27**: 268–317.

17. P. B. Batalden, F. Davidoff. What is "quality improvement" and how can it transform healthcare? *Qual Saf Health Care* 2007; **16**(1): 2–3.

18. M. Wakefield. To err is human: an Institute of Medicine report. *Prof Psychol Res Pract* 2000; **31**(3): 243.

19. H. Askitopoulou, A. N. Vgontzas. The relevance of the Hippocratic Oath to the ethical and moral values of contemporary medicine. Part I: the Hippocratic Oath from antiquity to modern times. *Eur Spine J* 2018; **27**(7): 1481–1490.

20. World Health Organization. Patient safety: making health care safer. 2017. https://apps.who.int/iris/handle/10665/255507 (accessed September 16, 2021).

21. World Health Organization. Global patient safety action plan 2021–2030: towards eliminating avoidable harm in health care. 2021. https://apps.who.int/iris/handle/10665/343477 (accessed February 10, 2022).

22. K. R. Steffner, K. A. McQueen, A. W. Gelb. Patient safety challenges in low-income and middle-income countries. *Curr Opin Anaesthesiol* 2014; **27**(6): 623–629.

23. World Bank. Delivering quality health services: a global imperative for universal health coverage. 2018. www.worldbank.org/en/topic/universalhealthcoverage/publication/delivering-quality-health-services-a-global-imperative-for-universal-health-coverage (accessed September 18, 2021).

24. C. J. L. Murray, M. Hanlon, J. Dieleman, et al. Financing global health 2012: the end of the golden age? 2012. www.healthdata.org/policy-report/financing-global-health-2012-end-golden-age (accessed September 19, 2021).

25. J. N. Agyeman-Duah, A. Theurer, C. Munthali, et al. Understanding the barriers to setting up a healthcare quality improvement process in resource-limited settings: a situational analysis at the Medical Department of Kamuzu Central Hospital in Lilongwe, Malawi. *BMC Health Serv Res* 2014; **14**: 1.

26. M. Letaief, S. Leatherman, L. Tawfik, et al. Quality of health care and patient safety in extreme adversity settings in the Eastern Mediterranean Region: a qualitative multicountry assessment. *East Mediterr Health J* 2021; **27**(2): 167–176.

27. S. Leatherman, L. Tawfik, D. Jaff, et al. Quality health care in extreme adversity: an action framework. *Int J Qual Health Care* 2019; **31**(9): G133–G135.

28. P. Varkey. *Medical Quality Management: Theory and Practice*, 2nd ed. Burlington, Jones & Bartlett Learning, 2010.

29. E. C. Nelson, J. J. Mohr, P. B. Batalden, et al. Improving health care, Part 1: the clinical value compass. *Jt Comm J Qual Improv* 1996; **22**(4): 243–258.

30. Institute for Healthcare Improvement. Model for improvement. 2012. www.ihi .org/resources/Pages/HowtoImprove/ default.aspx (accessed February 10, 2022).

31. B. Ruth, H. Gill, M. Claire, et al. Quality improvement: theory and practice in healthcare. 2008. www.england.nhs.uk/ improvement-hub/wp-content/uploads/ sites/44/2017/11/Quality-Improvement-Theory-and-Practice-in-Healthcare.pdf (accessed September 19, 2021).

32. A. K. Lawal, T. Rotter, L. Kinsman, et al. Lean management in health care: definition, concepts, methodology and effects reported (systematic review protocol). *Syst Rev* 2014; **3**: 103.

33. E. H. Wagner. Chronic disease management: what will it take to improve care for chronic illness? *Eff Clin Pract* 1998; **1**(1): 2–4.

34. G. J. Langley, R. D. Moen, K. M. Nolan, et al. *The Improvement Guide: A Practical Approach to Enhancing Organizational Performance*. Chichester, Wiley, 2009.

35. A. Aggarwal, H. Aeran, M. Rathee. Quality management in healthcare: the pivotal desideratum. *J Oral Biol Craniofac Res* 2019; **9**(2): 180–182.

36. V. de Jonge, J. Sint Nicolaas, M. E. van Leerdam, et al. Overview of the quality assurance movement in health care. *Best Pract Res Clin Gastroenterol* 2011; **25**(3): 337–347.

37. L. Desveaux, J. I. Mitchell, J. Shaw, et al. Understanding the impact of accreditation on quality in healthcare: a grounded theory approach. *Int J Qual Health Care* 2017; **29** (7): 941–947.

38. D. Greenfield, S. A. Lawrence, A. Kellner, et al. Health service accreditation stimulating change in clinical care and human resource management processes: a study of 311 Australian hospitals. *Health Policy* 2019; **123**(7): 661–665.

39. H. Brixi, E. Lust, M. Woolcock. Trust, voice, and incentives: learning from local success stories in service delivery in the Middle East and North Africa. 2015. https://open knowledge.worldbank.org/handle/10986/ 21607 (accessed February 10, 2022).

40. T. Fortune, E. Connor, B. Donalds. Guidance on designing healthcare external evaluation programmes including accreditation. 2015. https://login.isqua .org/navless/resources/resource/19 (accessed September 19, 2021).

41. A. M. Falstie-Jensen, S. B. Bogh, S. P. Johnsen. Consecutive cycles of hospital accreditation: persistent low compliance associated with higher mortality and longer length of stay. *Int J Qual Health Care* 2018; **30**(5): 382–389.

42. Y. A. Halasa, W. Zeng, E. Chappy, et al. Value and impact of international hospital accreditation: a case study from Jordan. *East Mediterr Health J* 2015; **21** (2): 90–99.

43. Health Care Accreditation Council. What we do. 2021. https://hcac.jo/en-us/About-Us/ What-We-Do (accessed September 23, 2021).

44. G. Scally, L. J. Donaldson. The NHS's 50 anniversary: clinical governance and the drive for quality improvement in the new NHS in England. *BMJ* 1998; **317**(7150): 61–65.

45. R. Waston. Clinical governance: a guide to implementation for healthcare professionals. *J Adv Nurs* 2001; **38**: 1.

46. Australian Commission on Safety and Quality in Health Care. National model clinical governance framework. 2017. www .safetyandquality.gov.au/sites/default/files/ migrated/National-Model-Clinical-Governance-Framework.pdf (accessed February 10, 2022).

47. S. Nicholls, R. Cullen, S. O'Neill, et al. Clinical governance: its origins and its foundations. *Clin Perform Qual Health Care* 2000; **8**(3): 172–178.

48. K. M. Walshe. Principles for best practice in clinical audit. 2002. www.nice.org.uk/ media/default/About/what-we-do/Into-practice/principles-for-best-practice-in-clinical-audit.pdf (accessed September 23, 2021).

49. A. Ettorchi-Tardy, M. Levif, P. Michel. Benchmarking: a method for continuous quality improvement in health. *Healthc Policy* 2012; **7**(4): e101–e119.

Chapter 27

Harnessing the Contribution of the Private Health Care Sector toward Public Health Goals

Dominic Montagu, A. Venkat Raman, and Malabika Sarker

Key Messages

- The private sector is very large in most low- and middle-income countries (L&MICs).
- Data on private provision should be regularly collected.
- Engagement with the formal private sector is needed to achieve universal health coverage (UHC).
- Engagement should include, but not be limited to, financing of privately provided services.

27.1 Introduction

In most countries, health care services are delivered by a mix of public and private sector providers. This is true despite the widespread perception in many L&MICs that both financing and delivery of health services is the responsibility of the government, with care provided from government facilities, either free at the point of care or subsidized. Health care provided by the public sector is seen both as a safety net and public entitlement. Being the stewards of the health system, governments are indeed responsible for the overall management of health care, including the education of health professionals, the provision of medical supplies, disease outbreak surveillance, monitoring quality of care, and the day-to-day provision of care by both public and private providers [1–3].

During the past few decades, some L&MICs have struggled to adequately finance and effectively manage the public health system, leading to a steady deterioration in their ability to provide quality health care, which in turn has increased the importance of, and reliance on, private provision as citizens increasingly seek care outside of government facilities [4, 5]. At the same time, countries with rapidly growing economies have seen a steady rise in demand for health care, outstripping the capacity of government facilities and leading to the expansion of private provision at all levels of care [6]. The rising purchasing power, the epidemiological shift of the burden of illness toward long-term management of noncommunicable diseases, aging populations, growing private investment in health care, ease of access to information, and higher levels of awareness and expectations among patients have all contributed to increasing the importance of private health care provision in many L&MICs [7].

27.2 Private Health Sector and Private Health Care Sector

The private health sector is diverse and includes aspects of health beyond care provision, such as blood banks, pharmaceutical imports and manufacturing, and diagnostic care [7]. Figure 27.1 attempts to capture this diversity under five broad areas: (1) private health care providers, (2) clinical support services, (3) support industries, (4) private medical and allied health professionals' educational institutions, and (5) organized interest groups and associations. In this chapter we focus only on the components of the private health sector (PHS) that provide care – from drug sellers to single-provider clinics to tertiary hospitals and everything in between. As a shorthand, we will use the term *private health care sector* or PHCS to refer to the delivery-related private sector unless specified otherwise.

The PHCS is not a homogeneous group of service providers. It ranges from informal caregivers using traditional or indigenous systems of medicine to the Western system of medicine. Moreover, the PHCS includes both "for-profit" and "nonprofit" groups. Polyclinics, nursing homes, specialty hospitals, and hospitals affiliated to medical colleges constitute various forms of private sector facilities. Further differentiation within the private sector exists according to the primary funding source (user fees, donations, government contracts, or insurance) and level of quality assurance (accredited or not, and by whom). While most private sector providers and facilities are independent, in a number of middle-income countries the proportion of "corporate" hospitals and hospital chains, while still small, is growing [8, 9].

The most significant subdivision within the PHCS is according to ownership and motivation. Not-for-profit providers are typically health facilities funded or managed by philanthropic, religious, or charitable trusts, and in some countries by external donors, and are termed nongovernmental organizations (NGOs). Although there are a small number of countries where religious hospitals provide up to one-quarter of facilities and care (notably the Philippines, Indonesia, Tanzania, and Benin), in most countries the

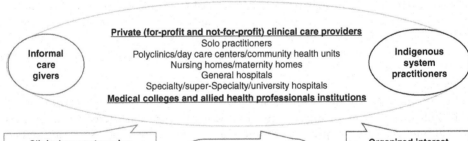

Figure 27.1 The PHS in L&MICs: providers and the ecosystem. *Source:* Adopted from A.Venkat Raman. Private health sector policy: a guidance document on private health sector in the national health policy. Policy brief (unpublished). WHO-Geneva. June 2020 (TRL90935)

private sector is overwhelmingly for-profit [10, 11]. This is particularly true for dispensing and outpatient diagnostic services, which are nearly always both private and for-profit – examples include pharmacies, drugs sellers, and laboratories for routine tests [12].

27.3 Characteristics and Attributes of the Private Health Care Sector

27.3.1 Evolution and Growth of Private Health Care Providers

In nearly all countries around the world, health care services trace their origins to private practitioners and charitable facilities. In sub-Saharan Africa, the backbone of health services under colonial rule were the mission hospitals and clinics [13]. In Mexico and much of Latin America, early hospitals were established by the Catholic Church [14]. Government prominence in care provision took over in some countries as part of larger political shifts as in the case of the former Soviet Union and countries in Eastern Europe, but has mostly made space for private care to exist in parallel [14]. In Vietnam, the government started allowing private medical services in the early 1990s, which have been growing rapidly since then [6, 15, 16].

Growth of private provision in recent decades has been rapid in many countries, particularly China and countries such as Kazakhstan or Tanzania, which were previously influenced by the statist models of the Soviet Union. However, health systems are slow to change, and the global data does not support a universally shared trend toward private sector growth. Two analyses of global household survey data in the past 15 years concur that private health care provision is growing in some countries, shrinking in others, and overall largely static as a proportion of all care provided [10, 17]. There are, nevertheless, some clear global commonalities – charitable care is less important now than 50 years ago, and for-profit care more significant. In nearly all countries private provision is much more predominant in urban settings, where patients are numerous and incomes are higher. Population density and greater wealth, for obvious reasons, makes the business of health care – whether in a pharmacy or a hospital – more attractive to providers, investors, and entrepreneurs.

27.3.2 Responsiveness of Private Health Care Providers

For patients, private providers are often popular because they are easy to access, have longer working hours, and shorter waiting times – critical to the working poor who cannot afford a day off from work to wait for medical treatment – and are responsive to the demands or unspoken expectations of patients, even if it is contrary to best medical practice. Antibiotics are available over the counter in most L&MICs and are widely overprescribed. In fact, many formal and informal primary care providers make most of their profit from sales of medicines [18]. Studies have shown that patients in all countries are more satisfied when they leave with some kind of treatment, even when that treatment, like antibiotics for a viral infection, may not be warranted [19, 20]. Private providers may be more or less skilled than their public counterparts; however, they are frequently more responsive to the preferences of their paying "customers" [21]. As a result, many patients hold to the unfounded assumption that private care is of higher clinical quality than public care.

27.3.3 Increase in Utilization of the Private Health Care Sector

While preventive care is arguably the most critical aspect of health services to overall population health, it is not what comes to mind for most when thinking of a health system. The health care delivery component of the PHCS is the most visible aspects of the overall health system. It absorbs the largest amount of financing, specialized staffing, oversight, and attention. Patients overwhelmingly think first of "care" – from a pharmacy or from a maternity center – when thinking about health systems. If care is affordable and good, the overall health system is working well. If it is not, then something is wrong and interventions are needed. For this reason, attention to the organization of care provision is central to understanding how a health system addresses population needs.

Household surveys across 70 L&MICs suggest that 67% of diarrhea and 63% of fever cases among children are attended to by private providers [22, 23]. While there is variation among the six regions of the World Health Organization, the private sector is important in all. It provides nearly 40% of all health care in pan-American, African, and Western Pacific Regions, 57% in the Southeast Asian Region, and 62% in the Eastern Mediterranean Region (EMR). In countries of the EMR, 81% of the poorest quintile seek services from the private sector [10]. Additionally, in Egypt, Pakistan, and India more than two-thirds of all outpatient care is provided by the private sector, while within hospitals and clinics data shows that in Egypt, Pakistan, and Bangladesh more than two-thirds of all institutional deliveries are provided by the private sector [10, 24].

Apart from medicine sales and clinical care, a wide range of clinical support service providers, such as laboratories, diagnostic centers, blood banks, pharmacies, and ambulance operators, exist predominantly in the private sector. In India and a few other countries, the majority of medical education and training institutions are run by the private sector [25, 26]. The private sector also dominates pharmaceuticals, biomedical equipment and devices, and clinical and nonclinical supplies.

27.3.4 Informality in the Private Health Care Sector

Informality characterizes much of care at the lower end of the spectrum. A high proportion of people in both rural areas and urban slums in L&MICs depend on the "services" rendered by unqualified providers categorized as "quacks," informal practitioners, and "faith-healers," all working for pay, albeit outside of the regulatory and quality assurance systems and/or government oversight [27, 28]. At the same time, informality does not imply a clear differentiation from services of formal care. The overlap exists clearly in a few areas of clinical care, notably in support for delivery of services, and is widespread in the sale of pharmaceuticals. Drug sellers serving lower-income communities are common, whether wholly unlicensed or licensed only for over-the-counter medicines, and these sellers frequently sell a wide range of Western medicines, which are normally prescription drugs and should only be sold by trained and licensed pharmacists. In some countries, especially in Asia, a significant proportion of private care providers are licensed practitioners of indigenous health systems of medicine (e.g., *Ayurveda, Tibb, Unani,* and homeopathy), and are not to be considered as part of the informal sector.

27.3.5 Expansion of Digital Technology in the Private Health Care Sector

In recent years there has been a growing number of social entrepreneurs and technology-based service providers (e.g., telemedicine, digital health, m-health, e-pharmacy) in the health care delivery domain. While these remain only a small section of the overall care sector, they have expanded during the COVID-19 pandemic due to lack of access to hospitals, pharmacies, and diagnostic facilities.

27.4 Harnessing the PHCS toward Public Sector Goals

27.4.1 Regulation of the PHCS

Private providers, both nonprofit and for-profit, are driven by many motivations, including the desire to cure, to ensure community betterment, to serve the needy, to achieve the highest possible level of quality, and to generate income and profit. Like their public sector counterparts, private providers respond to incentives, both positive and negative. They seek to make money, ensure and enhance their personal and institutional reputations, adhere to the tenets of science and rationality, be efficient, and more.

The regulation of private providers by governments seeks to encourage the best aspects of private care (entrepreneurial innovation and investment; responsiveness to the priorities of patients and clients; experimentation with new business models, opening hours, locations, and technologies) and deter the worst (conflict of interest as providers diagnose, treat, and sell medicines to patients; prioritizing the wealthy over the poor; over-treatment; or the focus on quality of "hotel services" rather than quality of "clinical services," the latter being frequently less visible to paying clients). Box 27.1 provides a simplified framework for regulation of PHS, which is equally relevant to public health care facilities.

Box 27.1 Framework for Regulating the Private (and Public) Health Sector

What Is Regulation?

The sustained use of various control mechanisms, including coercive measures, if needed, and/or incentives for influencing behavior to address health system issues or problems and to help attain desired health system objectives.

Why Regulate?

To change the behaviors and practices of the following:

Individuals – providers such as physicians, dentists, pharmacists

Institutions – health care facilities, associations of health professionals' education

Market – the pharmaceutical sector

Public – reckless driving, junk food, smoking

What to Regulate?

Quality – of care (patient safety, avoid medical negligence)

Price – of lab tests, medicines, consultations, procedure

Volume – supply of medical devices, diagnostics, services, etc.

Distribution – e.g., urban crowding of hospitals

Market – private insurance market; pharmaceutical sector

Demand – for unhealthy food, tobacco; supplier-induced demand (e.g., antibiotics, injections, etc.)

How to Regulate?

Coercive approach – legislation is a prerequisite; development of regulations and rules; standard setting; strengthening enforcement mechanisms (e.g., institutional – drug regulatory authority; individual – food inspectors); impose sanctions or penalties; monitoring and feedback

Incentive-based approach – financial incentives (tax subsidies, pay for performance, cash transfers [for population]; nonfinancial incentives – training, career advancement, social marketing)

Regulatory Tools (Some Examples)

Individual (professionals) – e.g., registration, certification, credentialing, privileging

Institutional – e.g., licensing, quality assurance, audit, accreditation

Who Should Regulate?

Government – regulatory authorities (e.g., Ministries of Health, food and drug authorities)

Independent bodies – medical, dental, and nursing councils; orders of allied health professionals; health care commissions; accrediting bodies

Professionals' associations – self-regulation, code of ethics

A broad understanding of the regulatory aspects of governance often includes efforts to ensure greater transparency and accountability, optimization of financial incentives and disincentives, and the generation and enforcement of a wide range of regulations regarding private practice in the medical fields. Typical regulatory dimensions involve ensuring providers are *registered* with the proper governmental body, that businesses, whether pharmacies or hospitals, are *licensed* to provide services, are *inspected* regularly, and are *staffed* by professionals who meet the training standards appropriate to their role. Standards exist in most countries that cover all aspects of care, such as the sourcing and storage of pharmaceuticals, the methods and frequency of equipment sterilization, and the annual recertification for practice of surgeons, anesthetists, and ambulance drivers. Professional organizations in many countries set the standards and certification requirements for practice by their members, and governments then require that those certifications are up to date. Commonly, the implementation of regulations is delegated to subnational entities such as the local district or state; however, many have limited capacity to enforce the regulations.

Regulations ultimately are the practical embodiment of national policies and legislation, as the latter are inherently more generic and broader. Some countries, such as the Philippines, Thailand, and South Africa, have encouraged and incentivized the growth of PHS as a policy, whereas in others private provision of care has grown indiscriminately, without regulatory supervision of physical standards, quality, tariffs, geographical location, or staffing norms, such as in Egypt, Nigeria, Pakistan, and Sudan. In most L&MICs, regulatory oversight is limited in scope and effectiveness. Often this is due to the complexity of regulatory issues, lack of local staffing, lack of clarity regarding oversight authority and guidance for enforcement, conflicting authorities between different branches or levels of government, and frequent challenges of corruption and weak management. While many aspects of governance in other sectors are highly visible and thus influenced by public opinion – air transport safety, for instance – most dimensions of health care are difficult for the public to assess, and so weak regulation of private providers can and often does endure.

The lack of regulation is problematic for two reasons: quality and cost. Health care transactions are highly idiosyncratic, meaning they are dependent on the needs and desires of the patient, which can vary greatly from person to person depending on age, sex, genetic makeup, personal, cultural, or religious preferences, comorbidities, ability to pay for care, or other factors. Health care transactions also stand out for the high level of differential information between the provider and the patient – a differential that exists in brain surgery or in treatment for pediatric fever. Many studies have shown that patients are extremely poor judges of clinical quality [19, 29–32], and the obvious challenges with comparison-shopping for clinical care (imagine trying to compare hospitals when seeking treatment for an urgent medical issue) leave patients at a disadvantage when trying to ensure both the quality of care and the appropriateness of costs.

Ensuring quality and affordability requires effective regulation in addition to other aspects of government payment or encouragement. Planning for how to inform, support, and enforce laws and standards is needed before governments can effectively make the shift from policy to legislation and regulation. Within different departments and levels of government this requires clarifying roles and authority. The importance cannot be over-stated, for in nearly all countries ensuring the effective regulation of private health provision is central to ensuring effective health system functioning.

Where governance systems are strong, regulators step in to ensure quality and often to set rules on pricing transparency. Where purchasers of care are large, well organized, and properly incentivized – whether governments or social health insurance systems or large private health insurance companies – they are able to negotiate strongly on the basis of large registered populations, and to demand standardized pricing, thorough documentation, and predictability of both quality and cost. Unfortunately, neither strong governance nor organized large purchasers are the norm in most L&MICs. The result is wide variation in quality and cost among private providers. Studies have shown that the resulting risks of poor treatment or family impoverishment due to medical costs fall most heavily on the poor [33–35].

27.4.2 Public–Private Engagement: First and Foremost

Government commitments to achieve UHC in recent years have led to growing attention to, and interest in active engagement with, private providers of health care in many L&MICs (see Chapter 28). In countries where one-third or half of all health services are provided by private hospitals, clinics, providers, and pharmacies, there is no way to UHC without engaging this component of the overall health system.

What that engagement looks like naturally varies. In papers and courses for the World Bank, the authors have previously described the four key approaches to engagement depending on governmental priorities, regulator and fiscal capacity, the organization and quality of private provision, and health-seeking preferences of the population [36]. These four approaches include prohibition, constraint, encouragement, or purchase, each responding to one or more identified market failures (Figure 27.2) [37]. *Prohibition* of the private sector is seldom effective: it requires strong governance and enforcement systems and implies the

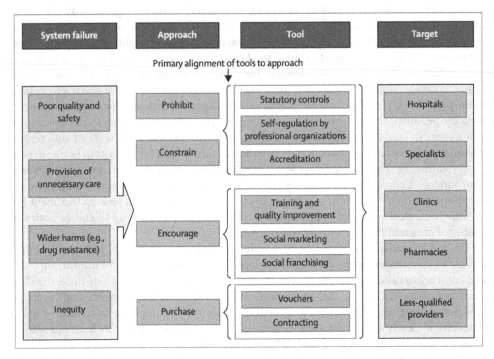

Figure 27.2 Approaches to private health care sector engagement. Reproduced from [37].

existence of public alternatives. Both are rare, and so effective prohibition is seldom appropriate or attempted. *Encouragement* and *constraint* are effectively two sides of the same coin – policy strategies toward the private sector effected by a mix of regulatory methods. The latter include strengthening or weakening the enforcement of licensure, registration, employment, oversight, and quality assessment rules along with related regulations on access to finance, data reporting standards, and referrals or other interactions with the public sector.

The strongest engagement method, providing the most scope for assuring quality and appropriate pricing and influencing public health-related benefits, is the fourth method noted above: *purchase*. The widespread adoption of UHC as a goal in many countries has led to an unprecedented expansion of government contracting and both direct and indirect purchasing of privately delivered health care from private providers (see Chapter 18). In some instances, such as in Ghana, Mexico, and Lesotho, this has been accomplished through direct government contracts to providers. More common has been the creation or expansion of national or social health insurance agencies that collect and disburse money quasi-independently from government and so are more easily able to maintain independent standards for pricing, provision, quality, and related norms, and to enforce these as a condition of payment eligibility among both private and public institutions (see Chapter 17). In Kenya, the Philippines, South Africa, and many other countries the expansion of social health insurance systems is facilitating private sector engagement, particularly for hospitals, nursing homes, and to a lesser extent clinics. Growing evidence confirms that this expansion is leading to increased facility-level quality accreditation and use of care by the poor and other previously excluded populations.

The experiences of OECD countries make clear that assuring these benefits in the future will require investment in oversight, accounting and claims reviews, and enforcement [38]. A similar engagement on a smaller scale has happened in many countries to support service or disease-specific services. Tuberculosis care, family planning, malaria testing and treatment, and some maternity services are often subsidized in the private sector, with free or below-cost medicines supplied to providers in order to increase access to goods and services critical to public health [39–41]. Distributing subsidized medicines and diagnostics holds less risk and requires less oversight than supporting the provision of wide-ranging clinical treatments. Experience with these less complex support programs is important in building positive relations between public and private actors, and in giving government regulators experiences in engagement that can provide a foundation for the more intensive work needed to purchase general services [42]. By the same token, contracting for deliveries, HIV/AIDS care, pediatrics, or a broad range of health care serving all ages, while more complex and expensive, can also provide more scope for purchasers to set and enforce conditions [43]. The conditions for payment can be set to complement regulatory goals and ensure that private actors meet quality and public benefit criteria. Examples could include requiring third-party quality accreditation for hospitals, or cold-chains for drug storage, sterilization standards, opening hours, patient records and privacy, and a host of other norms important for ensuring health care quality, for building patient confidence, and for increasing early health-seeking practices.

The government cannot be a passive participant in health provision, even when – perhaps especially when – provision is significantly undertaken by private providers and organizations. Engagement by policymakers and regulators cannot be limited to expanded financing alone. Engagement is a key precondition for governance and ensuring the safe and beneficial activities of the private health care sector within the larger health system. When coupled with effective regulation – with clear rules on licensure, quality, transparency, staff qualification, equipment standards, and a host of other issues, engagement through dialog and financial support can make the formal components of the private sector effective partners to advance UHC. Engagement and regulation are combined in the national health policies of some L&MICs.

27.4.3 Data Sharing and Information Compliance

The precondition for developing or refining strategies and policies toward the private sector must begin with accurate estimates of the number of private providers at different levels of care, their geographic distribution, and the range and volume of services they provide. In many L&MICs this first hurdle is still a bottleneck to good policies because accurate master facility lists do not exist. When that is the case, getting the count right must be a priority.

The informal private sector, by definition, is not compliant with licensure and registration standards, and does not report data to government purchasers, regulators, or into the broader public sector health information system [26]. For this reason, engagement must always prioritize formal private sector providers. Regulation and financial engagement are both predicated on good information: what services were provided, using what diagnostics, equipment, and medicines; how often, to whom, and with what outcome. While a system of reporting from government clinics and hospitals exists in most L&MICs and is reasonably well functioning in many, reporting from private providers at all levels is widely agreed to be poor. There are many reasons for this: reporting is onerous, it brings few or no benefits, and it opens providers to risks – of greater attention, accusations of providing unlicensed services, and demands for taxes or unofficial payments by government agents at all levels. In a growing number of L&MICs, national data information systems have made data reporting more standardized, faster, and easier [44]. This has not yet expanded to private providers.

It is clear that ensuring better data reporting will require the introduction of either new rules and enforcement, or new incentives. Health systems academics are currently hoping that expanding purchase agreements either directly from governments or indirectly through social health insurance agencies will provide enough incentive to overcome the real and perceived risks [45]. In the meantime, governments need to ensure registration of local businesses is in place for clinics, push for more effective clinical licensure verification, and advance dialogs with and self-regulation by private representative bodies, such as private hospital associations and private clinical specialist associations. These representative organizations are a key vehicle to increase awareness and adoption of electronic health information system reporting by private facilities and ensure the most accurate picture possible of where services are provided and by whom. Nationally representative surveys such as the USAID-supported Demographic Health Surveys (DHS), which are conducted every five years in over 40 countries around the world, can also provide some basic information to estimate private sector importance. This is only indicative, and encouraging better data sharing – through ease of engagement, ensuring nonpunitive uses, and financial incentives – is the key first step to effective governance.

27.4.4 Cost of Private Health Care

Privately delivered health care exists at the highest end of care in many L&MICs, including quite often the very best hospitals measured by clinical excellence, staff training and comprehensiveness of modern equipment and methods, patient–staff ratios, waiting times, and what are broadly characterized as "hotel services," meaning the comfort of patients before, during, and after care. These facilities charge rates in accordance with their standards and are highly priced by local and sometimes international norms. Private health care also, as noted above, dominates the lowest end of the health care spectrum, providing near-to-patient drug sales, diagnostics, outpatient services of all kinds, formal and informal clinical care, and more. These services range from very low-priced to over-priced – a challenge for patients because the unpredictability of costs is inherent to most medical care. Often comparable care is free in government facilities.

Higher-end hospitals in particular offer treatments that include high-end technologies and highly paid specialists not available in public facilities. This can both explain and probably justify high costs of care; and also create dangerous incentives for these specialists to conduct costly diagnostics or treatments in order to ensure the use of expensive technologies that in turn require patients to pay fee-based charges. In L&MICs, an unregulated PHS escalates health care costs, negatively affects quality and patient safety, equity, access, and health system priorities. In countries where PHS is a major service provider and where private out-of-pocket (OOP) payment is the mode of financing for accessing services, the economic consequences for poor households could be devastating. The share of OOP expenditure as a percentage of total health expenditure is estimated to be 78% in Afghanistan, 77% in Iraq, 67% in Pakistan, 63% in Sudan, and more than 63% in India.

In many instances the public and private clinicians are the same [46]. While numbers are hard to come by, studies in Angola, Indonesia, Peru, and elsewhere have reported dual public–private practice among clinicians to be "ubiquitous and unregulated" [47, 48]. While this raises concerns for many reasons, not least self-referrals as public doctors advise patients to visit their private clinic after hours, there is some evidence that the same provider, operating in both public and private clinics, gives better clinical care in private – due largely to spending more time with patients and asking more questions about their illnesses [46, 49]. The incentives to be responsive to patients can lead to positive outcomes as well.

27.5 Conclusion

The private sector represents a significant part of health care services in nearly all countries, sometimes the dominant part. Despite this, data collection, effective integration into referrals and reporting systems, and guarantees of quality and cost limits are all weak in most L&MICs. This needs to change, and it seems likely to. Public–private partnerships (see Chapter 28) are increasing along with integration of private providers into national data reporting systems, training programs, referral systems, and service payments either directly from government or through a social health insurance intermediary. There is a growing recognition that achieving the goal of UHC is possible only if the public and private sectors work together; and that governments can no longer ignore the role of the private sector in the country's health system. If properly engaged and regulated, the PHS can positively contribute to the population's health care needs and strengthen the overall health system of the country.

Regulation of private providers is a large part of the work of health departments and ministries in these countries. Private provision is not disappearing anywhere in the world, and so to ensure effective governance for UHC the private sector will need to be prioritized in L&MICs, for which a significant level of effort and investment in oversight and regulation needs to be made by Ministries of Health in these countries.

References

1. G. Lagomarsino, D. de Ferranti, A. Pablos-Mendez, et al. Public stewardship of mixed health systems. *Lancet* 2009; **374**(9701): 1577–1578.

2. World Health Organization. Engaging the private health service delivery sector through governance in mixed health systems. 2020. www.who.int/docs/default-source/health-system-governance/strategy-report-engaging-the-private-health-service-delivery-sector-through-governance-in-mixed-health-systems.pdf?sfvrsn=3 e870582_1 (accessed November 6, 2021).

3. World Bank. Healthy partnerships: how governments can engage the private sector to improve health in Africa. 2011. https://openknowledge.worldbank.org/handle/10986/2304 (accessed November 8, 2021).

4. S. K. Hooda. Growth of formal and informal private health care providers in India: structural changes and implications. *J Health Care Finance* 2017; **44**(2).

5. S. Davalbhakta, S. Sharma, S. Gupta, et al. Private health sector in India: ready and willing, yet underutilized in the Covid-19 pandemic – a cross-sectional study. *Front Public Health* 2020; **8**: 571419.

6. K. Hort, P. Annear. The growth of non-state hospitals in Indonesia and Vietnam: market reforms and mixed commercialised health systems. 2012. www.ssrn.com/abstrac t=2069757 (accessed November 5, 2021).

7. M. Mackintosh, A. Channon, A. Karan, et al. What is the private sector? Understanding private provision in the health systems of

low-income and middle-income countries. *Lancet* 2016; **388**(10044): 596–605.

8. R. Morgan, T. Ensor. The regulation of private hospitals in Asia. *Int J Health Plann Manage* 2016; **31**(1): 49–64.

9. A.Venkat Raman, J.W. Bjorkman. *Public–Private Partnership in Health Care in India*, London, Routledge, 2009.

10. D. Montagu, N. Chakraborty. Standard survey data: insights into private sector utilization. *Front Med (Lausanne)* 2021; **8**: 624285.

11. R. C. Kagawa, A. Anglemyer, D. Montagu. The scale of faith based organization participation in health service delivery in developing countries: systematic [corrected] review and meta-analysis. *PLoS One* 2012; **7**(11): e48457.

12. Z. U. Babar. Ten recommendations to improve pharmacy practice in low and middle-income countries (LMICs). *J Pharm Policy Pract* 2021; **14**(1): 6.

13. B. McPake. Hospital policy in Sub-Saharan Africa and post-colonial development impasse. *Soc Hist Med* 2009; **22**(2): 341–360.

14. J. L. León-Cortés, G. Leal Fernández, H. J. Sánchez-Pérez. Health reform in Mexico: governance and potential outcomes. *Int J Equity Health* 2019; **18**(1): 30.

15. S. Witter. "Doi Moi" and health: the effect of economic reforms on the health system in Vietnam. *Int J Health Plann* 1996; **11**(2): 159–172.

16. N. T. Chuc, G. Tomson. "Doi moi" and private pharmacies: a case study on dispensing and financial issues in Hanoi, Vietnam. *Eur J Clin Pharmacol* 1999; **55**(4): 325–332.

17. K. A. Grépin. Private sector an important but not dominant provider of key health services in low- and middle-income countries. *Health Aff (Millwood)* 2016; **35** (7): 1214–1221.

18. S. Siddiqi, S. Hamid, G. Rafique, et al. Prescription practices of public and private health care providers in Attock District of Pakistan. *Int J Health Plann Mgmt* 2002; 17 (1): 3–40.

19. R. Trivedi, K. Jagani. Perceived service quality, repeat use of health care services and inpatient satisfaction in emerging economy: empirical evidences from India. *Int J Pharm Healthc Mark* 2018; **12**(3): 288–306.

20. G. J. Young, M. Meterko, K. R. Desai. Patient satisfaction with hospital care: effects of demographic and institutional characteristics. *Med Care* 2000; **38**(3): 325–334.

21. A. Khattak, M. I. Alvi, M. A. Yousaf, et al. Patient satisfaction: a comparison between public & private hospitals of Peshawar. *IJCRIMPH* 2012; **4**(5): 713–722.

22. N. M. Chakraborty, A. Sprockett. Use of family planning and child health services in the private sector: an equity analysis of 12 DHS surveys. *Int J Equity Health* 2018; **17** (1): 50.

23. K. A. Grépin. Private sector an important but not dominant provider of key health services in low- and middle-income countries. *Health Aff (Millwood)* 2016; **35** (7): 1214–1221.

24. National Institute of Population Studies (NIPS). Pakistan Demographic and Health Survey, 2017–18. 2019. https://dhsprogram .com/pubs/pdf/FR354/FR354.pdf (accessed November 19, 2021).

25. N. M. Shah, W. R. Brieger, D. H. Peters. Can interventions improve health services from informal private providers in low and middle-income countries? A comprehensive review of the literature. *Health Policy Plan* 2011; **26**(4): 275–287.

26. M. Sudhinaraset, M. Ingram, H. K. Lofthouse, et al. What is the role of informal health care providers in developing countries? A systematic review. *PLoS One* 2013; **8**(2): e54978.

27. A. Solanki, S. Kashyap. Medical education in India: current challenges and the way forward. *Med Teach* 2014; **36**(12): 1027–1031.

28. A. Mahal, M. Mohanan. Growth of private medical education in India. *Med Educ* 2006; **40**(10): 1009–1011.

29. R. P. Rannan-Eliya, N. Wijemanne, I. K. Liyanage, et al. The quality of outpatient primary care in public and private sectors in Sri Lanka: how well do patient perceptions match reality and what are the implications? *Health Policy Plann* 2015; 30(Suppl. 1): i59–i74.

30. D. C. McFarland, M. J. Shen, P. Parker, et al. Does hospital size affect patient satisfaction? *Qual Manag Health Care* 2017; 26(4): 205–209.

31. R. Fayyaz, F. A. Ahmed, A. Abid, et al. The quality of patient care in oncology departments in Karachi, Pakistan: patients' perceptions. *Int J Health Care Qual Assur* 2020. doi: 10.1108/IJHCQA-12-2019-0201.

32. N. Aujla, Y. F. Chen, Y. Samarakoon, et al. Comparing the use of direct observation, standardized patients and exit interviews in low- and middle-income countries: a systematic review of methods of assessing quality of primary care. *Health Policy Plann* 2021; 36(3): 341–356.

33. J. Yadav, G. R. Menon, D. John. Disease-specific out-of-pocket payments, catastrophic health expenditure and impoverishment effects in India: an analysis of national health survey data. *Appl Health Econ* 2021; 19: 769–782.

34. E. W. Barasa, T. Maina, N. Ravishankar. Assessing the impoverishing effects, and factors associated with the incidence of catastrophic health care payments in Kenya. *Int J Equity Health* 2017; 16 (1): 31.

35. J. A. M. Khan, S. Ahmed, T. G. Evans. Catastrophic health care expenditure and poverty related to out-of-pocket payments for health care in Bangladesh: an estimation of financial risk protection of universal health coverage. *Health Policy Plan* 2017; 32(8): 1102–1110.

36. A. Harding, D. Montagu. Role of the private sector in health-care financing and provision. In B. Carrin, Q. Heggenhougen, eds., *Health Systems Policy, Finance, and Organization*. Geneva, Elsevier, 2009.

37. D. Montagu, C. Goodman. Prohibit, constrain, encourage, or purchase: how should we engage with the private health-care sector? *Lancet* 2016; 388 (10044): 613–621.

38. D. Montagu. The provision of private health care services in European countries: recent data and lessons for universal health coverage in other settings. *Front Public Health* 2021; 9: 636750.

39. B. Randive, V. Diwan, A. De Costa. India's conditional cash transfer programme (the JSY) to promote institutional birth: is there an association between institutional birth proportion and maternal mortality? *PLoS One* 2013; 8(6): e67452.

40. S. Tougher, Y. Ye, J. H. Amuasi, et al. Effect of the Affordable Medicines Facility-malaria (AMFm) on the availability, price, and market share of quality-assured artemisinin-based combination therapies in seven countries: a before-and-after analysis of outlet survey data. *Lancet* 2012; 380(9857): 1916–1926.

41. K. Lönnroth, M. Uplekar, V. K. Arora, et al. Public–private mix for DOTS implementation: what makes it work? *Bull World Health Organ* 2004; 82: 580–586.

42. B. McPake, K. Hanson. Managing the public–private mix to achieve universal health coverage. *Lancet* 2016; 388(10044): 622–630.

43. M. Lagarde, N. Palmer. The impact of contracting out on health outcomes and use of health services in low and middle-income countries. *Cochrane Database Syst Rev* 2009; 4: CD008133.

44. G. Karara, F. Verbeke, M. Nyssen. The role of hospital information systems in universal health coverage monitoring in Rwanda. *Stud Health Technol Inform* 2015; 216: 193–197.

45. World Health Organization. Social health insurance: sustainable health financing, universal coverage and social health insurance: report by the Secretariat. 2005. https://apps.who.int/iris/handle/10665/20302 (accessed November 18, 2021).

46. J. Das, A. Holla, V. Das, et al. In urban and rural India, a standardized patient study showed low levels of provider training and huge quality gaps. *Health Aff (Millwood)* 2012; 31(12): 2774–2784.

47. B. B. Báez-Montiel, E. Gutiérrez-Islas, M. Bolaños-Maldonado, et al. The odysseys of Ulysses: a study of tales in a normal working day of the family doctor in Paraguay, Mexico, Peru, and Spain. *Aten Primaria* 2014; **46**(2): 68–76. In Spanish.

48. D. Macaia, L. V. Lapão. The current situation of human resources for health in the province of Cabinda in Angola: is it a limitation to provide universal access to health care? *Hum Resour Health* 2017; **15** (1): 88.

49. J. Das, J. Hammer. Money for nothing: the dire straits of medical practice in Delhi, India. *J Dev Econ* 2007; **83**(1): 1–36.

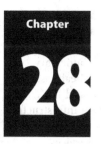

Chapter 28

Public–Private Partnership in Health Care Services

A. Venkat Raman

Key Messages

- Achieving universal health coverage (UHC) is not possible without mobilizing all the health sector resources, including the private health sector.
- Public–private partnership (PPP) is desirable as it could help improve much-needed health infrastructure, optimally manage existing health facilities, improve access to underserved groups, and reduce financial distress among the poor.
- There are several models and methods of engaging the private sector for a myriad of objectives, which should be considered while involving the private sector.
- Before embarking on PPP, governments should systematically plan to strengthen the policy, legal, and regulatory ecosystem; strengthen institutional mechanisms; establish organizational units and enhance their technical and managerial capacity; and create fiscal space for partnerships.
- PPPs are highly contextual and any search for a standard formula or a template that guarantees better outcomes is not realistic.
- To ensure that PPPs support the achievement of health equity central to UHC, there is a need to build consensus around the means and strategies of partnership and its objectives between public sector, private providers, and the community stakeholders.

28.1 Introduction

There is hardly a country in the world where health care is financed or provided entirely by the government. While promoting, maintaining, and restoring the health of its citizens is widely recognized as the responsibility of government, private capital and expertise are increasingly viewed as welcome sources to promote efficiency and innovation. What is less clear, however, is the appropriate balance of public and private resources in financing and managing health and how to ensure that the two work in unison. One such arrangement is PPPs, whereby governments are increasingly looking at the various options to solve larger problems in care delivery and wellness and to improve the health of their citizens [1].

The UN Sustainable Development Goals (SDGs) [2], especially Goal 17, reiterate that governments should find ways to effectively harness the private sector and "encourage and promote effective public–private, and civil society partnerships." Recognizing the importance of working with the private health care sector (PHS), the 63rd World Health Assembly (2010; Resolution #27) stated that "private providers play a significant and growing role in health care delivery across the world . . . engagement of [range of private] providers can lead to [their] constructive role in providing essential health services" [3]. The importance of collaboration, engagement, and partnership (with the private sector and civil society organizations) is considered essential to achieve UHC.

According to the World Bank, governments are increasingly facing budgetary constraints to invest in health infrastructure and improve access to quality health services and are therefore exploring PPPs to leverage resources, capital, capacity, and know-how from the private sector [4]. PPPs were traditionally restricted to developing infrastructure (such as transport and energy). However, during the past few decades PPPs have been increasingly deployed in social sectors, including in the delivery of health services.

28.2 Defining Public–Private Partnership

Public–private partnership as a policy option presumes that the health care needs of people could be met more effectively if both sectors worked together. Although widely used, the term "public–private partnership" often evokes an ideological response. Some consider PPP as covert privatization, whereas others view all forms of interaction between government and the private sector as PPP [5]. There is no single universally accepted definition of PPP. Some of these definitions, not restricted to the health sector, are given in Box 28.1.

Drawing from these definitions, the key characteristics of PPP in the health sector include collaborative efforts with mutually agreed obligations, accountability, and benefits;

Box 28.1 Selected Definitions of PPP

A long-term contractual arrangement between public (national, state, provincial, or local) and private entities through which the skills, assets, and/or financial resources of each of the public and private sectors are allocated in a complementary manner – thereby sharing the risks and rewards, to seek to provide optimal service delivery and good value to citizens. [6]

An agreement between the government and one or more private partners (which may include the operators and the financers) . . . within the agreement, the private partners deliver the service so that the service delivery objectives of the government are aligned with the profit objectives of the private partners . . . government specifies the quality and quantity of the service it requires from the private partner. Furthermore, the effectiveness of the alignment depends on a sufficient transfer of risk to the private partners. [7]

In the health sector, PPP is defined as

Variety of cooperative and contractual arrangements between the government and private sector in delivering public goods or services and/or securing the use of assets necessary to deliver public services. The structure of the partnership varies to take advantage of the expertise of each partner, so that resources, risks and rewards can be allocated in a way that best meets clearly defined public health needs. [8]

Collaborative effort and reciprocal relationship between the government or a public authority and a private organization with carefully structured, time-bound, formal agreements with clear terms and conditions, mutual commitments, with specified performance indicators for the production or delivery of specified set of health services. [5]

clear ownership and financing responsibilities; defined timeframe; shared risks; well-defined management structures; specified quality and performance indicators; efficient deployment of resources; and harmonizing public goods (health services) with private commercial interests.

PPPs should be based on certain foundational principles, such as: a sense of equality between partners (not a master–servant relationship); mutual trust (not by formal contract alone); recognition of mutual benefits (financial gain as a legitimate motive of the private sector); right to decisional autonomy; and a shared commitment toward public health objectives. Partnerships are therefore distinct from traditional procurement contracts. Viewed from the principal–agent perspective (see Chapter 4), partnerships can be seen as complete only if issues of information asymmetries, moral hazards, and adverse selection are clearly addressed by the partners (Box 28.2).

It is also critical to understand that PPP is not privatization or perpetual transfer of public assets to private ownership, nor the abdication of the government's role in the provision of health services. Even under PPP, the government continues to be responsible for ensuring health services for all, with more direct attention to socially and economically vulnerable populations by leveraging on its own, as well as private partners' resources. The key is to identify appropriate strategies that draw upon the respective strengths of the public and private sectors to achieve the overall objectives of the health system [11]. Private sector engagement should in general be aimed at enhancing five key attributes of health care provision that are related to improving access, equity, efficiency, quality and safety, and accountability (see Chapter 10).

Besides accruing mutual benefits, as specified in the formal partnership contract, PPPs in the health sector offer other benefits. There is evidence from case studies done in many countries that PPPs: (1) improve access to services for people in underserved areas or services

---

Box 28.2 Definitions of Key Terms in the Context of PPPs

- **Information asymmetry** [9] (also called information gap) refers to when one party (e.g., agent or private partner) in a transaction is in possession of more information than the other (e.g., principal or purchaser) on, for example, cost, quality, risks, and returns. In a health sector PPP transaction, for example, private health care providers can take advantage of the public sector purchaser because asymmetric information exists whereby the provider has more knowledge on the attributes of the service being provided than the purchaser.

- **Moral hazards** in the context of PPP occur both from the beneficiary's and the provider's perspective. The former happens when the beneficiary or users overconsume health care or engage in its frivolous use. The latter happens when the provider acts in their own self-interest, for example, by under-provision of services or reduced quality of care to cut costs in order to maximize benefits/revenue. The purchaser may not be able to monitor the activities of the agent on a day-to-day basis.

- **Adverse selection** in PPPs refers to a situation wherein the principal (purchaser) selects an agent (provider) who may not be the appropriate one to deliver the services at the required level of quality or efficiency. Adverse selection occurs due to misinterpretation of the ability of the agent by the principal or inability of the principal to diligently verify the skills and abilities of the agent at the time of selection or while under contract [10].

that are not available in the public facilities [12]; (2) prevent impoverishment among the uninsured who seek health services from the private sector paying out-of-pocket (OOP) [13]; (3) facilitate optimal utilization of public health facilities that are not functional due to shortages of staff, equipment, or other requirements [14]; (4) augment additional health infrastructure through private sector investment [15, 16]; and (5) facilitate greater regulatory oversight on the PHS [5, 17, 18]. A systematic review by Odendaal et al., however, revealed that private sector engagement, especially contracting out in child care services, reduces (individual) OOP spending but makes little difference in other service delivery outcomes [19].

Many countries around the world have rich experience or are in the process of implementing PPPs in the health sector. For example, the Organisation for Economic Co-operation and Development (OECD) countries have a long history of PPPs in health, ranging across contracting of private physicians for delivering primary care services, management contracts of public health facilities, and more complex PPPs to build and manage hospitals under the private finance initiatives, a model popularized in the United Kingdom [20–22].

28.3 Public–Private Partnership: Engagement Models

There are several models of engaging the PHS. Some regard PPPs in the health sector from a classical perspective, wherein hospitals and health facilities are constructed with private funds, while services are delivered by the government after the building is handed over post-construction or even by a private provider (the same one who built the facility or a new one). Such models include a combination of private finance initiatives (PFI) such as Design, Build, Finance, and Operate (DBFO); Build, Own, Operate/Lease, and Transfer (BOOT/BOT); and Rehabilitate, Operate, and Transfer (ROT) options. These models are usually used for constructing health facilities, hospitals, and medical colleges. Countries that need additional health infrastructure use these PPP models.

Others view PPP in health as having a wider scope and objectives. Unlike infrastructure (e.g., roads, ports, or energy), health services are more varied, complex, and relatively intangible. In countries where public health facilities such as primary care centers or hospitals are either nonfunctional or underutilized, or where certain specialized diagnostic services are not offered, PHS can be engaged to run the facility, through arrangements called *management contracts*, or to provide specific services such as laboratories, radio-diagnostics, dialysis, and specialty wards, through arrangements called *outsourcing contracts* or *colocation*.

Some governments use innovative financing options (e.g., vouchers, insurance arrangements, or pay-for-performance) to improve access to quality health services for vulnerable populations. Such arrangements with the PHS fall under the framework of purchasing arrangements. Options for engaging the private sector also exist in areas such as training and capacity building, research, advocacy, community mobilization, self-regulation, quality improvement, and social marketing. Private sector engagement is the meaningful inclusion of private providers for service delivery in mixed health systems, and requires that governments focus on governance of the whole health system – both private and public – to ensure quality of care and financial protection for patients, irrespective of where they seek care [23–25]. In summary, PPP models depend on the scope and objective of engaging the private sector. There are various models of PPP, which are depicted in Figure 28.1; several are elaborated in the following sections.

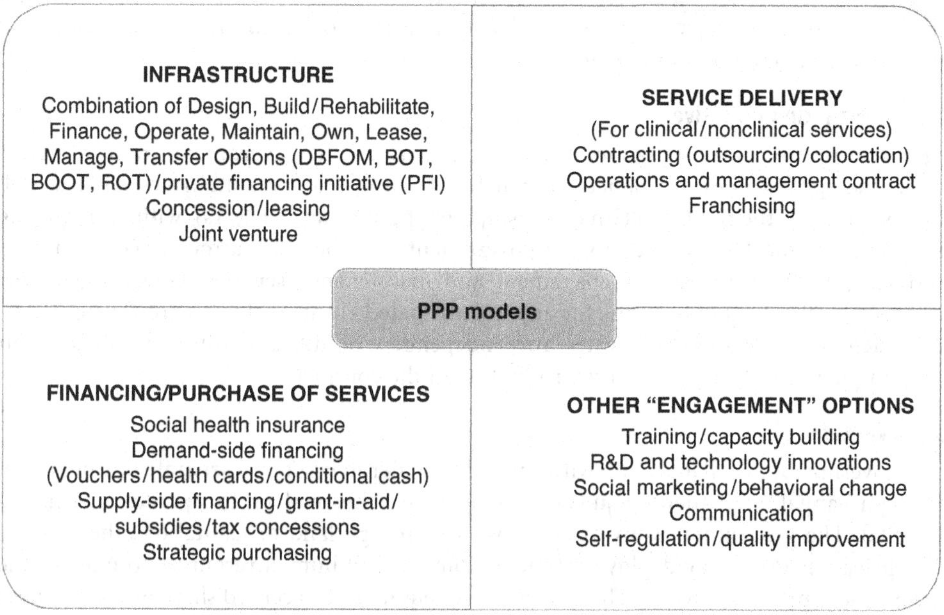

INFRASTRUCTURE
Combination of Design, Build/Rehabilitate,
Finance, Operate, Maintain, Own, Lease,
Manage, Transfer Options (DBFOM, BOT,
BOOT, ROT)/private financing initiative (PFI)
Concession/leasing
Joint venture

SERVICE DELIVERY
(For clinical/nonclinical services)
Contracting (outsourcing/colocation)
Operations and management contract
Franchising

PPP models

FINANCING/PURCHASE OF SERVICES
Social health insurance
Demand-side financing
(Vouchers/health cards/conditional cash)
Supply-side financing/grant-in-aid/
subsidies/tax concessions
Strategic purchasing

OTHER "ENGAGEMENT" OPTIONS
Training/capacity building
R&D and technology innovations
Social marketing/behavioral change
Communication
Self-regulation/quality improvement

Figure 28.1 Public–private partnership models in health sector. Modified from [11].

28.3.1   Infrastructure-Related PPP

Design, Build/Rehabilitate, Finance, Operate, Manage, and Maintain (Own and Transfer)

The private sector is invited to build hospitals or medical colleges (usually on government land) with their own or borrowed funds (or with partial funding from the government, called a viability gap fund [VGF]). The latter is a fixed grant (i.e., a proportion of total project cost) from the government to help projects that are economically justified but are not financially viable. VGF is in the form of capital subsidy to attract private sector players to participate.

The facility, once completed, is leased to the private partner for a fixed, and usually long-term, period; the government repays the private partner for the investment made in creating the asset, including interest. At the end of the lease period, control of the facility is transferred to the government. During the lease period, the private partner is responsible for managing the hospital and its infrastructure and the government may opt to provide the clinical services with its own staff and supplies. In some cases the private partner may be asked to provide clinical services in addition to maintaining the hospital support services. This is often termed an *integrated PPP*. The government may negotiate the purchase of certain services from the hospital on a long-term basis.

There are other options such as BOT, BOOT, ROT, and so on. Variations of these options are used to create or expand health infrastructure. Some are called "greenfield" projects, when investing in new asset creation; others are termed "brownfield" projects, when an existing health facility is redeveloped using a combination of the above options. In health infrastructure PPPs, risk sharing, performance (volume of services), and sources of revenue are critical issues. If the revenue is earned through user fees and the use of facility premises for other amenities (e.g., shops), it would be called a *concession*. If user fees are not the source of revenue, the government may pay the contractor for construction and operational management of the facility.

Private Financing Initiative

Prevalent in the United Kingdom, under the PFI model the government grants a private entity the right to mobilize finances; design, build, manage, and maintain a hospital, as well as in some cases the right to retain ownership for a period (say, 30 years), without requiring it to transfer the facility back to the government. The private partner is contracted to provide non-clinical facility management and maintenance services. Government may also assume financial obligations for any unanticipated events including contingent liabilities such as payment to the private entity independent of utilization of the facility, default on non-guaranteed loans, or early termination of the contract.

Joint Venture

The government in collaboration with a private partner may set up a separate business unit, through capital investment (equity) to build a new hospital or to operate an existing hospital. The government's investment may be through land or capital or other means. The private partner may deploy capital, equipment, and human resources to manage the hospital and provide services. The government's equity or its accrued share of the revenues is leveraged to purchase a certain volume of services. A private partner (or consortium of partners) may lead the joint venture through majority equity. The government may periodically infuse equity in the joint venture. This model is often used when the government is unable to invest or operate tertiary care hospitals on its own (Box 28.3).

28.3.2 Service Delivery-Related PPP

Management Contract

A government health facility, hospital, or asset is transferred to a private provider to manage, maintain, and deliver services. The government may transfer funds equivalent to

---

Box 28.3 Alzira Hospital, Valencia, Spain: Model of PPP

Hospital de La Ribera (University Hospital and Primary Care), Alzira, Valencia, Spain is one of the most widely cited hospital PPPs (also called "the Alzira model"). The partnership is to develop and manage an integrated health facility (a 300-bed university hospital, four health centers, and 46 primary care units) for a population of 250,000. The hospital provides a full range of services, including inpatient care, surgery, and other clinical services. All eligible residents of the province carry an electronic health care card. If a resident seeks care elsewhere, the private partner pays 100% of the costs of care to the government; if patients from other provinces come to Alzira, the government pays 85% of the tariff to the private partner. A single capitation payment per resident includes capital costs. The profit margin is capped at 7.5%. Ministry can impose a 12.5% penalty if the patient turnover rate exceeds a certain proportion. The success of this model spawned four more such PPPs in the province. The Alzira partnership model began in 1999 and has been operational for over 20 years.

Source: [26].

> **Box 28.4** Hospital Management Contract
>
> **Hospital Geral de Pedreira, São Paolo, Brazil:** In the late 1990s, the state of São Paolo financed, built, and equipped 16 new hospitals under a traditional public works contract and contracted several not-for-profit hospital operators, known as the Social Organization in Health (Organização Social em Saúde, or OSS), to operate the hospitals, including the provision of clinical and nonclinical services. The OSSs are obliged to treat all local residents and are not permitted to charge fees or treat private patients. The OSSs received a global fixed budget from the state upon fulfillment of specified patient volumes and predetermined quality parameters. Each OSS has autonomy over human resources, purchasing, and outsourcing, but not capital investments.
>
> *Source:* [27].

the budgetary allocation originally earmarked for the facility or a reimbursement of expenditure (within negotiated limits) along with service charges. This model is used when the government is unable to run a facility or the asset (e.g., mobile health van) due to constraints on human resources in remote areas or facilities that are not fully utilized. The duration of management contracts depends on the scope of services and the value of the contract. Management contracts for primary care facilities or mobile health vans may be of shorter duration, whereas for larger hospitals the duration might be longer, as it may entail capital investment and deployment of expensive resources, including specialist physicians (Box 28.4).

Colocation and Outsourcing

Private provider(s) are contracted to invest in setting up and operating a specialty unit or a ward of a hospital or to provide a specific set of clinical services inside a government-run hospital. Colocation, as this is often called, involves providing specialty clinical services in settings such as surgical wards and in vitro fertilization clinics within a public facility. Colocation allows a private partner to create specialty clinical service units within a government-run facility. When clinical support services, such as laboratory tests, high-end radio-diagnostics, radiotherapy, dialysis, blood banks, physiotherapy, or nonclinical support services such as laundry or catering are provided through private providers, such partnership arrangements are called *outsourcing contracts*. This model is useful when the government is unable to run such services efficiently or unable to invest in high-end technology.

Franchising

Franchising refers to the right to operate a new or existing facility or asset (e.g., pharmacy stores, birth delivery clinics, immunization centers), with the private contractor retaining a larger portion of the revenue and paying the remainder to the authority or government. The government may lend its name and legitimacy for "brand" purposes. The government may also subsidize or directly buy services exclusively from such privately managed branded clinics under a service agreement. However, the franchisee bears the commercial risk as regards revenue. There can be "full franchising" (all products and services offered in the networked clinics are standardized) or "fractional franchising" (only certain services that are standardized are to be delivered). In franchising, the key focus is on uniform quality standards and monitoring. Franchising could standardize the skills through uniform training and help improve cross-learning of innovations across the network.

28.3.3　Financing and Purchase of Services through PPP

Demand-Side Financing

Demand-side financing is a means whereby public (or sometimes donor) funds are provided to individuals or households to allow them to use the available health services. The most common forms are cash transfers and vouchers (see Chapter 5). From a PPP perspective, the government empanels a list of private providers who agree to provide a specific set of clinical services at a negotiated tariff. The target beneficiaries – that is, the individuals or households – are then issued purchase instruments such as vouchers, purchase coupons, or health cards to access those specified services free at the point of care from the designated private providers (Box 28.5). The beneficiaries receive the vouchers after preliminary screening by the responsible government department. In addition to a package of clinical services (e.g., antenatal care, deliveries, postnatal care, and immunization), the vouchers/cards may include cost of transport, hospitalization, and medicines. The government reimburses the provider based on the use of vouchers or other instruments. Demand-side financing instruments are commonly used to protect the poor from the financial burden of OOP spending while accessing services at private service delivery points. Another form of demand-side financing is *conditional cash transfers*, which aim to provide regular payments to low-income beneficiaries, on the condition that they comply with certain prerequisites (e.g., antenatal check-ups, institutional delivery, immunization, intake of nutritional supplements, and others).

Supply-Side Payments (Subsidies Financing)

The government offers payments or incentives directly to individual private providers for delivering a specific service in public health facilities. For example, private obstetricians are paid to perform birth deliveries in public hospitals. In public facilities where specialists are

---

Box 28.5 Vouchers for Birth Deliveries/Neonatal Care: Experience from Gujarat, India

Launched in 2005–2006 in the province of Gujarat, India the scheme called Chiranjeevi was aimed at improving access to institutional deliveries and emergency neonatal care for women from low-income families and socially marginalized groups. Beneficiaries received free services at the empaneled private clinics or hospitals. The government reimbursed the private providers on the basis of a pre-negotiated tariff for a package of 100 deliveries. There was no limit on the number of deliveries private clinics could conduct. The pregnant women were required to visit a government hospital for an initial antenatal check-up and to receive the beneficiary card/voucher. The scheme covered services such as one predelivery consultation, ultrasonography, lab tests, delivery (normal, complicated, or cesarean), blood transfusions, neonatal intensive care, food, and transportation. The beneficiary was not expected to bear any costs related to medicine and anesthesia. The scheme was expanded to cover neonatal care, emergency transportation, and care of low birth-weight babies from remote districts of the province.

Source: Venkatraman et al., unpublished report funded by DFID.

either unavailable or not needed on regular payroll, such contracting mechanisms allow continued service delivery. Tax subsidies (e.g., custom duty waiver for the import of high-end medical equipment), grant-in-aid to NGOs, and subsidies (e.g., land price) are other forms of incentives extended by the government to the PHS in exchange of certain specific services offered free to low-income families or patients referred by the government. These measures are different from the wider health care financing strategies addressed in Chapters 16–18.

Health Insurance and Strategic Purchasing

Private sector involvement is an important element of different models of health insurance, including large-scale social insurance programs offered in many L&MICs (see Chapter 17). The mode of financing, enrolment of beneficiaries, role of the government and the private sector, instruments to access services (e.g., premium, purchase, reimbursement), and regulatory and governance frameworks vary from country to country. In these situations, the government through a social security agency or an insurance provider strategically purchases services from a list of accredited or empaneled private providers in the form of a package of services, including hospitalization and medicines, with partial or full payment. Purchasing prevents high OOP payments at the point of service delivery, providing financial protection to the poor and vulnerable. Providers are paid either through fee-for-service based on the number and type of services provided, or through capitation based on the number of projected patients or population entitled to the package of services, or through other mechanisms or a mix of several methods. Strategic purchasing, under which the payment mechanisms are structured to maximize health outcomes at lower costs, with incentives for quality, is being increasingly employed by health insurance organizations (see Chapter 18).

28.3.4 Other Options for Involving the Private Health Sector

Social Marketing

The private sector is "hired" to use commercial marketing strategies such as branding, customer segmentation, advertising, or other strategies to change people's behavior toward health. It is widely used to market low-cost health products (e.g., contraceptives, insecticidal bed nets, oral rehydration solution, immunization) and influence behavior (e.g., against tobacco use, substance abuse, or unsafe sex). Besides mass and social media, social marketing can also harness health care providers for the purpose of behavioral change communication (BCC) – for instance, against overuse of antibiotics. Social marketing can be used with franchising (see above) for improving access and quality of care for disadvantaged populations in L&MICs (Box 28.6).

While there is a plethora of various PPP models, their appropriateness is highly dependent on contextual factors, such as the need, scope, and objectives of partnerships, the private sector's interest and resources, leadership and governance capacity in the government, and trust and relationship between partners, besides other factors such as duration, mutual obligations, and risk sharing.

28.4 Challenges to PPPs in the Health Care Sector

Despite growing recognition of the importance of engaging the PHS in advancing the goal of UHC and in improving health system performance, there is little consensus on how to

---

Box 28.6 Social Marketing of Contraceptives: DKT International in Pakistan

Using social marketing, subsidized contraceptives are distributed through easily accessible, neighborhood private utility units such as pharmacies, shops, kiosks, and even salons. In 2012, DKT International started a program in Pakistan to improve access to affordable contraceptives through social marketing for people living in rural and underserved areas, through a wide network of private outlets (small roadside shops, pharmacies, superstores, and branded health clinics). Advertisements were put on television and radio, motor rickshaws, and the walls of pharmacy stores. As a result of extensive promotion, the contraceptive prevalence rate rose from 9% in 1991 to 26% in 2012. By 2015, an estimated 300,000 unwanted pregnancies and 280,000 unsafe abortions were averted due to DKT Pakistan's efforts. DKT also launched the Dhanak clinics under a social franchising model to expand access to family planning services, including affordable contraceptives in rural areas. By 2015, more than 1,000 Dhanaks were established, providing services in all the provinces of Pakistan.

Source: [28].

---

implement this option. In many L&MICs, political and ideological positioning and discourse preclude an objective assessment of the merits and demerits of PPP, leading to a restrained response by governments. Weak governance combined with ineffective regulation of the private sector further raises suspicion about PPPs in health. For many countries, PPPs offer vast untapped potential, but they also involve complex challenges.

28.4.1 Strategic Challenges

According to the Asian Development Bank, some of the challenges with PPPs in the health sector include: (1) poor understanding of the concept of PPP; (2) weak institutional capacity of public sector agencies; (3) lack of political commitment to sustain PPPs; (4) informal working arrangements between partners; (5) limited sustainability of resources; (6) lack of or weak regulations and monitoring; and (7) prevalence of moral hazards and political influence and practices [29]. Box 28.7 identifies the major barriers to private sector engagement and PPPs in health in L&MICs based on an extensive literature review [1, 15, 26, 27, 29–34].

Despite its dominance in some countries and rapid expansion in others, few governments in L&MICs have an explicit policy regarding PHS. The absence of a PPP-related policy and a dedicated organizational unit within the Ministries of Health can undermine the confidence of private sector providers about the government's commitment toward PPP. Partnerships based on "relational contracts" by well-meaning bureaucrats are not sustainable. Inconsistent approaches to PPP deter private sector enthusiasm and necessitate a consensus-based policy that signals the government's long-term commitment to PPPs [34].

28.4.2 Operational Challenges

There are several operational challenges in the day-to-day management of PPPs, such as delayed payments, incomplete or poorly drafted contracts leading to varied interpretations and disputes, and the absence of key performance indicators (KPIs) to measure partnership outcomes. Delays in payment, a common phenomenon among service delivery contracts, often lead to disruption or reduction in the quality of services and breeds a culture of kickbacks and corruption. Ministry of Health representatives are generally not trained to

> **Box 28.7** Barriers to Effective PPPs in Health
>
> - Lack of explicit, long-term political and administrative commitment to private sector engagement
> - Inadequate information on the PHS and its characteristics
> - Absence of sector-specific policy, legal and regulatory framework, and guidelines for engaging the private sector
> - Absence of a dedicated organizational unit or weak technical and managerial capacity to design, implement, and manage PPP projects and schemes
> - Weak regulatory enforcement capacity or inadequate resources for oversight
> - Absence of dedicated budgetary allocation for private sector engagement resulting in payment delays and opportunities for corruption
> - Lack of dialog forums between the public and private sectors and perpetuation of popular antagonism and lack of trust between both the sectors

design, manage, and monitor partnership contracts. They are more comfortable with traditional procurement methods such as competitive tendering and selection of the lowest commercial bidder, a phenomenon called path dependency.

28.5 Approaches and Practical Steps for Operationalizing PPP

Governments that are seriously contemplating PPPs need to establish a dedicated unit within the Ministry of Health, with competent professionals and resources to conceive, design, and manage partnerships. Managing the relationship between public and private sector officials is a key enabler of well-functioning partnerships. A contract management framework with well-defined mechanisms for oversight, decision-making, coordination, and grievance redressal along with an information technology-based system helps in effectively managing partnerships. In recent years, performance-based contracting (PBC) has become the preferred mode of partnerships, especially in primary care service delivery. Under PBC, certain KPIs (outputs) are used to monitor and pay the private partner. A robust IT-based system to track the performance and payments is essential for its success.

We propose the following steps as an optimal pathway for operationalizing the PPPs:

1. **Generate political and stakeholder commitment:** In order to create more favorable political commitment, continued interaction, policy dialog forums, and stakeholder engagement strategies need to be explored. According to Taylor [35], politics is the main cause of failed PPP arrangements, perhaps due to electoral pressures and lack of bureaucratic buy-in. Bureaucracy tends to explore private sector partnerships as a possible solution to an immediate problem rather than a long-term policy option.

2. **Compile information on the private sector:** Detailed information on the size, distribution, and characteristics of the PHS, including its resources, costs, quality standards, and efficiency is critical for developing contextually appropriate partnership strategies. This should be complemented by a dedicated IT-based information system that monitors performance and tracks payments.

3. **Adopt a health sector-specific policy toward the PHS, including PPP:** The PPP policy should be complemented with guidelines and a legal framework for conceiving, designing, and managing partnerships. An evidence-informed PPP policy should reflect

the government's long-term commitment, provide stability and continuity, and pave the way for transactions in a professional manner. The policy should also provide for administrative and fiduciary commitment and enable stakeholders to understand why the country needs PPPs in health.

4. **Create legal and regulatory frameworks and oversight functions:** Legal and regulatory frameworks complemented with effective licensing and accreditation are imperative for PPPs. Regulatory enforcement requires staff, resources, and authority. Regulatory authority needs to be independent of the government, as the public health system is also subject to regulatory compliance. Partnership contracts can be used as an incentive for better regulatory compliance.

5. **Provide dedicated financial resources and set up accounting systems:** Dedicated budgetary support for PPPs or other forms of engagement is critical, especially for nonrevenue-generating PPP projects, where payment is a direct fiscal commitment by the government.

6. **Create organizational units and build institutional capacity:** The Ministry of Health and its officials need to organize and equip themselves for purchasing services from the private sector. PPPs in the health sector are more complex in terms of costs, quality, and outcomes. Transaction advisors can provide initial support, but in-house capacity is critical.

7. **PPP dialog platforms:** Popular discourse is often derisive about the private (for-profit) sector and equates PPPs with privatization. Building trust and overcoming suspicion is critical in creating a conducive ecosystem by establishing forums for dialog and encouraging objective, evidence-based debate on PPP in health. The private sector needs to organize itself into a more cohesive network and display its commitment to the country's health objectives, which encompass equitable access to quality care that is efficient and accountable.

References

1. Health Research Institute. Build and beyond: the r(evolution) of healthcare PPPs. 2010. www.pwc.se/sv/halso-sjukvard/assets/build-and-beyond-the-revolution-of-healthcare-ppps.pdf (accessed December 17, 2021).

2. UN General Assembly. Resolution adopted by the General Assembly on 25 September 2015. 2015. www.un.org/ga/search/view_doc.asp?symbol=A/RES/70/1&Lang=E (accessed November 18, 2020).

3. WHO. Resolutions. 2010. http://apps.who.int/gb/ebwha/pdf_files/WHA63-REC1/WHA63_REC1-P2-en.pdf (accessed October 18, 2020).

4. World Bank Group. Public–private partnerships in health: World Bank Group engagement in health PPPs. 2016. https://openknowledge.worldbank.org/handle/10986/25383 (accessed November 16, 2020).

5. A. Venkatraman, J. W. Björkman. *Public–Private Partnerships in Health Care in India: Lessons for Developing Countries.* London, Routledge, 2009.

6. Asian Development Bank. PPP guidance note on procurement. 2018. www.adb.org/sites/default/files/ppp-procurement.pdf (accessed October 14, 2020).

7. OECD. Recommendation of the Council on principles for public governance of public–private partnerships. 2012. www.oecd.org/governance/budgeting/PPP-Recommendation.pdf (accessed November 10, 2020).

8. H. Axelsson, F. Bustreo, A. Harding. Private sector participation in child health: a review

of World Bank projects, 1993–2002. 2003. https://openknowledge.worldbank.org/bitstream/handle/10986/13793/288590 Axelsson010Private0sector1whole.pdf?sequence=1&isAllowed=y (accessed October 19, 2020).

9. A. Bloomenthal. Asymmetric information. 2021. www.investopedia.com/terms/a/asymmetricinformation.asp#:~:text=% 22Asymmetric%20information%22%20is %20a%20term,being%20sold%20than%20 the%20buyer (accessed February 1, 2022).

10. F. Amagoh. Information asymmetry and the contracting out process. *TIJ* 2009; **14** (2): 1–4.

11. A. Venkatraman, J. W. Björkman. Public–private partnerships in healthcare. In E. Kuhlmann, R. H. Blank, I. L. Bourgeault, eds., *The Palgrave International Handbook of Healthcare Policy and Governance.* London, Palgrave Macmillan, 2015.

12. Joint Learning Network. Engaging the private sector in primary health care to achieve universal health coverage: advice from implementers, to implementers. 2016. www.jointlearningnetwork.org/wp-content/uploads/2019/11/EngagingPrivate SectorFinal.pdf (accessed December 17, 2021).

13. World Bank. Handshake : IFC's quarterly journal on public–private partnerships. 2016. https://documents.worldbank.org/en/publication/documents-reports/documentdetail/972481468315320373/handshake-ifcs-quarterly-journal-on-public-private-partnerships-3 (accessed December 17, 2021).

14. M. B. Baig, B. Panda, J. K. Das, et al. Is public private partnership an effective alternative to government in the provision of primary health care? A case study in Odisha. *J Health Manag* 2014; **16**(1): 41–52.

15. Institute for Global Health Sciences. PPPs in healthcare: models, lessons and trends for the future. 2018. https://globalhealthsciences .ucsf.edu/sites/globalhealthsciences.ucsf.edu/files/pub/ppp-report-series-business-model.pdf (accessed December 17, 2021).

16. L. Kostyak, D. M. Shaw, B. Elger, et al. A means of improving public health in low- and middle-income countries? Benefits and challenges of international public–private partnerships. *Public Health* 2017; **149**: 120–129.

17. UNECE. A preliminary reflection on the best practices in PPP in healthcare sector: a review of different PPP case studies and experiences. Working Paper. 2012. www .unece.org/fileadmin/DAM/ceci/images/ICoE/PPPHealthcareSector_DiscPaper.pdf (accessed December 16, 2020).

18. Global Health Group. Public financing partnerships to improve private sector health care: case studies of intermediary purchasing platforms. 2018. https://globalhealthsciences .ucsf.edu/sites/globalhealthsciences.ucsf .edu/files/pub/public-financing-partnerships_0.pdf (accessed October 17, 2020).

19. W. A. Odendaal, K. Ward, J. Uneke, et al. Contracting out to improve the use of clinical health services and health outcomes in low- and middle-income countries. *Cochrane Database Syst Rev* 2018; **4**(4): CD008133.

20. A. Mills, J. Broomberg. Experiences of contracting health services: an overview of the literature. 1998. https://apps.who.int/iris/handle/10665/64773 (accessed December 10, 2020).

21. R. England. Experiences of contracting with the private sector: a selective review. 2004. https://assets.publishing.service.gov.uk/media/57a08cd140f0b64974001476/Experience-of-contracting-with-the-Private-sector.pdf (accessed October 17, 2020).

22. G. A. Hodge, C. Greve. Public–private partnerships: an international performance review. *Public Adm Rev* 2007; **67**(3): 545–558.

23. World Health Organization. Strengthening private sector engagement for UHC. 2022. www.who.int/activities/strengthening-private-sector-engagement-for-uhc (accessed February 15, 2022).

24. L. Suchman, E. Hart, D. Montagu. Public–private partnerships in practice: collaborating to improve health finance

policy in Ghana and Kenya. *Health Policy Plan* 2018; **33**(7): 777–785.

25. Z. C. Shroff, K. D. Rao, S. Bennett, et al. Moving towards universal health coverage: engaging non-state providers. *Int J Equity Health* 2018; **17**(1): 135.

26. N. Sekhri, R. Feachem, A. Ni. Public–private integrated partnerships demonstrate the potential to improve health care access, quality, and efficiency. *Health Aff (Millwood)* 2011; **30**(8): 1498–1507.

27. Global Health Group. Public–private investment partnerships for health: an atlas of innovation. 2010. https://globalhealthsciences.ucsf.edu/sites/globalhealthsciences.ucsf.edu/files/pub/hsi-ppip-atlas.pdf (accessed October 15, 2020).

28. DKT International. No easy place to do family planning. 2020. https://2umya83uy24b2nu5ug2708w5-wpengine.netdna-ssl.com/wp-content/uploads/2011/04/DKT-Pakistan-White-Paper.pdf (accessed October 11, 2020).

29. Asian Development Bank. Guidebook on public–private partnership in hospital management. 2013. www.adb.org/publications/guidebook-public-private-partnership-hospital-management (accessed October 13, 2020).

30. E. Banzon, J. A. Lucero, B. L. Ho, et al. PPP options for universal health coverage in the Philippines. 2016. https://think-asia.org/handle/11540/6843 (accessed October 18, 2020).

31. Caribbean Development Bank. Public–private partnerships in the Caribbean: building on early lessons. 2014. www.caribank.org/publications-and-resources/resource-library/thematic-papers/public-private-partnerships-caribbean-building-early-lessons (accessed October 20, 2020).

32. KPMG. What works, the triple win: rethinking public private partnerships for universal healthcare. 2018. https://assets.kpmg/content/dam/kpmg/xx/pdf/2017/08/what-works-the-triple-win.pdf (accessed September 10, 2020).

33. B. O'Hanlon, A. Nakyanzi, V. Musembi, et al. Exploring partnership opportunities to achieve universal health access: 2016 Uganda private sector assessment in health. 2017. www.uhfug.com/wp-content/uploads/2019/08/Uganda-PSA-Report-2017.pdf (accessed December 20, 2020).

34. A. Venkatraman, G. La Forgia. PPP hospitals in India: a comparative analysis of purchasing arrangements and performance. 2013. https://link.springer.com/chapter/10.1057%2F978113 7384935_23 (accessed December 18, 2020).

35. R. Taylor. Mission difficult . . . but not impossible: making public–private partnerships work for the poor. 2010. https://openknowledge.worldbank.org/handle/10986/10570 (accessed October 18, 2020).

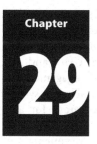

Chapter 29

Embedding People's Voice and Ensuring Participatory Governance

Lessons from the Thai Experience in Community Engagement

Walaiporn Patcharanarumol, Viroj Tangcharoensathien,
Somtanuek Chotchoungchatchai, Dheepa Rajan, and
Sameen Siddiqi

Key Messages

- Community participation and community engagement (CE) are essential pillars of strong people-centered governance and underpin universal health coverage (UHC) reforms.
- There is no single and universal definition of CE and the rationale for it has been described along at least two main perspectives, as intrinsically valuable and as an essential contributor to desired outcomes.
- The literature about CE includes consideration of its definitions, motivations, modalities, conditions, actions, and impact.
- The community can play a number of roles in health system strengthening, including in planning and priority-setting, program implementation, monitoring and evaluation, and in advocacy.
- The WHO identifies three roles for the community: as advocates, as co-creators of health and social services, and as self-carers and caretakers.
- Thailand provides a uniquely rich example of citizen engagement in the development of legislation and policies for UHC, illustrating the central role of leadership, transparency, accountability, and an enabling legal framework.
- Strong competencies are required in government and in people.

29.1 Introduction

Community participation and engagement have been identified as essential pillars of strong people-centered governance which underpins UHC reforms. In the declarations of Alma-Ata (1978) and Astana (2018), the core principles of CE have been repeatedly advocated for their positive impact on health. The "whole of society approach" proposed by WHO acknowledges the contribution and the important role played by different stakeholders, including individuals, families, and communities, in support of national efforts for disease prevention and control. The voice of communities is integral to driving the UHC agenda.

At the global level, 193 heads of state and/or their representatives made a policy commitment in September 2019 by adopting the United Nations Political Declaration of the High-level Meeting on Universal Health Coverage [1]. The Declaration highlights engagement with people and communities as pivotal for achieving UHC and the Sustainable Development Goals (SDGs): "we ... recognize that people's engagement ... and the inclusion of all relevant stakeholders is one of the core components of health system governance ... contributing to the achievement of universal health coverage for all." However, translating the commitment of engagement with people and communities into practice is complex and requires skills that are often lacking within governments and ministries. While many countries resort to single or occasional health sector events to engage with populations, communities, and/or civil society, few have managed to embed CE as a true *modus operandi* and as an integral element of health system operations.

This chapter builds on Chapter 11 and focuses on "how" CE can be implemented at the national and subnational levels. To do so, we first provide an overview of the evidence and outline some of the processes and strategies that have been shown to enable CE. We then turn to examples of effective CE and highlight the many lessons drawn from Thailand's efforts in this area. We review, in particular, Thailand's Universal Coverage Scheme's (UCS) participatory approach as a practical example and one of the myriad ways in which the voice of Thai's people has been embedded in legislation and operations to ensure that the governance of UCS is responsive to their needs. We lastly summarize the lessons learned for a proactive approach to CE in health.

29.2 Effective Strategies for CE: Drawing on Evidence

As mentioned in Chapter 11, there are at least two broad perspectives on the value and impact of CE. A social justice perspective that acknowledges that the process of engagement itself is valuable, and a more utilitarian perspective that considers CE as an essential contributor to other desirable outcomes [2]. In the latter case, CE has been linked to improved outcomes, improved quality of care, and more responsive services, as well as increased social capital, greater community empowerment, and improved health equity, among others. Overall, robust evidence to support these claims is limited, in large part because of the lack of consensus on the definition and conceptual construct of CE, and in part because CE is a fundamentally complex phenomenon which makes it impossible to fully capture its effective elements in isolation from the context in which they exist [3]. There is, therefore, no clear roadmap for CE that automatically leads to demand-driven and responsive health systems. Conversely, there are circumstances where the voices of the people, and specifically of the users of health services, are clearly absent from the planning, implementation, delivery, and evaluation of health-related policies and services, undermining the ability of health systems to be more responsive.

To help the transition from rhetoric to reality, Brunton et al. have proposed a useful conceptual framework that captures the complexity and diversity of CE based on a systematic review of the literature (Figure 29.1) [2]. The conceptual framework offers a taxonomy of definitions, rationale, motivations, modes of participation, conditions, actions, and impact along a spectrum of CE from being social justice-dominant to utilitarian-dominant. The framework can be used to inform which type of CE is needed in particular contexts and at each of the macro, meso, and micro levels of the system, while also providing examples of what activities or strategies can be used to implement CE.

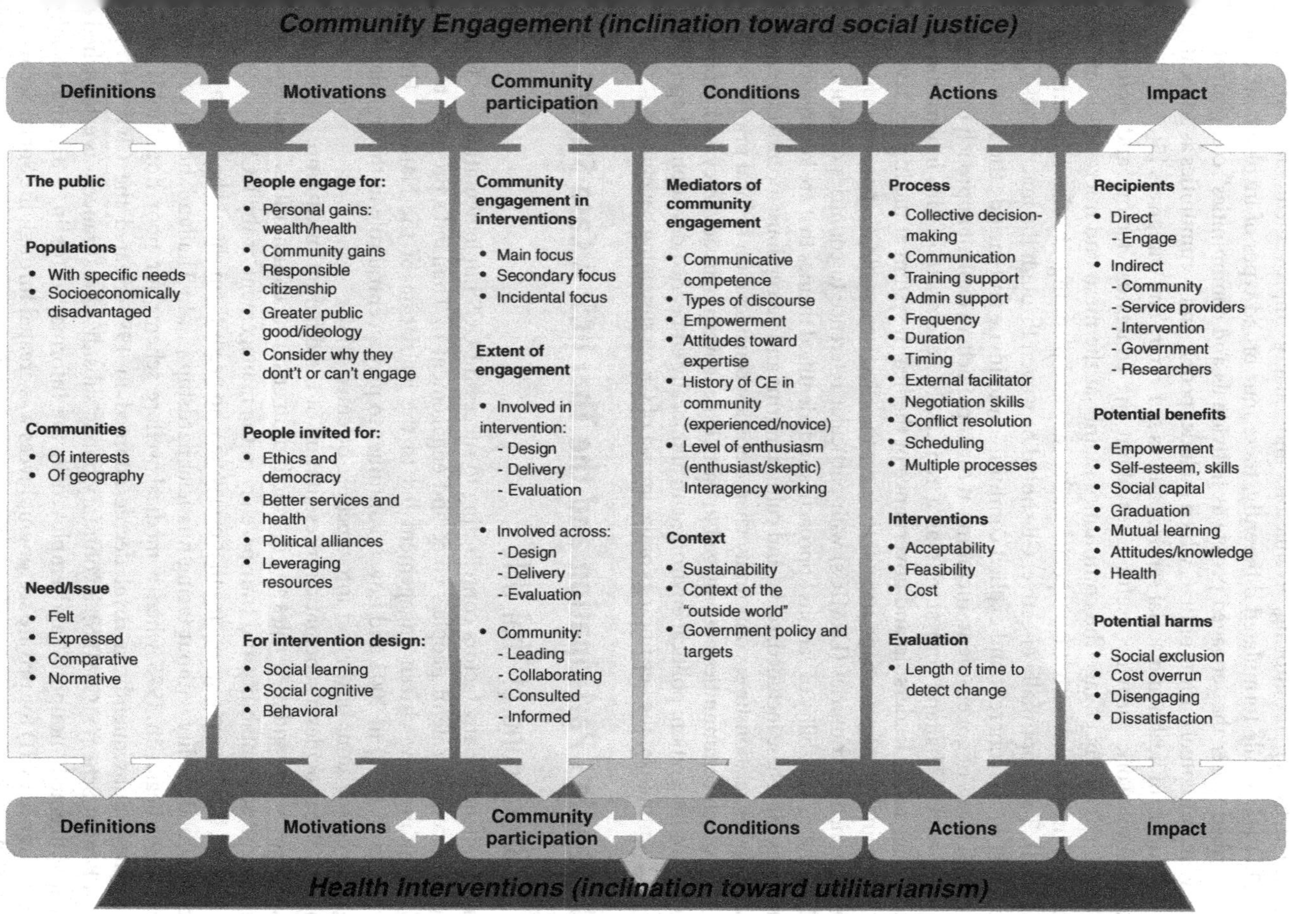

Figure 29.1 Community engagement in interventions: conceptual framework [2].

A taxonomy of community roles in health systems strengthening proposed by Sacks et al. is also potentially useful in implementing CE. It outlines four broad types of involvement and activity by the community: planning and priority-setting; program implementation (including service delivery); monitoring, evaluation, and quality improvement; and advocacy (Table 29.1) [4]. While formulated differently, these four broad types of involvement echo those described under the "engaged people as individuals and communities" component of the renewed conceptual outline of PHC which includes people and communities as advocates, as co-developers of health and social services and as self-carers and caregivers [5].

These frameworks provide useful clues about the contextual factors and potential activities to effectively engage the community mainly at the meso and micro levels of CE (although some of these activities, especially advocacy and planning, are also relevant at the macro level). To be optimally effective, CE should be woven through the macro, meso, and micro levels with a coherent and explicit commitment to invite and include the voice of the people at all levels of government, including at the top. Such an explicit approach to CE has been adopted by Thailand and stands as a remarkable exemplar of the integration of people's voice in the leadership and governance of the health system at the highest level.

A recent analysis of systematic reviews to assess the effectiveness of CE approaches in low- and middle-income countries (L&MICs) with particular reference to countries of South Asia examined the sustainability of various approaches and identified themes that are key to successful outcomes [6]. These included: social and cultural norms and perceptions; incentives; gender roles and power relationships; community characteristics; consideration of local priorities; the process by which communities are engaged to participate; government advocacy and support; health system integration; political environment; and locally embedded development agencies. Table 29.2 summarizes the key findings of the impact of CE on sustaining benefits.

29.3 People's Participation and the Thai UCS: A Case Study

29.3.1 Background of Thai UHC

Among Thailand's many factors contributing to successful UCS implementation, we focus here on the central role of people's voice and engagement in Thailand's progress toward UHC, including how citizen engagement led to the legislation of the National Health Security Act (NHSA) in 2002 and how it continues to play a central role in the translation of legislative provisions of the Act into a people-oriented UHC.

Figure 29.2 provides a schematic representation of the different institutions, organizations, and key actors and their roles and interactions in ensuring communities' engagement, and enhanced accountability and transparency in the management of the UCS.

Universal health coverage means that everyone who needs them should be able to access services of good quality without facing financial hardship [3]. In Thailand, health reforms toward UHC began in 1975 when a medical welfare scheme for poor households was implemented. Subsequently, a royal decree adopted in 1980 created the Civil Servant Medical Benefit Scheme (CSMBS), a voluntary public subsidized insurance was established for people deemed "nonpoor" and employed in the informal sector in 1983, and social health insurance (SHI) for private sector employees was created through the Social Security Act in 1990. Despite these various government efforts to expand coverage to different population groups, 30% of the population remained uncovered. In 2001, reform under the NHSA combined the medical welfare scheme for the poor and the voluntary public

Table 29.1 Illustrative community roles in health systems strengthening

Planning and priority setting
- Participate in planning (identification of objectives and formulation of sequential action steps).
- Health outreach activities, selection of community-level health agents, and evaluation of performance at various levels of the health system.
- Determine fair and just distribution of profits or program benefits.
- Provide support and incentives for community health workers (CHWs and community volunteers) to perform interpersonal counseling, especially for home care and key family practices and referral.
- Contribute or subsidize labor, land, produce, cash, and other resources to support locally appropriate health services, health agents, and disadvantaged populations.

Program implementation
- Families and extended community members serve as primary caregivers of children and patients.
- Community agents (such as CHWs) serve as peer educators and close-to-community health providers.
- Community leaders communicate support for health interventions.
- Community leaders and members plan and implement multisectoral activities that address health conditions of daily life (such as water, sanitation, and others).
- Utilize behavior change communication strategies to accelerate the uptake and proper use of health products, vaccines, and technologies.
- Utilize local communication channels to diffuse health-related information.
- Develop and support collective systems for emergency transport.
- Establish community-based health insurance (CBHI) schemes, though CBHI is neither financially sustainable nor has the capacity to expand to UHC [7, 8].

Monitoring, evaluation, and quality improvement
- Collect vital events information, identify and prioritize health problems based on accessible local data.
- Problem-solving when the health situation changes and anticipate future health threats.
- Use data to guide community dialogs and to take collective action.
- Participate in various processes (participatory action research, community scorecards) to hold donors, researchers, and health care providers accountable.

Advocacy
- Organize local leadership and governance structures with viable support networks and intergroup collaboration to ensure that health services and the care provided in health facilities meet community needs, are patient-centered, meet the quality of care standards, and are accountable to the community.
- Have oversight of or engage in government resource allocation decisions so the basic health services receive priority, patients are protected from financial risk, and there are minimal disruptions in health service provisions.
- Access and leverage government and other resources to support the community's health priorities.
- Advocate for UHC including access to health care for all.
- Build a relationship of trust between the community and the health system to maximize utilization of health services and continuity of care.

Source: [4].

Table 29.2 Effectiveness of CE approaches for sustaining benefits in L&MICs: findings from a systematic review

Theme	Context	Action
Social and cultural norms, knowledge, and perceptions	Knowledge and perceptions were key influences on individual participation Low levels of education and knowledge can be barriers to participation Important role for health education	Investigate social and cultural norms, knowledge, and perceptions, and use findings to inform culturally appropriate behavioral change communication interventions as the foundation of CE Consider how to address varying levels of health education needs
Gender roles and power relationships	Female involvement as CHWs is an enabler for better service uptake and enhances women's capacity as CHWs	Consider local factors that may facilitate or hinder CE of women and those from marginalized groups
Community characteristics	Take account of economic status, accessibility (including user fees), and rural vs. urban implementation as these influence adequacy of CE	Tailor programs to geographical, sociocultural, and health system problems to suit urban and rural contexts
Consideration of local priorities	Consider issues related to health, development, economic significance, and enhancing "community fit"	Identify community needs and priorities and consider how CE responds to these priorities
Process by which communities are engaged to participate	Need for community mobilization in support of CE Local recruitment of CHWs ensures community representation for better positioning in communities Level at which decision-making occurs may influence CE	Achieve balance between local and higher responsibilities that harness grassroots knowledge and incorporate locally derived strategies for CE Use locally appropriate and inclusive recruitment processes that involve and reflect characteristics of communities
Government advocacy and supportive political environment	Supportive policymaking and political commitment is key to legitimizing CE programs Consider political environment in design of programs	Secure government advocacy and support for CE Ensure the design of frameworks for CE consider political environment and regional approaches to CE
Health system integration	Close integration or embedding in health system is an enabler for CHWs Close relations between health committees, workers, and management is important for sustainability	Integrate or embed approaches within the broader health system to support CE
Financial and human resources	Provision of training and regular supportive supervision of CHWs Intensive training that is relevant, sufficient, and of high quality is important	Ensure adequate training and supervision of volunteers and staff at all levels and commit to longer-term capacity-building

Table 29.2 (cont.)

Theme	Context	Action
		Ensure financial and human resources to build managerial, organizational, and technical capacity at community level
Locally embedded development agencies	Although not without challenges, involvement of NGOs in CE can be beneficial and sometimes essential	Embedded NGOs should be engaged to contribute resources to support CE

Source: [6].

subsidized insurance, and extended coverage for the remaining uninsured population with the establishment of the UCS, while CSMBS and SHI continued to operate their own systems.

Hence, the UCS refers to three public health insurance schemes that provide full coverage through a comprehensive benefit package to Thailand's 70 million population, with no copayment and a relatively low level of household health spending [4, 9].

These achievements resulted from a vision of ensuring availability of health services, especially primary health care, through four decades of public investment in health systems. The 2002 reform ensured financial risk protection for the whole population. The pivotal role played by the civil society organizations (CSOs) in driving Thailand's progress toward UHC and in its implementation is rife with important lessons, as described below.

29.3.2 Legislation: A Foundation for CE and Participatory Governance

Communities were fully engaged in the legislative process through CSO representatives who submitted "citizen versions" of the draft legislation and participated in the negotiation of the text of the Act. A number of progressive legal provisions were accepted in the final Act adopted by the House of Representatives and the Senate, which ensured citizen engagement in UCS operations and responsive UCS governance.

Citizen Engagement Leading up to the NHSA

The Constitution of 1997 and the Thai leadership in 2001–2002 were instrumental in laying the foundations for the participation of the Thai people in their health system and its progress toward UHC. Legislative provisions on participatory governance embedded in Article 170 of the 1997 Constitution and Article 133 of the 2017 Constitution [10] promote citizen participation in the "initiative process" (a form of direct democracy where citizens can propose legislation) through submission of draft laws for consideration by legislative bodies. In 2001, the launch of the UCS prompted Thai citizens to exercise their constitutional rights and submit such draft bills. Its main contents were included in the NHSA in 2002 [11]. The fact that the first Secretary-General of the National Health Security Office (NHSO) and most of its members were physicians who had previously worked in rural areas was critical in engaging citizens and CSOs in the legislative process. CSOs, notably the

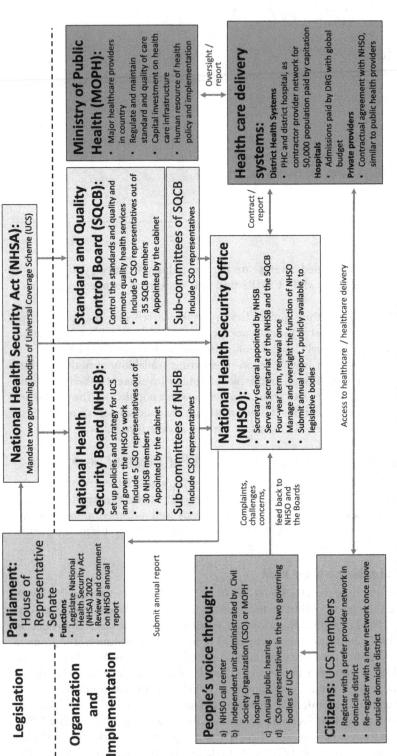

Legislation

Organization and Implementation

Parliament:
- House of Representative
- Senate

Functions
- Legislate National Health Security Act (NHSA) 2002
- Review and comment on NHSO annual report

National Health Security Act (NHSA):
Mandate two governing bodies of Universal Coverage Scheme (UCS)

Ministry of Public Health (MOPH):
- Major healthcare providers in country
- Regulate and maintain standard and quality of care
- Capital investment on health care infrastructure
- Human resource of health policy and implementation

Standard and Quality Control Board (SQCB):
Control the standards and quality and promote quality health services
- Include 5 CSO representatives out of 35 SQCB members
- Appointed by the cabinet

Sub-committees of SQCB
- Include CSO representatives

National Health Security Board (NHSB):
Set up policies and strategy for UCS and govern the NHSO's work
- Include 5 CSO representatives out of 30 NHSB members
- Appointed by the cabinet

Sub-committees of NHSB
- Include CSO representatives

National Health Security Office (NHSO):
- Secretary General appointed by NHSB
- Serve as secretariat of the NHSB and the SQCB
- Four-year term, renewal once
- Manage and oversight the function of NHSO
- Submit annual report, publicly available, to legislative bodies

Health care delivery systems:

District Health Systems
- PHC and district hospital, as contractor provider network for 50,000 population paid by capitation

Hospitals
- Admissions paid by DRG with global budget

Private providers
- Contractual agreement with NHSO, similar to public health providers

Oversight / report

Contract / report

Submit annual report

People's voice through:
a) NHSO call center
b) Independent unit administrated by Civil Society Organization (CSO) or MOPH hospital
c) Annual public hearing
d) CSO representatives in the two governing bodies of UCS

Complaints, challenges concerns, feed back to NHSO and the Boards

Access to healthcare / healthcare delivery

Citizens: UCS members
- Register with a prefer provider network in domicile district
- Re-register with a new network once move outside domicile district

Figure 29.2 Key actors and their accountability framework in management of the Universal Coverage Scheme.

Consumer Protection Foundation, worked closely with "reformists in the Ministry of Public Health" on the scope and contents of the draft bill that was submitted to the House of Representatives for consideration, supported by signatures of more than 50,000 eligible voters as required to amend the Constitution of the Kingdom of Thailand [12].

Gradually the Thai people acquired a full sense of ownership over UCS and successfully protected it from threats of political instability and interference due to the frequent turnover of governments. Between 2001 and 2011, the UCS not only survived but thrived, despite a decade of volatile politics that saw 7 governments, 6 elections, and 1 coup d'état, 10 health ministers who chaired the National Health Security Board (NHSB), and 6 permanent secretaries who head the Ministry of Public Health. This was largely due to the core principles of people's engagement and continued ownership of UCS.

Citizen Engagement Enabled by the NHSA

Reflecting the commitment to continued engagement that had led to the NHSA, the content of the Act itself embedded engagement, participation, empowerment, and responsiveness as the core principle of UCS operation and implementation, and deliberately established processes to include the voice of grassroots organizations beyond the conceptualization of the NHSA. Table 29.3 highlights how the various articles of the Act enable CE [13].

29.3.3 Translating Legislation into Modes of Engagement

Moving from legislation to implementation, the following three examples outline how Thailand's legislative provisions related to CE and citizens' participation is operationalized and specifically how the voices of citizens are heard through a call center (note that during the COVID-19 pandemic the call center was renamed a "contact center" as it played a larger and significant role in patient navigation and active support), annual public hearings, and CSO representation in the UCS governing board.

Complaint through Call Center: Ensuring Access and Voices Are Heard

The NHSA aims to ensure that UCS beneficiaries can not only access and use services, but that their voices are also heard and concerns addressed. Operationally, this is achieved through a mandate to oversee the standard and quality of health facilities and to manage complaints through 24-hour call centers present at the national, provincial, and hospital levels and supported and overseen by the NHSO. Complaints at all three levels are closely monitored to ensure the centers operate well [14].

Deliberative Process of Public Hearing: Ensuring Citizens' and Providers' Voices Are Heard and Actions Taken

Since 2004, the NHSO has been mandated to hold annual general public hearings with health care providers, local governments, technical experts, academia, and citizens. These hearings reinforce the responsiveness of UCS to both citizens and health care providers, and offer a forum to systematically acknowledge achievements and listen to the problems and challenges faced at the local level. Public hearings with health care providers are critical as they are major partners in the provision of services. Problems and challenges faced by either stakeholders are reported to the NHSB, where policy and management responses are taken to rectify the challenges.

Table 29.3 Contents of NHSA 2002 which enable community engagement and responsive Universal Coverage Scheme governance

Articles in NHSA 2002 relevant to responsiveness and empowerment	Principle highlighted
Article 6. *Citizens need to register* with provider network of their choice, change of registration is permitted anytime as needed	Mutual accountability combined with citizen autonomy, choice of provider, and flexibility to reregister
Article 13(4). National Health Security Board (NHSB) membership, five (5) out of a total thirty (30) members of the Board are CSO representatives chosen among themselves from the nine CSO constituencies	Active civil society engagement in governance, with a strong voice in the design and operation of UCS, representing different vulnerable or marginalized groups
Article 18(13). NHSB mandates the NHSO to conduct annual *general public hearing* with health care providers and citizens	Societal dialog offers citizens and health care providers the opportunity to express concerns through public hearing that enables overcoming access barriers to coverage schemes
Article 26(8). NHSO is mandated to oversee the standard and quality of services provided by health facilities and *manage citizens' complaints*	Quality focus, accountability, and responsiveness to citizens
Article 46. Criteria of payment to provider needs to respond to the public hearing as mandated by Article 18(13)	Provider payment methods sensitive to citizens' preferences
Article 48(8). Five members of *Quality and Standard Board* are representatives from CSO, chosen among themselves from the nine CSO constituencies	Civil society participation in quality monitoring and oversight
Article 50(5). The Quality and Standard Board has *mechanisms to ensure that citizens' complaints and voices are heard* and solutions are provided, including independent units (from providers) where citizens can voice their problems	Forum and processes well established and responsive to citizens' concerns/complaints

CSO Representatives on the NHSB and QSB

As part of the governance of UCS, citizens are empowered through CSOs that are well represented on the NHSB and the Quality and Standard Board (QSB), occupying 19% and 14% of membership positions, respectively. Such a high level of representation has been deliberately included in the Act to empower citizens and give them a prominent voice in the governance of UCS.

The experience of the last two decades has conclusively shown that the CSO representatives on the two Boards have contributed toward critical decisions related to budget approval and the introduction of new benefit packages. CSO representatives are well accepted by the Boards and their contribution is recognized by all. The diverse backgrounds of the CSO representatives matter as they have experience in the health sector, come from

Table 29.4 Examples of community engagement in Thai Universal Coverage Scheme

Needs	Interventions	Groups in the community
Ensuring access and use of health services	Complaint management • National level: call center • Provincial level: provincial CSO complaint center • Hospital level: complaint center	Citizens, CSO, health care providers
Ensuring citizens' and providers' voices are heard and actions are taken	Deliberative process of annual public hearing	Citizens, CSO, health care providers
Influencing the decision of the Boards	CSO representatives in the NHSB and QSB	CSO representatives

academia, are strong supporters of consumer protection, and some are former executives of the MOPH.

Table 29.4 summarizes the three examples of CE, including specific needs, corresponding interventions to address these, and the community groups engaged in the Thai UCS. The effectiveness of CE in influencing policies and practices related to the overall Thai health system reform [13], the UC benefit package [15], the impact of UC on health status [16, 17], and equity [18] has been corroborated by multiple studies.

29.4 Lessons Learned from the Thai and Other CE Experiences

Thailand's UCS and similar experiences have proven that engaging people as individuals and communities is feasible when certain conditions and features are in place, as described here.

29.4.1 Leadership and Clear Commitment at All Levels

As mentioned in previous chapters, effective engagement, like all aspects of health system strengthening, begins with a clear and collective vision, and effective leadership. This is true regardless of whether engagement is sought at the macro, meso, or micro levels. The Thai experience provides a compelling example of the importance of leadership and vision.

29.4.2 Transparency and Accountability to Enable Sustained Engagement

In keeping with the ongoing cultivation of engagement, processes that operationalize transparency and accountability can enable sustainable engagement. For example, the NHSO uses live streaming broadcast of monthly Board meetings and submits a publicly available annual report (including audited financial status, service utilization, and performance) to the Cabinet and Parliament demonstrating transparency in using public resources. This demonstration of transparency and accountability protects the organization against political interference, allowing it to stand firm in safeguarding public interests in the middle of political conflicts.

29.4.3 Legal Frameworks Are Key

Legal frameworks are key to meaningful citizen engagement, to overcome entrenched sociopolitical power relations and amplify the voices of those generally unheard. WHO's *Handbook on Social Participation for Universal Health Coverage* identifies three pivotal areas where legal provisions can facilitate more effective social participation: (1) representation and selection processes; (2) roles and responsibilities; and (3) funding modalities [19]. They are reflected below with regards to the NHSA:

1. Representation and selection. The adequate representation of CSOs on various subcommittees under the NHSB and the QSB effectively confers countervailing power to underrepresented populations that fall under CSO constituencies and comprise the marginalized and vulnerable groups, including people living with HIV, people with disabilities, and ethnic minorities [13]. To our knowledge, it is the only Thai law that provides CSO representation in the governance of the UCS that significantly boosts accountability [15].

2. Roles and responsibilities. The legislative provision in the NHSA pertaining to the NHSB and its duties are clear and specific [13], and ensures that community-based organizations operating in the nonprofit space, as well as health care providers, are consulted through annual public hearings and included in planning, monitoring, and decision-making processes of the Board.

3. Funding modalities. The Community Health Fund receives equal contributions from NHSO and the local government or municipality, and is managed locally at the subdistrict level [16] to deliver actions such as preventive health interventions, public health awareness campaigns, clubs for the elderly, traffic accident prevention campaigns, and local health-specific trainings. Program activities are selected with community input, demonstrating how the formal institutionalization of a budgetary mechanism through legislation can promote CE and ownership.

29.4.4 Strong Capacities Are Required on Both the Government and People's Side

Implementation capacity is as important as legislative provision. A legal framework alone cannot guarantee genuine participation when capacities on both the government (including power and attitude) as well as the people's sides are not sufficient to engage. WHO's social participation handbook distinguishes three dimensions of capacity needs for effective social participation: (1) skills in recognizing other partners; (2) communication skills; and (3) leadership and organizational skills. We analyze them in detail below with regards to the UCS's participatory platforms.

1. *Recognition skills for government* include understanding the added value participation offers to policymaking. The fact that citizens and CSOs publicly stood firm and were successful in protecting and increasing the UCS budget despite the government's initial intent to scale it down has been a great learning experience for NHSO senior management on the value of civic participation.
   Recognition skills for populations, communities, and civil society include perceiving one's needs, strengths, and weaknesses, as well as those of the community, with capacities for internal dialog and coordination. Thai civil society is generally well organized and highly

educated, with a fairly supportive health sector landscape in terms of funding and capacity assistance. The Thai Health Promotion Foundation is financed through a 2% additional surcharge on alcohol and tobacco, and the funds are channeled to support CSOs' capacity-building and operations on preventive and community health [17]. In addition, various government health institutions – such as the National Health Commission Office – work closely with CSOs and communities by providing capacity training to them. Taken together, investments in civil society capacity and Thailand's long-term vision has allowed for meaningful, mutually beneficial engagement in participatory spaces.

2. *Communication skills.* Government cadres need to prepare participatory events with nuanced and adapted information, minimizing jargon and technical terminology. At the same time, policymakers must know how to take in information expressed as lived experiences from starkly different perspectives and "translate" it into policy-relevant material for internal government uptake. NHSO's longstanding experience with public hearings and its interaction with civil society through its Boards has helped build its staff capacity for communication over time. Investment in CE platforms over more than two decades is bearing fruit.

Thai CSOs have developed a high degree of professionalism over the past two decades, cementing their legitimacy and position in policy circles. Many of them work closely with research partners, which contributes to evidence-based policy formulation and advocacies, though many of them are working at the operational level, notably related to HIV/AIDS campaigns. The health reform movement of the early 2000s helped shape a funding and policy landscape that has nurtured organic growth and increased the capacities of the civil society and given it a solid and credible voice in policy matters. Civil society's capacities have also been built due to repeated exposure to participatory processes and engagement at multiple platforms with decision-makers in Thailand.

3. *Leadership and organizational skills.* Policymakers require leadership and organizational skills in creating, managing, and sustaining participatory spaces, as these are hard to come by in the public health sector. The NHSO, as well as staff in Thailand's autonomous health institutions, has acquired this over time by advising the government and having regular exposure to and practice in social participation mechanisms.

29.5 Conclusion: What Lessons for Beyond the Thai Context?

The UCS illustration offers valuable lessons for other countries about participatory and responsive governance in their paths toward UHC. First and foremost, this well-documented experience demonstrates that many aspects need to converge for CE to become institutionalized at different levels of the health system, from policy to operations, including an enabling legal framework, adequate capacity of the government and citizens, sustained political will, and a pervasive commitment to participation.

One of the major challenges of CE is the bureaucratic mindset and unequal power relation which often prevents bureaucrats from recognizing and developing the skills of communities. In Thailand, a mandatory five years in rural service for health professionals since 1972 had exposed young professionals to rural poor, rural health services, and CE early in their careers. When these young professionals became high-level MOPH administrators, a narrow mindset was minimal. Another valuable insight is the need for a long-term perspective with participatory activities, as citizens and communities need time to build capacities, and activities mature and become fine-tuned and adapted to policy needs over time.

In the current COVID-19 crisis, countries with a high level of citizen engagement and trust in government institutions, either political or in the health sector, performed better in pandemic containment [20, 21]. This indicates the acute need for closer ties between decision-makers and the people they serve. Yet such ties cannot be created or strengthened during a pandemic, they must be nurtured and cultivated slowly and steadily over time. When an acute need arises, these ties can be effectively leveraged for mounting the emergency response, and during normal times continue to provide an overall steer toward a responsive health system.

References

1. United Nations. Political declaration of the High-Level Meeting on Universal Health Coverage: moving together to build a healthier world. 2019. www.un.org/pga/73/wp-content/uploads/sites/53/2019/07/FINAL-draft-UHC-Political-Declaration.pdf (accessed August 19, 2022).

2. G. Brunton, J. Thomas, A. O'Mara-Eves, et al. Narratives of community engagement: a systematic review-derived conceptual framework for public health interventions. *BMC Public Health* 2017; **17**(1): 944.

3. V. Haldane, F. L. H. Chuah, A. Srivastava, et al. Community participation in health services development, implementation, and evaluation: a systematic review of empowerment, health, community, and process outcomes. *PLoS One* 2019; **14**(5): e0216112.

4. E. Sacks, R. C. Swanson, J. J. Schensul, et al. Community involvement in health systems strengthening to improve global health outcomes: a review of guidelines and potential roles. *Int Q Community Health Educ* 2017; **37**(3–4): 139–149.

5. World Health Organization, United Nations Children's Fund (UNICEF). A vision for primary health care in the 21st century: towards universal health coverage and the Sustainable Development Goals. 2018. https://apps.who.int/iris/handle/10665/328065 (accessed February 9, 2022).

6. G. Pilkington, S. Panday, M. N. Khatib, et al. The effectiveness of community engagement and participation approaches in low and middle income countries: a review of systematic reviews with particular reference to the countries of South Asia.2017. www.researchgate.net/publication/326742746_The_effectiveness_of_community_engagement_and_participation_approaches_in_low_and_middle_income_countries_a_review_of_systematic_reviews_with_particular_reference_to_the_countries_of_South_Asia (accessed December 14, 2021).

7. R. Fadlallah, F. El-Jardali, N. Hemadi, et al. Barriers and facilitators to implementation, uptake and sustainability of community-based health insurance schemes in low- and middle-income countries: a systematic review. *Int J Equity Health* 2018; **17**: 13.

8. T. Lavers. Towards universal health coverage in Ethiopia's "developmental state"? The political drivers of health insurance. *Soc Sci Med* 2019; **228**: 60–67.

9. D. Hughes, S. Leethongdee. Universal coverage in the land of smiles: lessons from Thailand's 30 Baht health reforms. *Health Affairs* 2007; **26**(4): 999–1008.

10. Somdet Phra Paramintharamaha Bhumibol Adulyadej Sayammintharathirat Borommanatthabophit. Constitution of the Kingdom of Thailand. 2017. http://web.krisdika.go.th/data/outsitedata/outsite21/file/Constitution_of_the_Kingdom_of_Thailand.pdf (accessed December 14, 2021).

11. W. Patcharanarumol, V. Tangcharoensathien, S. Limwattananon, et al. "Good health at low cost" 25 years on: what makes a successful health system.

2011. https://ghlc.lshtm.ac.uk/files/2011/10/ Policy-Briefing-No5-Thailand.pdf (accessed December 14, 2021).

12. Somdet Phra Paramintharamaha Bhumibol Adulyadej Sayammintharathirat Borommanatthabophit. Constitution of the Kingdom of Thailand. 1997. https://dl .parliament.go.th/bitstream/handle/lirt/42 6419/2540_Thai_Constitution.pdf?sequen ce=1 (accessed August 19, 2022).

13. National Health Security Office. National Health Security Act B. E. 2545. 2002. https:// eng.nhso.go.th/view/1/National_Health_ Security_Act_B.E.2545/EN-US (accessed February 17, 2022).

14. V. Tangcharoensathien, D. Pichetkul, W. Patcharanarumol. Listen to the voice of citizens: implementing a call centre in Thailand's Universal Coverage Scheme. *Sophia J Asian Afr Middle East Stud* 2020; **38**: 21–29.

15. K. Kantamaturapoj, A. Kulthanmanusorn, W. Witthayapipopsakul, et al. Legislating for public accountability in universal health coverage, Thailand. *Bull World Health Organ* 2020; **98**(2): 117–125.

16. U. Saengow, T. Phenwan, A. Laohaprapanon, et al. Challenges in implementation of community health fund in Thailand. 2019. https://discovery

.dundee.ac.uk/en/publications/challenges- in-implementation-of-community-health- fund-in-thailand (accessed December 14, 2021).

17. S. Pongutta, R. Suphanchaimat, W. Patcharanarumol, et al. Lessons from the Thai Health Promotion Foundation. *Bull World Health Organ* 2019; **97**(3): 213–220.

18. World Health Organization. The triangle that moves the mountain: nine years of Thailand's National Health Assembly (2008–2016). 2017. https://apps.who.int/ iris/handle/10665/260464 (accessed December 14, 2021).

19. World Health Organization. *Voice, Agency, Empowerment: Handbook on Social Participation for Universal Health Coverage.* 2021. www.who.int/publications-detail- redirect/9789240027794 (accessed December 14, 2021).

20. R. Falcone, E. Colì, S. Felletti, et al. All we need is trust: how the COVID-19 outbreak reconfigured trust in Italian public institutions. *Front Psychol* 2020; **11**: 561747.

21. V. Gopichandran, S. Subramaniam, M. J. Kalsingh. COVID-19 pandemic: a litmus test of trust in the health system. *Asian Bioeth Rev* 2020; **12**(2): 1–9.

30
Achieving Health-Related Sustainable Development Goals
Role of Health Systems Strengthening

Rehana A. Salam, Jai K. Das, and Zulfiqar A. Bhutta

Key Messages

- The interrelatedness between SDG 3 – ensure healthy lives and promote wellbeing – and other health-related SDGs calls for a multisectoral approach to maximize synergies in reaching SDG targets.
- Low- and middle-income countries (L&MICs) could benefit from robust health systems research to assess the existing gaps and challenges, followed by a customized approach for improvement based on country needs.
- Internal capacity development is needed for L&MICs not only to enhance the health workforce, but also for institutional capacity and for workforce across sectors.
- Stakeholder engagement is key to understanding the context, setting purpose, and shaping influence.
- Countries need to significantly increase resource allocation to health and cross-sectoral initiatives to address health and the underlying determinants of health.

30.1 Introduction

Toward the end of the Millennium Development Goal (MDG) period in 2015, much progress was reported in the domains of global under-five mortality, maternal mortality, births attended by skilled health personnel, and burden and intervention coverage for HIV, malaria, and tuberculosis [1]. The progress was, however, largely inequitable, with lack of access to basic services across and within countries; gaps in intervention coverage between the poorest and the richest; and persistent gender inequalities [1]. The MDG era highlighted the indispensable role of strong political commitment and data to meet the demands for the new development agenda [1].

In 2015, the United Nations General Assembly replaced the MDG framework with the Agenda for Sustainable Development, which comprises 17 universal Sustainable Development Goals (SDGs), encompassing 169 targets and 231 indicators [2]. The 17 goals are far broader in their scope than the MDGs were, and are anticipated to be achieved by 2030. Out of these, SDG 3 aims to, "Ensure healthy lives and promote wellbeing for all at all ages" [3].

The Global Burden of Diseases, Injuries, and Risk Factors Study 2015 (GBD 2015) conducted a baseline assessment and analysis of 33 health-related SDG indicators documenting historical trends between 1990 and 2015 to inform roadmaps and provide a benchmark for monitoring the health-related SDG indicators [4]. This analysis suggested that from 2000 to 2015 there has been progress in the use of modern contraception, in universal health coverage (UHC) tracer interventions with reduction in under-five and neonatal mortality, and moderate improvements in the incidence of HIV and tuberculosis. However, hepatitis B incidence decreased only minimally, and childhood overweight considerably worsened. The analyses also suggested that factors like income, education, and fertility could act as drivers of health improvement, but that additional investment in other areas is needed to ensure sustainability beyond the MDGs [4]. These findings provide a reference point for measuring the progress on SDGs and highlight the fact that achieving equitable coverage at the population level will require renewed focus on a spectrum of factors besides those captured by direct health indicators.

Since the introduction of the SDGs there has been a lot of evidence pointing to the interrelatedness of all the SDG targets [5–10]. SDG 3 focuses directly on health; however, since health is affected by a multitude of factors, SDG 3 is inevitably connected to other SDGs, including most notably: SDG 2, end hunger, achieve food security and improved nutrition, and promote sustainable agriculture; SDG 4, ensure inclusive and equitable quality education and promote lifelong learning opportunities for all; SDG 5, achieve gender equality and empower all women and girls; SDG 6, ensure availability and sustainable management of water and sanitation for all; SDG 10, reduce inequality within and among countries; and SDG 12, ensure sustainable consumption and production patterns [11]. Accordingly, there are 33 overarching health-related indicators across all the SDGs, including better education for girls; tackling child malnourishment; ensuring access to safe water; and tackling ambient air pollution, to highlight a few. The health-related SDGs and the associated indicators are summarized in Table 30.1.

The integrative nature of the relationship between SDG 3 and other SDGs calls for an integrated implementation to maximize synergies between the various SDG targets. According to the United Nations Sustainable Development Goals Report 2020, the current pace of global progress is not sufficient to meet many of the health-related SDG targets [12]. With the ongoing COVID-19 pandemic, the progress is anticipated to slow further. Access to health care has been further restricted due to unprepared health facilities, with some being closed during the early stages of the pandemic and in other cases populations being afraid to seek health care services to avoid exposure to COVID-19. Health systems in many L&MICs have been unable to cope with the surge in demand for health care due to lack of health care workers, medical equipment, and supplies. With an estimated 71 million people pushed back into extreme poverty in 2020 [12], progress toward UHC has become increasingly vital in these challenging times. With less than a decade to achieve the SDGs, much effort is needed in L&MICs to make considerable improvements toward the SDG targets.

30.2 Framework for Analysis and Attainment of SDGs

In order to assess the implementation of health-related strategies and progress toward health-related SDG targets in L&MICs, Aftab et al. [13] developed a framework comprising nine domains (Figure 30.1), which represent political, technical, and institutional conditions that determine whether and to what extent health-related SDG targets and indicators are achieved.

Based on this analytical framework, the implementation modalities adopted at national level to achieve health and health-related SDGs were examined through a systematic review and multicountry case studies [13, 14]. The systematic review included 32 studies, of which

Table 30.1 Health-related SDG indicators

SDG	Health-related SDG indicators
Goal 1: End poverty in all its forms everywhere	Disaster related deaths (1.5.1 same as Indicators 11.5.1 and 13.1.2)
Goal 2: End hunger, achieve food security and improved nutrition, and promote sustainable agriculture	Stunting (2.2.1) Wasting (2.2.2a) Overweight (2.2.2b)
Goal 3: Ensure healthy lives and promote wellbeing for all at all ages	Maternal mortality ratio (3.1.1) Skilled birth attendance (3.1.2) Under-five mortality (3.2.1) Neonatal mortality (3.2.2) HIV (3.3.1) Tuberculosis (3.3.2) Malaria (3.3.3) Hepatitis B (3.3.4) Neglected tropical diseases (3.3.5) NCDs (3.4.1) Suicide (3.4.2) Alcohol (3.5.2) Road injuries (3.6.1) Family planning need met, modern contraception (3.7.1) Adolescent birth rate (3.7.2) UHC – service coverage (3.8.1) UHC – financial protection (3.8.2) Air pollution mortality (3.9.1) WASH mortality (3.9.2) Poisons (3.9.3) Smoking (3.a.1)
Goal 5: Achieve gender equality and empower all women and girls	Intimate partner violence (5.2.1)
Goal 6: Ensure availability and sustainable management of water and sanitation for all	Water (6.1.1) Sanitation (6.2.1a) Hygiene (6.2.1b)
Goal 7: Ensure access to affordable, reliable, sustainable, and modern energy for all	Household air pollution (7.1.2)
Goal 8: Promote sustained, inclusive, and sustainable economic growth, full and productive employment, and decent work for all	Occupational risk burden (8.8.1)
Goal 11: Make cities and human settlements inclusive, safe, resilient, and sustainable	Disaster related deaths (11.5.1; same as Indicators 1.5.1); and Disaster risk reduction related (13.1.2) Mean PM2.5 (11.6.2)

Table 30.1 (cont.)

SDG	Health-related SDG indicators
Goal 13: Take urgent action to combat climate change and its impacts	Disaster related (13.1.2, 1.5.1 and 11.5.1)
Goal 16: Promote peaceful and inclusive societies for sustainable development, provide access to justice for all, and build effective, accountable, and inclusive institutions at all levels	Violence (16.1.1) War (16.1.2)

24 provided information at the national level and 8 provided information for multiple countries or regions. Based on the findings of the review, a series of consultative meetings were conducted with representatives from 15 countries across five regions, assessing the evidence on early achievements, gaps and challenges, and opportunities for the implementation of health-related SDGs [14]. Consultations included a diverse set of participants from the health sector, related public sectors, civil society organizations, academia, and development partners. In the following section we have used the nine domains of the framework to assess how best to incorporate the health and health-related SDGs into the national policy agenda of L&MICs.

30.2.1 Political Commitment

A key factor behind progress in the implementation of health and health-related SDGs appears to be high-level political commitment at the national level, with alignment of the health-related SDGs to existing development strategies and plans [15]. There is evidence that governance-specific interventions, including civil society participation and engaging community members with health service structures and processes, can lead to tangible improvements in health as well as better service uptake and quality of care [13, 14]. Leadership capacity development and mentoring are central for effective governance. There is evidence that complex leadership programs blending skills development, mentoring, and promotion of teamwork bring about improvements in service quality, management, competence, and motivation [16]. Findings from the aforementioned systematic review and consultative meetings suggest that many L&MICs are focusing on key SDGs based on national priorities and available capacity and resources, which commonly include health, but not all health-related goals [14].

30.2.2 Institutional Setup

It is essential to make efforts to strengthen existing institutions and establish new ones to reach underserved populations in order to achieve positive health outcomes and take a leap toward the SDG targets. Health institutions in many L&MICs have not adapted to the epidemiological transition and are still focused on basic health care requirements [17]. An analysis from the GBD 2016 data suggests that about 15 million excess deaths from 61 conditions occurred in L&MICs in 2016 [18]. After excluding deaths that could be

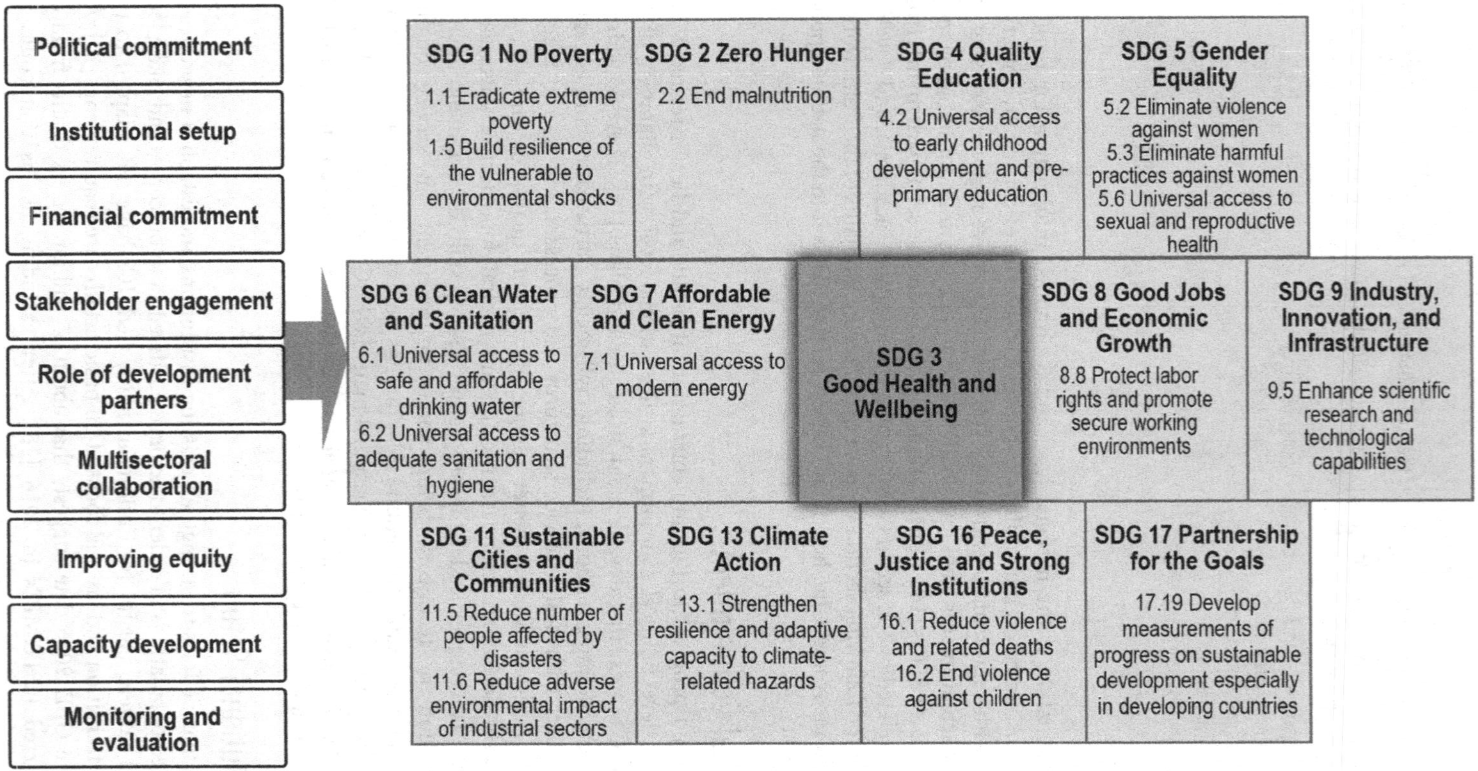

Figure 30.1 The analytical framework for assessing the implementation of health and health-related SDGs and their targets [13].

prevented through public health measures, around 8 million excess deaths were amenable to health care, of which 5 million were estimated to be due to receipt of poor-quality care and about 3 million to nonutilization of health care [18]. A recent analysis suggests that L&MICs appear to rely on existing institutions and implementation is overseen or led by multiagency structures such as planning commissions, cabinet committees, inter-ministerial forums, and parliamentary committees [13]. One of the key challenges faced by L&MICs is a lack of institutional mechanisms for coordination between national and subnational agencies [13]. L&MICs require a redesign of their health service delivery models, with a blend of existing and newer institutions established for the explicit purpose of maximizing health outcomes rather than geographical access to services alone [17]. As explained in the introductory section, SDGs are interconnected such that impact on health-related SDGs requires intersectoral interventions rather than mere provision of health services. Health systems should be adapted to maximize intersectoral collaboration and optimize intervention design to achieve the health-related SDG targets.

30.2.3 Financing

There is a need for investments in the existing health financing systems of L&MICs in order to achieve health and health-related SDG targets [19]. In the era of SDGs, funding constraints appear to be a major challenge for many countries as they contend with the negative impact of limited financial resources, high dependence on donor funding/external assistance, inadequate mainstreaming of SDGs in subnational planning and/or budgeting, and the deleterious effect of climate change on economic productivity and human capacity, as well as high levels of debt to international financial institutions [13]. A recent projection from 67 countries representing 95% of the total population in L&MICs estimates that between 2016 and 2030 an additional US$274 billion spending on health is needed per year to make progress toward the SDG 3 targets, while US$371 billion would be needed to reach health system targets in the ambitious scenario [19]. All countries will need to strengthen investments in health systems to expand service provision in order to reach SDG 3 targets. In view of anticipated resource constraints, each country will need to prioritize equitably, plan strategically, and cost realistically its own path toward SDG 3, including UHC [19]. Health financing alone will not lead to the achievement of SDGs and convergence with optimal benefits from investments in other SDGs will be needed to maximize the impact on health indicators in L&MICs [20].

30.2.4 Stakeholder Engagement

Given the integrated nature of the relationship between health and other SDGs, meaningful involvement of all stakeholders is particularly important. The recent report by the United Nations Department of Economic and Social Affairs (UNDESA) and the United Nations Institute for Training and Research (UNITAR), Stakeholder Engagement and the 2030 Agenda, identifies "major groups" and "other groups" of stakeholders [21]. The "major groups" include women, children, indigenous people, nongovernmental organizations (NGOs), local authorities, workers and trade unions, business and industry, the scientific and technological community, and farmers. "Other stakeholders" include local communities, educational and academic entities, faith groups, foundations and private philanthropic organizations, migrants and their families, older persons, parliamentary networks and associations, persons with disabilities, and volunteer groups. At the global level, "major groups and other stakeholders" is the terminology used to refer to the participation of diverse sectors at intergovernmental deliberations, and both of these groups have been granted comprehensive participatory opportunities in the High-Level Political Forum on Sustainable Development through the UN General Assembly Resolution. Maher and Buhmann [22] suggest that stakeholder engagement can be maximized with a bottom-up approach as it allows for nonstate actors to "meaningfully" engage with stakeholders as opposed to merely listening. Findings from a recent systematic review suggest that the stakeholders most commonly involved in SDG implementation include the private sector, think tanks and academia, development partners, and civil society organizations [13]. Moreover, some governments are collaborating with development partners and UN agencies to support planning at the national level, institutional development, and capacity-building. National and regional think tanks and multilateral agencies are facilitating experience sharing between regional countries in Southeast Africa, South Asia, and Latin America [13].

30.2.5 Role of Development Partners

The health and health-related SDGs offer enormous opportunities for partnerships and collaborations, and SDG 17 highlights the potential role partnerships and collaborative governance could play at all levels, from global to local. There is a need for close engagement with development partners in terms of financial and technical assistance; however, they should not be allowed to lead the SDG agenda in countries. Besides the development partners, high-income countries can play a significant role in supporting L&MICs governments in building capacities, finances, and implementation. Findings from a recent systematic review suggest that bilateral and multilateral agencies are actively supporting health and related areas, and regional development banks are actively involved in South Asia and Africa [13]. A multicountry case study suggested that development partners led by United Nations Development Programme and multilateral organizations such as the World Bank and bilateral donors, especially the United States Agency for International Development, are active in this regard [14]. Findings from these studies also suggest that L&MICs face challenges such as poor coordination between development partners and development partner priorities taking precedence over government priorities [13].

30.2.6 Multisectoral Collaboration

The SDGs call for an interlinked and integrated approach toward global and national betterment, which requires that multiple sectors collaborate and work synergistically rather than in silos to achieve the SDG targets. Multisectoral collaboration can include national and international partnerships between national governments, local authorities, international institutions, business, civil society organizations, foundations, philanthropists, social impact investors, scientists, and citizens [23]. However, what sort of partnerships are required in which domains is not always clear. For L&MICs it has become imperative to comprehend where multisectoral collaboration will be most effective, how to ensure efficiency, and what factors enable these collaborations to contribute to transformative change [24]. Existing evidence suggests that L&MICs can benefit from various sectors contributing toward the SDG agenda; for example, nutrition, women's health, and child health [24–27]. In order to achieve these targets, multisectoral collaboration including with universities and civil society are needed to help governments increase their capacity to implement health-related SDGs. A recent systematic review suggests that in L&MICs, the most commonly used mechanism for multisectoral collaboration includes cabinet/inter-ministerial committees and secretariats, interdepartmental committees and units, and parliamentary committees [13]. Findings from a country case study suggest that some countries have taken more comprehensive approaches, such as health-in-all-policies and social-determinants-of-health approaches [14]. However, some challenges in multisectoral collaboration include inadequate coordination between national and subnational agencies for multisectoral work, and inadequate empowerment of local governments [13].

30.2.7 Improving Equity

Equity is central to the SDG 2030 agenda, and achieving health equity will require actions not merely on health but also on the social determinants of health, including: income, food, nutrition, education and lifelong learning, water and sanitation, decent work, fair employment, and aspects of the built and natural environment [28]. A commitment to equity also requires a renewed focus on vulnerable groups and disaggregated data to monitor access to required services by these vulnerable groups. In order to improve equity, L&MICs need to improve intersectoral collaboration whereby governments work with other sectors in a coherently stated strategy [28]. National policies focusing only on domestic factors rather than having a broader view of the global economy might not be effective in reducing country-level inequities [29]. Evidence suggests that combined policy interventions focusing on improved education and spatial integration could reduce inequity. Findings from a systematic review suggest that L&MICs are increasingly focusing on population groups most impacted by adverse determinants of health, such as women, children, elderly, people with disabilities, sexual minorities, indigenous peoples, and migrants [13, 14]. However, deliberate efforts to disaggregate data to monitor access and impact across marginalized and disadvantaged groups are required [13].

30.2.8 Capacity Development

The current numbers and capacity of the health workforce in L&MICs is insufficient and there is a need to build its existing capacity and improve its competencies [17]. Evidence from successful health care workforce models suggests that task shifting and skills-mix models can be successfully adopted by L&MICs to address the existing shortage of health care workers [16]. In addition to the health workforce, there is also a need to develop institutional capacity and to train other cadres of workers related to the various domains of health-related SDGs. Capacity-building of workers in cross-cutting areas directly or indirectly related to health would lead to enhanced implementation. Existing capacity-building challenges include SDG costing and budgeting, gender mainstreaming, monitoring and evaluation, policy formulation, technical capacity, and management of statistical information [13]. Recent analysis suggests that there is very limited evidence to guide action in the domain of capacity development [13, 14]. Findings from a multicountry case study suggest that capacity assessment to identify gaps in SDG implementation has not been considered adequately in L&MICs, with only a few sporadic capacity-building initiatives in some countries, mostly with the support of UN agencies [14].

30.2.9 Monitoring and Evaluation

There is a need to monitor and track progress in order to modify and refine programs targeting SDGs. This would require standardized metrics to measure the progress of countries consistently and reliably on SDG targets and specifically the 33 health-related SDG indicators. The routine health information systems in L&MICs function suboptimally due to lack of skills, poor technology, and inadequate processes and investments resulting in weak data collection and deficient analysis and use. Furthermore, health information systems in most L&MICs do not capture the health-related SDG indicators and need to be reconfigured to capture data on all health-related SDGs during regular surveys. Barriers to robust implementation and use of electronic health records and District Health Information Software (DHIS) include restricted ownership by end-users, scarce training on data skills, lack of motivation and engagement by overburdened health workers, large numbers of indicators required, and inadequate functionality of electronic platforms [17]. A recent analysis suggests that in many L&MICs, defining priority goals, targets, and indicators is still underway [13, 14]. Findings from a multicountry case study suggest that challenges commonly faced by L&MICs include poor baseline data; inadequate data management infrastructure and capacity; a focus on data gathering and management with limited analysis and use; missing private sector data in national data management systems; inconsistent availability of data to frequently monitor progress; poor data reliability; lack of disaggregated data; misalignment between national and subnational targets; inadequate funding for data collection and monitoring; exclusive focus on population survey data and inadequate use of routine administrative data; limited technical capacity and infrastructure for data collection and management; and heavy reliance on donors for data collection [13].

30.3 How Health Systems Contribute to and Benefit from Actions on Health-Related and Other SDGs

Health systems can vastly contribute to and benefit from interventions for achieving the SDGs, including nonhealth-related ones, due to their interrelatedness. A preferred approach is to move beyond the *health-only perspective* to a more inclusive and multi-sectoral approach. There has been a lot of global discussion around establishing "quality health systems" rather than "health systems" alone. The Lancet Health Commission on High Quality Health Systems in the SDG era evaluated the quality of care available to people in L&MICs and highlighted that the existing health care is "often inadequate" and of poor quality, and is even worse for the poor segments of society [17]. Accordingly, eight million lives could be saved annually in L&MICs if high-quality health systems were put in place. The Commission proposed a conceptual framework for forming high-quality health systems, based on three key domains: foundations, processes of care, and quality impacts (Figure 30.2). The framework incorporates health system functions, user experience, and population health needs and experience, which form the core of the primary health care approach (Chapter 2) [17]. L&MICs could benefit from robust health systems research to assess the existing gaps and challenges, followed by a customized approach for improvement based on country needs.

Unstable political environment, incoherent policy and planning, and lack of prioritization are common challenges faced by L&MICs [13]. Governments need to demonstrate strong political will to prioritize SDGs, especially the health-related SDGs within

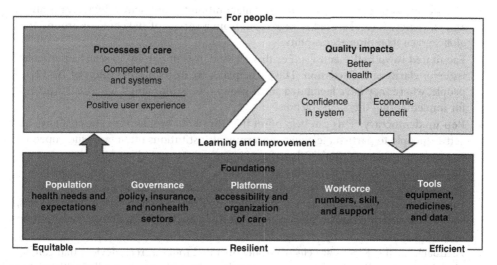

Figure 30.2 A high-quality health system framework [17].

countries [15]. Clear mechanisms should be devised for consultation and integration across various sectors, including civil society and academia. By working together these sectors could bring critical pressure to bear and secure resources for evidence-based action. Political commitment to SDGs should be translated into effective programs utilizing the "Health in All Policies" approach, which integrates and articulates health considerations into policymaking across sectors to improve the health of communities and its people (see Chapter 37). Implementation capacities should be strengthened at national, subnational, and district levels, with a strong focus on reaching the most vulnerable and marginalized populations. Robust interagency governance arrangements also need to be established to enhance accountability and liability in health systems under normal circumstances, as well as in humanitarian situations [17].

Financing for SDGs in L&MICs is either incorporated into existing funded plans or occurs through SDG-specific budgeting and tracking [15]. In some instances, additional funding is mobilized by increasing domestic taxation, subsidization, or through collaboration with development partners, including UN agencies, and in some instances the private sector. Existing evidence of successful financing models suggests focusing on equitable distribution and improvement in health outcomes of the population, with increased public spending on health [16]. External aid, if well utilized, can also improve health outcomes and health equity, depending on the aid delivery approach [16].

Stakeholder engagement is key – be it at the governance level, financing, or multisectoral involvement. Engagement at any level involves understanding the context, scoping the project, understanding the people, setting the purpose, and shaping influence. Multiple innovative approaches have evolved over time, which can be utilized to engage stakeholders in sectors other than health. A few of the innovative approaches highlighted in the recent UNDESA and UNITAR training reference material for effective stakeholder engagement for the 2030 agenda include [21]:

- **Crowdsourcing:** This seeks to harness collaboration for problem-solving, innovation, and efficiency. It can be used to seek input from a variety of stakeholders around the globe, given its online accessibility.
- **Facilitated town hall meetings:** For this method, it is important to select a particular issue for clarity and discussion. The participants are divided into groups of 10–12 people, where they have facilitated small-group discussions about a particular process for implementing the 2030 Agenda.
- **Pop-up democracy:** This can help offset the "threshold problem" or the challenge of getting people to participate, which government institutions often face when opening engagement processes. Rather than expecting people to attend meetings in areas and buildings that might be unfamiliar or too far away from where they live, pop-up democracy is an attempt to reach the furthest behind by bringing the stakeholder engagement method to the stakeholders. Pop-up democracy can take different forms, such as inserted or modular interventions, food as a medium of exchange, pop-up shops, or activist spaces.
- **Feedback kiosks:** Kiosks are electronically operated touch-screen devices that can be placed in any public space (e.g., bus terminals, train stations). They allow citizens to provide feedback and answer survey questions about SDG priorities in their neighborhoods.

Common stakeholder engagement challenges in L&MICs include unclear roles for various stakeholders; deficient involvement and/or coordination with the government; limited involvement of the private sector, civil society, research institutions, and community; and lack of resources to maintain well-structured collaborations and fair representation [15]. Figure 30.3 highlights the 10 components of the stakeholder engagement strategy suggested in UNDESA and UNITAR 2020's "Stakeholder Engagement and the 2030 Agenda: A Practical Guide" [21].

Besides engagement, monitoring and tracking progress on key SDG indictors is essential. L&MICs need to transform their data collection measures into agile new surveys and real-time measures of health and health-related SDG indicators. Digital health, in the form of m-health and telehealth, offers a unique opportunity to use a relatively low-resource platform for data collection, monitoring, and evaluation [30, 31]. Global development partners can provide assistance for health information systems such as civil and vital registries, routine data systems, and routine health system surveys; and they can promote capacity-building of relevant national and regional institutions (see Chapters 8 and 22) [17].

More recently, the COVID-19 pandemic has challenged the capacity and emergency preparedness of health systems all across the globe [32]. With one-third of the timeline to achieve the SDGs already passed and insufficient progress on the set indicators, COVID-19 threatens to reverse the progress of health-related SDG indicators. The COVID-19 pandemic has fast become one of the greatest global health challenges, posing not only health but political, financial, and technical challenges. Global experts agree that the pandemic has exposed inherent weaknesses in our preparedness and response, with the existing health systems being grossly overwhelmed by the pandemic (see Chapter 34) [33, 34]. Although the COVID-19 scenario is ongoing and there is much more to learn from the evolving scenario, van Zanten and van Tulder [35] suggest that the SDG agenda provides three "logics" that could help transform toward sustainable societies: (1) a governance logic that sets goals, adopts policies, and tracks progress to steer impacts; (2) a systems (nexus) logic that

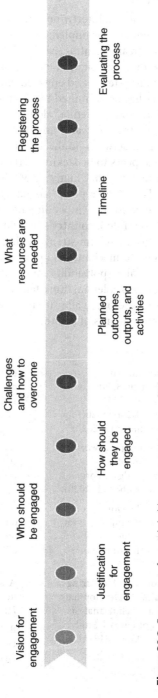

Figure 30.3 Components for a stakeholder engagement strategy [21].

manages SDG interactions; and (3) a strategic logic that enables (micro-level) companies to develop strategies that impact (macro-level) policy goals.

30.4 Way Forward

The SDGs are interdependent and intertwined, and achieving SDG 3 targets might not be possible if SDG-specific programs are implemented in silos. During the first five years of the SDG era, L&MICs from South and Central Asia and East Africa have demonstrated growing political commitment, with augmentation of multisectoral institutional arrangements, strengthening of monitoring systems, and engagement of development partners to accelerate implementation. There has been limited involvement of nonstate stakeholders such as civil society representatives and academia, along with the lack of capacity development initiatives, communication strategies, and any additional domestic financing for implementing SDGs [15]. The link between nonhealth SDGs and integrated multisectoral strategies for implementation appears to be lacking [14].

The bigger challenge remains that many L&MICs vary greatly in their approaches to implementing the SDGs. The WHO report, "Changing Mindsets: Strategy on Health Policy and Systems Research," called for the embedding of research into health systems processes [36, 37]. Embedding research into a country's individual health systems will help generate customized solutions for health system strengthening in the specific country's perspective (see Chapter 14). Appropriate mechanisms are needed for consultation and integration, grounded in notions of social responsibility and sustainability, to bring together various actors, including civil society, academia, think tanks, and the private sector. Countries will need to significantly increase resource allocation to health and cross-sectoral initiatives to address health and the determinants of health.

References

1. United Nations. The Millennium Development Goals report 2015. 2015. www.un.org/millenniumgoals/2015_MDG_Report/pdf/MDG%202015%20rev%20(July%201).pdf (accessed November 12, 2020).

2. United Nations. Transforming our world: the 2030 Agenda for Sustainable Development. 2015. https://sdgs.un.org/2030agenda (accessed November 11, 2020).

3. M. P. Kieny, H. Bekedam, D. Dovlo, et al. Strengthening health systems for universal health coverage and sustainable development. *Bull World Health Organ* 2017; **95**(7): 537–539.

4. GBD 2015 SDG Collaborators. Measuring the health-related Sustainable Development Goals in 188 countries: a baseline analysis from the Global Burden of Disease Study 2015. *Lancet* 2016; **388**(10053): 1813–1850.

5. J. Tosun, J. Leininger. Governing the interlinkages between the Sustainable Development Goals: approaches to attain policy integration. *Glob Chall* 2017; **1**(9): 1700036.

6. M. Stafford-Smith, D. Griggs, O. Gaffney, et al. Integration: the key to implementing the Sustainable Development Goals. *Sustain Sci* 2017; **12**(6): 911–919.

7. G. Dörgő, V. Sebestyén, J. Abonyi. Evaluating the interconnectedness of the sustainable development goals based on the causality analysis of sustainability indicators. *Sustainability* 2018; **10**(10): 3766.

8. P. Pradhan, L. Costa, D. Rybski, et al. A systematic study of sustainable development goal (SDG) interactions. *Earth's Future* 2017; **5**(11): 1169–1179.

9. B. Mainali, J. Luukkanen, S. Silveira, et al. Evaluating synergies and trade-offs among Sustainable Development Goals (SDGs): explorative analyses of development paths in

South Asia and Sub-Saharan Africa. *Sustainability* 2018; **10**(3): 815.

10. M. Nilsson, E. Chisholm, D. Griggs, et al. Mapping interactions between the sustainable development goals: lessons learned and ways forward. *Sustain Sci* 2018; **13**(6): 1489–1503.

11. R. M. Fernandez. SDG3 good health and well-being: integration and connection with other SDGs. In W. Leal Filho, T. Wall, A. M. Azul, et al., eds., *Good Health and Well-Being: Encyclopedia of the UN Sustainable Development Goals.* Cham, Springer.

12. United Nations. The Sustainable Development Goals Report. 2020. www.un.org/sustainabledevelopment/progress-report/ (accessed November 11, 2020).

13. W. Aftab, F. J. Siddiqui, H. Tasic, et al. Implementation of health and health-related sustainable development goals: progress, challenges and opportunities – a systematic literature review. *BMJ Glob Health* 2020; **5**(8): e002273.

14. S. Siddiqi, W. Aftab, F. J. Siddiqui, et al. Global strategies and local implementation of health and health-related SDGs: lessons from consultation in countries across five regions. *BMJ Glob Health* 2020; **5**(9): e002859.

15. Z. A. Bhutta, S. Siddiqi, W. Aftab, et al. What will it take to implement health and health-related sustainable development goals? *BMJ Glob Health* 2020; **5**(9): e002963.

16. S. Witter, N. Palmer, D. Balabanova, et al. Health system strengthening: reflections on its meaning, assessment, and our state of knowledge. *Int J Health Plann Manage* 2019; **34**(4): e1980–e1989.

17. M E. Kruk, A. D. Gage, C. Arsenault, et al. High-quality health systems in the Sustainable Development Goals era: time for a revolution. *Lancet Glob Health* 2018; **6** (11): e1196–e1252.

18. M. E. Kruk, A. D. Gage, N. T. Joseph, et al. Mortality due to low-quality health systems in the universal health coverage era: a systematic analysis of amenable deaths in 137 countries. *Lancet* 2018; **392**(10160): 2203–2212.

19. K. Stenberg, O. Hanssen, T. T. Edejer, et al. Financing transformative health systems towards achievement of the health Sustainable Development Goals: a model for projected resource needs in 67 low-income and middle-income countries. *Lancet Glob Health* 2017; **5**(9): e875–e887.

20. World Health Organization. Towards a global action plan for healthy lives and well-being for all: uniting to accelerate progress towards the health-related SDGs. 2018. https://apps.who.int/iris/handle/10665/311667 (accessed November 18, 2020).

21. UNDESA, UNITAR. Stakeholder engagement and the 2030 Agenda: a practical guide. 2020. https://sustainabledevelopment.un.org/StakeholdersGuide (accessed October 13 2020).

22. R. Maher, K. Buhmann. Meaningful stakeholder engagement: bottom-up initiatives within global governance frameworks. *Geoforum* 2019; **107**: 231–234.

23. Y. Blomstedt, Z. A. Bhutta, J. Dahlstrand, et al. Partnerships for child health: capitalising on links between the sustainable development goals. *BMJ* 2018; **360**: k125.

24. S. Kuruvilla, R. Hinton, T. Boerma, et al. Business not as usual: how multisectoral collaboration can promote transformative change for health and sustainable development. *BMJ* 2018; **363**: k4771.

25. K. Rasanathan, S. Bennett, V. Atkins, et al. Governing multisectoral action for health in low- and middle-income countries. *PLoS Med* 2017; **14**(4): e1002285.

26. V. Tangcharoensathien, O. Srisookwatana, P. Pinprateep, et al. Multisectoral actions for health: challenges and opportunities in complex policy environments. *Int J Health Policy Manag* 2017; **6**(7): 359–363.

27. E. de Leeuw. Engagement of sectors other than health in integrated health governance, policy, and action. *Annu Rev Public Health* 2017; **38**: 329–349.

28. M. Marmot, R. Bell. The Sustainable Development Goals and health equity. *Epidemiology* 2018; **29**(1): 5–7.

29. C. L. McNamara. Relieving the tension between national health equity strategies and global health equity. *Scand J Public Health* 2019; **47**(6): 608–610.

30. Y. M. Asi, C. Williams. The role of digital health in making progress toward Sustainable Development Goal (SDG) 3 in conflict-affected populations. *Int J Med Inform* 2018; **114**: 114–120.

31. O. Olu, D. Muneene, J. E. Bataringaya, et al. How can digital health technologies contribute to sustainable attainment of universal health coverage in Africa? A perspective. *Front Public Health* 2019; **7**: 341.

32. D. Blumenthal, E. J. Fowler, M. Abrams, et al. Covid-19: implications for the health care system. *N Engl J Med* 2020; **383**(15): 1483–1488.

33. Lancet Public Health. Will the COVID-19 pandemic threaten the SDGs? *Lancet Public Health* 2020; **5**(9) :e460.

34. S. Khetrapal, R. Bhatia. Impact of COVID-19 pandemic on health system & Sustainable Development Goal 3. *Indian J Med Res* 2020; **151**(5): 395–399.

35. J. A. van Zanten, R. van Tulder. Beyond COVID-19: applying "SDG logics" for resilient transformations. *J Int Bus Stud* 2020; **3**(4): 451–464.

36. World Health Organization. Changing mindsets: strategy on health policy and systems research. 2012. www.who.int/alliance-hpsr/alliancehpsr_changingmindsets_strategyhpsr.pdf (accessed November 15, 2020).

37. A. Ghaffar, E. V. Langlois, K. Rasanathan, et al. Strengthening health systems through embedded research. *Bull World Health Organ* 2017; **95**(2): 87.

The Determinants of Health Systems

Upstream Approach to Addressing Health and Social Inequities

31

Samer Jabbour, Carine Naim, Nyambura Muriuki, and Fadi Martinos

---

Key Messages

- Political, economic, sociocultural, and environmental determinants influence health systems in profound ways and should be central in health system thinking.
- Health systems also impact determinants in myriad ways, which can be negative (e.g., expending energy and producing waste, or exposing households to financial catastrophe and impoverishment); or positive (e.g., improving productivity of the population and contributing to economic growth and development).
- Addressing structural determinants in health system thinking, planning, and practice requires a multipronged strategy that includes focusing on tackling inequities; removing misconceptions about health determinants among health workers; easing the path to health system work on health determinants; engaging concerned communities; evaluating innovations to address health determinants; and focusing on intersectoral collaboration.
- Tackling health inequities, which in turn affects social and economic inequities, is perhaps the most impactful intervention health workers can do to address the structural determinants operating within the health system.

31.1 Introduction

Just as there are determinants of health of individuals and communities, there are determinants of health systems, which we term structural determinants. These determinants are similar to the social determinants of health (SDH) but include an even wider set of factors than SDH, such as politics, governance, and history, in addition to "typical" SDH such as social environment, economic systems, and power structures. This chapter explores how structural determinants affect health system organization and performance directly and indirectly. While such determinants are many, this chapter focuses on a limited set of determinants that are particularly relevant for health workers[1] in low- and middle-income countries (L&MICs). It addresses the imperative for considering

---

[1] In this chapter, *health workers* refer to the clinical and nonclinical cadres working within and outside the health sector (e.g., technology, government administration), whose job is to protect and improve the health of their communities as per the 2006 WHO report "Working Together for Health."

structural determinants in health systems thinking, including the objectives of addressing health inequities, reviews ways of integrating determinants in health system work, and examines the role of selected determinants in impacting health system performance, drawing on examples from L&MICs.

31.2 The Case for Integrating Structural Determinants in Health Systems Thinking

A health system does not operate in a vacuum. Rather, it is heavily influenced by factors such as the history of a country, its power structures, its economic configuration, and its social interactions. These factors shape the health system and influence its evolution and what it delivers for people. National-level factors are evidently important but factors operating beyond the national boundaries also influence the health system, as has become apparent during the COVID-19 pandemic and discussions of vaccine nationalism.

While the chapter focuses on the impact of determinants on health system organization and performance, we must note that health systems are not merely at the receiving end of determinants; health systems also shape and influence such determinants in many ways (Figure 31.1). For example, improving quality of health care and targeting health services to address social exclusion can increase productivity and improve macroeconomic performance, availing more resources for the health system and completing a virtuous cycle. These are examples of interventions *within* the health system, but health workers can also intervene on structural determinants *outside* the health system – for example, targeting issues such as poor housing [1]. These examples illustrate the potential impact of health workers when they advocate for addressing determinants. Conversely, these also highlight the hefty cost of ignoring such structural determinants in health system work, rendering health system strengthening efforts shallow and shortsighted. In practice, health workers are consistently confronted with adverse determinants of health and may or may not recognize their impact. It is important to make such consideration explicit and systematic.

31.3 Key Structural Determinants of the Health System

The chapter focuses on five sets of structural determinants (Figure 31.1), selected based on the availability of supporting evidence linking them with the health system, their implications for policy or program interventions, their relevance for equity, and tacit knowledge about the influence of such determinants in L&MICs. They include politics and governance; economy, livelihoods, and poverty; climate change and disasters; social and organizational culture; and wars and conflicts.

31.3.1 Politics and Governance

A country's health system is influenced by its political system, governance, and by contested politics, whether through elections or violence (Figure 31.2). Governance affects every health system pillar and function through six general pathways: the form of authority, institutional arrangements, political values, citizen participation, corruption, and informal governance channels. The impacts of conflict, violence, and instability are discussed separately later in the chapter.

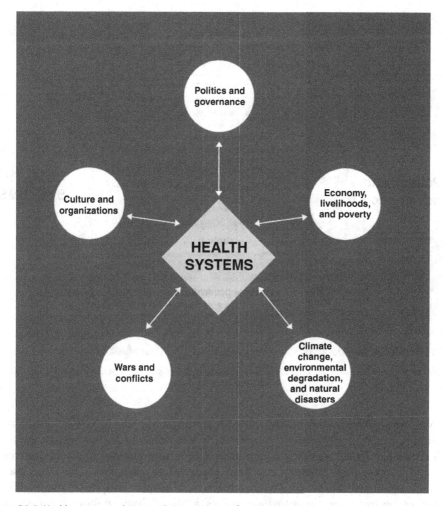

Figure 31.1 Health systems and structural determinants influence each other.

Form of Authority

Evidence regarding the influence of politics on health systems is complex and sometimes contradictory. Autocracies might curtail health promotion programs if they find them a threat, but can succeed in introducing health system measures that have populist appeal. For instance, they provide large-scale employment in the public sector but can hide early detection of infectious disease spread, thus jeopardizing public health [2–4]. Democratic regimes spread health-promoting resources more widely than autocratic ones because they must satisfy a broader support base [5]. Evidence from sub-Saharan Africa shows that democracy is associated with increased public health spending related to strengthened political competition and accountability mechanisms which guarantee citizens' welfare, political, and civil rights [6].

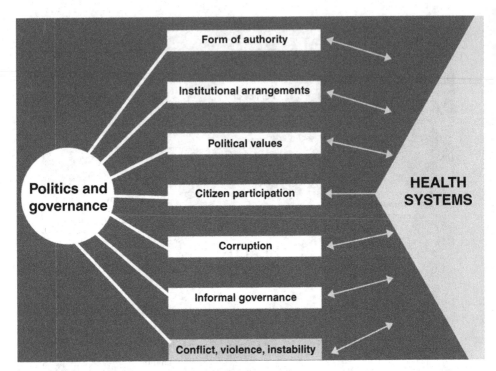

Figure 31.2 Interactions and influences between politics and governance as a determinant of health systems.

With most democracies in L&MICs still gaining root, the impact of democracy in promoting equitable distribution of services is not usual. In the context of the recent COVID-19 pandemic, the simple autocracy–democracy typology has been less revealing, and a three-part typology has been proposed to distinguish the responses by different countries. Some countries achieved a coherent response and significant degree of *control* over the situation; others achieved basic policy *consensus* about how to proceed; and in a third group policy *chaos* prevailed, with extensive conflict over policy goals and measures [7].

Political Values

Political values greatly influence health systems. Egalitarian systems favoring redistributive economic and social policies avail more service delivery for the poor while neoliberal regimes reduce social cohesion and produce greater income inequality, therefore impeding access to health care services. Countries that enshrined the right to health in their constitution, such as Ukraine and Slovakia, were better able to institutionalize equitable health system reforms [8].

Institutional Arrangements

The literature is not conclusive on the most effective framework for authority delegation, processes, and distribution of power in improving health system performance [9]. Comparisons between centralized arrangements, where a central, federal, or national state agency operates health departments across a territory, and decentralized ones, where local health departments plan and deliver services independently from the state, yield mixed findings [8]. The failure of centralized structures to respond comprehensively to local needs, and of decentralized ones to address issues of coordination and equity, suggests the need for a mix of centralized and decentralized frameworks in a hybrid or shared health system (see Chapter 10).

Citizen Participation

The weight of citizens in elections and their engagement in national and local affairs can greatly influence health system decisions. When health policies are a product of citizen participation, health systems tend to be more inclusive and distribute resources more fairly [10]. The extent to which a government fosters citizen participation at critical stages of policy development determines public ownership (see Chapters 11 and 29) [11]. This potential is not actualized in most L&MICs, although it has recently become a driving electoral mobilizer in some L&MICs, as seen in the 2019 elections in India where universal health coverage (UHC) was an important issue [12]. There are many constraints to citizen participation, including, for example, the perpetual dominance of the tribal and feudal systems, often as a legacy of colonial times, weak legal frameworks, ineffectual committees at the state and district levels, restricted financial disclosures, distrustful relationships with policymakers and providers, weak patient complaint systems, and low use of service charters [13, 14]. Increasingly, there are some promising experiences in L&MICs, such as citizen juries in Thailand which have proven to be an effective model for public participation in health policy [15]. Similarly, Tunisia went through a "societal dialog" benefiting from the "Citizen Jury" process for health system reforms and development of a national health policy for 2030. The experience highlighted the need for a legal framework to ensure the sustainability of such an approach [16]. Participatory health councils cover 98% of Brazil's population, operating at all levels of government and bringing together different social groups to monitor its health system. Despite this large reach and potential, issues of governance, such as agenda manipulation, delays in decision-making, and a lack of legal authority, transparency, training, monitoring, and inclusiveness have hindered the impact of councils on health policy [17, 18].

Control of Corruption

Corruption in its different forms undermines the legitimacy of state agencies, weakens the moral fiber of the state and society, reduces governance effectiveness, and redirects official activities. Corruption takes many forms, including nepotism, cronyism, bribery, irregularities in public purchasing and oversight, informal payments, and rent-seeking behavior (Box 31.1). Corruption rewards poor behavior, promotes untrustworthy leaders and staff, and deters legitimate and fruitful foreign and donor relationships, providing an adequate environment and culture for corruption to grow further (see Chapter 19) [19]. Corruption encourages aid fragmentation, reduces its effectiveness, and hinders overall health-related aid. Donors may avoid public sectors with weak governance, assuming corruption is less endemic in the private sector [20]. While channeling funds to the nonprofit private sector improves access to health care, there is no evidence to show that it is more effective than the public one [20].

> **Box 31.1** Forms of Corruption
>
> **Nepotism:** Using power or influence to favor relatives or friends.
>
> **Cronyism:** Appointing friends and associates to influential positions, even if they are not qualified.
>
> **Informal payments:** Monetary or in-kind transactions between a health service user and a service provider for services that are officially free of charge, typically in the public sector.
>
> **Rent-seeking:** This refers to when an entity seeks to gain wealth through the health system without contributing to productivity or quality.

Informal Governance

Actors and activities that exert influence on the health system outside the formal political system potentially undermine state-based health system strengthening efforts [21]. *Globally*, multilateral institutions such as the UN, World Trade Organization, International Monetary Fund, World Bank, and even the G7, which is not a formal institution, can greatly affect domestic health system governance and policies through their economic and bargaining power. This power is decisive in small, indebted countries. Global donors influence public health budget priorities and shape health and social policy and practice under the umbrella of public sector reform (see Chapter 35).

Locally, informal entities that have special interests can also shape the health system. Access to policymaking, resource allocation, and government institutions by special interest groups can result in patronage and nepotism and detract from the health system's ability to fulfill its public service role [4]. Religious organizations are significant providers of health services, and some have explicit political activities alongside their religious and social ones. Preferential provision of health services to select groups can deepen geographic inequalities and social inequities, hamper national integration efforts, and undermine the accountability of providers to beneficiaries [4]. This creates a real challenge for rights-based health work [22]. The complexity of the health system, high public spending, market uncertainty, information asymmetry, and other factors render the system susceptible to perpetuation of new forms of corruption. These factors play out at any time, especially during periods of violence, conflict, and instability when political and social tools for control of corruption are weakened.

31.3.2 The Economy, Livelihoods, and Poverty

The relationship between the economy and the health system is complex, multifaceted, bidirectional, context-dependent, and is often influenced by political factors (Figure 31.3; see also Chapter 36) [23, 24]. In general, better economic performance avails more resources for health systems strengthening, which can translate into improved health outcomes. These effects, typically seen in the long term, are hard to separate from the effects of factors such as improved water, sanitation, and nutrition. Short-term effects, and their translation into health outcomes, are more mixed and depend on context.

Poor economic performance undermines health system development due to reduced health sector financing, scaled-back services, and attrition of skilled health workers. This compounds the effects of loss of health coverage due to unemployment at a time when loss of

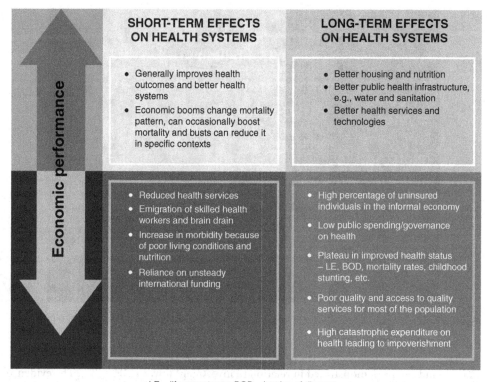

SHORT-TERM EFFECTS ON HEALTH SYSTEMS	LONG-TERM EFFECTS ON HEALTH SYSTEMS
• Generally improves health outcomes and better health systems • Economic booms change mortality pattern, can occasionally boost mortality and busts can reduce it in specific contexts	• Better housing and nutrition • Better public health infrastructure, e.g., water and sanitation • Better health services and technologies
• Reduced health services • Emigration of skilled health workers and brain drain • Increase in morbidity because of poor living conditions and nutrition • Reliance on unsteady international funding	• High percentage of uninsured individuals in the informal economy • Low public spending/governance on health • Plateau in improved health status – LE, BOD, mortality rates, childhood stunting, etc. • Poor quality and access to quality services for most of the population • High catastrophic expenditure on health leading to impoverishment

LE – life expectancy; BOD – burden of disease

Figure 31.3 Economic performance influences health systems.

income and livelihoods and impoverishment worsen health determinants, such as housing and nutrition, and create new health risks and needs for health services [20]. Economic hardship often pushes more people to work in the informal economy, where they do not have social security, safety nets, or protected access to health care [4]. With large informal economies characterized by prominent subsistence sectors and reliance on rent-seeking activities, many L&MICs struggle and become dependent on international assistance. Weak domestic tax revenue infrastructure results in limited opportunities to mobilize domestic resources, calling for international funding to fill funding gaps, including for the health sector.

Neoliberal economic policies[2] and trade liberalization, now widely adopted in many L&MICs, also strain health systems in various ways. Such policies reduce oversight in the context of limited regulatory capacity, increase out-of-pocket expenditures, create two-tier health systems according to the ability to pay, and encourage brain drain of skilled health workers. The results are increased health care costs and inequalities in access to health care [20].

Conversely, health systems are crucial for macro- and micro-economic development. Investments in health systems extend the economic benefits of general investments in health

---

[2] Neoliberalism is contemporarily used to refer to market-oriented reform policies such as eliminating price controls, deregulating capital markets, lowering trade barriers, and reducing, especially through privatization and austerity, state influence in the economy.

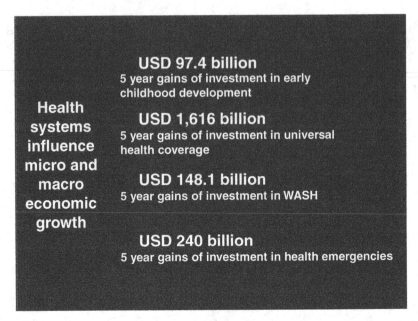

Figure 31.4 Expected economic gains of investing in global health and health systems (2019–2023) [27].

[25, 26] and can be demonstrated in relation to investment toward UHC [27]. The evidence is consistent across both high-income countries and L&MICs [25–29]. Health policymakers in L&MICs must support more research to demonstrate the economic case of investing in the health system (Figure 31.4).

31.3.3 Climate Change, Environmental Degradation, and Natural Disasters

Climate change is increasingly recognized as an important structural determinant of health systems. Health systems are the first line of defense against climate change-related ill-health, needing to provide protection, offer support, and treat and prevent diseases and outbreaks. With acute severe climate events, health systems can experience devastation, with damage to facilities and utilities, loss of staff, and supply chain interruptions [30]. The loss of health care services is perhaps the most significant climate change-related health system risk that communities face [31]. Climate-related health system disruptions disproportionally affect vulnerable people who are dependent on quick access to health services at the time they need them most.

Strengthening health systems to better manage the impact is a centerpiece of the health adaptation to climate change and is reflected in the WHO Operational Framework for Building Climate Resilient Health Systems (Figure 31.5) [32] and the Sendai framework (2015–2030) adopted at the Third UN World Conference on Disaster Risk Reduction in March 2015.

Health system adaptation to climate change requires system-level reforms. Most important is building the response, mitigation, and preparedness capacities for service delivery, whether at the level of workers, facilities, or the whole system. Preparation for acute events

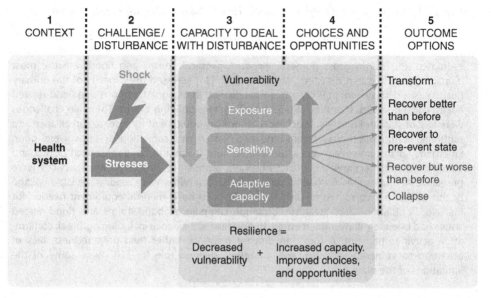

| 1 CONTEXT | 2 CHALLENGE/ DISTURBANCE | 3 CAPACITY TO DEAL WITH DISTURBANCE | 4 CHOICES AND OPPORTUNITIES | 5 OUTCOME OPTIONS |

Figure 31.5 Conceptual framework for resilience [32].

means anticipating damages, population displacement, and community health needs and planning appropriate responses. These responses include arranging alternate health-essential resources, including food, water, electricity, and emergency transportation, and ensuring the availability of health workers who are well trained to address the presenting health needs using well-established protocols.

Health systems in L&MICs struggle to address climate-change related risks due to low adaptive capacity, which needs to be scaled up [30, 33]. Essential public health functions (see Chapter 32) must be adapted for climate change [34]. Examples include setting up surveillance systems, training health workers on health aspects of climate change, such as investigation of infectious disease outbreaks, and developing communication strategies to inform the public and policymakers about the health impacts of climate change.

31.3.4 Social and Organizational Culture

In all parts of the world, societal constructs shape health systems and how they do or do not function. Racism, segregation, biases, and stigma – whether acknowledged or not – are reflected in where and how health system structures are set up, who is recruited as staff, which users are included or excluded, and what services are rendered, with profound implications for health and social equity [36]. Racialization (i.e., linking social meanings to certain biological or phenotypic features) and stigmatization (i.e., associating stereotypes with racialized groups) within the health system promote unequal power dynamics and discrimination. They work together to sustain hierarchies that affect access to health resources, undermine health care provision for racialized and stigmatized groups, and lead to more health inequalities.

Health system structures develop cultures of their own, with a range of factors, beyond race, affecting the nature and performance of health systems. Paramount is the

Box 31.2 Health System Challenges to Addressing Severe Climate Events in Vietnam

Vietnam is among the world's most disaster-prone countries and is significantly affected by climate change. Between 1994 and 2014, natural disasters led to over 13,000 deaths and an estimated 1% loss in gross domestic product. Tropical storms and floods are the most damaging and frequent disasters. Van Minh et al. [35] assessed the capacity of the primary health care (PHC) system in PhuVang, a rural district, to respond to storms and flood-related health consequences, based on WHO's health system building blocks. The main challenges were lack of staff and funding. In addition, laboratory equipment for disease surveillance and outbreak confirmation was insufficient, and water and sanitation systems were poor. Emergency plans, however, were established before storm and flood seasons at district and commune health facilities. At district hospitals, ambulance and emergency services were prepared. At the commune health station, first-aid services were readily available. Village health worker networks had medicines, supplies, and basic medical equipment needed for first aid. Population-based health information campaigns about storms and flood-related issues had been regularly implemented, but disease surveillance including outbreak confirmation activities had not. A focus on disaster response rather than preparedness, lack of attention to vulnerable groups, and a vaguely defined role for PHC were some of the limitations of the plan.

organizational culture, since it affects every level from policymaking to health care provision. Approaches to staff recruitment, assessment of performance, and mediation of interactions among staff and with users all impact the health system. A culture of blame, not sharing information, and manipulation are common in health systems in many L&MICs. These attributes potentially limit organizational effectiveness and likely contribute to low levels of motivation, job satisfaction, and productivity, and high attrition rates.

Health workers in L&MICs can explicitly consider, systematically describe, and change these attributes. Examples include moving from a culture of blame to one of fairness and learning, or from a control-based model that assumes that staff need constant monitoring, to commitment-based management, which assumes that staff perform better when supported and given discretion. Health workers can challenge restrictive gender norms, patriarchy, privilege, and power hierarchies within the health system to improve health provision and outcomes for disadvantaged groups, such as women and gender minorities. Equitable and rights-based policies and practices change the "soul" of the health system and can positively impact broader social attitudes. For example, through advocacy for victims of gender-based violence (GBV) and female genital mutilation (FGM), health workers can change broader cultural attitudes toward issues such as gender and the roles of women, human rights, and age of consent.

31.3.5 Wars and Conflicts

Perhaps no structural determinants have the same profound implications for health systems as do wars and conflicts, and more broadly instability. The Uppsala Conflict Data Program recorded 54 active state-based conflicts in 2019, including 7 wars, the highest number since 1946 [38]. Africa, with its fragile health systems, shouldered much of the burden, with 25 conflicts. Many of the current conflicts, as in Syria and the Democratic Republic of the Congo, are protracted and difficult to resolve. More than two billion people live in settings

Box 31.3 Transforming Health System Organizational Culture in South Africa [37]

South Africa is in a process of strengthening PHC to provide universal coverage. Developing organizational capacity is key in this process and includes addressing values, norms, relationships, communication, and use of power within the health system. After realizing that toxic organizational cultural values dominated by hierarchies, blame, and command and control approaches were restricting learning and limiting staff performance and engagement, the Western Cape Department of Health began a participatory process to achieve a just, commitment-based organizational culture identified with caring, competence, accountability, integrity, responsiveness, and respect. The transformation of organizational culture was possible through a participatory process that focused on leadership style, communication, and building relationships by means of cultural value assessments, feedback, coaching, and action learning in a cooperative inquiry group. After 18 months of participatory action, cultural entropy was substantially decreased.

affected by conflict, violence, and fragility that exacerbate existing challenges of all other determinants discussed thus far, particularly poverty, climate change, exclusion, and inequalities.

Political stability, not advocated here at the expense of rights and equity, increases government effectiveness and public health spending [6]. In contrast, wars and conflicts affect health systems in myriad ways [39, 40]. The effects can be indirect, due to the demands of the humanitarian emergency, such as massive displacement, widespread impoverishment, and increased health needs, as seen in Iraq, Syria, Venezuela, and Yemen, and the need to rely on unpredictable external funding as in Afghanistan [41]. Direct consequences are also numerous, including: destruction of health facilities, health worker attrition, reduced financing for core health system functions, reduced access to health service delivery and medicines and technologies, and a fragmented governance structure.

But health systems are not merely collateral victims of conflict; they can also be frontlines. Weaponization of health care now characterizes many conflicts, as currently in Ukraine and ongoing in Syria [42]. This might include: attacks on health care facilities, targeting health workers and driving them to leave; criminalizing the delivery of medical care to those perceived to be a threat; forcing health workers to engage in activities that violate medical ethics; and obstructing humanitarian health assistance. In Pakistan, militant groups have targeted and killed polio workers [43]. These practices, which constitute grave violations of international law, deprive people of essential health care. The WHO adopted Resolution WHA65.20 in 2012, urging action to protect health care workers from attacks, and launched a Surveillance System for Attacks on Health Care (SSA) to monitor such occurrences. Health workers and human rights monitors have documented attacks on health care, using innovative social media tools such as WhatsApp [44].

Health systems, specifically health workers, have potentially important roles in addressing wars and conflicts. In the *pre-conflict stage* there is recognition of how health professionals can leverage their knowledge, networks, and credibility to promote conflict prevention and peacebuilding [45]. Attention to this area in health system work remains very limited, but evidence is accumulating regarding the use of the health system as a key theater of "Peace through Health" interventions [45, 46]. The crucial role of health workers *during conflict* is well recognized in mitigating the impact of shocks and stressors on health system functioning and responding to the health needs of affected populations.

Box 31.4 Post-Conflict Health System Rebuilding in Northern Uganda

Between 1986 and 2005, Northern Uganda suffered a protracted armed conflict, leading to large population displacement, health system disruption, and closure of subdistrict health centers. Health professionals fled rural areas and conflict zones for larger trading centers and more stable districts. A growing, and better-paying, NGO sector distorted the health labor market by attracting many skilled health personnel. With the return of peace from mid-2006 onwards, the government attempted to draw health workers back to the public sector through benefits such as access to paid study leave and job security, but the NGO sector remained more attractive. Staffing rural areas, particularly where the security situation remained tenuous, became a serious challenge. Innovative solutions included separate postings for married couples within districts, task-shifting to fill staffing gaps, bonded training opportunities, and recruiting potentially high-performing future staff while still in training [50].

Humanitarian organizations have acknowledged the need for more "localization," whereby local health and humanitarian providers take the lead in program planning, design, and implementation, and receive commensurate funding, yet early assessment indicates that these reforms still have a long way to go [47, 48].

Health workers also have a critical role in the *transition, early recovery, and post-conflict phases*, during which more than one-third of all conflict-attributable maternal deaths and half of all child deaths occur [49]. Interventions in the immediate post-conflict period can affect the long-term trajectory of health system development. Priority areas include addressing health needs of impoverished and often traumatized communities, developing mechanisms to identify vulnerable households, adapting financing schemes to plan for universal coverage, strengthening district-level institutions and local governance capacity to coordinate and reinforce ownership, and strengthening national institutional capacity. Sadly, health systems strengthening efforts do not adequately address transitional and post-conflict settings, which remain woefully under-researched [49].

31.4 Incorporating Structural Determinants in Health System Planning and Programs: Toward a Strategic Approach

Considering the massive impact of structural determinants on health systems, we argue for a multipronged strategy for health systems in L&MICs to meaningfully incorporate such determinants in systems thinking, planning, and practice to affect health and equity.

The first strategy focuses on influencing how structural determinants play out within the health system. Health workers in L&MICs would have limited credibility outside the health system if they did not put their own houses in order. A primary objective here is tackling inequities within the health system. There is growing literature, and evidence, on what health systems can do to address inequities within existing structures and functions [51–54]. Health equity impact assessment and health equity plans are two tools to improve equity within the health system. Labonté advocates for the adoption of different health system roles to address equity; and stresses that equity-based health reforms are inherently political (Table 31.1; see also Chapter 36) [53].

Table 31.1 Addressing inequity: five health system roles

Educator/ watchdog	Resource broker	Community developer	Partnership developer	Advocate/ catalyst
Elevate awareness on health practices that are considered risk or protective factors. Monitor these factors and their impact on health status	Mobilize organizational resources by making them available to those working on health determinants	Develop and support the capacities of health staff, programs, and organizations working on health determinants	Mobilize private, public, and nonprofit partnerships and other stakeholder partnerships to address health determinants	Advocate policy statements that shape health determinants, at the governmental levels (e.g., ministries, parliament, and others)

Adapted from [53].

The second strategy is removing misconceptions about what structural determinants mean for health systems. Many health workers perceive that addressing such determinants is too difficult and too political, and is outside their scope of practice and potential influence. Through education, advocacy, and skill-building, health workers can see that many of the decisions they make daily, e.g., reconfiguring service delivery in poor neighborhoods, are shaped by structural determinants and their perceptions of them.

The third strategy is expanding the path to health system work on structural determinants. We must acknowledge critical gaps. The literature on the subject remains limited. Relevant health system case studies and interventions are still few. The pathways and mechanisms linking interventions on structural determinants with health system outcomes are hard to elucidate. There are no practical guides on how to address adverse structural determinants meaningfully and pragmatically through health system design and interventions. Serious work should start with addressing these gaps and generating evidence from implementation research and practice about what works.

The fourth strategy is engaging concerned communities (see Chapters 11 and 29). Addressing structural determinants begins with and leads naturally to participatory approaches whereby affected communities and mobilized groups drive priority setting, program design, intervention delivery, and outcome assessment. More public participation increases civic awareness, fosters health democracy, and can reduce health inequities through inclusion, transparency, and accountability.

The fifth strategy is incorporating and evaluating innovations in health system design to better address the structural determinants. The call by Palakshappa et al. urging the formal incorporation of health determinants into what would be "learning health systems" [55] – systems that mainstream health determinants in data collected and actions taken in a continuous feedback loop – is one example. Another example comes from addressing SDH in PHC [56]. Such innovations need sound design based on change theory; careful planning; engaging concerned communities and grassroots health workers to ensure local relevance and appropriateness; unbiased monitoring throughout implementation; and evaluation of their perception, efficacy, and cost-effectiveness.

The last strategy focuses on intersectorality [57, 58]. Work on structural determinants has little chance of succeeding without intersectoral collaboration, which can strengthen health systems and reduce inequities. The intersectoral interventions developed within the *Disease Control Priorities* third edition (DCP3) project are helpful [58] (see Chapter 15). The evidence for intersectoral work is growing [58]. In India, under the "National Rural Health Mission," a US$12.1 billion cross-sectoral investment over seven years in states and districts with poor health and demographic indicators helped improve health indicators compared with comparison states and districts. "Convergence" with nonhealth ministries was central to addressing SDH [59].

31.5 Conclusion

Political, economic, sociocultural, and environmental determinants unequivocally affect health systems. In turn, health systems impact such determinants – for example, improving social equity through advancing health equity. This chapter discusses how politics and governance, socioeconomic factors, climate change and disasters, organizational culture, and wars and conflicts influence health systems. Addressing structural determinants through health system work requires a multipronged strategy: tackling how determinants play out within the health system to produce inequities; removing misconceptions among health workers that they cannot influence such determinants; incorporating and evaluating innovations in health system design to address determinants; engaging concerned communities; and advancing intersectoral collaboration.

References

1. J. Koeman, R. Mehdipanah. Prescribing housing: a scoping review of health system efforts to address housing as a social determinant of health. *Popul Health Manag* 2021; 24(3): 316–321.

2. F. M. Burkle. Declining public health protections within autocratic regimes: impact on global public health security, infectious disease outbreaks, epidemics, and pandemics. *Prehosp Disaster Med* 2020; 35(3): 237–246.

3. V. Geloso, G. Berdine, B. Powell. Making sense of dictatorships and health outcomes. *BMJ Glob Health* 2020; 5(5): e002542.

4. R. Batniji, L. Khatib, M. Cammett, et al. Governance and health in the Arab world. *Lancet* 2014; 383(9914): 343–355.

5. S. Wigley, A. Akkoyunlu-Wigley. The impact of regime type on health: does redistribution explain everything? *World Polit* 2011; 63(4): 647–677.

6. I. Dianda. Do political factors affect government health spending? Empirical evidence from sub-Sahara African Countries. 2020. https://pdfs.semanticscholar.org/4541/9c8352cc69c5b380ea632373753f74b6113a.pdf (accessed July 18, 2021).

7. R. Rich. COVID-19 under democracy and autocracy. 2021. https://polisci.rutgers.edu/publications/student-faculty-publications/366-covid-19-under-democracy-and-autocracy/file (accessed January 8, 2022).

8. H. Matsuura. Exploring the association between the constitutional right to health and reproductive health outcomes in 157 countries. *Sex Reprod Health Matters* 2019; 27(1): 1599653.

9. A. Dwicaksono, A. M. Fox. Does decentralization improve health system performance and outcomes in low- and

middle-income countries? A systematic review of evidence from quantitative studies. *Milbank Q* 2018; **96**(2): 323–368.

10. S. Cinaroglu. Politics and health outcomes: a path analytic approach. *Int J Health Plann Manage* 2019; **34**(1): e824–e843.

11. J. A. Kiendrébéogo, B. Meessen Ownership of health financing policies in low-income countries: a journey with more than one pathway. *BMJ Glob Health* 2019; **4**(5): e001762.

12. K. Chalkidou, N. Jain, F. Cluzeau, et al. Modicare post-election: recommendations to enhance the impact of public health insurance on UHC goals in India. 2019. www.cgdev.org/sites/default/files/modicare-post-election-recommendations-enhance-impact-public-health-insurance-uhc-goals.pdf (accessed August 26, 2022).

13. K. Bolsewicz Alderman, D. Hipgrave, E. Jimenez-Soto. Public engagement in health priority setting in low- and middle-income countries: current trends and considerations for policy. *PLoS Med* 2013; **10**(8): e1001495.

14. D. C. Ogbuabor, O. E. Onwujekwe. Implementation of free maternal and child healthcare policies: assessment of influence of context and institutional capacity of health facilities in South-east Nigeria. *Glob Health Action* 2018; **11**(1): 1535031.

15. K. Chuengsatiansup, K. Tengrang, T. Posayanonda, et al. Citizens' jury and elder care: public participation and deliberation in long-term care policy in Thailand. *J Aging Soc Policy* 2019; **31**(4): 378–392.

16. H. Ben Mesmia, R. Chtioui, M. Ben Rejeb. The Tunisian societal dialogue for health reform (a qualitative study). *Eur J* 2020; **30**(Suppl. 5): ckaa166-1393.

17. J. C. Kohler, M. G. Martinez. Participatory health councils and good governance: healthy democracy in Brazil? *Int J Equity Health* 2015; **14**: 21.

18. M. G. Martinez, J. C. Kohler. Civil society participation in the health system: the case of Brazil's Health Councils. *Global Health* 2016; **12**(1): 64.

19. P. J. García. Corruption in global health: the open secret. *Lancet* 2019; **394**(10214): 2119–2124.

20. D. S. Richard, K. Hanson. *Health Systems in Low- and Middle-Income Countries: An Economic and Policy Perspective.* Oxford, Oxford University Press, 2012.

21. S. Abimbola, L. Baatiema, M. Bigdeli. The impacts of decentralization on health system equity, efficiency and resilience: a realist synthesis of the evidence. *Health Policy Plan* 2019; **34**(8): 605–617.

22. S. Jabbour, A. El-Zein, I. Nuwayhid, et al. Can action on health achieve political and social reform? *BMJ* 2006; **333**(7573): 837–839.

23. M. T. Ruiz-Cantero, M. Guijarro-Garvi, D. R. Bean, et al. Governance commitment to reduce maternal mortality: a political determinant beyond the wealth of the countries. *Health Place* 2019; **57**: 313–320.

24. A. B. Frakt. How the economy affects health. *JAMA* 2018; **319**(12): 1187–1188.

25. World Health Organization. Making the economic case for investing in health systems: what is the evidence that health systems advance economic and fiscal objectives? 2018. https://apps.who.int/iris/handle/10665/331982 (accessed July 18, 2021).

26. G. Yamey, N. Beyeler, H. Wadge, et al. Investing in health: the economic case. Report of the WISH Investing in Health Forum 2016. *Salud Publica Mex* 2017; **59**(3): 321–342.

27. World Health Organization. Investing global, investing local: supporting value for money towards the health SDGs. 2018. www.who.int/docs/default-source/investment-case/value-for-money.pdf (accessed August 19, 2021).

28. Bruegel. The macroeconomic implications of healthcare. 2018. www.bruegel.org/2018/08/the-macroeconomic-implications-of-healthcare/#:~:text=Health%2Dcare%20systems%20matter%20for,in%20output%2C%20employment%20and%20research.&text=Health%2Dcare%20systems%20also%20influence,influence%20on%20overall%20macroeconomic%20outcomes (accessed July 19, 2021).

29. World Health Organization. Economic and social impacts and benefits of health systems: report. 2019. https://apps.who .int/iris/handle/10665/329683 (accessed July 14, 2021).

30. K. L. Ebi, P. Berry, D. Campbell-Lendrum. Health system adaptation to climate variability and change. 2019. https://gca .org/wp-content/uploads/2020/12/Health SystemAdaptationToClimateVariability andChange_0.pdf (accessed July 18, 2021).

31. G. C. Benjamin. Shelter in the storm: health care systems and climate change. *Milbank Q* 2016; **94**(1): 18–22.

32. World Health Organization. Operational framework for building climate resilient health systems. 2015. www.who.int/ publications/i/item/operational- framework-for-building-climate- resilient-health-systems (accessed August 19, 2021).

33. V. Ridde, T. Benmarhnia, E. Bonnet, et al. Climate change, migration and health systems resilience: need for interdisciplinary research. *F1000Res* 2019; **8**: 22.

34. H. Frumkin, J. Hess, G. Luber, et al. Climate change: the public health response. *Am J Public Health* 2008; **98**(3): 435–445.

35. H. Van Minh, T. Tuan Anh, J. Rocklöv, et al. Primary healthcare system capacities for responding to storm and flood-related health problems: a case study from a rural district in central Vietnam. *Glob Health Action* 2014; **7**: 23007.

36. C. D. Cogburn. Culture, race, and health: implications for racial inequities and population health. *Milbank Q* 2019; **97**(3): 736–761.

37. R. Mash, A. De Sa, M. Christodoulou. How to change organisational culture: action research in a South African public sector primary care facility. *Afr J Prim Health Care Fam Med* 2016; **8**(1): e1–e9.

38. T. Pettersson, M. Öberg. Organized violence, 1989–2019. *J Peace Res* 2020; **57**(4): 597–613.

39. R. Thompson, M. Kapila. Healthcare in conflict settings: leaving no one behind. 2018. www.wish.org.qa/wp-content/uploads/ 2018/11/IMPJ6078-WISH-2018-Conflict- 181026.pdf (accessed August 13, 2021).

40. B. S. Levy, W. S. Victor. *War and Public Health*. Oxford, Oxford University Press, 2008.

41. J. R. Acerra, K. Iskyan, Z. A. Qureshi, et al. Rebuilding the health care system in Afghanistan: an overview of primary care and emergency services. *Int J Emerg Med* 2009; **2**(2): 77–82.

42. F. M. Fouad, A. Sparrow, A. Tarakji, et al. Health workers and the weaponisation of health care in Syria: a preliminary inquiry for The Lancet–American University of Beirut Commission on Syria. *Lancet* 2017; **390**(10111): 2516–2526.

43. Z. A. Bhutta. What must be done about the killings of Pakistani healthcare workers? *BMJ* 2013; **346**: f280.

44. M. Elamein, H. Bower, C. Valderrama, et al. Attacks against health care in Syria, 2015–16: results from a real-time reporting tool. *Lancet* 2017; **390**(10109): 2278–2286.

45. W. H. Wiist, S. K. White. *Preventing War and Promoting Peace: A Guide for Health Professionals*. Cambridge, Cambridge University Press, 2017.

46. N. Arya, J. S. Barbara. *Peace through Health: How Health Professionals Can Work for a Less Violent World*. Boulder, Kumarian Press, 2008.

47. P. B. Spiegel. The humanitarian system is not just broke, but broken: recommendations for future humanitarian action. *Lancet* 2017; **17**: 31278-3.

48. D. V. Canyon, F. M. Burkle Jr. The 2016 World Humanitarian Summit Report Card: both failing marks and substantive gains for an increasingly globalized humanitarian landscape. *PLoS Curr* 2016; **8**. doi: 10.1371/currents.dis. a94dd3e2f84d0a5abc179add7286851c.

49. T. Martineau, B. McPake, S. Theobald, et al. Leaving no one behind: lessons on rebuilding health systems in conflict- and crisis-affected states. *BMJ Glob Health* 2017; **2**(2): e000327.

50. R. M. Ayiasi, E. Rutebemberwa, T. Marttineau. Understanding deployment policies and systems for staffing rural areas in Northern Uganda during and after the conflict: synthesis report: ReBUILD consortium. 2016. www.rebuildconsortium.com/resources/under standing-deployment-policies-and-systems-for-staffing-rural-areas-in-northern-uganda-during-and-after-the-conflict-synthesis-report/ (accessed July 13, 2021).

51. L. Gilson, J. Doherty, R. Lowenson, et al. Challenging inequity through health systems. Final Report. Knowledge Network on Health Systems. 2007. https://research online.lshtm.ac.uk/id/eprint/7136/ (accessed July 18, 2021).

52. R. Mador. Health system approaches to promoting health equity. Discussion Paper. 2010. www.bccdc.ca/pop-public-health/ Documents/HealthSystemApproaches_ FINAL.pdf (accessed July 19, 2021).

53. R. Labonté. Health systems governance for health equity: critical reflections. *Rev Salud Publica (Bogota)* 2010; **12**(Suppl. 1): 62–76.

54. M. Ford-Gilboe, C. N. Wathen, C. Varcoe, et al. How equity-oriented health care affects health: key mechanisms and implications for primary health care practice and policy. *Milbank Q* 2018; **96**(4): 635–671.

55. D. Palakshappa, D. P. Miller Jr. G. E. Rosenthal. Advancing the learning health system by incorporating social determinants. *Am J Manag Care* 2020; **26**(1): e4–e6.

56. M. Marmot. Addressing social determinants of health in primary care. 2018. www.aafp.org/dam/AAFP/ documents/patient_care/everyone_ project/team-based-approach.pdf (accessed July 19, 2021).

57. N. López, V. L. Gadsden. Health inequities, social determinants, and intersectionality. 2016. https://nam.edu/health-inequities-social-determinants-and-intersectionality/ (accessed August 13, 2021).

58. D. A. Watkins, R. Nugent, H. Saxenian, et al. Intersectoral policy priorities for health. In D. T. Jamison, H. Gelband, S. Horton, et al., eds., *Disease Control Priorities: Improving Health and Reducing Poverty*, 3rd ed. Washington, DC, International Bank for Reconstruction and Development and the World Bank, 2017.

59. A. M. Prasad, G. Chakraborty, S. S. Yadav, et al. Addressing the social determinants of health through health system strengthening and inter-sectoral convergence: the case of the Indian National Rural Health Mission. *Glob Health Action* 2013; **6**: 1–11.

Chapter 32

Integrating Essential Public Health Functions in Health Systems
Ensuring Health Security

Jose M. Martin-Moreno, Beatriz Lobo-Valbuena, and Alejandro Martin-Gorgojo

---

Key Messages

- Essential public health functions (EPHF) are the primary responsibility of the state and are fundamental for achieving public health goals through collective action.
- There are several EPHF frameworks that have core and enabling functions, which should be integrated within health systems. The preferred approach is to identify the framework that best suits the local context.
- International Health Regulations (IHRs) are the legally binding set of regulations meant to prevent the international spread of diseases, and are closely related to EPHF.
- EPHF focus on building capacity for public health nationally, while IHRs respond to the obligations of public health globally.
- Investing in public health and ensuring well-performing EPHF is an obligation and an ethical and moral imperative of governments in every country.

32.1 Introduction

Health systems include all organizations, institutions, and resources whose primary aim is to produce health [1]. In contrast to clinical disciplines that deliver more obvious and sometimes more spectacular care at the individual level, public health contributes to protecting and improving health through sustained and often less noticeable action at the population level. Historically, public health has not received the same attention, funding, and recognition, despite being acknowledged as a discipline that can decidedly impact the health and wellbeing of populations both locally and globally.

Essential public health functions are the indispensable set of actions, under the primary responsibility of the state, that are fundamental for achieving the goal of public health, which is to improve, promote, protect, and restore the health of the population through collective action [2]. The importance of EPHF is most acutely recognized in the context of crisis and health emergencies, but their full contribution to health system goals requires sustained attention and investment that ensures the promotion of health, prevention of illness and injury, and the mitigation of health threats during ordinary times, as well as during health emergencies.

32.2 The Scope of Public Health

Winslow, in 1920, defined public health as

the science and the art of preventing disease, prolonging life, and promoting physical health and efficiency through organized community efforts for the sanitation of the environment, the control of community infections, the education of the individual in personal hygiene, the organization of medical and nursing service for the early diagnosis and preventive treatment of disease, and the development of the social machinery which will ensure to every individual in the community a standard of living adequate for the maintenance of health. [3]

A more contemporary definition of public health adapted from Acheson states it to be, "the art and science of promoting and protecting health and preventing illness through the organized efforts of society" [4]. Over the past decades, our growing understanding of social and structural determinants of health have broadened the scope of public health, highlighting its intersection with clinical practice as well as education, environment, transportation, and industrial sectors and urban development [5]. The broad scope of public health can be a source of confusion and conflict among stakeholders (including policymakers and the general population), and sometimes makes it difficult to translate into practice [6].

In 2020 the American Public Health Association helped address this challenge by proposing 10 essential public health services (EPHSs) categorized into the three domains of *assessment, policy development,* and *assurance.* These have recently been revised to have *equity* placed at the center [7]. This provides a framework for public health to protect and promote the health of all people in any given community that has a logical sequence from the identification of needs (assessment), to the development of a set of related interventions (policy development), followed by their systematic evaluation (assurance; Table 32.1) [7]. These are not unique, as other countries and national public health associations have also outlined the services included under the remit of public health, and the means to assess their performance, each according to their unique socioeconomic and cultural contexts, with highly diverse results across countries [8].

Table 32.1 EPHS as proposed by the American Public Health Association

Domains		Essential public health services
Assessment		• Assess and monitor population health.
		• Investigate, diagnose, and address health hazards and root causes.
Policy development		• Communicate effectively to inform and educate.
		• Strengthen, support, and mobilize communities and partnerships.
		• Create, champion, and implement policies, plans, and laws.
	Equity	• Utilize legal and regulatory actions.
Assurance		• Enable equitable access.
		• Build a diverse and skilled workforce.
		• Improve and innovate through evaluation, research, and quality improvement.
		• Build and maintain a robust organizational infrastructure for public health.

32.3 The Evolution of EPHF

32.3.1 Early Initiatives: The 1990s

In 1997, in the context of renewed commitment to "Health for All" for the twenty-first century, WHO encouraged the identification of public health *functions* deemed to be essential to allow health systems to respond to the evolving health needs through public health *services* [9]. In 1998, an international consensus on the main characteristics of these functions was reached [10]. This was the public health community's first comprehensive attempt that identified nine different public health roles and responsibilities, being a notable achievement given the challenges inherent in the increasingly broad definition of public health (Box 32.1).

32.3.2 EPHF Regional Initiatives

Subsequently, practical adaptations were made in different regions of the world by the regional offices of WHO, as well as by other organizations [11, 12]. Concurrent efforts were also made to identify public health stakeholders and assess their training needs to provide

---

Box 32.1 EPHF: Results of a 1998 Delphi Study

1. **Prevention, surveillance, and control of infectious and noncommunicable diseases:** injury prevention, disease surveillance, disease outbreak control, vaccination.

2. **Monitoring of the health situation:** assessment of population needs and risks to determine which subgroups need services, evaluation of the effectiveness of public health functions, evaluation of the effectiveness of promotion, prevention, and care programs, surveillance of the determinants of health, and surveillance of morbidity and mortality.

3. **Health promotion:** promotion of community involvement in health; provision of health education and information for health and life skills enhancement at school, home, work, and in community settings; institution and maintenance of links with decision-makers, policy and other sectors, and the community to advocate for health promotion and public health.

4. **Occupational health:** creation of standards for occupational safety and health.

5. **Environmental protection:** food quality and safety control; vector control; water, air, and soil protection; pollution control, including radiation risks; consideration of environmental issues in development policies, programs, and projects.

6. **Public health legislation and regulation:** establishment of health legislations, regulations, and administrative procedures; ensuring environmental health protection legislation; health inspection and authorization; enforcement of health legislations, regulations, and administrative procedures.

7. **Public health planning and management:** management and planning of health policy; use of levels of scientific evidence in the development and implementation of public health policies; preservation and improvement of the quality of health services; public health research and health systems analysis; international cooperation in health.

8. **Specific public health services:** school health services, disaster relief missions, public health laboratory services.

9. **Health for vulnerable and at-risk populations:** early childhood care, maternal and child health, and family planning.

Source: [9].

guidance to actors from a variety of professions and scientific disciplines, ultimately to advance contemporary thinking and contribution to public health [13].

Three regional initiatives deserve particular attention. First, the WHO Regional Office for the Americas, also called the Pan American Health Organization (PAHO), published in 2002 a book titled *Public Health in the Americas: Conceptual Renewal, Performance Assessment, and Bases for Action* [14]. This publication analyzed the context in which public health is perceived and practiced, and discussed the extent to which the functions that are essential to promoting and preserving the public's health are being implemented in the American Region. Box 32.2 lists the 11 EPHF recognized in the Americas, as defined by PAHO.

Subsequently, the European region, co-led by one of the authors of this chapter, reorganized the list of essential public health *actions* for Europe to include aspects of governance, financing, and human resources. Other functions, such as *occupational and environmental health*, were grouped under broader headings, in this case of *health protection* [15]. In Europe, the word *Operation* replaced *Function* in order to draw a clear distinction between the essential public health operations (EPHO) and the functions of the health system framework published earlier in the *World Health Report 2000* [1]. The health system functions are also commonly called building blocks. Furthermore, a new operation – *Communication* – was included in response to the increasing relevance of the Internet and social media, ushered in by the information and communication technology (ICT) revolution of the 2000s [16].

The list of 10 EPHO of the European Regions Framework (Figure 32.1) reflects the *core public health services* related to disease prevention, health promotion, and health protection. Furthermore, it includes the *supportive health system operations* that enable services to be delivered properly. All the details and conceptual and instrumental references of this tool are in the public domain [15].

A third notable initiative is that of the WHO Eastern Mediterranean Regional Office, co-developed by one of the editors of this book [17]. Some of the particularly useful contributions of this initiative, whose outcomes are summarized in Figure 32.2, include: (1) the development of a glossary of terms; (2) methods used that employed

---

Box 32.2 Eleven EPHF as Defined by PAHO

1. Monitoring, evaluation, and analysis of health status
2. Public health surveillance, research, and control of risks and threats to public health
3. Health promotion
4. Social participation in health
5. Development of policies and institutional capacity for planning and management in public health
6. Strengthening of institutional capacity for regulation and enforcement in public health
7. Evaluation and promotion of equitable access to necessary health services
8. Human resources development and training in public health
9. Ensuring the quality of personal and population-based health services
10. Research in public health
11. Reducing the impact of emergencies and disasters on health

Source: [2].

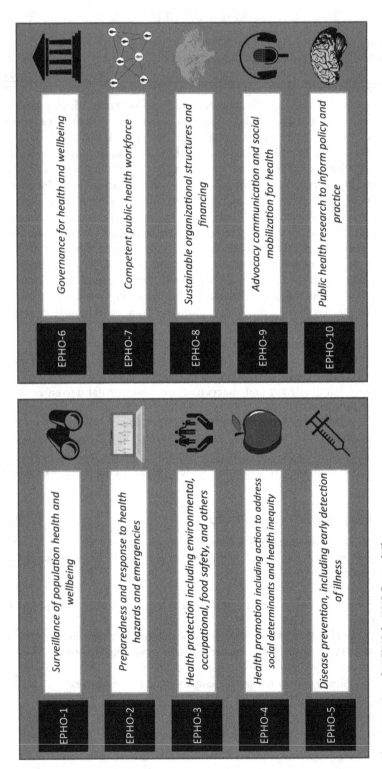

Figure 32.1 List of 10 EPHO for WHO Europe [15].

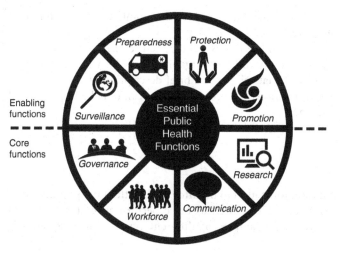

Figure 32.2 Summary of the EPHF in the WHO Eastern Mediterranean Region [17].

three assessment pathways (a two-tiered assessment process, a self-assessment, and a joint external assessment); (3) the involvement of a national team from the early stages and throughout the process; and (4) the systematic use of WHO and other relevant tools.

32.3.3 EPHF Global Initiatives

In addition to the efforts of WHO regional offices, several global organizations have also developed EPHF frameworks. For instance, the World Bank proposed a framework for EPHF which was adapted by countries to meet their specific needs [18]. Similarly, the Global Charter for the Public's Health, jointly produced with the World Federation of Public Health Associations, WHO, and multiple other stakeholders, is a comprehensive and flexible framework that includes public health functions and services and offers a set of tools, definitions of services, and enabler functions, which can help public health professionals and organizations to develop policies, take action, and promote the conditions for healthy living [19, 20].

A recent concept similar to EPHF proposed by economists is called the Common Goods for Health. These are population-based functions or interventions that require collective financing and governance and contribute to health and economic progress with a clear economic rationale based on market failures. These interventions focus on (1) public goods, which by definition are nonrival and nonexclusionary; or (2) have large social externalities [21, 22].

32.4 Core and Enabling EPHF: Two Sides of the Same Coin

The frameworks described above have many similarities and some differences that reflect their unique circumstances. There is no single "best" framework, and a preferred approach might be to identify and adapt the framework that best suits the national or local context in which it is applied. Nevertheless, some important inferences can be drawn: (1) it is useful to segregate the EPHF into core and enabling functions as the two sets are complementary; (2) it is important to consider the usefulness of the assessment tools and related documents in the local context; and (3) while self-assessment is a good starting point, it should be followed by independent assessment of EPHF.

In addition, terms such as: *functions, operations, actions,* and *services* in the context of EPHF have been used interchangeably by different organizations. We will use the term *functions* unless otherwise specified. What follows is a brief description of the essential – core and enabling – public health functions. The core functions can only be implemented when the enabling EPHF are in place.

32.4.1 "Core" EPHF

Surveillance

Surveillance refers to the means and tools used to monitor the health of the population as a whole or that of subgroups of interest, as well as basic performance standards and reporting systems. Box 32.3 provides examples of different types of disease surveillance [23].

Monitoring, Preparedness, and Response to Emergencies

This function refers to the systems and procedures needed to prepare for and respond to a public health emergency. More specifically:

- **Monitoring** includes: (1) identifying, and predicting priorities in biological, chemical, and physical health risks in the workplace and the environment; (2) risk assessment procedures and tools to measure environmental health risks; (3) release of accessible information and the issuance of public warnings; and (4) planning and activation of interventions aimed at minimizing health risks.
- **Preparedness** for the management of emergency events includes: (1) formulation of suitable action plans; (2) development of systems for data collection and prevention and

---

> **Box 32.3** Types of Surveillance for Monitoring Population Health
>
> - **Active surveillance:** a system employing staff members to regularly contact health care providers or the population to seek information about health conditions.
> - **Passive surveillance:** a system by which a health jurisdiction receives reports submitted from hospitals, clinics, public health units, or other sources.
> - **Routine health information system:** a passive system in which regular reports about diseases and programs are completed by public health staff members, hospitals, and clinics.
> - **Categorical surveillance:** an active or passive system that focuses on one or more diseases or behaviors of interest to an intervention program.
> - **Integrated surveillance:** a combination of active and passive systems using a single infrastructure for collecting information on multiple diseases or behaviors of interest to several programs (e.g., gathering information on multiple infectious diseases and injuries at health facilities).
> - **Syndromic surveillance:** an active or passive system that uses case definitions based entirely on clinical features without clinical or laboratory diagnosis (e.g., surveillance of cases of diarrhea rather than cholera, or "rash illness" rather than measles).

control of morbidity; and (3) the application of an integrated and cooperative approach with various authorities involved in management.

- **Response** ensures that there is capacity to: (1) perform gap analysis; (2) develop and implement national or subnational action plans to prevent, detect, and respond to public health threats, taking into account the most likely events; and (3) in the event of an emergency execute activities that reduce the public health impact of emergencies and disasters through intrasectoral, intersectoral, and interinstitutional collaboration.

Health Protection

Health protection at a minimum includes environmental, occupational, and food safety. Its scope involves having a legal and regulatory framework for health protection in areas such as environmental health, occupational safety, radiation safety, consumer product safety, and others. It also includes supervision and monitoring, enforcement mechanisms, and management and mitigation of risks.

Disease Prevention, Including Early Detection of Illness

This refers to those public health services that are offered to prevent disease, to detect it as early as possible, and to ensure that patients can live with and manage morbidity, maintaining the highest possible quality of life. *Primary prevention* concerns taking measures before getting the disease, such as health promotion activities and vaccinations. *Secondary prevention* is the subset that involves early detection and management of disease. It includes population-based disease screening programs. *Screening* refers here to a process or test to identify a disease before the appearance of symptoms, applied to an eligible population in an agile, acceptable, and efficient manner, such as screening for breast cancer.

Health Promotion

Health promotion is the process of enabling people to increase control over, and improve, their health [24]. It often works through interventions that include intersectoral action to address some of the most important and complex threats to public health, including exposure to behavioral risk factors and the underlying social determinants that undermine health inequity. These challenges require inputs from broad coalitions of different actors through whole-of-government and whole-of-society approaches (see Chapter 37). Examples include improving physical activity by providing parks, walkways, and bicycle routes for promoting health.

32.4.2 "Enabling" EPHF

Governance for Health

The EPHF are primarily the responsibility of the state, and hence require good governance to be effectively discharged or implemented. In its broadest sense, governance would include, among others, a vision for public health, encouraging stakeholder participation, ensuring accountability and transparency, and having the capacity to monitor and evaluate. It also means that the Ministries of Health function as stewards of the health system and protect public health. Conversely, measuring EPHF can help assess the performance of the national health authority or the Ministries of Health and indirectly ascertain the quality of health system governance.

Organizational Structures and Financing

This function ensures sustainable organizations and financing for public health to provide efficient, effective, and responsive services. It promotes coordination, integration, and sufficient funding for long-term sustainability of the "core" EPHF. Ultimately, this contributes to building strong public health institutions in the country.

Public Health Workforce

It is vital to educate, manage, and govern a fit-for-purpose public health workforce. In addition to ensuring the competency of public health experts who have the primary responsibility for the planning and implementation of public health measures, it is also important that the entire workforce works toward impacting public health by having the required public health skills and knowledge to carry out their duties. In other words, while only a limited proportion of the workforce is qualified as public health professionals, the entire workforce should be oriented toward and understand the importance of good public health.

Information, Communication, and Social Mobilization for Health

Every public health program should have a communication strategy as its integral component. This may entail communication campaigns or innovative Information and Communications Technology (ICT) tools that enable channels for effective communication with the relevant stakeholders, such as communities, patients, or providers. The communication and social mobilization component should be well organized to build partnerships with media and marketing firms or to interact with civil society. Importantly, the communication and social mobilization interventions should be regularly evaluated for impact assessment.

Public Health Research

Implementing the core functions is an exercise that needs to be regularly monitored and hence requires concurrent public health and implementation research to generate evidence and continuously inform public health policy, programs, and practice (see Chapters 14 and 23).

32.5 EPHF: Methodological and Implementation Challenges

32.5.1 Methodological Approaches to Assessing EPHF

A review conducted by the authors in 2016 revealed that EPHF assessments, using a variety of approaches, have been completed and published in English language in as many as 100 countries [8]. Assessment questionnaires and other data collection methods have primarily been done in the context of research, such as those used in countries of the European Union, Australia, India, and Sri Lanka. In contrast, assessments have also been done as part of country evaluation strategies by the World Health Organization (WHO) or the Centers for Disease Control and Prevention (CDC) in order to inform policies to strengthen public health functions.

An important issue in the application of different frameworks for assessing EPHF is the variation in methodology followed in different contexts and countries. In most instances, the evaluation is self-administered and is based on a template that is completed by technical staff of Ministries of Health. In this approach there is a tendency to underreport existing gaps and challenges, especially when the results are to be presented to high-level policymakers or to Parliament. On the other hand, a more exaggerated picture is sometimes presented when the purpose is to secure funds from an external agency. Independent external assessment by a team of qualified experts, as was done in countries of the Eastern Mediterranean by WHO, is perhaps the most suitable model for countries to adopt [25].

32.5.2 Anchoring EPHF within Health Systems

Health systems and public health are highly interdependent. However, the scope of public health goes beyond the health system because of the whole-of-society and multisectoral factors that influence health. At the same time, health systems provide a sound basis and a platform for implementation of public health interventions (see Chapter 1). Hence, it is imperative that EPHF are well integrated within health systems in order not to drift into a set of ineffective actions. Once EPHF are firmly anchored within health systems they can potentially influence population health through actions within the health system, as well as at the multisectoral level. Finally, each EPHF is truly essential and if implemented in isolation of the others or in a fragmented manner, the collective health impact cannot be maximized [8].

32.5.3 Central Role of Governments in EPHF: Responding to the COVID-19 Pandemic

Governments have a central role in the implementation of EPHF and in ensuring health security. *Health security* encompasses all activities required to minimize the danger and impact of acute public health events that endanger the collective health of populations living across geographical regions and international boundaries [26]. Investing in enabling, effective, and safe public health interventions is of enormous value. Public health contributes to improving the quality of life, life expectancy, control of infectious diseases, and prevention of cancer and cardiovascular diseases, and other chronic conditions. Hence, governments can play a major leadership role by mobilizing the necessary resources from within public budgets and investing in EPHF, thereby promoting and protecting public health and ensuring health security.

Box 32.4 presents the European experience of the application of the EPHO in countries in response to the ongoing COVID-19 pandemic.

Box 32.4 The Case of COVID-19 and EPHO: The European Experience

The case of COVID-19 illustrates the role of the EPHO in Europe [27]. Following the European model previously specified [16], the importance of the surveillance of population health (EPHO-1) was clear, whereas the monitoring and response to health hazards and emergencies (EPHO-2) were at the heart of the challenge. Equally relevant are the other essential operations, such as communication and social mobilization for health (EPHO-9); the operation related to the goal of finding solutions for effective vaccines (EPHO-10 and 5); health protection actions, including environmental, occupational, and food safety actions (EPHO-3); and promotion of population health and wellbeing, with the focus on tackling inequalities and the broader social and environmental determinants (EPHO-4). All this could only be possible with the support of the enabling EPHO, such as the proper health governance for health, reliable infrastructure, and financing to ensure the resources and viability of public health interventions, and the responsibility to ensure a competent workforce (EPHO-6, 7, and 8).

32.6 EPHF and IHRs

All EPHF frameworks foster health security; however, their impact is primarily to strengthen public health at the national level. A similar set of legally binding regulations are the IHRs [28]. Their remit, however, is to prevent, protect against, control, and provide a public health response to the international spread of diseases in ways that are commensurate with and restricted to public health risks, and which avoid unnecessary interference with international traffic and trade [28]. While the two are complementary and well aligned with each other, IHR implies an international and global dimension for action, while EPHF have a national purview. Through IHR, countries have agreed to shape their capacities to detect, assess, and report public health incidents. IHR also include specific measures at airports, ports, and ground crossings to limit the spread of health risks to neighboring countries. Table 32.2 provides a summary of the seven main areas of work of IHR.

Table 32.2 IHR (2005) main areas of work

Area of work	Goal
1. Foster global partnerships	WHO, all member countries, and all relevant sectors must be aware of the new rules and collaborate to provide the best available technical support and, where needed, mobilize the necessary resources for effective implementation of IHR (2005).
2. Strengthen national disease prevention, surveillance, control, and response systems	Each country assesses its national resources in disease surveillance and response and develops national action plans to implement and meet IHR requirements.
3. Strengthen public health security in travel and transport	Permanent public health measures and response capacity at designated airports, ports, and ground crossings in all countries to minimize the risk of international spread of disease.
4. Strengthen WHO global alert and response systems	Coordinated response to international public health risks and public health emergencies of international concern (PHEIC) should be ensured in a timely and effective manner.
5. Strengthen the management of specific risks	Systematic international and national management of the risks known to threaten international health security, such as influenza, yellow fever, SARS, COVID-19, poliomyelitis, and risk arising from chemical and radioactive substances.
6. Sustain rights, obligations, and procedures	New legal mechanisms as set out in the Regulations are fully developed and upheld. All professionals involved in implementing IHR (2005) have a clear understanding of, and sustain, the new rights, obligations, and procedures laid out in the Regulations.
7. Conduct studies and monitor progress	Indicators are well known and collected regularly to monitor and evaluate IHR (2005) implementation at national and international level. WHO Secretariat reports on progress to the World Health Assembly. Specific studies are defined to facilitate and improve implementation of the Regulations.

Modified from [29].

Despite the binding nature of IHR, which was approved as the governing framework for global health security to make the world more secure, the progress on IHR implementation has left a lot to be desired [30]. In order to bridge the weaknesses, WHO has committed to helping countries embed IHR in their national health sector planning processes and health systems strengthening initiatives [31].

An assessment tool called the Joint External Evaluation (JEE) has been developed by WHO [32] to help countries analyze and develop IHR capacities. The JEE process is extremely useful in identifying critical gaps within health systems, not only in human but also in animal and environmental systems following the *one health approach*, and prioritizes actions to improve preparedness and response capacities. It is a voluntary and multisectoral process, conducted under the supervision and with the support of WHO. It aims to comprehensively assess a country's capacity in the areas of prevention and reduction of the likelihood of outbreaks and other public health hazards, detection of threats, and provision of a rapid and effective response, including multisectoral and national and international coordination and communication. In addition, WHO offers several other supporting sources on health systems strengthening terminologies [33], dynamics and control of disease outbreaks [34], and processes for emergency preparedness [35] to help countries prepare for IHR.

The JEE process is followed by the development of a clear roadmap outlining activities for the implementation of IHR in the country that includes expression of the commitment and active role of the government, engagement in resource mobilization at the national level, and the provision or management of international funds for the implementation of IHR [29]. In addition, areas that need attention are the appointment of a national IHR focal point and coordination with different IHR stakeholders through an established mechanism for the sharing of information, mapping of potential hazards in the country, and the development of a public health preparedness and response plan. This should be further complemented by an action plan for training to strengthen capacity for disease prevention, surveillance, risk assessment, control, and response.

32.7 EPHF, IHR, and Health System Strengthening Interrelations and Health Security

The EPHF, IHR, and health systems strengthening (HSS) do not constitute three separate sets of policies, each of which is interdependent in terms of leadership, funding, resources, and services. In fact, they must be closely aligned while planning on all aspects related to alert and emergency preparedness that blends contemporary global thinking with local implementation if "health security" is to be ensured. In other words, it is vital to embed the IHR and EPHF simultaneously in the national health planning processes and HSS efforts to achieve the dual goal of universal health coverage (UHC) and health security. Figure 32.3 illustrates how EPHF and IHR working within the wider canvas of health systems, public health, and multisectorality can contribute to the goals of UHC and health security.

32.8 Conclusion

The epidemiological and demographic transitions, influence of social determinants, and the increasing recognition of climate change impacts on population health are some of the key imperatives to strengthen public health in all countries of the world. The EPHF framework

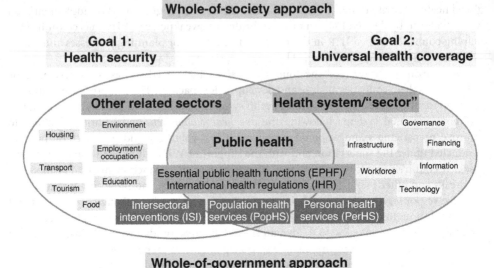

Figure 32.3 Conceptual links between health systems, health security, UHC, public health functions, IHR actions, other sectors, and the whole-of-society approach.

offers the most coherent and evidence-informed approach to assess, plan, and prepare for strengthening public health in countries. This requires an organized approach that is well integrated within the health system so that the necessary infrastructure, personnel, and financial resources – as well as other EPHF enablers – are available to support implementation of the "core" EPHF.

Strengthening IHR will complement EPHF implementation at the national level, and at the same time meet the obligations at the global level to prevent the international spread of diseases and health hazards. Similar to EPHF, IHR must also be integrated within the health system for a meaningful impact. The frailty of global public health has been well illustrated by the COVID-19 pandemic, which has exposed faultlines within health systems and public health in many countries, irrespective of their income status, and has shown the need for better preparedness to ensure global and national health security (see Chapter 34).

There is no room to be regretful tomorrow for the decisions that are made today, for now there is no excuse for not investing in public health and EPHF. Investing in public health is no longer a mere option; rather, it is an obligation and an ethical and moral imperative of governments in every country, rich or poor, to ensure well-performing EPHF.

References

1. WHO. *The World Health Report 2000: Health Systems: Improving Performance*. Geneva, WHO, 2000. www.who.int/whr/2000/en/whr00_en.pdf (accessed April 29, 2021).

2. Pan American Health Organization/World Health Organization (PAHO/WHO). Public Health in the Americas: conceptual renewal, performance assessment, and bases for action. 2002. https://iris.paho.org/handle/10665.2/2748 (accessed January 20, 2022).

3. C. E. Winslow. The untilled fields of public health. *Science* 1920; **51**(1306): 23–33.

4. D. Acheson. *Public Health in England: The Report of the Committee of Inquiry into the Future Development of the Public Health Function*. London, The Stationary Office, 1998.

5. A. J. Viseltear. History of the medical care section: emergence of the medical care section of the American Public Health Association, 1926–1948. *Am J Public Health* 1973; **63**(11): 986–1007.

6. R. Beaglehole, R. Bonita. *Public Health at the Crossroads: Achievements and Prospects*, 2nd ed. Cambridge, Cambridge University Press, 2004.

7. American Public Health Association. 10 essential public health services. 2020. www.apha.org/what-is-public-health/10-essential-public-health-services (accessed April 11, 2021).

8. J. M. Martin-Moreno, M. Harris, E. Jakubowski, et al. Defining and assessing public health functions: a global analysis. *Annu Rev Public Health* 2016; **37**: 335–355.

9. D. W. Bettcher, S. Sapirie, E. H. T. Goon. Essential public health functions: results of the international Delphi study. 1998. https://apps.who.int/iris/bitstream/handle/10665/55726/WHSQ_1998_51_1_p 44-54_eng.pdf;sequence=1 (accessed January 20, 2022).

10. D. W. Bettcher, S. Sapirie, E. H. Goon. Essential public health functions: results of the international Delphi study. *World Health Stat Q* 1998; **51**(1): 44–54.

11. WHO Regional Office for the Western Pacific. Essential public health functions: a three-country study in the Western Pacific Region. 2003. https://iris.wpro.who.int/handle/10665.1/5437 (accessed April 28, 2021).

12. Population Health and Wellness Ministry of Health Services of the Province of British Columbia. A framework for core functions in public health. 2005. www.health.gov.bc.ca/library/publications/year/2005/core_functions.pdf (accessed April 22, 2021).

13. J. Pommier, O. Grimaud. Essential public health functions: history, definition and potential applications. *Sante Publique* 2007; **19**(Suppl. 1): S9–S14.

14. Pan-American Health Organization. *Public Health in the Americas: Conceptual Renewal, Performance Assessment, and Bases for Action*. Washington, DC, Pan-American Health Organization, 2002. https://iris.paho.org/handle/10665.2/2748 (accessed April 21, 2021).

15. World Health Organization Regional Office for Europe. The 10 essential public health operations. 2022. www.euro.who.int/en/health-topics/Health-systems/public-health-services/policy/the-10-essential-public-health-operations (accessed January 20, 2022).

16. WHO Regional Office for Europe. Self-assessment tool for the evaluation of essential public health operations in Europe. 2015. www.euro.who.int/__data/assets/pdf_file/0018/281700/Self-assessment-tool-evaluation-essential-public-health-operations.pdf (accessed April 22, 2021).

17. A. Alwan, O. Shideed, S. Siddiqi. Essential public health functions: the experience of the Eastern Mediterranean Region. *East Mediterr Health J* 2016; **22**(9): 694–700.

18. P. Khaleghian, M.D. Gupta. Public management and the essential public health functions. 2004. https://openknowledge.worldbank.org/bitstream/handle/10986/14785/wps3220Publicmgt.pdf?sequence=1&isAllowed=y (accessed January 20, 2022).

19. B. Borisch, M. Lomazzi, M. Moore, et al. Update on the Global Charter for the Public's Health. *Bull World Health Organ* 2018; **96**(6): 439–440.

20. WFPHA. Global Charter for the Public's Health. 2016. www.wfpha.org/the-global-charter-for-the-publics-health (accessed April 30, 2021).

21. A. Soucat. Financing common goods for health: fundamental for health, the foundation for UHC. *Health Syst Reform* 2019; **5**(4): 263–267.

22. World Health Organization. Common goods for health. www.who.int/docs/

default-source/health-financing/common-good-for-health/common-goods-for-health-definition.pdf?sfvrsn=b5c9a9f8_2#:~:text= Definition%3A%20Common%20Goods%20 for%20Health,health%20and%20economic %20progress%3B%202 (accessed January 24, 2022).

23. P. Nsubuga, M. E. White, S. B. Thacker, et al. Public health surveillance: a tool for targeting and monitoring interventions. 2006. www.ncbi.nlm.nih.gov/books/ NBK11770 (accessed January 24, 2022).

24. World Health Organization. The 1st international conference on health promotion, Ottawa. 1986. www.who.int/ teams/health-promotion/enhanced-wellbeing/first-global-conference#:~:text= The%20first%20International%20 Conference%20on,health%20movement%20 around%20the%20world (accessed January 20, 2022).

25. World Health Organization. Assessment of essential public health functions in countries of the Eastern Mediterranean Region assessment tool. 2017. https:// applications.emro.who.int/dsaf/EMRO Pub_2017_EN_19354.pdf?ua=1 (accessed January 4, 2022).

26. World Health Organization. Health security. 2022. www.who.int/health-topics/health-security#tab=tab_1 (accessed January 4, 2022).

27. J. M. Martin-Moreno. Facing the COVID-19 challenge: when the world depends on effective public health interventions. SEEJPH 2020; 14. doi: 10.4119/seejph-3442.

28. WHO. International Health Regulations (2005), 3rd ed. 2016. http://apps.who.int/ iris/bitstream/10665/246107/1/978924158 0496-eng.pdf?ua=1 (accessed April 12, 2021).

29. WHO. International Health Regulations (2005): areas of work for implementation. 2007. www.who.int/ihr/finalversion9 Nov07.pdf (accessed April 23, 2021).

30. L. O. Gostin, R. Katz. The International Health Regulations: the governing framework for global health security. Milbank Q 2016; 94(2): 264–313.

31. H. Kluge, J. M. Martín-Moreno, N. Emiroglu, et al. Strengthening global health security by embedding the International Health Regulations requirements into national health systems. BMJ Glob Health 2018; 3(Suppl. 1): e000656.

32. WHO. Joint external evaluation. 2022. www.who.int/emergencies/operations/ international-health-regulations-monitoring-evaluation-framework/joint-external-evaluations (accessed January 20, 2022).

33. WHO. World Health Organization health systems strengthening glossary. 2011. www .who.int/healthsystems/Glossary_January 2011.pdf (accessed April 23, 2021).

34. WHO. Disease outbreaks. 2016. www .who.int/topics/disease_outbreaks/en (accessed April 8, 2021).

35. WHO. Community Emergency Preparedness: A Manual for Managers and Policy-Makers. Geneva, WHO, 1999. https:// apps.who.int/iris/bitstream/handle/10665/ 42083/9241545194.pdf;jsessionid=204A4 A60D07C70ED69406147662F2408? sequence=1 (accessed April 12, 2021).

Engaging in a Health Care Recovery Process

33

Enrico Pavignani

Keep your nose in the wind and your eye along the skyline.[1]

Key Messages
• Shifting the focus toward the side magnified by a severe crisis will sharpen the analysis: from state to society, from hardware to software, from health care supply to demand, from official to informal, from within borders to across borders, and from forms to functions. This change of perspective will give qualitative information its right weight. The diversity of the health care arena must be recognized, and tailored measures be taken in light of it.
• Economics, social sciences, demography, history, and geography offer generous insights for the health recovery operator. Exploring the political economy of the recovery process will identify threats, as well as suggest opportunities for health gains. Communication and negotiation skills, which are as important as technical ones, are required to turn political factors to advantage.
• Engaging in a health recovery process requires alertness to events, sensitivity to context, flexibility, and acceptance of risk. Unexpected events must always be expected, and be promptly recognized, discussed, and acted upon. Capable and autonomous analysis hubs must feed decision-makers with action-oriented information.
• Parsimonious priorities, modest expectations, and preparedness for reversals are key to progress. Vigilant care is needed to anchor strategies and interventions to foreseeable capacity and resource constraints, with capacity being a more serious limitation than resources. Arrangements for the long haul must be made, and bumpy progress foreseen.

Health recovery after a severe disruption is a complex, confusing, and surprising process, shaped by numerous actors and multiple forces. At the end of a recovery cycle, old and new health needs are expressed and addressed in novel ways. Some pre-existing health problems may have been tackled by recovery-oriented measures, others may have worsened, and new ones emerged. The expectations of people, the desires of policymakers, and the projections of planners may differ widely. Achieving a common understanding of recovery should take precedence on formulating detailed plans that are often left unimplemented. *In other words, the process will be more important than the content.*

This chapter highlights the interplay of forces, dilemmas, and interventions shaping recovery processes in a long-term perspective. Recovery necessarily involves a complex array of ambiguities, controversies, pitfalls, and reversals that are reflected in this chapter,

---

[1] From *Jeremiah Johnson*, a film directed by Sidney Pollack (1972).

which eschews recommendations or ready-made "solutions." Best practice has to be looked for in the methods adopted – and adapted to each unfolding process.

Situation analysis, debate, and *intervention* – the three main components of a health recovery process – are discussed in Sections 33.2, 33.3, and 33.4, respectively. In real life they occur concomitantly and affect each other. For this reason, no linear or cyclical depiction of the health recovery process is proposed, as neat distinctions would misrepresent the blurriness of actual events, as well as of the related responses.

Section 33.1 calls attention to the diversity of crisis contexts, and in turn to the variety of health recovery processes. Section 33.2 is devoted to exploring the health care arena and highlighting the benefits of complex thinking. Section 33.3 focuses on the need to promote an informed discussion among stakeholders. Without such an exchange of ideas, decision-makers might proceed in isolation, motivated by their own agendas at the expense of a fulsome picture. Section 33.4 suggests empirical principles to guide decision-makers, followed by advice on negotiating strategies and designing interventions, as well as sequencing them. Specific aspects of recovery are commented upon.

33.1 Contextualizing Health Recovery

Health recovery may take place in the aftermath of sudden shocks, following protracted stresses, or a combination of both. For instance, the economic decline may undermine the capacity of a health system to respond to an epidemic. Such disturbances impact societies and their health systems, which acquire new characteristics as they recover amid changed circumstances.

A **shock** refers to a disruption in an otherwise continuous trajectory. If the disturbance is transient and amenable to control, the health system may bounce back to its original state. If the shock induces fundamental changes, a restorative response may not be sufficient. Embracing change in the pursuit of systemic gains becomes a better option. Conversely, **stress** is an enduring and pervasive change, which can disrupt the health system or not, depending on the response. A resilient health system (see Table 33.3) can reconfigure itself to respond to stress. A vulnerable one will fall apart, reacting in ill-adaptive ways [1].

Disruption does not mean termination. By limiting or eroding their operations, many health systems survive repeated shocks and stresses. Some stresses are easily recognizable, while others are subtle, becoming apparent only when investigated. Table 33.1 presents a sample of possible shocks and stresses.

Rather than a technical exercise managed by rational planners, health recovery is always an intensely political process:

> politics is not a perfidious activity, but an inherent and necessary ingredient of all human endeavor arising out of the real differences among men over what they consider important, and their willingness and ability to strive for what they believe in. [2]

The health care arena is shaped by powerful external determinants, which need to be correctly identified and understood to negotiate favorable trade-offs. Health recovery options must be appraised in light of the main political drives. The prevailing political faction will impose its health care model, regardless of its merit or appropriateness in the post-crisis environment. Therefore, even promising approaches risk being sidelined if they are associated with losing factions. Tact is needed to preserve valid innovations against the political tide.

The political tensions and controversies of the transition period, which color even the best-intentioned health care-related decisions, must be defused. Rational, efficiency-, and

Table 33.1 Shocks and stresses

Shocks	Stresses
Political/economic collapse, sometimes endogenous, as in the case of the Soviet Union, or induced by external intervention (e.g. Iraq). In both cases, health recovery has been sluggish, tortuous, and unfinished.	*Protracted conflict or endemic violence* such as in Somalia and South Sudan. In many instances, "health recovery" is a misnomer because these health systems had never functioned properly.
Political uprising challenging the pre-existing order, which included state-led health care provision (e.g., Syria and Libya). Inconclusive conflict impedes a political settlement, and hence health recovery. Internal fragmentation may induce disconnected processes.	*Environmental, demographic, economic, and social pressures* exceeding health systems' capacity to respond effectively. Yemen presented this conflation of stresses of deepening severity before its implosion into unrestrained war.
Disaster, sometimes natural but often compounded by human factors. Recurring disasters have tortured Haiti, against a backdrop of poverty, environmental degradation, violence, and misrule.	*Health care decline* due to shrinking resources, caused by misrule (e.g., Venezuela) or sanctions (e.g. Iran). Restoring pre-existing resource levels implies a political and economic turnaround.
Epidemics, such as Ebola or COVID-19, may shake a health system. Even if it rebounds to its pre-existing state, reforms addressing the detected vulnerabilities may gain political support.	*Health spending inflation* skews allocative decisions in favor of demanded services. Savings may be pursued at the expense of performance, undermining public health programs and the response to new threats and needs. Overall efficiency may suffer as a result.
Destabilization may be induced by turmoil in neighboring countries, as with a sudden inflow of refugees and/or foreign fighters. Cluster crises encompassing several countries are common: African Great Lakes, Lake Chad, and the Levant being among the prominent ones.	*Deliberate reforms,* such as ideology-driven privatization, may erode health systems' capacity. Botched/stalled reforms may perturb the old health system without attaining the intended configuration.

equity-oriented strategies have to accommodate politically motivated decisions, such as job-creation schemes and grievance-appeasing investments. The distance separating health care systems segregated by longstanding frontlines must be reduced, through a difficult but necessary dialog.

33.2 Exploring Health Care Arenas as They Have Evolved under Shocks and Stresses

There's a hard lesson learned by every practitioner in a full-scale societal emergency – whether famine, war, massacre or epidemic: first, pause and think. Critical reflection is never, ever a luxury. Every post-disaster assessment contains the regret that there was a rush to action on the basis of assumptions that turned out to be incomplete, and expertise that turned out to be partial, short-cutting consultation and reflection. [3]

33.2.1 Making Sense of the Messy Recovery Process

This is akin to "drawing a map while traveling." Carrying out a health system analysis is frequently overlooked by hard-pressed actors, or it takes place for fundraising purposes – for instance, before a donor conference – to be subsequently shelved. Collecting updated and relevant information and circulating it among stakeholders supports the development of a shared picture of the health care arena to inform decisions. The identification of the most conspicuous knowledge gaps can orient research toward policy-relevant issues (see Chapter 23). Bringing together disconnected pieces of information into a coherent whole is essential for the generation of genuine intelligence.

33.2.2 Methodological Considerations in Analyzing Health Systems

A *complexity lens* is needed to conduct a robust health systems analysis [4]. The messy health field emerging from severe crisis is better understood as an arena or stage, with multiple actors entering or leaving, collaborating or squabbling, playing according to the script or improvising [5]. The health care arena is a complex adaptive system (see Table 33.3) embedded in a multifaceted, evolving societal system. These health care spaces should be considered as mirrors of their respective societies and histories, which explains to a large extent the recurrent failure of outsiders to engineer best-practice reforms [6].

Indeed, "health systems are not simply static technical constructs that are reducible to predefined health systems 'building blocks' (i.e., services, systems, products) or 'essential service packages'. On the contrary . . . health systems are also dynamic social constructs that are highly sensitive to the transitional forces of social, economic, and political change of which they form a vital subset" [7].

Moreover, multiple *wicked problems* will challenge stakeholders (see Table 33.3). Such problems lack a straight, "scientific," conclusive solution. Responses to them may generate ambiguous outcomes and severe side-effects, depending on context and process. "Because wicked problems are in essence 'expressions of diverse and conflicting values and interests,' the process of working with them is fundamentally social" [8]. Viewing a health care arena in crisis as a laboratory of diverse experiments carried out in unforgiving conditions by assorted players offers opportunities to be seized and lessons to be learned.

Fully embracing a complexity-oriented approach has fundamental implications for planning. For instance, "a large part of the information needed for implementation is generated along the way, making it essential that plans are more adaptive to unfolding realities." "If not everything can be foreseen, the reluctance to invest in detailed up-front planning is not a failure or a lack of professionalism ('not knowing what to do') but a prudent – and efficient – attitude when faced with limited insights" [9].

The behavior of the health system during the crisis provides crucial indications about vulnerabilities and strengths, likely to be carried over to the recovery phase. Ideally, the recovering health system should become resilient to future shocks, whose nature, timing, and intensity cannot be predicted. The reserves of resources and capacity that might be available to withstand future shocks and stresses should be appraised. "Global health discourse and action appears biased in favour of hardware – building resilience is sometimes seen as demanding more money, more health workers, more hospitals, better surveillance systems." "However, health system resilience is more about software than hardware" [10]. *Software aspects* must be studied alongside the hardware that usually gets the most attention. *Tangible software* includes information, spare capacity, interfaces, flexible funding, and international connectedness. *Intangible software* refers to trust, alertness, communication, initiative, reputation, and commitment – factors frequently overlooked with serious consequences.

Other disciplines such as social sciences, economics, geography, and history must expand the narrow biomedical perspective that usually dominates standard analyses. For instance, communicable diseases cannot be successfully managed on pure epidemiological grounds, as starkly demonstrated by the ongoing COVID-19 pandemic.

Neat binary constructs, such as public–private, legal–illegal, emergency–development, or domestic–foreign should be applied with caution, because reality usually escapes them. Most complex patterns tend to lie along a spectrum between one pure form and its opposite. For instance, health services are frequently delivered through a mix of public and private inputs and arrangements.

Due attention should be paid to the demand side (see Table 33.3) of health care to better reflect the perspective of users. Demand is determined by many factors, including cost, access, acceptability, quality, and communication. Otherwise, unjustified and unsustainable supply-inspired investments will occur.

Widely held views must be verified before being accepted as facts. Frequently, they are factoids or "social facts" (see Table 33.3). The limited access to the field by stakeholders interacting within fenced circles facilitates the circulation of unproven beliefs. Their persistence grants them the status of evidence, even when solid data is available to challenge these widely held views.

33.2.3 Patterns and Trends

The new health care landscape is reshaped by violence, destruction, impoverishment, migration, fragmentation, urbanization, and privatization. Protracted stress irreversibly transforms society as well as health care needs. Demography is affected by differential mortality across population groups and selective migration. Traditional livelihoods are frequently abandoned, with large portions of the population traumatically urbanized.

Turmoil disrupts and fragments health care provision. Emergency health care may expand, whereas essential services suffer. In response to violence or disease the public, and in turn the politicians, accord priority to hospital care, which absorbs most of the resources and capacity, worsening inequalities in access to health services.

Trends are more instructive than singular values and should be looked for or thoroughly assembled. A worrisome trend should ring an alarm bell, even if the related snapshot indicator suggests otherwise. Trends may be unavailable due to disarray, as well as the deliberate obfuscation of inconvenient facts. Particularly misleading are *"fossil"* figures, frequently referred to year after year without being updated.

33.2.4 Localized/Transborder Crises

These demand adapted recovery strategies. Turmoil diversifies health care arenas, inducing the development of *local health systems,* shaped by geographical, political, military, economic, or ethnic factors. Such a patchwork must be recognized, alongside the political uncertainties and tensions shaping it.

Transborder health care provision is prominent in many protracted crises [11]. Within the Middle Eastern crisis complex, Lebanon, Jordan, and Turkey have evolved into big exporters of health services for large numbers of Iraqi, Syrian, or Yemeni patients. Together, state resources, aid flows, charities, and households finance health care for refugees, as well as transient travelers. Protracted crises encompassing multiple countries reconfigure supply and demand in ways that should be thoroughly considered from a recovery perspective.

The transborder dimension of disease transmission must also be incorporated in effective response strategies, which are usually state-centric. Official controls are often put in place on the front stage while large population movements occur across porous borders on the backstage. The collaboration between political formations demanded by disease control is undermined by their rivalries, exacerbated by panic and political expediency.

33.2.5 Stakeholders (Internal and External) with Respective Agendas

The recovering health care arena is frequently overcrowded and fragmented. Coordinating interventions between multiple actors is a constant concern. In fast-moving circumstances, a thorough stakeholder analysis (see Table 33.3) requires hard work sustained over time (see Chapter 13). Care is needed to capture influential stakeholders located outside the country, alongside those active within it. The views of some stakeholders frequently absent from formal and informal coordination circles must be gathered. These include the diaspora, private providers, businesses, charities, de-facto rulers, and non-Western donors.

Mapping stakeholders at the national and supra-national levels is the first step, to be complemented by similar studies in peripheries marked by neglect, violence, impoverishment, or grievance. Ethnically divided or stratified societies are the stage for diverse stakeholders living side by side within the same location.

Where external assistance is large and influential, aid networks involve global health partnerships, official donors, international agencies, charities, and private benefactors. Some players without a country presence act remotely, while others provide health services or support indigenous operators. Beneficiaries used to dealing with aid agencies may adopt imaginative strategies to maximize advantages. Eventual outcomes result from multiple transactions, thereby challenging efforts to track funds or determine the eventual outcome.

The analysis of health care arenas in crisis is covered in detail by Pavignani and Colombo [12].

33.3 Encouraging an Informed Debate, Linked to Contextual Patterns

Multiple factors influence the choices of stakeholders and the nature of recovery. Depending on the country's outlook, choices should diverge quite markedly. Unfortunately, the same "traveling models" [13] are adopted time and again during the recovery process, in disregard of the present and future country context. Such decontextualized interventions are likely to fail in the health care arena, as in any other field.

In most cases, the governance setup is uncertain, with rulers unsure of their tenure and ready to renege on commitments if expedient. Enlarging the debate about recovery to include stakeholders outside the incumbent government is essential to sharpen the main ideas, as well as to increase the odds that future decision-makers will keep the course.

Threats and *opportunities* in the recovery environment will be perceived differently by stakeholders. Hospital investments will please politicians, doctors, contractors, and urban residents, whereas they will alarm progressive health planners. Privatization will be promoted by free-market proponents, but will raise serious concerns in equity-oriented circles. Expanding health care provision in underserved opposition strongholds might be resisted by the central government, or otherwise be promoted by it to gain political support. A policy vacuum – a common occurrence during a political transition – may look like an opportunity to promoters of imported "solutions," but like a threat to advocates of indigenous approaches. Therefore, controversies must be expected and managed, accepting trade-offs when opportune.

In many environments emerging from profound disruption, stakeholders will have to grapple with multiple issues. Some of them are related to the population, others to health service delivery.

33.3.1 Challenges Related to Population

- *The health care needs of displaced people set* in motion by improving security conditions demand tailored, assorted responses. The uncertainty related to the eventual settlement requires flexible supply options, such as mobile services, temporary facilities, assisted referrals, and financial support (mostly cash-based). Unearmarked funding will be needed to respond to unpredictable, fast-changing needs.

- *The chronic disease burden is usually exacerbated by the crisis.* The legacy of disability and mental distress among the population requires adapted responses that integrate medical and social services. A backlog of inadequately managed noncommunicable diseases must be addressed. Such population health needs will persist over decades, with huge social, financial, health care, and assistance implications, which should be considered in any recovery plan.

- *Slum populations are often dramatically inflated by the crisis.* Rural violence swells peri-urban settlements (e.g., Darfur), whereas urban fighting destroys them (e.g., Syria and Iraq). Refugees disperse across cities (e.g., Lebanon). "The humanitarian response in middle-income countries often intersects with the rising needs of urban poor. Fuelled by increased population mobility, humanitarians are increasingly forced to respond to violence and exclusion from basic services in urban centres" [14].

- *Marginalized communities should not be neglected,* so that recovery is equitable. Disadvantaged groups are often invisible to decision-makers and overlooked by health data. Marginalization may be due to social, ethnic, religious, economic, or livelihood factors. Nomads, minorities, inhabitants of distressed peripheral regions, and displaced people are among the population groups requiring special attention and innovative delivery approaches.

33.3.2 Challenges Related to Health Service Delivery

- *Communicable diseases require special attention during the transition,* when routine programs have not yet developed solid roots, and transmission may be hastened by resettlement. Investing early in communicable-disease surveillance and control across frontlines and borders can foster collaboration and nurture management capacity.

- *The urban landscape reshaped by crisis generates new and diverse social configurations.* Physical investments in health facilities will respond to such restructuring, either in a planned way or through dispersed decisions. Urban growth demands novel health care delivery models – a policy issue of relevance in societies shaken by population growth, environmental deterioration, economic decay, violence, and migration.
- *The new realities of health care provision* must be considered while rethinking the new health system. New health service delivery model(s) better adapted to future context(s) will have to be experimented with. Affordability should be prominent among decision-making criteria, considering the impoverishment caused by the crisis.
- *The changes in health care provision may have become entrenched.* Informal charges, dual practice, and other coping strategies are frequently condemned as "corruption." Whereas certain predatory practices impact negatively on health care, others keep health staff active and in place, despite unpaid or paltry salaries. Forbidding these practices without altering their causes will inevitably lead to their clandestine persistence.
- *The recovery of the whole health care system needs to be financed.* In many cases, the health care demand of an impoverished and unhealthy population can be satisfied only through externally financed subsidies; managing such financial inflows to good effect calls for strategic clarity, active data collection, and negotiation capacity. Financing and expenditure estimates are desirable, but usually unavailable. Cost figures computed in the midst of a crisis tell little about the actual operating costs of recovered health services. But approximate recurrent expenditure figures may help temper rushed investment decisions. Given that actual health expenditures tend to vastly exceed projections, caution in choosing service delivery models and setting standards is in order. "It is better to have a lean health service functioning according to plan, than a service designed to be fatter but losing weight rapidly from resource starvation" [15].
- *A surge of investment in physical infrastructure is common*, particularly in contested situations where external allies jostle for political dominance [16]. Facts on the grounds are associated with political and business calculations, powerful enough to escape rational plans. An inefficient and unsustainable health care network, weakened by health spending inflation as witnessed in Lebanon [17], is a common outcome. Investments and resource allocation patterns during and after the crisis must be managed through active monitoring and negotiation within a system-wide perspective, to avoid the "white-elephant syndrome" exemplified in post-disaster Haiti by donor-financed hospitals [18].
- *The derelict health workforce must be revived*, within a global labor market of increasing openness. The process must be congruent with other recovery directions, so that future health workers match emerging service delivery models, financing strategies, and governance setups. Integrating health workers segregated by frontlines and borders, trained under dissimilar programs, and used to practicing under diverse contract regimes, constitutes a key step toward recovery. Pressures to quickly train large contingents of low-skilled workers should be opposed, while upgrading the skills of active workers and training of underrepresented categories should be given precedence.
- *The circulation of affordable medicines of proven quality must be promoted* in an environment of poor regulation and lax law enforcement. Quality controls must be put in place with the backing of power-holders. The urge to resuscitate the pre-crisis

pharmaceutical production capacity needs to be managed, to contain wasteful investments and ensuing high recurrent-cost commitments and/or high retail prices.

Such a daunting array of challenges will intimidate stakeholders, who may be tempted to pick low-hanging fruits to demonstrate their agency, or fall back on magic bullets in the hope that many problems will recede as recovery progresses. By attracting most attention, fashionable policy options may impede a comprehensive analysis. To counter such a risk, an informed discussion encompassing the whole health care arena must focus on the relative priority of the main issues and of the related responses.

Ambitious plans with long timeframes should be discarded in favor of modest measures of growing ambition, which may provide concrete returns. The inadequacy of conventional health planning increases in crowded health care arenas, where official health authorities enjoy limited clout.

33.4 Supporting Positive Health Recovery Processes, While Containing Harmful Drives

33.4.1 Empirical Principles to be Adopted

- *Alertness to events, sensitivity to context, flexibility, and acceptance of risk* are all preconditions for the formulation of realistic health recovery strategies, which must remain *in progress* as long as the context remains fluid – often for decades. For a full discussion see Pavignani and Colombo 2016 [21].

- *Harnessing facts on the ground* in the pursuit of sector-wide returns demands a cold appraisal of their benefits, side-effects, and opportunity costs, and in turn the ability to foster a productive discussion about them with the parties concerned. For instance, the unplanned investments in epidemiological surveillance and response spurred by Ebola and COVID-19 in poor countries should be sustained, provided they focus on threats of local relevance, and do not starve other services of capacity and resources.
- *Thinking strategically* takes precedence over writing "strategic" plans. It entails identifying key weaknesses and vulnerabilities, selecting those that can realistically be addressed, mobilizing stakeholders, raising resources and focusing sustained efforts on the chosen measures [22]. The usual proliferation of "priorities" must be resisted, so that scarce capacity does not spread thin and serious gaps remain.
- *"Never let a crisis go to waste"* [23]. The vulnerabilities unveiled by the shock may lead to reconsidering previously ignored warnings. Adaptation and innovation encouraged by stress may provide models for the design of strengthened health systems. But these precious opportunities may go unnoticed and be forgotten. Seizing existing opportunities requires intelligence, operational and networking capacity, flexible funding, and risk-taking.
- *No-regret interventions* can provide tangible results even if the political environment becomes unfavorable, or the recovery process stalls. Self-contained measures, once entrenched, may offer firm foundations for later initiatives of greater scope. *For example*: putting in place an efficient pharmaceutical procurement mechanism, which ensures the availability of quality medicines at affordable cost, offers immediate benefits. It may be later absorbed into the revamped health system, even if the health choices made by stakeholders change.

33.4.2 Health Recovery Requires Adapted Management Capacity

This is crucial to delivering health services under harsh political and financial constraints, within an uncertain and unstable institutional perspective. The weakening of central state structures may have facilitated the emergence of local management capacity. The problem-solving skills acquired during the crisis by field managers constitute a big asset for the building of management structures of broader scope.

Too often, normative policies and plans surpass the existing management capacity and fail the implementation test. Most recovery strategies include management strengthening among their pillars, which often leads to the establishment of unresponsive and stifling formal structures. However, a sophisticated management architecture may be premature in the fluid transition period. Instead, flexible procedures, management autonomy, spare capacity, and sound intelligence are key to responding to events.

33.4.3 Realistic Goals, Contextualized Strategies, and Effective Measures

These must all be negotiated with assorted stakeholders, public and private, formal and informal, central and peripheral. If the recovering country attracts foreign attention, due to geopolitical calculations or development potential, the health policy discussion may become cacophonic. International models are promoted by incoming advisors without much consideration of their suitability to the context. Given the inadequacy of the knowledge base and the prevailing uncertainty, any recovery strategy must be considered as tentative and evolutionary, to be monitored and adapted to changing circumstances.

33.4.4 The Desirability and Feasibility of Health Reforms Must be Appraised

This must be done in consideration of prevailing conditions. Political and technical acumen is needed to gauge the need for change against the strengths that should be preserved. Outsiders will press for radical reforms, whereas many insiders will be conservative. A convergence of professional, political, business, and aid forces, overriding family practice models in favor of tertiary care, needs to be resisted (as described in Kosovo) [24].

The health reform experience of the countries born out of the dissolution of the Soviet Union is rich in lessons for would-be reformers. Incentives must be harnessed in the pursuit of policy objectives. Efficiency gains are needed to free resources to sustain equity and improved effectiveness. "In many cases, pre-transition performance problems have been exacerbated by half thought-out reforms that coexist with the remnants of the old system; moving forward will require creativity and political will" [2].

33.4.5 Sequencing Interventions

This entails a thorough scrutiny of the main issues to be addressed, their logical hierarchy, the knowledge held of each issue, the political and technical feasibility of different measures under consideration and their effectiveness in the given context, and the timeframe such measures need to produce effects (Table 33.2).

33.4.6 Management Tools

Management tools intend to optimize external assistance, as well as mobilize local capacity and resources. Thorough scrutiny of what has remained in place is needed before introducing a new management arrangement. Some management structures will be irredeemable, while others could be revived with adequate backing. For instance, budget support could bear promise in underfunded health systems maintaining core administrative operations. In other settings, resources must be protected from rapacious state bodies. Incentive-based interventions have clear limitations where the verification of results is constrained.

As a rule, large and sophisticated management mechanisms tend to be cumbersome, and hence ill-suited to fluid, unpredictable contexts where swift adaptation is at a premium. Management tools introduced in the field in response to concrete problems have a better record. By patient experimentation, the successful ones can be strengthened and merged with others. See the Liberia Health Sector Pool Fund [26] and the Zimbabwe Health Transition Fund [27].

33.4.7 Intervening at the Local Level

Intervening at the local level within a broad recovery strategy may offer better returns than grand national designs, which may remain on paper or be poorly implemented. Moreover, firmly grounded interventions offer opportunities for experimenting with diverse approaches and changing track as needed [28]. When tackling wicked problems, such an open-ended

Table 33.2 Rationale for sequencing interventions

Sequence	Interventions	Examples
First batch: tackling pressing issues at the start of a recovery process, or even before if possible	Measures targeting well-understood issues, with affordable capacity and resource requirements, and likely to bear fruit within a fairly short time span. Many technical problems fall into this category. Working on such issues will shed light on capacity, obstacles, and opportunities, and on the measures to be taken.	• Addressing the backlog of services derailed by an epidemic • Removing substandard medicines from the market • Containing iatrogenic contagion boosted by degraded working environment and practices
Second batch: issues needing patient experimentation and contextual adaptation	Poorly known issues, without clear solutions and often politically risky, need to be clarified before action is taken. Addressing their main determinants may be required. A range of measures must be tested on a small scale, to learn hands-on what works and what does not.	• Raising the uptake of health services by a marginalized community, by lowering deep-rooted demand barriers, alongside scaling up supply
Third batch: issues requiring thorough work before action is taken, due to their complex and multidisciplinary nature	Interventions entailing long-term efforts, with potentially severe side-effects. Recognizing such issues as symptoms of underlying problems calls for structural correction, rather than superficial mending. For instance, instead of being expanded, hospitals overloaded during an epidemic may need to be protected by strengthened primary services.	• Strengthening the health workforce requires protracted investments and involves other domains beyond health • A study on banning dual practice in Palestine concluded that it might outweigh its benefits, and would be unsustainable and unenforceable

Source: [25].

approach is mandatory. Promising local experiences are prone to be missed by decision-makers discussing lofty strategies without meaningful contributions from the ground.

33.4.8 Investing in the Quality of Care

Recovery processes are often marked by expansive drives, privileging hardware and quantitative expansion over strengthening management and support systems. While market, fiscal, and technical considerations recommend the prioritization of quality over quantity, political and economic pressures act in the opposite direction. Decision-makers should keep in mind that "simply scaling up interventions in weak health systems that deliver poor-quality services is likely to waste precious resources and fail to show the anticipated improvements in health" [29]. Improving quality of care demands well-designed and sustained interventions, which pay attention to the many factors contributing to it.

33.5 Concluding with a Cautionary Word

Given the multiple vulnerabilities affecting most countries stricken by severe crisis, their risk of relapsing into trouble after a few years of recovery is high. Therefore, engaging in a health recovery process is a gamble, to be taken humbly. Interventions should be geared toward mitigating vulnerabilities, or at least not introducing new ones. Aid dependency, siloed programs, and efficiency-pursuing cuts have all compromised the response to threats in settings as diverse as Afghanistan, Liberia, and Italy. The study of their tortuous trajectories should protect decision-makers from the allure of linear narratives, ready-made solutions, and missions accomplished. But these rarely admitted lessons risk being buried in deference to vested interests: "To the extent that recognition of mistakes is suppressed, so is learning" [30].

Box 33.2 Seven Best Resources on Health Recovery

F. de Weijer. A capable state in Afghanistan: a building without a foundation? 2013. www.wider.unu.edu/publication/capable-state-afghanistan (accessed January 27, 2022).

Government of Liberia, Ministry of Health and Social Welfare. Country situational analysis report. 2011. www.healthresearchweb.org/?action=download&file=CountrySituational AnalysisReport.pdf (accessed January 27, 2022).

J. Grundy, Q. Y. Khutb, S. Oumc, et al. Health system strengthening in Cambodia: a case study of health policy response to social transition. *Health Policy* 2009; **92**: 107–115.

J. Kutzin, M. Jakab, C. Cashin. Lessons from health financing reform in central and eastern Europe and the former Soviet Union. *Health Econ Policy Law* 2010; 5(2): 135–147.

A. R. Noormahomed, M. Segall. The public health sector in Mozambique: a post-war strategy for rehabilitation and sustained development. 1994. http://whqlibdoc.who.int/hq/1994/WHO_ICO_MESD.14.pdf (accessed January 27, 2022).

S. Stasse, D. Vita, J. Kimfuta, et al. Improving financial access to health care in the Kisantu district in the Democratic Republic of Congo: acting upon complexity. *Glob Health Action* 2015; **8**: 25480.

W. Van Lerberghe, A. Mechbal, N. Kronfol. The collaborative governance of Lebanon's health sector: twenty years of efforts to transform health system performance. 2018. www.moph.gov.lb/userfiles/files/Programs%26Projects/PSO/The-Collaborative-Governance-of-Lebanons-Health-Sector.pdf (accessed January 27, 2022).

Table 33.3 Definitions of selected concepts used in the chapter

Term	Definition/key issues	Source/suggested reading
Arena framework	It *"focuses on multiple actors rather than on international agencies, analyses processes rather than projects, and premises the analysis on social negotiation rather than planned interventions."*	[5]
Demand for health care	It is determined by many factors, including cost, access, acceptability, quality and communication. Demand may be *potential* (often described as need), or *expressed*, which leads to the actual use of health services. Individual and population demands may take different forms. Demand may be induced by supply.	[31]
Complex adaptive system	It is composed of many elements interacting dynamically across networks. Their components are linked by feedback loops. Interactions may be nonlinear. Complex systems are far from stable, they adapt and change. System-wide properties emerge. Components may be ignorant of the system as a whole.	[4]
Health spending inflation	National health spending growing faster than the respective economic growth rate. *"Rising health care costs exert pressure on every country and threaten the sustainability of the world's health care systems. In other words, health expenditures account for an ever-increasing share of total economic output, and payers have to allocate a larger share of their incomes to pay for health services."*	[32]
Resilience	*"Resilience is more than bouncing back."* "Health systems are resilient when they adapt and transform to support the continued delivery of good quality services and wider action to address emerging health needs appropriately. Within	[10]

	a complexity paradigm, nurturing resilience is about creating the conditions that enable system's effectiveness; i.e, that enable desirable emergent future states by feeding the natural, bottom-up dynamics of emergence and innovation, rather than by imposing simple and mechanistic, cause and effect type solutions to current problems."	
Safe-fail experiment	"Small actions designed to test ideas to deal with a problem where it is acceptable for these interventions to fail.' The learning obtained in this low-risk way is particularly valuable in uncertain conditions, present and future.	[09]
Social fact	"things that are deemed to be 'true' because they are widely believed to be true."	[33]
Stakeholder analysis	"Stakeholder analysis is an approach, tool or set of tools for generating knowledge about actors – individuals or organizations – to understand their behaviour, intentions, interrelations and interests; and for assessing the influence and resources they bring to bear on decision making and implementation processes."	[34]
Supply of health care	This results from the inputs, such as funding, personnel, medicines, and facilities, used in producing health care. Supply is determined by many factors, including costs, regulation, incentives, service mix, productivity, and quality. The common assumption that if health services are made available they will be used by patients is not always warranted. Decision-makers, planners, and funding bodies tend to focus on the supply side of health care, neglecting the demand side.	[31].

Table 33.3 (cont.)

Term	Definition/key issues	Source/suggested reading
Transition	A broad term, used to describe social, political, military, and/or economic change processes. The period between all-out civil war and recovery may be described in this way. The adoption of a market economy to replace Soviet central planning is another example. Most transitions are protracted, open-ended processes, punctuated by frequent reversals and ambiguous results.	
Wicked problem	A "class of social system problems which are ill-formulated, where the [available] information is confusing, where there are many clients and decision makers with conflicting values, and where the ramifications in the whole system are thoroughly confusing ... [such that] proposed 'solutions' often turn out to be worse than the symptoms." Wicked problems are contrasted with tame problems, typical of sciences and engineering, which have – at least in principle – clear formulation and definite solutions.	[8].

References

1. M. Leach, I. Scoones, A. Stirling. Governing epidemics in an age of complexity: narratives, politics and pathways to sustainability. *Glob Environ Change* 2010; **20**(3): 369–377.

2. B. J. Mott. The politics of health planning. II: the myth of planning without politics. *Am J Public Health Nations Health* 1969; **59**(5): 797–803.

3. A. de Waal. Thinking critically in a pandemic: reinventing peace. 2020. https://sites.tufts.edu/reinventingpeace/2020/04/06/thinking-critically-in-a-pandemic (accessed December 17, 2021).

4. D. De Savigny, T. Adam, eds. *Systems Thinking for Health Systems Strengthening.* Geneva, WHO, 2009. https://apps.who.int/iris/bitstream/handle/10665/44204/9789241563895_eng.pdf?sequence=1 (accessed December 15, 2021).

5. D. Hilhorst, M. Serrano. The humanitarian arena in Angola, 1975–2008. *Disasters* 2010; **34**(Suppl. 2): S183–S201.

6. J. van Olmen, B. Marchal, W. Van Damme, et al. Health systems frameworks in their political context: framing divergent agendas. *BMC Public Health* 2012; **12**: 774.

7. J. Grundy, Q. Y. Khut, S. Oum, et al. Health system strengthening in Cambodia: a case study of health policy response to social transition. *Health Policy* 2009; **92**(2–3): 107–115.

8. W. N. Xiang. Working with wicked problems in socio-ecological systems: awareness, acceptance, and adaptation. *Landsc Urban Plan* 2013; **110**: 1–4.

9. R. Hummelbrunner, H. Jones. A guide for planning and strategy development in the face of complexity. 2013. https://odi.org/en/publications/a-guide-for-planning-and-strategy-development-in-the-face-of-complexity (accessed December 19, 2020).

10. E. W. Barasa, K. Cloete, L. Gilson. From bouncing back, to nurturing emergence: reframing the concept of resilience in health systems strengthening. *Health Policy Plan* 2017; **32**(Suppl. 3): iii91–iii94.

11. O. Dewachi, M. Skelton, V. K. Nguyen, et al. Changing therapeutic geographies of the Iraqi and Syrian wars. *Lancet* 2014; **383**(9915): 449–457.

12. E. Pavignani, S. Colombo. UHC2030 Technical Working Group on UHC in Fragile Settings. 2019. www.uhc2030.org/fileadmin/uploads/uhc2030/Documents/About_UHC2030/UHC2030_Working_Groups/2017_Fragility_working_groups_docs/UHC2030_Guidance_on_assessing_a_healthcare_arena_under_stress_final_June_2019.pdf (accessed December 18, 2020).

13. J. P. Olivier de Sardan, A. Diarra, M. Moha. Travelling models and the challenge of pragmatic contexts and practical norms: the case of maternal health. *Health Res Policy Syst* 2017; **15**(Suppl. 1): 60.

14. J. Whittall. The "new humanitarian aid landscape." Case study: MSF interaction with non-traditional and emerging aid actors in Syria 2013. 2014. www.almendron.com/tribuna/wp-content/uploads/2019/08/the-new-humanitarian-aid-landscape.pdf (accessed December 18, 2020).

15. M. Segall. Health sector planning led by management of recurrent expenditure: an agenda for action-research. *Int J Health Plann Manage* 1991; **6**(1): 37–75.

16. C. S. Hamieh, R. M. Ginty. A very political reconstruction: governance and reconstruction in Lebanon after the 2006 war. *Disasters* 2010; **34**(Suppl. 1): S103–S123.

17. K. Sen, A. Mehio-Sibai. Transnational capital and confessional politics: the paradox of the health care system in Lebanon. *Int J Health Serv* 2004; **34**(3): 527–551.

18. F. Chabrol, L. Albert, V. Ridde. 40 years after Alma-Ata, is building new hospitals in low-income and lower-middle-income countries beneficial? *BMJ Glob Health* 2019; **3**(Suppl. 3): e001293.

19. S. Witter, B. Hunter. Do health systems contribute to reduced fragility and state-building during and after crises? What does it mean and how can it be enhanced? 2017. www.rebuildconsortium.com/resources/do-health-systems-contribute-to-reduced-

fragility-and-state-building-during-and-after-crises (accessed June 3, 2022).

20. T. K. Al Hilfi, R. Lafta, G. Burnham. Health services in Iraq. *Lancet* 2013; **381**(9870): 939–948.

21. E. Pavignani, S. Colombo. Strategizing in distressed health contexts. In G. Schmets, D. Rajan, S. Kadandale, eds., *Strategizing National Health in the 21st Century: A Handbook*. Geneva, WHO, 2016.

22. W. Van Lerberghe, A. Mechbal, N. Kronfol. The collaborative governance of Lebanon's health sector. twenty years of efforts to transform health system performance. 2018. www.moph.gov.lb/userfiles/files/Programs%26Projects/PSO/The-Collaborative-Governance-of-Lebanons-Health-Sector.pdf (accessed January 19, 2022).

23. D. Kolie, A. Delamou, R. van de Pas, et al. "Never let a crisis go to waste": post-Ebola agenda-setting for health system strengthening in Guinea. *BMJ Glob Health* 2019; **4**(6): e001925.

24. V. Percival, E. Sondorp. A case study of health sector reform in Kosovo. *Confl Health* 2010; **4**: 7.

25. J. Alaref, J. Awwad, E. Araujo, et al. To ban or not to ban? Regulating dual practice in Palestine. *Health Syst Reform* 2017; **3**(1): 42–55.

26. J. Hughes, A. Glassman, W. Gwenigale. Innovative financing in early recovery: the Liberia Health Sector Pool Fund. Center for Global Development. 2012. https://core.ac.uk/reader/6719070 (accessed December 18, 2020).

27. P. Salama, W. Ha, J. Negin, et al. Post-crisis Zimbabwe's innovative financing mechanisms in the social sectors: a practical approach to implementing the new deal for engagement in fragile states. *BMC Int Health Hum Rights* 2014; **14**: 35.

28. S. Stasse, D. Vita, J. Kimfuta, et al. Improving financial access to health care in the Kisantu district in the Democratic Republic of Congo: acting upon complexity. *Glob Health Action* 2015; **8**: 25480.

29. A. K. Rowe, D. de Savigny, C. F. Lanata, et al. How can we achieve and maintain high-quality performance of health workers in low-resource settings? *Lancet* 2005; **366**(9490): 1026–1035.

30. R. L. Ackoff, H. J. Addison, S. Bibb. *A Little Book of f-Laws. 13 Common Sins of Management*. Bridport, Triarchy Press, 2006.

31. T. H. Tulchinsky, E. Varavikova. *The New Public Health*, 2nd ed. Amsterdam, Elsevier, 2009.

32. W. C. Hsiao. Why is a systemic view of health financing necessary? *Health Affairs* 2007; **26**(4): 950–961.

33. P. Andreas, K. M. Greenhill. Introduction: the politics of numbers. In P. Andreas, K. M. Greenhill, eds., *Sex, Drugs and Body Counts: The Politics of Numbers in Global Crime and Conflict*. New York: Cornell University Press, 2010.

34. Z. Varvasovszky, R. Brugha. A stakeholder analysis. *Health Policy Plann* 2000; **15**(3): 338–345.

Chapter 34

Health System Response to the COVID-19 Pandemic
Fault Lines Exposed and Lessons Learned

Arush Lal, Victoria Haldane, Senjuti Saha, and Nirmal Kandel

Key Messages

- The COVID-19 pandemic emphasized the importance of maintaining routine health services while mitigating the acute impact of the pandemic – in low- and middle-income countries (L&MICs) and high-income countries (HICs) alike.
- The pandemic highlighted the importance of bringing together health security and universal health coverage (UHC) as complementary goals of the health system, to be achieved by leveraging a range of essential public health functions, strengthening primary health care, and enhancing risk management capacities.
- This calls for building resilient health systems by operationalizing systems thinking and aligning with the wider Sustainable Development Goals (SDGs) through a multisectoral approach.
- The omnipresent public health gaps in the health systems of L&MICs call for innovative approaches for a more effective response.

Health system strengthening is what we do; universal health coverage, health security and healthier populations are what we want. [1]

34.1 Introduction

Around the world, COVID-19 continues to pose major challenges for countries' health systems. From policymakers to community health workers (CHWs), all have had to respond to a rapidly spreading, novel disease outbreak while maintaining access to routine and essential health services – amid mounting socioeconomic pressures. This underscores two overarching goals for the health system: health security and UHC. The Director-General of WHO characterized these in 2017 as "two sides of the same coin" [2], and several reports and initiatives highlighted the importance of health systems as foundational to achieving them [3, 4].

The experience with COVID-19 in L&MICs and HICs suggests that global attention does not necessarily lead to the better-directed investments required to support equitable and resilient health systems for all communities. By contextualizing the impact of the pandemic on health systems around the world – as well as specific aspects of health systems in mitigating the crisis – emerging fault lines and novel lessons offer salient insights into how to achieve both HSc and UHC, as well as accelerate progress across the SDGs and wider social and political goals.

It is critical to understand the broader implications of health systems thinking in reforming the way public health professionals approach their work. The COVID-19 pandemic has demonstrated at least two important lessons when it comes to strengthening health systems: (1) there is no single "cookie-cutter" approach for designing and reforming health systems because different health systems respond to crises differently; and (2) the way we strengthen health systems must be significantly more comprehensive and robust if we hope to better prevent, detect, and respond to future health emergencies while advancing the equity agenda of UHC by leaving no one's health behind.

At the time of publication, the COVID-19 pandemic is still ongoing. The world has now faced 5–7 waves of transmission, and new variants continue to emerge. More than one year after the initial roll-out of vaccines, people in HICs are being offered their second booster (fourth dose), while less than 11% of people in low-income countries have received at least one dose [5].

34.2 The Spread and Impact of COVID-19 on Health Systems

In the two years since the first cases of SARS-CoV-2 (the scientific name of the virus responsible for COVID-19) were reported in December 2019, what started as a seemingly innocuous outbreak has become a major pandemic that threatened all aspects of life in every country across the world. In addition to killing millions globally, the 2020 report of the Global Preparedness Monitoring Board estimated the cost of COVID-19 to reach US$21 trillion [6]. Another estimate by the International Monetary Fund contends that COVID-19 could cost the world US$28 trillion over the period 2020–2025 [7]. Diverse domestic and international responses – and missed opportunities along the way – offer important health systems insights for better preventing and responding to future outbreaks while safeguarding Health for All.

34.2.1 COVID-19 and Its Impact on Health Security

The World Health Organization has warned that "pandemics, health emergencies and weak health systems not only cost lives but pose some of the greatest risks to the global economy and security faced today" [8]. The ongoing COVID-19 pandemic has proven this point, demonstrating that all countries are vulnerable to public health threats.

Around the world, nations struggle to develop coordinated, multisectoral response plans and overcome the institutional barriers that prevent coherent national strategies. Risk communication and early warning alert systems have been inadequate; laboratory and surveillance networks are weak; data systems are misaligned while an "infodemic" fuels misinformation; health workers are limited and often left without critical personal protective equipment (PPE); and there is inadequate infection prevention and control measures [9].

This is true regardless of income level. Several HICs that had initially scored high in health security assessments (see Box 34.1) failed to curb transmission, while many L&MICs leveraged recent experience with infectious disease outbreaks to mitigate the impact of the pandemic despite lack of lifesaving resources. In addition, some countries, such as Vietnam and Thailand, saw rising cases after early "success," while other countries, such as the United Kingdom and United States, have struggled to rapidly respond due to poor leadership and complacency [10].

For health systems traditionally designed along vertical, disease-centered silos, the resulting fragmentation in health security core capacities (as well as fragmentation between primary care and emergency preparedness functions) has hampered the ability to effectively

---

Box 34.1 Defining Health Security (HSc)

Health security is defined as the activities required, both proactive and reactive, to minimize vulnerability to acute public health events that endanger the collective health of populations living across geographical regions and international boundaries [8]. Accordingly, this involves the core capacities required to prevent, detect, and respond to infectious disease threats of international concern – including public health interventions such as scaling up surveillance, laboratories, food and animal safety, and risk communication. Rooted in the legally binding International Health Regulations (IHR) – see Chapter 32 – these capacities are critical tools to support a robust response to health emergencies, or better yet, avoid an outbreak altogether by leveraging emergency risk management capacities and essential public health functions (EPHFs) [8].

---

respond to the ongoing pandemic. The lack of alignment between national and global actors has weakened health system efficiency and increased competition for scarce resources, ultimately undermining multisectoral response plans and sidelining the wider socioeconomic impacts of health emergencies on communities [11].

The recent rise of variants amid relaxed public health measures and the inequitable scramble to secure doses of vaccines – often at the expense of international solidarity – have put all countries at greater risk, even those with high vaccine coverage. The emergence of global mechanisms to help mitigate these inequities, such as the Access to COVID-19 Tools (ACT) Accelerator and its COVAX facility, highlights the inadequacy of national responses. The subsequent failure of international partners to deliver on these promises similarly points to shortcomings that are important to consider for those who design health systems [12].

Political decision-makers and senior officials in all sectors should see COVID-19 as a salient reminder to proactively invest in emergency preparedness and risk management capacities. Meanwhile, the crisis is an urgent call to support and protect vulnerable and marginalized populations who are most at risk during health crises, through financial and social protection programs. World leaders must break the cycle of "panic and neglect," and instead build health systems that can ensure health security by embedding risk management capacities and financing for public health preparedness into the national health system at large, and primary health care (PHC) in particular, well before the next pandemic or health emergency.

34.2.2 COVID-19 and Its Impact on UHC

The importance of "Health for All" and UHC has been well documented over decades. Even prior to the pandemic, commitments for UHC were largely off-track [13]. Half the world's population lacks access to essential health services, and millions are pushed into poverty each year due to out-of-pocket spending on health [14]. Additionally, governments have neglected the foundational investments in health systems, forgoing critical financing in quality health facilities, sufficient health workers, and interoperable health information systems [15]. Government officials and community leaders alike have grappled to remedy the worsening inequities and deteriorating health outcomes as a result of the crisis. COVID-19 continues to disproportionately impact already-vulnerable populations, including racial and ethnic minorities, refugees, and LGBTQ+ groups. Women and girls have been routinely sidelined in response and recovery plans, and marginalized groups have been left behind when trying to access COVID-19 tools, from vaccines and tests to basic resources like oxygen and hospital beds [16]. Without urgent reform and investment in health systems that prioritize dignified and quality health services for all, UHC will remain out of reach and societies will remain vulnerable to worsening health outcomes.

Particularly in L&MICs, the absence of social safety nets and affordable, accessible health services for individuals and communities, which are made vulnerable by adverse determinants of health, have meant that there is little in place to protect these populations during the COVID-19 pandemic. As a testament to this, 90% of countries have reported ongoing disruptions to essential health services a year into the pandemic, further underscoring how health emergencies can impact the health of communities and cause long-term harm at a population level [17].

Foundational UHC-focused health systems' investments are needed not only to support equity in access but equally to ensure resiliency in the face of new and emerging crises, particularly through a strong PHC approach. The success of the latter relies on investing in adequate models of care, physical infrastructure, medicines and health products, purchasing and payment systems, and digital technologies for health.

34.3 Public Health Gaps and Innovations in L&MICs While Responding to COVID-19

Health systems in L&MICs continually struggle to provide quality health care or catalyze needed innovation to support evidence-based policy decisions. Often, they are trapped in a vicious cycle, where limited resources lead to inadequate data required to attract new resources. International funds for health research are usually provided for (or limited to) short-term "studies" that are designed such that data unidirectionally flows from the Global South to the Global North, with limited attention to local community involvement or development [18].

Policymakers in L&MICs have to juggle many competing priorities as resources are scarce. Hence, public health challenges in L&MICs are manifold, often due to gaps in health systems. For instance, most L&MICs in South Asia underspend on health – Bangladesh spends 2.3%, Pakistan 3.2%, and India 3.5% of their GDPs on health, with their respective governments' contributing one-third of the health expenditure at the most [19]. In terms of service provision, Bangladesh has 0.8 hospital beds per 1,000 people (India has 0.5 and Pakistan has 0.6), in comparison to 2.5 in the UK [20]. With increasing GDP and life expectancy, the burden of noncommunicable diseases is expected to rise, exacerbating existing challenges in already-fragile health systems.

Amid overburdened health services, many L&MICs are routinely forced to redirect valuable limited resources away from other endemic diseases. While also experienced in HICs, the inability to provide regular care due to the redirection of resources is most acutely felt in least-resourced settings. For example, during the Ebola outbreak in West Africa more people died from untreated malaria than from Ebola [9]. In Bangladesh, a study depicted the indirect impact of the pandemic on the health of neonates requiring hospitalization during COVID-19 by showing that a high proportion of deaths was caused by otherwise preventable diseases [21]. It has been reported that tuberculosis notifications dropped by 25–30% in three high-burden countries (India, Indonesia, and the Philippines) in 2020 due to the pandemic, likely leading to undiagnosed and untreated tuberculosis [22].

Against the backdrop of resource-constrained health systems and limited research capacity, the COVID-19 pandemic has presented a unique global crisis forcing each community to act locally – regardless of how few resources were available. Communities in L&MICs have instrumentalized local health system innovations, creatively leveraging existing limited resources for maximal output. For example, many countries in Southeast Asia, Latin America, and Africa have quickly adapted existing laboratory infrastructure for COVID-19 diagnostics as well as genomic surveillance to track variants (Box 34.2). Indeed, the speed and efficiency of sequencing efforts in several L&MICs was applauded by international media, who noted that countries with far fewer resources, such as Bangladesh, Sri Lanka, and Suriname, process samples faster than the United States [23].

The COVID-19 pandemic has provided concrete evidence that, when given the resources, L&MICs have both the expertise and intelligence required to fight infectious diseases through local communities. Many of the solutions to tackle COVID-19 have been driven by the urgent need to address the acute local and global crises, and have relied on the creative recycling of existing technologies, without multimillion-dollar investments in new innovations.

34.4 Health System Responses to the COVID-19 Pandemic

As the widespread transmission of COVID-19 during 2020 has persisted into 2021 and 2022, health systems have faced an increasingly difficult task: providing care for growing numbers of COVID-19 patients and delivering large-scale vaccination programs against the virus, while ensuring continuity of essential health services for all.

Box 34.2 Spotlight on L&MICs Public Health Innovations

Pakistan [24]

- Built live dashboards for real-time monitoring of spatial and temporal distribution of cases
- Delivered all patient reports electronically through SMS to minimize population mobility
- Enabled patients to easily access information through telephone hotlines
- Enabled people to register for vaccines using locally built registration apps

Bangladesh [18]

- Used undergraduate and graduate student volunteers to run training programs across the country to rapidly increase testing capacity
- Leveraged local reagent and supply vendors to address supply chain gaps by bypassing the need to import supplies from different parts of the world
- NGOs and private laboratories quickly stepped in to increase testing and genomic surveillance capacity
- The Expanded Program of Immunization (EPI) and the local WHO office leveraged their expertise and networks to distribute vaccines and transport samples for COVID-19 testing from all over the country to urban testing laboratories

Despite being comparatively well resourced, health systems in HICs have been overwhelmed by successive waves of COVID-19 infections. In these countries the pandemic has disproportionately impacted the most vulnerable, including those living in congregate settings and working in crowded conditions, those with precarious employment, and racial and ethnic minority communities [25]. Indeed, communities with least access to care and social protection have been most at risk of long-term impacts.

A similar pattern has played out in many L&MICs, where already under-resourced and fragmented health systems have faced the combined challenges of responding to the pandemic, managing pre-existing crises like HIV/AIDS, and maintaining essential health services mainly through primary care (e.g., maternal and antenatal services, and routine immunizations) [26]. Notably, responses to COVID-19 to protect lives and livelihoods were not defined by a country's income level, but rather the political will to sustain resilient and comprehensive health systems and ensure robust technical coordination at both the national and subnational levels.

Previous high-profile health emergencies, including Ebola virus disease, severe acute respiratory syndrome (SARS), and Middle East respiratory syndrome coronavirus (MERS), have shaped our understanding of health systems resilience (see Chapters 32 and 37) to emerging infectious disease threats. While these crises catalyzed the uptake of EPHF and IHR core capacities (see Chapter 32) as important health systems functions to prevent, detect, and respond to health emergencies, limited resources and fragmented health agendas have meant that other health systems elements, such as diverse and adequate health workers and accessible and affordable primary care services, have been neglected. The COVID-19 pandemic has made clear that health systems resilience is only possible when systems thinking is operationalized to holistically consider the entire health system and not just capacities related to core public health activities.

Three key elements of health systems resilience have characterized COVID-19 national responses: (1) supporting system-wide public health functions of surveillance, testing, contact tracing, and quarantine; (2) adapting health system capacity and strengthening the health workforce; and (3) preserving medical supplies and health service delivery. These are detailed below.

34.4.1 Supporting Core Public Health Functions

When responding to an emerging infectious disease outbreak, core public health functions – as part of the general EPHF – can reduce community transmission. These include surveillance, testing, contact tracing, and quarantine. These approaches have evolved over time in many countries and jurisdictions. By reducing transmission and preventing widespread outbreaks, health system capacity can be preserved, and the health and wellbeing of communities safeguarded.

Surveillance

During the ongoing COVID-19 pandemic, health systems with strengthened surveillance functions used "real-time" epidemiological data to inform decision-making, which was key in operationalizing a public health response, and to plan for bed capacity and health workforce deployment. For example, Vietnam launched an online COVID-19 reporting system allowing for real-time, countrywide epidemiological monitoring [27].

Testing

Throughout COVID-19, countries used a mix of testing strategies (active and passive testing), including establishing testing sites in communities (e.g., pharmacies, local public spaces, or food markets); drive-through testing centers; and mobile "rapid response" teams to reach remote or marginalized communities. For example, Thailand relied on existing rapid response teams established during avian influenza outbreaks, and Peru created new teams responsible for COVID-19. The testing and response infrastructure required the support of an equally robust laboratory system, which needed to be rapidly mobilized. In Uruguay a network of 24 laboratories known as "The COVID-19 diagnostic lab network" was quickly established, resulting in a fivefold increase in diagnostic capacity between March and May 2020 [28].

Contact Tracing

In response to COVID-19, both HICs and L&MICs used digital technologies to support contact tracing efforts in addition to more traditional contact tracing strategies. Digital contact tracing included proximity tracing mobile applications (e.g., Trace Uganda [29], COVID Alert SA in South Africa [29], careFIJI [30], HaMagen in Israel [31], Stopcoronavirus in Russia [32], Aarogya Setu in India [33]) or QR scanning and other electronic log entry systems (e.g., NZ COVID Tracer in New Zealand [34], KI Pass in South Korea [35], SafeEntry in Singapore [36], or Thai Chana in Thailand [37]).

Quarantine

The mitigation of COVID-19 transmission required people who met various contact criteria to quarantine, either in dedicated facilities or at home, with in-person or telehealth check-ins, or without external enforcement measures. Vietnam implemented a "four tier" approach that applied a continuum of measures based on exposure to COVID-19 [28].

Broader Public Health Measures and Community Engagement

In order to preserve health system capacity, these public health functions were supported by broader public health and social measures throughout the COVID-19 pandemic. These included mask-wearing policies, school and workplace closures, restrictions on gathering and movement, and border closures [38].

34.4.2 Adapting Health System Capacity

It is important to ensure onward care for individuals diagnosed with COVID-19. As cases have surged, many countries, including L&MICs, have created temporary treatment centers. These centers have cared for patients with mild to moderate COVID-19 and eased the pressure on hospital beds. For example, in China, 16 rapidly built sites added 13,000 beds in Wuhan [39]. Other health system responses have included developing makeshift hospitals (often established in conjunction with the armed forces), converting large public infrastructure (e.g., convention centers or arenas) into isolation facilities, and transforming existing hospital wards into ICUs. Notably, these rapidly established care sites have required palliative care capacity, clear discharge planning, and integration within the existing health system to ensure high-quality care, pointing to the importance of health systems thinking in responding to a crisis [40].

Globally, countries have actively recruited, trained, and reallocated health workers, including trainees, to respond to COVID-19. For example, Brazil has allowed final-year medical students to directly enter clinical practice [41]. Many health systems have further incentivized recruitment and retention by providing additional financial support (e.g., hazard pay or bonuses) to health workers. In Argentina, financial incentives were granted to health care workers in the public and private sectors who were exposed to patients with COVID-19. In some HICs such as New Zealand, health workers have had access to additional mental health support to mitigate burnout [42]. However, health worker shortages continue to limit global efforts to expand the health workforce, highlighting the need to support and protect current health workers, including those employed in informal caregiving roles. L&MICs may not be able to invest adequately in health workers; therefore, governments need to bring in other sectors, including academia, civil societies, and private sectors, to meet this demand.

34.4.3 Preserving Medical Supplies and Health Service Delivery

Significant efforts have been made locally and globally to preserve medical supplies during the COVID-19 pandemic. Ongoing shortages of test kits, PPE, medicines, and oxygen have hindered health systems' ability to safely provide care [43]. Many L&MICs have strengthened domestic research, development, and production of these supplies. Additionally, countries have established policies prohibiting medical supply export, while relaxing import licensing requirements. Some countries have relied on purchasing consortia to secure medical supplies. For example, the PAHO Strategic Fund is one of the only pooled procurement mechanisms facilitating access to all types of medicines and supplies serving Latin America and the Caribbean, ranging from COVID-19 tests to treatments for hypertension and neglected tropical diseases [44].

As COVID-19 has disrupted health service delivery, strategies to ensure ongoing access to essential health services has been critical, and has largely relied on sustaining primary care services and supporting health workers. In some countries, primary care centers and workers have been integrated into the pandemic response. In Uganda, for example, CHWs were recruited to provide COVID-19 education, identify suspected cases, and refer positive cases to higher levels of care [45]. In both HICs and L&MICs, telemedicine has been used for routine consultations and prescription refills [46]. See Box 34.3 on selected health system options used to enhance health system response to the COVID-19 pandemic.

Box 34.3 COVID-19 Has Demonstrated How Health Systems Can Better Support Health Security and UHC through Coordinated Efforts Across All Health Systems Building Blocks before and during Crises

- Invest in pandemic planning and training for all health workers, including primary care providers and CHWs, and ensuring health workers' physical, mental, and economic protection.
- Increase health system capacity and maintain system functioning by creating temporary treatment centers, enhancing capacity for critical care especially in secondary hospitals.
- Strengthen supply chains and ensure adequate access to medical supplies through purchasing consortia.
- Ensure that public health functions, including surveillance, testing, contact tracing, and quarantine are proactive, comprehensive, integrated throughout the health system, grounded in human rights, and co-developed with communities.

34.5 Multisectoral Engagement for HSc and UHC

The world has witnessed many public health events that have emerged locally and spread globally, like the fast-moving COVID-19 pandemic, which has demonstrated that health systems capacities are insufficient to deliver an effective response to severe and large-scale public health emergencies at subnational and national levels. Inability to confront such crises undermines the twin goals of ensuring HSc and UHC.

Evidence suggests that while the return on investment for preparedness is high, financing for HSc remains at a bare minimum [47]. The COVID-19 pandemic has led to ever-growing economic impact, with trillions of dollars in costs to countries and millions of people pushed into poverty [48]. According to a recent systematic review, the cost of preparedness ranges from US$1.6 billion to US$43 billion annually [49], and the 2020 report of the Global Preparedness Monitoring Board has estimated that the cost of preparedness is in the order of US$5 per person per year (around $40 billion globally). An analysis of IHR annual reporting data conducted in the context of COVID-19 showed that countries vary widely in their ability to prevent, detect, and respond to outbreaks, including operational readiness (Figure 34.1) [50]. This serves as a stark reminder that countries are only as strong as the weakest health system in our interconnected world, and emphasizes the need to invest in well-functioning and adaptable health systems while equally working toward aligning and integrating health emergencies preparedness and response into health system strengthening efforts by incorporating national action plans for IHR or health security (e.g., NAPHS) into comprehensive national health strategic plans.

34.5.1 Challenges and Opportunities

The challenges to multisectoral action are more visible and acute in L&MICs, where institutions are frequently weak and fragmented – even within the health sector – which

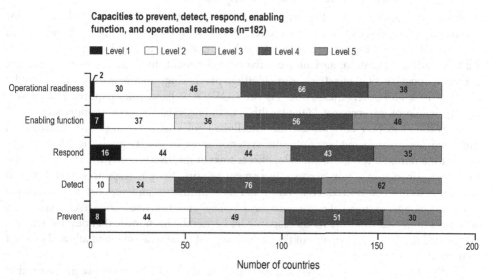

Figure 34.1 Health security capacities in the context of the COVID-19 pandemic: an analysis of IHR annual report data from 182 countries [50].

undermines coordination. From a governance perspective, diverse factors influence the success of multisectoral action. These factors include high-level political commitment, incentives that enable either competition or collaboration between agencies, and the extent to which there is common understanding about the problem among actors. The root causes of the challenges include poor governance entrenched in political and administrative irregularities, widespread clientelism, lack of citizen voice, weak social capital, lack of trust, and lack of respect for human rights. These are compounded by governments' poor capacity for the management of public funds and low levels of transparency and accountability [51]. Finally, the traditional view of the Ministries of Health to function as Ministries of Health Care still prevails in most L&MICs, and requires a paradigm shift toward a more holistic view of their role as stewards of the health systems. While these presented significant challenges during the pandemic, some countries nevertheless overcame these impediments to successfully launch multisectoral responses to COVID-19.

The WHO "health systems for health security" framework offers guidance on how countries can align the capacities required for the IHR with components of health systems and other sectors to enable multisectoral, multidisciplinary, and effective management of health emergencies [52]. The framework complements existing concepts and tools to build capacity in HSc, and covers different types of risks arising from biological and nonbiological hazards and events. For example, the application of the framework to the COVID-19 pandemic has uncovered the pandemic's disproportionate impact on vulnerable communities as a result of preventable risk factors, economics, and social determinants [53].

Even with optimal IHR capacities, health systems alone cannot guarantee timely, whole-of-society, and efficient prevention, detection, and response to public health emergencies such as COVID-19. Indeed, beyond the IHR and health systems components, capacities resting with other sectors are required to ensure a true multisectoral approach to HSc and UHC.

34.5.2 Multisectoral Responses during COVID-19

National policies in sectors other than health have a major impact on the risk factors for diseases. Health gains can be achieved much more readily by influencing public policies in sectors that directly impact determinants of health, such as the environment, transport, trade, taxation, education, agriculture, urban development, food, and energy. Increasing evidence suggests that effectively anticipating, preventing, and managing acute public health events and emergencies, such as the COVID-19 pandemic, requires a whole-of-society, whole-of-government, "One Health," and multilevel engagement approach.

COVID-19 further emphasized the interlinked roles of leadership, governance, and financing, both within and beyond health systems, in responding to public health emergencies. At the national level, this includes efforts toward multisectorality, where health is the focus of coordinated action across government sectors. Several responses have featured decision-making committees comprising multiple ministries and supported by scientific advisory groups to translate evidence into policy and practice. Conversely, countries without a multisectoral COVID-19 response had generally been those that devalue science, minimized the potential impacts of the pandemic, had delayed action, and allowed distrust to undermine efforts [9].

Without focused attention on socioeconomic needs, pandemic response measures that aim to preserve health system capacity often exacerbate pre-existing vulnerabilities in communities, further bolstering health inequities within populations, for example globally and across nations. Key strategies to reduce vulnerabilities include financial and food supports. Globally, many individuals have been unable to comply with public health measures that would limit their ability to earn an income. In response, some countries have financially supported individuals and families through cash transfers, debt relief, or wage subsidies. In Latin America, many workers are informally employed with little social protection [54]. In response, Argentina, which has had lengthy lockdowns, temporarily suspended evictions and banned rent increases [55]. Additionally, the social safety nets were expanded to include food distribution to an estimated 296 million people who were at risk of food insecurity by April 2021 [56]. Other countries, such as Sri Lanka, implemented price caps on essential food items [57].

34.5.3 Developing Multisectoral Health Systems

Careful consideration of diverse sectors is required to ensure the readiness of health systems for enhanced HSc and UHC. For example, as illustrated in Figure 34.2, the infection prevention and control (IPC) measures needed to deliver essential health services are only made possible through continuous support from multiple sectors. While IHR capacities define the specific requirements for IPC across multiple sectors, their implementation requires that the health system provides an enabling environment with the relevant IPC protocols, training, and governance in place, as well as adequate and effective operationalization. This implementation requires support from sectors such as water and sanitation for adequate hygiene, and the power sector for continuous energy supply to operate medical devices, and industry and transportation sectors for maintained provision of logistics and supplies through timely production and transportation. Box 34.4 summarizes some lessons from multisectoral actions during public health emergencies.

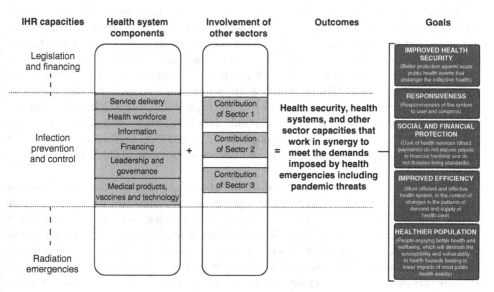

Figure 34.2 Building health systems for health security capacities to meet the demands imposed by health emergencies. Adapted from [58].

> **Box 34.4** Lessons for Multisectoral Action during Public Health Emergencies
>
> 1. Adopt a whole-of-government approach to ensure adequate translation of evidence into effective and cohesive policy and practices.
> 2. Provide financial and social support for individuals and families to ensure they are able to adhere to public health measures.
> 3. Ensure health systems are responsive to user needs and concerns at all stages of health emergencies.
> 4. Manage scarce health resources efficiently when they are diverted, disrupted, or limited during emergencies.

Only when the entire health sector works in synergy to meet the demands of health emergencies and other public health threats can communities, countries, and a globalized world prevent a future pandemic and ensure accessible health services for all people, including the most vulnerable. These should be aligned with the strategic levers and pillars for PHC operationalization (see Chapter 2), including political leadership, governance frameworks, funding and allocation of resources, and engagement of communities [15].

34.6 Moving Forward: Lessons Learned from the COVID-19 Pandemic for Future Health Systems Thinking

The COVID-19 pandemic has made clear that health is a fundamental human right. Everyone, everywhere should be protected from threats to public health and be able to access the health services they need. Therefore, strengthening health systems is the most efficient and sustainable way to simultaneously achieve both HSc and UHC.

This chapter demonstrates how designing health programs and policies for specific diseases or interventions actually weakens health systems during crises as it duplicates initiatives and fragments resources. The experience of managing COVID-19 has demonstrated that health practitioners should focus on strengthening health systems in a cross-cutting and holistic way. The COVID-19 pandemic has underscored that primary care anchored in a PHC-oriented health system is the most cost-effective way to bring affordable, good-quality health care to communities – as the foundation of strong health systems to mitigate inequities and build resilience. Not only does PHC, when optimally implemented, safeguard vulnerable and marginalized populations, it also cultivates trust in local health services, thereby supporting more rapid compliance with public health measures during outbreaks like COVID-19.

This chapter also showed how countries that have integrated preparedness and strategic response to COVID-19 into their health systems through measures such as scaling up testing, training epidemiologists for contact tracing, establishing national health emergency frameworks, and strengthening leadership coordination mechanisms have been better able to protect health, societies, and economies during the pandemic. COVID-19 continues to have profound social, political, and economic impacts on L&MICs and HICs. Health systems that support health security and UHC better reflect the social contracts between governments and citizens. Ultimately, strengthening health systems is essential to achieve

Box 34.5 Summary of Lessons for Health Practitioners to Strengthen Health Systems Post-COVID-19

- Equity should be a core principle for health system strengthening efforts, including addressing systemic barriers to quality and affordable health care through targeted policy interventions.
- Resilience should be a key objective for sustainable health systems, and health services and systems should be prepared for and withstand future threats. This often further supports economic and social resilience of communities.
- Health practitioners should work within their organizations and roles to end the "panic and neglect" cycle by investing in the foundations of health systems.
- Domestic stakeholders should push their governments to scale up public financing to develop health systems, as well as to ensure accountability and transparency of spending toward this.
- All health actors must carefully evaluate their roles in contributing toward the wider health system by better coordinating health policies and investments for both HSc and UHC.
- Multisectoral action is needed within and beyond the health sector to foster healthy lives and societies for all, including designing health systems that integrate investments in PHC, health service delivery, EPHFs, and emergency risk management with wider health interventions.

the wider economic, social, and political benefits of health, and to accelerate progress on other SDGs, from climate change to gender equality.

34.7 Conclusion

Over the course of this chapter we have covered the various challenges and opportunities for health systems strengthening exposed by the COVID-19 pandemic. The rapid and sustained spread of COVID-19 has underscored the need for rapid and coordinated response measures for both HSc and UHC. Socioeconomic impacts have highlighted an inequitable, chronic lack of protection for vulnerable and marginalized populations. Insights from diverse countries, ranging from L&MICs to HICs, emphasized the importance of resilient health systems in dealing with public health shocks. Examples of innovations in resource-constrained settings offer new ways to combat persistent gaps in public health. And robust evidence has made a compelling case to move away from siloed local and global health approaches toward multisectoral, whole-of-society initiatives to sustainably strengthen health systems that better address future health crises and protect the right to Health for All. Some lessons for health practitioners from the response to the COVID-19 pandemic are summarized in Box 34.5.

References

1. J. Kutzin, S. P. Sparkes. Health systems strengthening, universal health coverage, health security and resilience. *Bull World Health Organ* 2016; **94**(1): 2.

2. T. A. Ghebreyesus. All roads lead to universal health coverage. 2017. www .who.int/news-room/commentaries/detail/ all-roads-lead-to-universal-health-coverage (accessed June 18, 2021).

3. M. P. Kieny, H. Bekedam, D. Dovlo, et al. Strengthening health systems for universal health coverage and sustainable development. *Bull World Health Organ* 2017; **95**(7): 537–539.

4. United Nations. Universal Declaration of Human Rights. www.un.org/en/about-us/ universal-declaration-of-human-rights (accessed December 13, 2021).

5. Our World in Data. Coronavirus (COVID-19) vaccinations. 2022. https://ourworldin data.org/covid-vaccinations (accessed February 16, 2022).

6. World Health Organization. *A World in Disorder: Global Preparedness Monitoring Board Annual Report 2020*. Geneva, WHO, 2020. www.gpmb.org/docs/librariesprovi der17/default-document-library/annual-reports/gpmb-2020-annualreport-en.pdf? sfvrsn=bd1b8933_36 (accessed February 16, 2022).

7. G. Gopinath, A. Long. Uneven and uncertain ascent. IMF Blog. 2020. https:// blogs.imf.org/2020/10/13/a-long-uneven-and-uncertain-ascent/ (accessed June 19, 2021).

8. World Health Organization. Health security. 2021. www.who.int/health-topics/ health-security/#tab=tab_1 (accessed June 4, 2021).

9. Independent Panel for Pandemic Preparedness and Response. COVID-19: make it the last pandemic. 2021. https:// theindependentpanel.org/mainreport (accessed June 10, 2021).

10. S. L. Dalglish. COVID-19 gives the lie to global health expertise. *Lancet* 2020; **395** (10231): 1189.

11. A. Lal, N. A. Erondu, D. L. Heymann, et al. Fragmented health systems in COVID-19: rectifying the misalignment between global health security and universal health coverage. *Lancet* 2021; **397**(10268): 61–67.

12. A. D. Usher. Health systems neglected by Covid-19 donors. *Lancet* 2021; **397**(10269): 83.

13. World Health Organization, World Bank. Tracking universal health coverage: 2021 global monitoring report – conference edition. 2021. https://cdn.who.int/media/ docs/default-source/world-health-data-platform/events/tracking-universal-health-coverage-2021-global-monitoring-report_ uhc-day.pdf?sfvrsn=fd5c65c6_5&down load=true (accessed January 29, 2022).

14. World Bank, WHO. Half the world lacks access to essential health services, 100 million still pushed into extreme poverty because of health expenses. 2017. www.who.int/news/item/13-12-2017-world-bank-and-who-half-the-world-lacks-access-to-essential-health-services-100-million-still-pushed-into-extreme-poverty-because-of-health-expenses (accessed June 4, 2021).

15. A. Lal, H. C. Ashworth, S. Dada, et al. Optimizing pandemic preparedness and response through health information systems: lessons learned from Ebola to COVID-19. *Disaster Med Public Health Prep* 2022; **16**: 333–340.

16. S. Bali, R. Dhatt, A. Lal, et al. Off the back burner: diverse and gender-inclusive decision-making for COVID-19 response and recovery. *BMJ Glob Health* 2020; **5**(5): e002595.

17. World Health Organization. COVID-19 continues to disrupt essential health services in 90% of countries. 2021. www .who.int/news/item/23-04-2021-covid-19-continues-to-disrupt-essential-health-services-in-90-of-countries (accessed June 19, 2021).

18. S. Saha, M. Pai. Can COVID-19 innovations and systems help low- and middle-income countries to re-imagine healthcare delivery? *Med (N Y)* 2021; **2**(4): 369–373.

19. World Bank. Current health expenditure (% of GDP). 2021. https://data.worldbank .org/indicator/SH.XPD.CHEX.GD.ZS? view=map (accessed May 30, 2021).

20. World Bank. Hospital beds (per 1,000 people). 2021. https://data.worldbank.org/ indicator/SH.MED.BEDS.ZS (accessed June 10, 2021).

21. S. Saha, A. N. U. Ahmed, P. K. Sarkar, et al. The direct and indirect impact of SARS-CoV-2 infections on neonates:

a series of 26 cases in Bangladesh. *Pediatr Infect Dis J* 2020; **39**(12): e398–e405.

22. M. Pai. It's time to use Covid-19 innovations and systems to reimagine TB care. 2020. www.forbes.com/sites/madhukarpai/2020/10/22/time-to-tap-covid-19-innovations–systems-to-reimagine-tb-care (accessed February 23, 2021).

23. E. Cohen. Much of US data to catch newest coronavirus variants is several months old. 2021. www.cnn.com/2021/01/10/health/old-coronavirus-sequences/index.html (accessed February 8, 2022).

24. Government of Pakistan. COVID-19 health advisory platform. 2022. https://covid.gov.pk (accessed January 26, 2022).

25. R. E. Glover, M. C. I. van Schalkwyk, E. A. Akl, et al. A framework for identifying and mitigating the equity harms of COVID-19 policy interventions. *J Clin Epidemiol* 2020; **128**: 35–48.

26. T. Roberton, E. D. Carter, V. B. Chou, et al. Early estimates of the indirect effects of the Covid-19 pandemic on maternal and child mortality in low-income and middle-income countries: a modelling study. *Lancet Glob Health* 2020; **8**(7): e901–e908.

27. S. A. Balajee, O. G. Pasi, A. G. M. Etoundi, et al. Sustainable model for public health emergency operations centers for global settings. *Emerg Infect Dis* 2017; **23**(13): PMC5711308.

28. J. B. Nuzzo, D. Meyer, M. Snyder, et al. What makes health systems resilient against infectious disease outbreaks and natural hazards? Results from a scoping review. *BMC Public Health* 2019; **19**(1): 1310.

29. COVID-19, Online Resource and News Portal. COVID Alert SA app. 2021. https://sacoronavirus.co.za/covidalert (accessed January 26, 2022).

30. S. Turaga. careFIJI COVID-19 tracing app now available to download. 2020. www.fijivillage.com/news/careFIJI-COVID-19-tracing-app-now-available-to-download-5f4xr8 (accessed January 26, 2022).

31. Ministry of Health. HaMagen 2.0. 2021. https://govextra.gov.il/ministry-of-health/hamagen-app/download-en (accessed January 26, 2022).

32. Moscow Times. Russia develops coronavirus contact-tracing app. 2020. www.themoscowtimes.com/2020/11/17/russia-develops-coronavirus-contact-tracing-app-a72068 (accessed January 26, 2022).

33. Government of India. Aarogya Setu. 2021. www.aarogyasetu.gov.in (accessed January 26, 2022).

34. Unite against COVID-19. NZ COVID Tracer app. 2021. https://covid19.govt.nz/prepare-and-stay-safe/keep-up-healthy-habits/keep-track-of-where-youve-been/nz-covid-tracer-app (accessed January 26, 2022).

35. J. H. Kim, J. A. An, S. J. Oh, et al. Emerging COVID-19 success story: South Korea learned the lessons of MERS. 2021. www.exemplars.health/emerging-topics/epidemic-preparedness-and-response/covid-19/south-korea (accessed February 8, 2022).

36. Singapore Government Agency. SafeEntry. 2021. www.safeentry.gov.sg (accessed January 26, 2022).

37. Bangkok Post. New anti-Covid phone app for use when entering shops. 2020. www.bangkokpost.com/thailand/general/1918092/new-anti-covid-phone-app-for-use-when-entering-shops (accessed January 26, 2022).

38. L. Tian, X. Li, F. Qi, et al. Harnessing peak transmission around symptom onset for non-pharmaceutical intervention and containment of the Covid-19 pandemic. *Nat Commun* 2021; **12**(1): 1147.

39. S. Chen, Z. Zhang, J. Yang, et al. Fangcang shelter hospitals: a novel concept for responding to public health emergencies. *Lancet* 2020; **395**(10232): 1305–1314.

40. L. Oliver. Providing end-of-life care in a Nightingale hospital. *Br J Nurs* 2020; **29**(17): 1044–1045.

41. Reuters. Brazil to hire more doctors to fight coronavirus, including Cubans. 2020. www

.reuters.com/article/us-health-coronavirus-brazil-cuba-idUKKBN21340F (accessed June 10, 2021).

42. HealthCare New Zealand. Free mental wellbeing support for frontline health workers. 2020. www.healthcarenz.co.nz/wellbeing-services (accessed June 10, 2021).

43. T. Burki. Global shortage of personal protective equipment. *Lancet Infect Dis* 2020; **20**(7): 785–786.

44. PAHO. PAHO Strategic Fund minimizes disruption of critical medications and supplies during COVID-19. 2020. www.paho.org/en/news/26-10-2020-paho-strategic-fund-minimizes-disruption-critical-medications-and-supplies-during (accessed October 26, 2020).

45. V. Haldane, Z. Zhang, R. F. Abbas, et al. National primary care responses to COVID-19: a rapid review of the literature. *BMJ Open* 2020; **10**(12): e041622.

46. A. Blandford, J. Wesson, R. Amalberti, et al. Opportunities and challenges for telehealth within, and beyond, a pandemic. *Lancet Glob Health* 2020; **8**(11): e1364–e1365.

47. S. Lo, S. Gaudin, C. Corvalan, et al. The case for public financing of environmental common goods for health. *HS&R* 2019; **5**(4): 366–381.

48. G20 High Level Independent Panel on Financing the Global Commons for Pandemic Preparedness and Response. A global deal for our pandemic age. 2021. https://pandemic-financing.org/report (accessed February 17, 2022).

49. L. Clarke, E. Patouillard, A. J. Mirelman, et al. The costs of improving health emergency preparedness: a systematic review and analysis of multi-country studies. *EClinicalMedicine* 2022; **44**: 101269.

50. N. Kandel, S. Chungong, A. Omaar, et al. Health security capacities in the context of COVID-19 outbreak: an analysis of International Health Regulations annual report data from 182 countries. *Lancet* 2020; **395**(10229): 1047–1053.

51. V. Tangcharoensathien, O. Srisookwatana, P. Pinprateep, et al. Multisectoral actions for health: challenges and opportunities in complex policy environments. *Int J Health Policy Manag* 2017; **6**(7): 359–363.

52. S. Chungong, L. B. T. Choupe, J. Nuzzo. Health systems for health security: strengthening prevention, preparedness and response to health emergencies. 2021. www.researchgate.net/profile/Nirmal-Kandel/publication/351613177_Health_systems_for_health_security_-_Strengthening_prevention_preparedness_and_response_to_health_emergencies/links/60a08626458515c26595d63c/Health-systems-for-health-security-Strengthening-prevention-preparedness-and-response-to-health-emergencies.pdf (accessed June 18, 2021).

53. E. J. Williamson, A. J. Walker, K. Bhaskaran, et al. Factors associated with COVID-19-related death using OpenSAFELY. *Nature* 2020; **584**(7821): 430–436.

54. International Labour Organization. Employment and informality in Latin America and the Caribbean: an insufficient and unequal recovery. 2021. www.ilo.org/wcmsp5/groups/public/–americas/–ro-lima/–sro-port_of_spain/documents/genericdocument/wcms_819029.pdf (accessed February 17, 2022).

55. S. Allin, V. Haldane, M. Jamieson, et al. Comparing policy responses to COVID-19 among countries in the Latin American and Caribbean Region. 2020. https://openknowledge.worldbank.org/handle/10986/35002 (accessed June 19, 2021).

56. C. Béné. Resilience of local food systems and links to food security: a review of some important concepts in the context of COVID-19 and other shocks. *Food Secur* 2020; **12**: 805–822.

57. Government of Sri Lanka. Part 1: Section (I) – general government notifications. Colombo. 2020.

58. World Health Organization. *Health Systems for Health Security: A Framework for Developing Capacities for International Health Regulations, and Components in Health Systems and Other Sectors That Work in Synergy to Meet the Demands Imposed by Health Emergencies.* Geneva, WHO, 2021. www.who.int/publications/i/item/9789240029682 (accessed February 16, 2022).

Chapter 35

Understanding the Global Health Architecture

Toward Greater "Donor" Independence

Agnès Soucat and Richard Gregory

Key Messages

- The global aid architecture comprises multiple players that provide international assistance for health, plus the modalities by which assistance is provided both globally and in countries.

- The three groups of actors involved include bilateral donors (countries); multilateral donors (international organizations, development banks, and partnerships); and nongovernmental agencies (philanthropic foundations, nongovernmental organizations), and now the private sector.

- Types of assistance includes financial aid (grants and/or concessional loans); aid in-kind (e.g., medicines and other health commodities); and technical cooperation.

- Although aid has contributed to incredible progress in many countries, the ways in which it is provided can create challenges. Key issues with development aid include lack of predictability, fragmentation, and delays in implementation.

- In low-income countries (LICs), externally funded programs can shift government priorities and health aid can be largely fungible, displacing domestic funding toward other sectors.

- Global health governance includes decision-making and oversight at multiple levels for individual agencies in their work with countries, and for collective action to address global health issues. It is inherently political and not always related to financing needs.

35.1 Background: From the Great Escape to the Great Convergence

Throughout their history, human beings have faced a fate of low life expectancy, driven by high child and maternal mortality and the devastating impact of communicable diseases. Epidemics regularly hit high-density populations, sometimes decimating entire populations. The Black Plague in thirteenth-century Europe and the Middle East led to population decline by about 40% [1]. The spread of smallpox and measles in the Americas may have killed close to 100 million people in the fifteenth and sixteenth centuries [2].

Toward the end of the nineteenth century and throughout the twentieth, humans broke out of the 300,000-year fate, moving to a new normal of low child mortality, low fertility, and longer life expectancy driven by better hygiene and nutrition. Helped by the emergence of new technologies such as vaccines, anesthetics, and then antibiotics, and later by access to family planning, part of the world succeeded in escaping the millennial human fate and created this new normal: the demographic transition which contributed to improvements both in human populations' health and economic development. Nobel Prize laureate Angus Deaton called this incredible progress of humanity "the Great Escape" [3], in which the rich world started distinguishing itself from the developing world by its low child mortality, low fertility, good nutritional status, and high life expectancy, in addition to higher income.

This new normal has become an inspiration for the progress of humanity, while at the same time unveiling increasingly visible and unacceptable inequalities. As the UN system was created in 1945 and WHO in 1948, the new global community placed great hopes in fostering humanity's progress and prosperity. As affordable lifesaving technology became increasingly available, all countries assembled in the World Health Assembly in 1978 in Alma-Ata and agreed that "Health for All" (HFA) was achievable, aiming to reach that goal by 2000 through a primary health care (PHC) approach [4]. Since then, the call for PHC has expressed itself through different forms, including through a longstanding debate on alternative strategies of selective [5] versus comprehensive PHC [6], but always with the primary goal of redressing the inequality in health and access to services between the richer and the poorer worlds.

The international community claimed success in achieving some of the targets associated with the HFA goal by declaring universal access to childhood immunization by 1990 [7]. The World Bank also endorsed the goal of universal health in 1993, making the case for investing in basic health services as a way to improve health in low- and lower middle-income countries and contribute to economic development [8] – calling for more development aid to go to health. The commitment culminated in the adoption of the Millennium Development Goals (MDGs), several of which were health goals, with an accompanying sharp increase in development aid for health between 2000 and 2015 [9]. With increasing economic evidence about the benefits of investing in health, the 2013 Lancet Commission on "Investing in Health" championed a "Grand Convergence," supporting policies that would lead all countries to reach low child and maternal mortality and foster health promotion and disease prevention [10].

35.2 The Global Aid Architecture and the Key Players Involved

The "global aid architecture" comprises the different players that provide international assistance for health, plus the mechanisms and modalities by which assistance is provided – both globally and in countries. Broadly, there are three groups of actors: bilateral donors (countries), multilateral donors (international organizations, development banks, and partnerships), and nongovernmental agencies (philanthropic foundations, NGOs, and, increasingly, the private sector). Assistance includes financial aid (grants and/or concessional loans); aid in-kind (e.g., medicines and other health commodities); and technical cooperation. Assistance may be provided directly to a country or indirectly via one or more implementing partners. In different contexts, the same player may act as a funder, an implementer, or both. Traditional categories are increasingly blurred as new models of support and partnerships emerge and evolve.

There are differences between development partners that are engaged in lending, granting, and technically assisting countries, and the strengths and limitations of each. Different agencies have different "theories of change" guiding their assistance and provision of different services. For instance, WHO, UNICEF, UNFPA, and to some extent the World Bank provide technical assistance and capacity building. UNICEF, UNFPA, the World

The **UNDP** is the largest UN development assistance program. It was formed in 1965 to help countries eliminate poverty and achieve sustainable human development, using an approach to economic growth that emphasizes improving the quality of life of all citizens while conserving the environment and natural resources for future generations. This is reflected in its continued focus on social, economic, and environmental determinants of health. In recent years, the UNDP has also opted to become the primary recipient of funds from the GHIs such as GFATM to support program implementation of priority health programs in eligible countries.

The **WHO** was established on April 7, 1948. Its predecessor, the *Health Organization*, was an agency of the League of Nations. The WHO's primary role is to direct and coordinate international health within the UN system. Its mission is to promote health, keep the world safe, and serve the vulnerable. It provides global guidance on norms and standards; advises national Ministries of Health; and detects and responds to global health emergencies.

The **UNFPA**, created in 1960, is a UN agency aimed at improving reproductive and maternal health worldwide [1]. Its mission is to ensure that every pregnancy is wanted, every childbirth is safe, and every young person's potential is fulfilled.

More recent additions to the UN health family include the **Joint UN Programme on HIV/AIDS (UNAIDS)**, which leads global efforts to end AIDS as a public health threat, and **UN Women**, the global champion for gender equality.

The World Bank Group and the Regional Development Banks

The **World Bank Group (WBG)** works to help nations build healthier, more equitable societies and to improve fiscal performance and country competitiveness. It supports the world's poorest countries with IDA concessional financing. The IDA's purpose is to promote economic development and raise standards of living in the less developed areas of the world by providing financing on flexible terms, including grants and interest-free loans and loans. The International Bank for Reconstruction and Development (IBRD) is the lending arm of the World Bank.

The **regional development banks** provide financial and technical assistance for development in L&MICs within their regions. They include the African Development Bank (AfDB), the Asian Development Bank (ADB), the European Bank for Reconstruction and Development (EBRD), and the Inter-American Development Bank (IDB).

Global Health Initiatives

GAVI is an international organization that was created in 2000 to improve access to new and underused vaccines for children living in the world's poorest countries. GAVI brings together public and private sectors with the shared goal of creating equal access to vaccines for children, wherever they live.

The **GFATM** is an international financing and partnership organization that was created in 2002 to attract, leverage, and invest additional resources to end the epidemics of HIV/AIDS, tuberculosis (TB), and malaria, in support of the attainment of the related MDGs [1].

The **Global Financing Facility for Women, Children and Adolescents (GFF)**, housed at the World Bank, was created in 2015, in support of low- and lower middle-income countries to scale up access to affordable, quality care for women, children, and adolescents. It aims to mobilize additional funding through the combination of grants from a dedicated multi-donor GFF Trust Fund, financing from IDA and IBRD, and additional domestic and external resources. Table 35.1 summarizes some of the main categories of the multilateral donors and their roles in the global aid architecture in health.

35.2.3 Nongovernmental Agencies

Philanthropic foundations have long been important players in the development assistance landscape. For example, the **Rockefeller Foundation** (founded in 1913), **Ford Foundation** (1936), and **Hewlett Foundation** (1966) have long histories of supporting health programs, with multibillion US dollar endowments. Other charitable organizations are known for championing specific health issues. **Rotary International** has played a leading and sustained role in the global fight to end polio, and since 1986, the **Carter Center** (founded by former US President Jimmy Carter) has led the global campaign to eradicate Guinea worm disease. **Bloomberg Philanthropies** fund health promotion, particularly reducing tobacco use and traffic injuries.

The **Bill & Melinda Gates Foundation (BMGF)** is an American private foundation established in 2000 and reported to be the largest private foundation in the world, holding US\$46.8 billion in assets [12]. The primary goals of the foundation are to enhance health care and reduce extreme poverty across the globe, and to expand educational opportunities and access to information technology in the United States. The scale of the foundation and the way it seeks to apply business techniques to giving makes it one of the leaders in venture philanthropy [13]. It has paved the way for other foundations from the world of business and technology.

A huge range of NGOs play crucial roles as both program implementers and advocates at all levels of the health architecture. Their scale ranges from small grassroots community organizations to major voices on the global stage. Prominent international NGOs such as **Oxfam** and **Save the Children** deliver health programs in many countries around the world and raise (and spend) billions of dollars each year. NGOs such as **Médecins Sans Frontières (MSF)** and the **Red Cross and Red Crescent Movement** are especially important actors in humanitarian response and fragile settings, where government capacity to deliver health services to marginalized and vulnerable communities is often extremely limited.

In recent years the private sector has increasingly been acknowledged in global health discussions as including important funders and providers. This spans multiple contexts from private involvement in funding partnerships, to the private sector's role in developing and manufacturing medicines and health commodities, to (for-profit and not-for-profit) provision of health services. Efforts have been made to provide guidance on governance of the private sector [14] and to better reflect the importance of private sector contributions and principles for good practice [15]. Several organizations such as the **World Economic Forum** (the international organization for public–private cooperation) and the **Aga Khan Development Network** (a network of private, nondenominational development agencies) have taken particular interest in mobilizing the private sector to complement more traditional health and development actors.

35.2.4 Partnerships, Initiatives, and Alliances

Many health partnerships and initiatives exist to foster collaboration or to focus on specific issues, across the different players in the health architecture. Examples include **Roll Back Malaria, Stop TB,** the **Partnership for Maternal, Newborn and Child Health,** the **Non-Communicable Diseases Alliance,** and the **UHC2030,** which aim to provide an overall

Table 35.1 Main categories and roles of key multilateral players in the global aid architecture in health

Agency	Mandate	Key focus areas and modalities	Norms and standards	Technical assistance	Capacity building	Procurement of commodities	Country grants	Concessional lending	Market rates lending
WHO	Established in 1948 to direct and coordinate international health within the United Nations system	Provide global guidance on norms and standards, advise national Ministries of Health, and detect and respond to global health emergencies	XXX	XXX	XXX	X	X		
UNICEF	Address the long-term needs of children and women, particularly in developing countries	Strengthening PHC, operational delivery of programs (especially in fragile settings), and commodity procurement		X	XX	XXX	X		
UNFPA	Improve reproductive and maternal health worldwide	Support reproductive health advocacy, policy guidance, and supply of family planning commodities		X	XX	XX	X		

Table 35.1 (cont.)

Agency	Mandate	Key focus areas and modalities	Norms and standards	Technical assistance	Capacity building	Procurement of commodities	Country grants	Concessional lending	Market rates lending
World Bank and other development banks	Help nations build healthier, more equitable societies and to improve fiscal performance and country competitiveness	International Development Association (IDA) concessional financing to poorer countries, plus International Bank for Reconstruction and Development (IBRD) for lending		X	X	XXX	XXX	XXX	XXX
GAVI	Improve access to new and underused vaccines for children living in the world's poorest countries	Bring together public and private sectors and provide grant financing to countries				XXX	XXX		
GFATM	Attract, leverage, and invest additional resources to end the epidemics of HIV/AIDS, tuberculosis and malaria	Bring together public and private sectors and provide grant financing to countries				XXX	XXX		

platform and movement for strengthening health systems toward shared UHC goals. Most of these partnerships and alliances include many of the key global health agencies and players described throughout this chapter. Collectively these partnerships can both support global coordination and help provide a focus for country implementation. In some instances they are found to contribute to complexity and fragmentation across the health architecture.

35.3 A Rapid Increase of Development Aid at the Onset of the Twenty-First Century

At the onset of the twenty-first century, access to health services increased in L&MICs, largely owing to economic growth and poverty reduction, and was supported by international development assistance (aid). Between 2002 and 2018, the GDP of L&MICs increased by 4% per annum on average, thereby multiplying health spending six times, with domestic spending on health reaching US$600 billion in 2018 in these countries (Box 35.1) [16]. The commitments of the development aid community also grew and development assistance increased steadily over the MDGs era (2000–2015), going from more than US$5 billion per year in 2002 to more than US$25 billion in 2018 (Figure 35.2). The largest increase was for disease control, mostly HIV, with only a fraction allocated to health systems, health security, and emergency preparedness.

In 2018, more than half of development assistance for health was channeled to middle-income countries, including significant amounts to upper middle-income countries such as China (US$818 million) and South Africa (US$3.1 billion) (Figure 35.3).

Although aid has contributed to incredible progress in many countries, the ways in which it is provided can create challenges for countries. Key issues with development aid include lack of predictability, fragmentation, and delays in implementation. Looking across the commitments and disbursements of Official Development Assistance (ODA) for health shows that aid commitments and disbursements increased in the four Ebola-impacted countries (Guinea, DRC, Sierra Leone, and Liberia) in response to the crisis, but most of the increase happened after the epidemic was over. In Liberia, aid subsequently declined to pre-crisis levels (Figure 35.4).

Overall, aid has systematically tended to crowd-out public spending (Figure 35.5), particularly in LICs. Between 2000 and 2018, as health aid increased, it substituted for

---

Box 35.1 Domestic Health Spending and Official Development Assistance

Domestic health spending includes domestic resources, both public and private, including household spending.

Official development assistance (ODA) is defined as flows to countries and territories on the Development Assistance Committee (DAC) List of ODA Recipients [17] and to multilateral development institutions that are:

1. provided by official agencies, including state and local governments, or by their executive agencies; and
2. concessional (i.e., grants and soft loans) and administered with the promotion of the economic development and welfare of developing countries as the main objective.
   The DAC list of countries eligible to receive ODA is updated every three years and is based on per capita income.

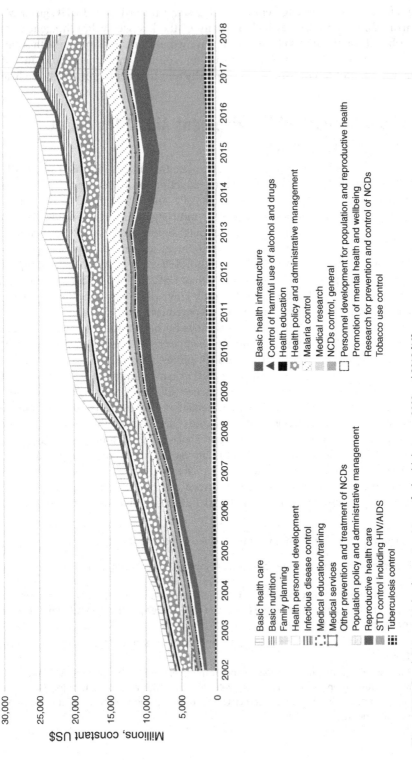

Figure 35.2 Steady increase in development assistance for health between 2000 and 2018 [18].

Total Development Assistance for Health Recipient Countries (2014–2018)

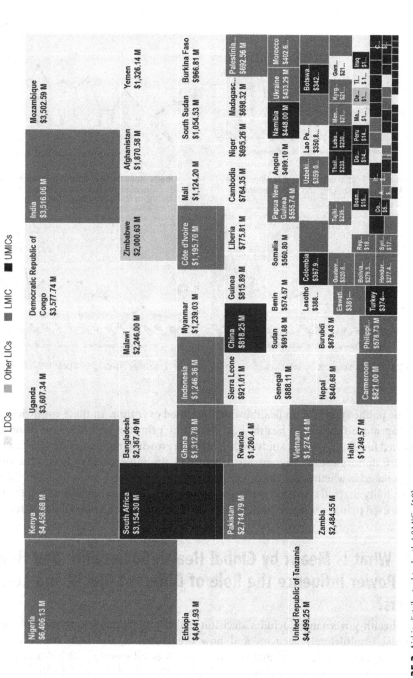

Figure 35.3 Aid is distributed to both L&MICs [18].

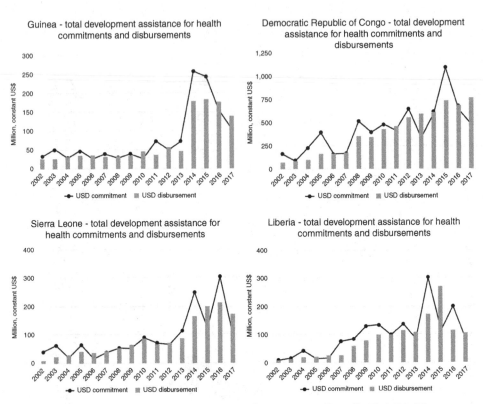

Figure 35.4 Commitments and disbursements in West African countries affected by Ebola [19–22].

domestic public spending on health, which declined over time. In these countries, aid does not bring more funding to health, but influences priorities in health spending through earmarked funding. A recent study highlighted the growing fragmentation of aid, with more and more donors using different instruments in the same country [23]. One persistent concern raised is whether aid effectively promotes the goals of donors, or *fungibility*; that is, the possibility that aid is used in ways not intended by donors when disbursing the funds. It could be used to lower taxes, to fund projects in a different sector, or sometimes for personal gain.

35.4 What Is Meant by Global Health Governance and How Does Power Influence the Role of Different Global and Local Players?

Global health governance includes decision-making and oversight at multiple levels for individual (multilateral) agencies and how they work in and with countries, and for collective action to address global health issues. It is inherently political and not always related to financing needs. If it is to be effective, it should respond to the needs of the countries it serves, and ultimately be accountable to people and communities.

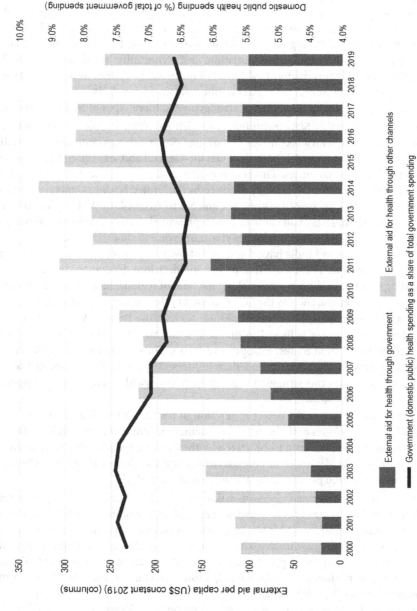

Figure 35.5 When external aid increased, health priority in domestic budget allocations declined [24].

With so many players and agencies, global health governance is complex. Specific roles and boundaries are unclear, with vast overlap between the mandates of the various agencies. Yet the nature and mandate of each of these institutions de facto shape this governance and its effectiveness and constraints. For example, WHO tends to focus on political coordination, providing norms and standards and overall technical guidance mainly for L&MICs. It also keeps a role in emergencies and some specific programs such as smallpox and polio eradication. Other agencies are known for strengths in specific areas: UNICEF for implementation capacity, including in fragile settings and for large humanitarian programs, and for driving universal immunization, nutrition, and community-based services; UNFPA for family planning and reproductive health; GAVI for making vaccines available; and GFATM for making medicines available for AIDS, tuberculosis, and malaria.

In today's global health governance arrangements, three types of institutions emerge:

- First, the UN Member State institutions in which governance is based on the *one country one vote principle*, with a broad-based sharing of power between countries. This is directly the case for WHO, in which both the Director-General and six regional directors are directly elected by countries. This is also indirectly the case for the UN funds (UNICEF, UNFPA, etc.), which are ultimately overseen by the United Nations General Assembly and associated bodies, such as the Economic and Social Council. In WHO's World Health Assembly the interests of all countries are represented on an equal basis, although it is argued that the governance modalities give more voice to small countries at the expense of large ones. China and India have the same voting power as small countries of fewer than one million people. This means that power and decisions depend on diplomacy and building effective coalitions – often along the lines of regional blocs or groups of countries with shared interests, such as the G77 coalition of developing countries [25].

- Second is agencies based on shareholding, such as the Bretton Woods institutions where decision power is linked to financial contributions, with a major role being played by the United States, Europe, and Japan. Since agencies have primary accountability to their boards and shareholders rather than the countries they support, countries can struggle to get their voices heard or ensure that support responds to their needs.

- Third is governance of the newer generation of institutions such as the GFATM and GAVI, which includes both donor and implementing constituencies and also the private sector. Decisions here tend to be driven by the funding agencies that have contributed the most, mostly Ministries of Foreign Affairs and Development Aid in high-income countries and large private foundations such as the BMGF.

The picture of power and decision-making across the above three categories remains complex. That said, some of these dynamics are shifting as countries become less dependent on external support and more able to engage with international partners on their own terms. There remains a further asymmetry when it comes to people and communities who should ultimately benefit from this support and ensure that agencies are answerable to them. This reinforces the importance of social participation mechanisms and involving community organizations in local decision-making.

More broadly, an important movement is emerging to "decolonize" global health [26]. This explicitly recognizes and challenges historical legacies and power imbalances. It calls for better representation in decision-making, listening to more diverse voices, and questioning who sets the agenda for policy and implementation.

35.5 What Ministries of Health, Finance, and Planning in L&MICs Can Do to Reduce Dependence on and Dominance of Donors and Development Partners

With such a large and diverse group of donors and development partners, fragmentation of country support is a painful reality. The onus of coordination often falls on the governments of recipient countries, who bear high transaction costs; those countries with the greatest need of external assistance may have the least capacity to manage and coordinate it. Since the early 2000s, countries and agencies have worked to address these issues. Many have committed to support mechanisms of harmonization and alignment based on seven behaviors [27] for effective health cooperation (Figure 35.6), signed the UHC2030 Global Compact, or are signatories to the SDG 3 Global Action Plan. Joint assessment tools are available to support the goal of one plan, one budget, one report. Yet progress on this objective is slow.

The issues themselves are evolving. Fewer countries are as aid-dependent as they were 10 years ago. Only 31 countries were listed as LICs in 2020. This can lead to more power and flexibility for recipient countries to choose which agencies to enter into partnerships with and on what terms. Conversely, as agencies push to be more "strategic" or "catalytic" in their investments, additional competing and distorting influences can be an unintended consequence. The limited capacity of poorer countries is often captured to serve the objectives of specific programs. Externally funded programs can shift government priorities by paying higher wages than governments or supplementing government wages with bonuses. With money chasing a limited workforce, it is no wonder that health aid proves largely fungible, displacing domestic funding toward other sectors [28]. Asymmetry of power and capture of specific donor programs by special interests within the country are difficult to overcome.

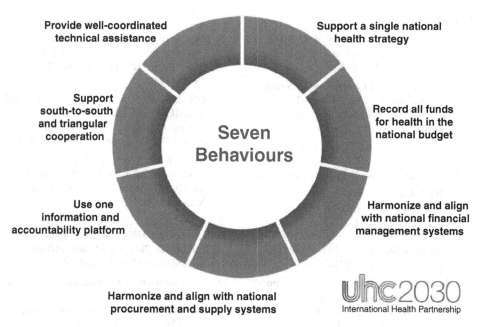

Figure 35.6 Seven behaviors for international development partners to change in support of UHC.

The fundamental principles are still to promote country leadership and ensure external support is aligned with national strategies and plans. An inclusive process of regular policy dialog with all relevant stakeholders in health is important to promote this. While difficult to enforce, some countries have seen success with compacts that set out the terms of collaboration or convene all partners around support for the national health strategy or UHC roadmap. Those countries that are becoming wealthier and approaching transition from external finance should plan at an early stage for a coherent approach to sustaining essential health services, including by making the case for domestic resources for the health sector as a whole [29].

Ultimately, upstream reforms are needed in the way donors provide incentives to international agencies. The MDGs' focus on results to some extent led to a "results cartel" [30]. Narrowly defining results for each agency makes it more difficult to promote coherence, while also neglecting the economic, societal, and behavioral determinants of results. If Member States and donors can make a consistent case across the health architecture for responsive and flexible ways of working, and investments in health systems, countries will have a better chance of directing agencies and donors toward collective action for more sustainable outcomes.

35.6 Conclusion

The global aid architecture is complex and numerous players are involved, including UN organizations, bilateral donors, GHIs, and charities. The COVID-19 pandemic has shed light on the weaknesses of these arrangements, which are often fragmented and uncoordinated. Empirical evidence shows no clear relations between aid flows and countries' needs for financing. Aid also mostly substitutes for domestic funding in LICs and may undermine the building of collective financing of national institutions. To make the best out of health aid, countries need to prioritize health in their national budgeting processes and identify specific areas for donors to intervene to complement domestic financing.

References

1. S. K. J. Cohn. Epidemiology of the black death and successive waves of plague. *Med Hist Suppl* 2008; **27**: 74–100.

2. Centers for Disease Control and Prevention. Smallpox: history of smallpox. 2021. www .cdc.gov/smallpox/history/history.html (accessed March 14, 2021).

3. A. Deaton. *The Great Escape: Health, Wealth, and the Origins of Inequality.* Princeton, Princeton University Press, 2013.

4. WHO. Declaration of Alma-Ata International Conference on Primary Health Care, Alma-Ata, USSR, September 6–12, 1978. www.who.int/ publications/almaata_declaration_en.pdf (accessed March 10, 2021).

5. J. M. Walsh, K. S. Warren. Selective primary health care: an interim strategy for disease control in developing countries. *N Engl J Med* 1979; **301**: 967–974.

6. M. Cueto. The origins of primary health care and selective primary health care. *Am J Public Health* 2004; **94**(11): 1864–1874.

7. UNICEF. Why a world summit for children? A UNICEF perspective. 1990. www.cf-hst .net/unicef-temp/Doc-Repository/doc/ doc349374.PDF (accessed March 11, 2021).

8. World Bank. World development report 1993: investing in health. 1993. https://doi .org/10.1596/0-1952-0890-0 (accessed March 11, 2021).

9. United Nations Development Programme. End poverty: Millennium Development Goals and beyond 2015. www.un.org/millennium goals (accessed March 11, 2021).

10. D. T. Jamison, L. H. Summers, G. Alleyne, et al. Global health 2035: a world converging within a generation. *Lancet* 2013; **382**(9908): 1898–1955.

11. OECD. Development finance data. 2020. www.oecd.org/dac/financing-sustainable-development/development-finance-data (accessed February 15, 2022).

12. Bill & Melinda Gates Foundation. Foundation fact sheet. 2022. www.gatesfoundation.org/about/foundation-fact-sheet (accessed February 17, 2022).

13. OECD Development Centre. Venture philanthropy in development dynamics, challenges and lessons in the search for greater impact. 2014. www.oecd.org/dev/Venture%20Philanthropy%20in%20Development-BAT-24022014-indd5%2011%20mars.pdf (accessed February 17, 2022).

14. World Health Organization. Strengthening private sector engagement for UHC. 2022. www.who.int/activities/strengthening-private-sector-engagement-for-uhc (accessed January 20, 2022).

15. International Health Partnership. Private sector contributions towards universal health coverage. UHC2030 private sector constituency statement. 2019. www.uhc2030.org/fileadmin/uploads/uhc2030/Documents/Key_Issues/Private_Sector/UHC2030_Private_Sector_Constituency_Joint_Statement_on_UHC_FINAL.pdf (accessed January 20, 2022).

16. World Health Organization. Global report on global spending on health: a world in transition. 2019. www.who.int/health_financing/documents/health-expenditure-report-2019/en (accessed March 11, 2021).

17. OECD. DAC list of ODA recipients. 2021. www.oecd.org/dac/financing-sustainable-development/development-finance-standards/daclist.htm (accessed February 9, 2022).

18. World Health Organization. Country planning cycle database: from whom to whom. 2021. https://extranet.who.int/countryplanningcycles/fwtw-healthda (accessed February 15, 2022).

19. World Health Organization. From whom to whom: Liberia. 2021. https://extranet.who.int/countryplanningcycles/fwtw-recipient/LBR (accessed February 15, 2022).

20. World Health Organization. From whom to whom: Sierra Leone. 2021. https://extranet.who.int/countryplanningcycles/fwtw-recipient/SLE (accessed February 15, 2022).

21. World Health Organization. From whom to whom: Democratic Republic of Congo. 2021. https://extranet.who.int/countryplanningcycles/fwtw-recipient/COD (accessed February 15, 2022).

22. World Health Organization. From whom to whom: Guinea. 2021. https://extranet.who.int/countryplanningcycles/fwtw-recipient/GIN (accessed February 15, 2022).

23. M. Piatti, A. Hashim, S. Alkenbrack, et al. Are development partners using government systems? 2021. https://blogs.worldbank.org/health/are-development-partners-using-government-systems (accessed January 20, 2022).

24. World Health Organization. Global health expenditure database. 2022. https://apps.who.int/nha/database (accessed February 15, 2022).

25. G77. The Group of 77 at the United Nations. 2021. www.g77.org/doc (accessed February 9, 2022).

26. S. Abimbola, M. Pai. Will global health survive its decolonisation? *Lancet* 2020; **10263**: 1627–1628.

27. UHC 2030. 7 behaviours for effective development cooperation. 2022. www.uhc2030.org/what-we-do/working-better-together/harmonised-approaches-to-health-systems-strengthening/7-behaviours-for-effective-development-cooperation (accessed February 9, 2022).

28. World Health Organization. New perspectives on global health spending for universal health coverage. 2017. www.who.int/health_financing/topics/resource-tracking/new_perspectives_on_global_health_spending_for_uhc.pdf (accessed February 17, 2022).

29. WHO. Sustainability, transition from external financing and health system strengthening technical working group. 2030. www.uhc2030.org/what-we-do/working-better-together/uhc2030-technical-working-groups/sustainability-transition-from-external-financing-and-health-system-strengthening-technical-working-group (accessed March 11, 2021).

30. Y. Rajkotia. Beware of the success cartel: a plea for rational progress in global health. *BMJ Glob Health* 2018; 3(6): e001197.

Chapter 36

Political Economy of Health Reforms in Low and Middle Income Countries

Vivian Lin

Key Messages

- Health system development, reform, and transformation is as much a social and political intervention as it is technical.
- Political economy analysis is central to the successful formulation of health policies and plans and ensuring their effective implementation.
- Political economy analysis can help to identify potential barriers and facilitators for policy and system change.
- Political economy analysis is relevant through all stages of the policy cycle.

36.1 What Is Political Economy (and Politics of Health) and Its Relevance to Health?

Political economy is a field of study about the relationship between economics and politics. It examines how economic and political forces combine to affect public policies, especially with regards to the distribution of costs and benefits across society. Political economy is concerned with how power and resources are distributed and contested, and ultimately how equity and wellbeing of the population of a country are affected as a result of these structural forces.

The political economy of health, as a field of study and policy advocacy, grew rapidly in the 1970s with studies and political activism in the United Kingdom [1], the United States [2–5], Latin America [6, 7], and Africa [8] that sought to explain the disparities in health care access and the socioeconomic differential in health status across society. Such studies examined the profit and power of hospitals, specialist doctors, and the pharmaceutical industry, and provided explanations for why health care policies supported a two-tier health system and left some impoverished due to health care costs. The application of the political economy framework to studies of disparities in health status within and across countries pointed to exploitation by profit-seeking industry, especially in the context of weak regulatory protection for workers and the environment, resulting in environmental and occupational health disasters and the dumping of hazardous products in developing countries (a term being replaced by low- and middle-income countries [L&MICs]) [9, 10].

Political economy analysis (PEA) thus helps to explain why inequities exist; why certain policy choices are made; and why making policy change can be difficult. In the twenty-first century, while successive attempts to improve health systems and health equity have fallen short of hopes and expectations in many countries, the value of PEA has become increasingly recognized to explain why technical blueprints have not been implemented or are not workable. Conversely, with PEA, health system reform proposals may become more practicable, acceptable, and feasible, with a recognition that reform is a journey rather than a technical fix.

This chapter focuses on health reforms in L&MICs and on how political economy framework and analysis can help explain the current state of health systems and what can be done in the face of structural challenges. The chapter starts with a brief description of a framework for political economy and offers explanations of why structural reforms in health are frequently shaped by political considerations. Specific examples are offered on how priority-setting and resource allocation decisions may be the result of political expediency. Finally, suggestions are made about the measures that can be taken to minimize political obstacles so that evidence-informed decisions become more possible.

36.2 A General Framework for Political Economy

There are many models that try to explain the factors that affect health and health inequalities. The political economy of health models from the 1970s provided early intellectual foundation for the work of the Commission on Social Determinants of Health (CSDH) [11]. From the social epidemiology perspective, the CSDH framework places emphasis on individual, household, and community levels of health and refers only broadly to the socioeconomic and political context at the macro level. The framework recognizes the key elements of the socioeconomic and political context as comprising governance, macroeconomic policies, social policies (labor, market, housing, and land), public policies (health, education, and social protection), and culture and values. Figure 36.1 points to where interventions would need to occur to address these social determinants. The fact that interventions at all levels require policy considerations means that attention must be paid to the political and economic factors that shape decision-making. However, the social determinants of health model typically does not offer the policy analysis that is required for action.

Models of health determinants based on political economy, however, do not necessarily point to specific health care policy and system interventions, possibly because social determinants may have a greater effect on health outcomes and health inequities than health care. From the viewpoint of health policy and health care system interventions, the required analytical framework focuses more squarely on political actors and institutions and on the financing and organization of health systems [12]. Thus, a framework for understanding system change enables the analysis of the structural factors, the institutions, and the actors that are involved in the health system, political system, and economic system of a country.

Analyses rooted in political economy of health [13] put more emphasis on how health and health inequalities are shaped by socioeconomic inequalities, and particularly by political power and resources, labor markets, and welfare/redistributive policies. A stronger focus on policy intervention would point attention to the impact of electoral behavior, labor movement density, employment policies, coverage and expenditure of social policies and public services, and wealth and income distribution, on health equity.

In PEA, understanding actors and power must be accompanied by an understanding of finances. Evans [14] brings actors and financing together in a simple equation where total

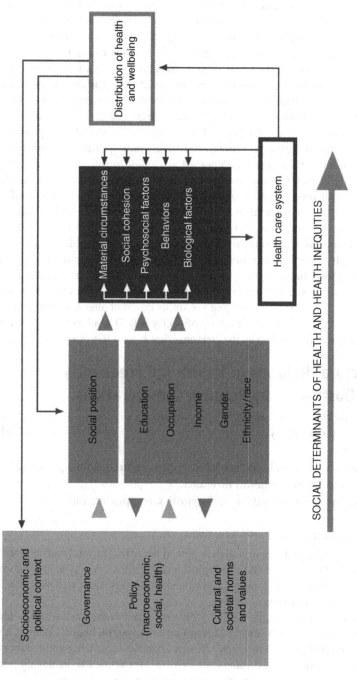

Figure 36.1 Commission on Social Determinants of Health conceptual framework [11].

revenues in a system equal total expenditures, and equal total incomes of all actors/institutions. In other words, there is a finite amount of money in a system, so the incomes of some actors are the expenditures of other actors. In other words, if one set of actors gain, others lose. This perspective cuts across the complexities of other models to point to the essential elements of political economy. It also explains why change is difficult and how people and parties who understand how money flows can maximize the benefits for themselves.

Policy outcomes always reflect an interplay between structural forces and actions on the part of actors (or agency), hence health systems are the result of historical decisions and actions (i.e., they are path-dependent). That is to say that prior decisions shape current ones; and the prevailing political environment and particular circumstances at a given time determine subsequent political developments and next steps [15]. Alford [16] points to the importance of structural interests (corporate rationalists, monopolists, or community advocates) in shaping policy debates and outcomes. At any point in time, however, health policy reflects the coming together of interest groups, ideas, values and ideology, and the exercise of power [17, 18]. It reveals how underlying competing rationalities – exemplified by research evidence, community expectations, and political imperatives – need to align for policy adoption. Kingdon [19] suggests that political will and "windows of opportunity" explain the moment when particular policy solutions are agreed upon to address particular policy problems. The wide array of health policy problems at any given moment results in the *status quo*, without momentum for policy change. The complexity of policymaking, the complexity of health systems, and the underlying political economy of health policy and financing systems inevitably means that changing the status quo is challenging. Experience shows that such change requires a combination of: (1) political leadership, (2) social movement, and (3) evidence, referred to as the "triangle that moves the mountain"[20].

36.3 Why Structural Reforms in Health Are Frequently Influenced and Obstructed by Political Considerations

Reform implies deliberate change, and any change, by definition, disrupts existing interests. The core stakeholders of the health system whose interests may be positively or negatively affected by the change are:

- health service providers – hospitals and specialist doctors being the most powerful;
- health financiers – government or health insurance;
- producers of medical products – medicines, diagnostics, equipment, and other technologies; and
- health care users – patients and families/caregivers.

In countries that have federal structures or a high degree of decentralization (such as Brazil, Pakistan, India, China, Indonesia, and the Philippines), the change process is more complex, with an increased number of stakeholders and entrenched interests, as well as political, legal, and other governance frameworks.

When health system change is implemented with new money, the status quo is less affected even if new services and actors may be brought into the system, because there is not a redistribution of existing resources. However, reforms aimed at increasing equity, accessibility, quality, and responsiveness (including specific measures related to achieving universal health coverage [UHC]) require the redistribution of resources, increased productivity, and new service models. The system changes required to improve the experiences of users are commonly counterbalanced by the resistance of stakeholders who benefit from the existing system, including providers and producers. Reforms also entail behavioral change likely to elicit resistance. System change that requires the redistribution of resources and power is particularly challenging, as system insiders who know how the system operates can use that knowledge to their advantage. As Evans [21] shows, when limited resources circulate in a health system they are distributed or allocated in the system according to the roles of various actors (Figure 36.2).

Those who understand the rules that govern finances are well positioned to manipulate the system. Those with access to existing resources have the strongest stakes in the status quo; they include manufacturers and distributors of medicines/diagnostics/equipment, senior specialists, senior managers of tertiary hospitals, and health insurance companies. In any expansionary system, these stakeholders are also more likely to advocate for policies that maximize their gain.

Dual practice by physicians is another example of insiders exercising their power within the system to make money. A review of dual practice in South and East Asia, where health service uptake is increasing, particularly in the private sector, found that it can improve access and the range of services offered. Nevertheless, weakly regulated dual practice can negatively affect public health service access, quality, efficiency, and equity, as doctors split their time between public and private work to maximize their income and other benefits. The regulatory capacity required to ensure that the advantages of a combined private practice do not threaten the provision of adequate public services are often missing in L&MICs. Effective regulation of dual practitioners not only accommodates public sector providers' private work but also encourages adequate provision of public services [22].

Those who benefit the most financially can manipulate the rules to maximize their profits. They can also work with the political system to change the rules to further benefit themselves, through lobbying and political donations. Those with financial interests can also be linked to government and political elites in other ways. They may come from the same social background or be related through kinship and family bonds. They may also come to have their roles in financially profitable institutions through political patronage, including board and other employment arrangements. In other words, power, position, and finances are often interrelated if not intertwined [23–25].

In developing policy, the government needs to weigh the costs and benefits of change with attention to who wins and who loses. Political policy (see Section 36.4) is not the same as health policy; while health policy advocates consider technical solutions to address efficiency and equity [16, 18], policymakers are concerned about voter support and trading off the interests of different sectors. The assessment of a policy's political costs and benefits often has greater effect on decisions than its economic considerations and population benefits.

36.4 How Political Expediency Influences Priority-Setting Decisions in Health That Are Frequently Related to Allocation of Resources or Can Lead to Policy Implementation Failure

Political considerations affect health policy decisions in numerous ways. Case studies in high-income countries and L&MICs point to similar dynamics in political economy,

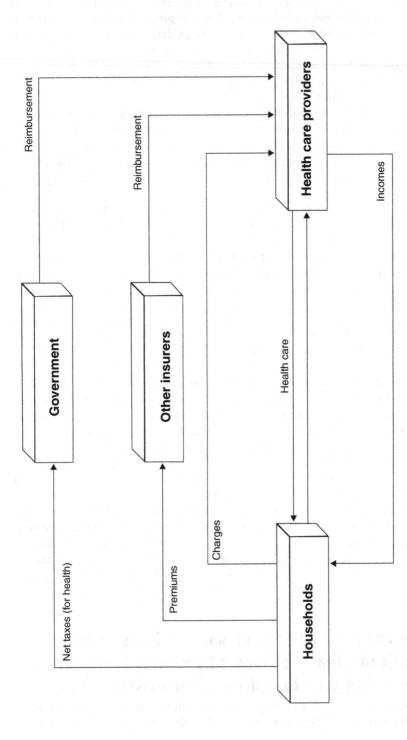

Figure 36.2 Health system income and expenditure distribution [21].

regardless of specific circumstances and issues. Seven types of examples are offered below based on key political influences in health policymaking.

1. **Ideology and values** can be barriers to public health policy development and implementation. For example, despite protective national laws in support of human rights in South Africa, violations continue against people living with HIV [26]. This is attributed to implementation failures at the community level due to incomplete dissemination efforts and limited enforcement [27]. Globally, women and girls are the most affected by HIV, yet they continue to report higher levels of human rights violations than men living with HIV [28]. In general, discrimination impacts access to education and health services (e.g., due to the requirement for authorization by husbands or parents), and results in violence against women. Despite the recognized benefits of such human rights laws, lack of investment in scaled up rigorously evaluated interventions using standardized measures inhibits good policymaking, and calls for increasing the body of evidence on the effectiveness of such laws globally, including how to overcome the barriers to implementation [27].

   The Programme of Action resulting from the 1994 International Conference on Population and Development (ICPD) in Cairo [29] recognized that the rights of women and girls, and empowerment and gender equality, are all cornerstones of population and development programs, and a prerequisite to sustainable development, yet gender inequity and exploitation continue [30]. Key issues in women's reproductive health are still unaddressed globally and have become yet more urgent, given high rates of child marriage, preventable maternal deaths, and pervasive violence against women – which is even worse in the context of regional conflicts and environmental emergencies. The continuing belief that untempered global production and consumption is a measure of human achievement [30] continues to be a barrier to good policymaking.

2. The desire for **domestic revenue sources**, together with international commercial interests, can be a barrier to good health policy. China is the world's largest producer of tobacco, and despite 1.2 million people dying in China annually from smoking and the country experiencing the highest tobacco-related burden of disease globally, a representative from the State Tobacco Monopoly Administration (STMA) was included in the delegation to negotiate the Framework Convention on Tobacco Control (FCTC). Furthermore, despite the inclusion of the minister of health on the delegation, the central role of the Ministry of Trade in the negotiations, together with an explicit statement by the government that the treaty should not undermine the important status of the tobacco industry in China's national economy, undermined the process of good health policymaking [31].

3. **Industry lobbying and vested commercial interests** also impact good public health policy. For example, the power of international pharmaceutical companies in negotiation of free trade agreements has significant implications for the capacity of policymakers to secure core features of good pharmaceutical policy recognized internationally. A review by Gleeson et al. [32] examined four large regional trade agreements: Trans-Pacific Partnership Agreement (TPP), Comprehensive and Progressive Agreement for Trans-Pacific Partnership (CPTPP), Comprehensive Economic and Trade Agreement (CETA), and US–Canada–Mexico Agreement (USMCA). Typically, pharmaceutical companies pushed for extended intellectual property protection, limited tendering in procurement processes, and applied pressure

to speed up approval processes, all of which impact access, quality, and price of medicines.

4. **Professional interests** may work against good policy. For example, as briefly mentioned above, many countries allow doctors to practice in the public as well as the private sectors (dual practice). Dual practice is recognized as a threat to the efficiency, quality, and equity of health services, especially in the public sector. Various policies adopted by some countries to minimize adverse impacts of dual practice include: bans on dual practice, attempts to limit hours worked or prices charged in the private sector, permission for limited hours of private practice in public facilities, and incentives to work only in the public sector [33, 34]. Public–private partnerships (PPPs) are common in the health sector (see Chapter 28); in Vietnam, for example, PPPs have led to staff investing in their own hospitals [35]. Evaluations of the effectiveness of such PPPs are skewed by nonindependent studies [36], with positive findings likely resulting from poor-quality studies financed by organizations promoting PPPs.

5. **Political promises** are another factor that can impact good policymaking. In the case of the Malaysian government, the commitment not to raise the copayment above 1 ringgit for primary care has had a positive impact on equity of access in the country's health system [37], but was detrimental for meeting the rising cost of care and the financing needs of the health sector. Similarly, the commitment of the Philippines' government in 1998 to the national insurance scheme (Philhealth) and the use of Health Technology Assessment (HTA) has resulted in the subsidization of high-cost treatments that are not cost-effective.

6. **Program funding and structures** can run counter to good policymaking by creating rigidities. For example, global health initiatives, such as the Global Alliance for Vaccines and Immunizations (GAVI) [38], have limited ability to expand their scope to address other health issues or to adopt different approaches. As a result, they can distort the prioritization of funding, resulting in money going to existing programs rather than those needed to respond to other health priorities [39] such as: improving water, sanitation and hygiene (WASH); protection from dangerous products (e.g., smoking, alcohol, and unhealthy diets); threats to adolescents' health (e.g., road injury, HIV, and suicide); and reducing the threat of antimicrobial resistance.

7. **Nationalism versus international solidarity for public goods** has remained a challenge for epidemics and pandemics. Good public health policy to provide more equitable access to COVID-19 vaccines would facilitate creative equitable international cooperation through a multilateral framework for supporting stringent regulatory reviews and innovative low-cost manufacturing and supply chains. Vaccine solidarity could not be achieved due to vaccine nationalism in the case of the COVID-19 vaccines [40].

The COVAX facility was established to enable equitable and fair distribution of COVID-19 vaccines, especially in resource-poor settings. However, some countries took positions that have prevented achieving this noble objective. Examples of such behaviors include: (1) leveraging influence to disparage vaccines produced by other countries; (2) distributing vaccines to other countries without review by a stringent regulatory authority as defined by WHO; (3) some vaccine-producing countries having restricted distribution to within their own borders; and (4) allowing the dissemination of anti-science aggression and disinformation, which has contributed to vaccine hesitancy. Vaccine nationalism means that many low-income countries may not achieve sufficient supply of COVID-19 vaccines until 2023 or 2024, and also undermines regulation of vaccine effectiveness and monitoring of adverse effects.

36.5 What Measures Can be Taken to Minimize Political Obstacles and Barriers in Favor of Evidence-Informed Decisions

For health analysts who are focused on research evidence and committed to evidence-based decision-making, the ever-present influence of political and economic forces at the macro level can be overwhelming, annoying, and feel insurmountable. However, understanding the political economy allows navigating the policy system successfully, developing realistic policy proposals and implementing them smoothly, and strengthening the technical rationality (rather than political rationality) in policymaking. There are, therefore, two critical measures to be taken to minimize political barriers to support evidence-informed decisions: (1) doing PEA to understand the barriers and facilitators; and (2) knowing how to engage with policy and political processes.

A starting point for considering how best to engage with policymaking is to undertake PEA, which aims to situate policy interventions within an understanding of the prevailing political and economic processes in society. Such an analysis will consider structures, institutions, and actors, and how they interrelate – more specifically, the incentives, relations, and distribution and contestation of power between different groups and individuals. The analysis should take account of history to explain the present circumstances as well as to foreshadow potential facilitators and barriers for change. Such an analysis is not solely a desk review, but can engage with stakeholders, so as to ascertain support for more politically feasible and therefore more effective policies; and set and manage realistic expectations of what can be achieved, over what timescale, and the risks involved.

PEA can and should be done both for the health sector and at the appropriate level of government – national and subnational in a decentralized system. At the political level there is a need to understand both the role of political institutions and actors in health policy-making as well as understanding who the health policy actors are (within and outside government). At the same time, there is a need for the technical analysis of financing, organization, and regulation of the health system, and its performance in relation to access, quality, equity, efficiency, and accountability.

At the macro/national level, PEA aims to understand the political dimensions of policy development. Key questions to ask that help identify constraints, risks, and opportunities include[41]:

- What is the underlying nature of the governance regime?
- Who holds power and in whose interests is it used?
- Who has access to power and positions of political power?
- What is the nature of the political settlement and the social contract?
- How do laws reinforce and sustain equality or subordination?

More specifically, mapping should be done (by those with relevant skills) about: (1) political structures and how they function; (2) key formal and informal institutions, their relations, and the imperatives for these institutions; (3) key players and alliances who drive or oppose reform, their relations, and incentives for their actions; and (4) how do decision-making processes actually work, what drives decision-making, and what is the information base for decision-making. In addition, it is important to have a historical understanding of how political and policy processes have evolved, and how they have been informed or shaped by the social, economic, and cultural environment. Whether community trust in governance institutions and political decision-makers is gaining or waning may also be an important factor to be understood.

Following a macro-level political analysis, similar analysis needs to be done for the health sector. In relation to health reform, the core issue to understand is the relations or lack thereof between the key health and health system performance issues and the positioning of the key stakeholders. Questions should be asked about key players (including state and nonstate actors), components (such as hospitals, primary health care, and prevention activities), and key functions (such as financing, planning, and regulation) of the system. Specific questions should cover:

- Who are the key players, what are their big issues, and what is their capacity to make themselves heard?
- What are the power dynamics among these players, and what are their networks and constituents?
- Who are the main proponents and antagonists for health reform, and what are their motivations?
- What roles have they played in the recent history of health system change or proposals for change?
- What are the values and ideologies that inform their actions and views?

Beyond understanding the ecosystem of stakeholders, the institutional decision-making processes need to be well understood. It is important to map: (1) the roles and responsibilities of different agencies at central and local levels; (2) the key decision processes and timeframes for decision-making, such as budget and legislation; (3) the nature of bureaucratic politics, budget politics, and leadership politics that influence the formal institutional decision-making processes; (4) how institutions interface with beneficiaries and interest group politics; and (5) who is party to decision-making and what information base informs decisions. Again, knowledge of the history of health reform attempts is invaluable in helping to understand the positioning and behavior of various institutions.

Beyond the broad sector analysis, a further step is to analyze the political economy surrounding the specific priority issues that have prompted the health reform, be that cost and efficiency, quality of care, equity of access, supply shortages, disease outbreaks, and so on. A similar process of analysis should be used to understand the broader context – for example, mapping of the institutional and governance issues of key actors and their behaviors, the drivers that constrain or support change, and other relevant factors. It is particularly useful to understand both repeated failures to address similar reform objectives and the circumstances surrounding previous successes. Understanding the contexts for specific decisions can help reveal and differentiate the more universal drivers in decision-making from the contingent factors at a point in time.

There are a variety of PEA frameworks in use or promoted by various development assistance donors, such as the former UK Department for International Development and the World Bank. The new institutional economics thinking that underlies PEA approaches is not without its critics. Some argue PEA frameworks focus too narrowly on casting actors as rational, utility-maximizing individuals, neglecting the role of prevailing ideas or ideologies, and issues of power, agency, and coalitions [42]. Some suggest that PEA frameworks fail to systematically incorporate the impact of gender on power relations [43]. These critiques do not go to the heart of the importance of PEA, but they do suggest that no one framework is perfect and all frameworks should only be adopted as reference points.

Knowledge of how to engage with and analyze policy and political processes are equally important. Political economy dimensions are important for health reform, as reform proposals by definition mean change from the status quo – that is, reforms have: redistributive implications, impacts on money for different stakeholders and extent of government intervention, if not electoral implications. It is natural to expect that getting reforms adopted would be a challenging policy and political process. For proponents of progressive change, the key question is how to engage effectively with the political process to make sure reforms can be adopted and implemented. This requires an understanding of both the formal governance processes and the informal processes for change.

At the formal level, it is useful to use the model of the policy cycle [44], map the specific steps involved, map the stakeholders, and consider the constraints and facilitators at each stage (Figure 36.3). Appropriate strategies to address these factors can be developed for each stage of the cycle. While every political system works differently, and policy processes are typically quite messy, a policy cycle approach can help clarify the analytical tasks as well as the political engagement processes.

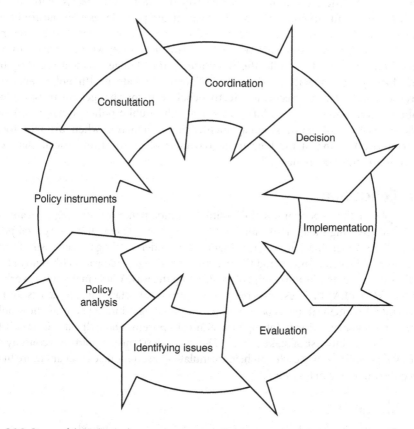

Figure 36.3 Stages of the policy cycle.

Given that policy processes are fundamentally political processes, each stage of the policy cycle will need to take account of stakeholder interests and positions (see Chapter 13). As importantly, for the reform to succeed, stakeholder engagement will be necessary. This starts with agreement about priority issues to be addressed. Different types of evidence – and how the evidence is framed and communicated – can play a very important role in bringing stakeholders to a shared understanding. A variety of forms of evidence, from diverse disciplines, will also be important for stakeholders to agree that policy analysis has been sufficiently comprehensive and robust. The selection of policy instrument will rest on strong analysis of options and potential impacts, covering distribution of costs and benefits, community acceptability, as well as implementation feasibility.

Maintaining stakeholder engagement is important through the remaining part of the policy cycle, especially in order to prevent implementation failure. Health reforms represent a complex system change. Implementation failure could occur due to many reasons and a PEA can lead to a better understanding of which actors and institutions are likely to be barriers. Reasons for implementation failure commonly include [45, 46]: insufficient budget, changed political priorities, perverse commercial incentives, stakeholder opposition, and poor planning and execution skills. While the latter aspects may be more easily addressed from a technical perspective, the former set of issues are typically related to political economy.

The global political economy is particularly relevant for L&MICs who are reliant on donor support for implementation. Because of the path-dependent nature of health system development, and the complex set of stakeholder interests in any health system, health reform is difficult. While PEA can plan a stepwise approach to a long journey, time is needed to build the foundations for change. Critical building blocks include having the capacity to generate and communicate health policy and system research (see Chapter 14); securing effective coalitions for change, ensuring leadership of policy entrepreneurs with ability to navigate the public policy system; and setting up platforms for stakeholders' engagement. These elements, when brought together with an understanding of the long-term dynamics of political and social change, can build constituents for change.

36.6 Conclusion

The interplay between economics and politics is fundamental to devising relevant health policies and ensuring their endorsement and subsequent implementation. Several political considerations underpin health reforms that require understanding the interests of multiple stakeholders. PEA helps understand the structural challenges facing a health reform process and offers measures to minimize impediments along the way. While many frameworks exist to undertake a PEA, their essence revolves around understanding the actors and their power, and the structural forces between them. In this regard understanding how political expediency influences priority setting in health is important and helps minimize obstacles arising out of the interest of stakeholders. Hence, understanding political economy at the various stages of the policy cycle can help formulate relevant policies that are more likely to succeed during implementation.

Acknowledgment

The research assistance of Bronwyn Carter is gratefully acknowledged.

References

1. V. Navarro. *Class Struggle, the State, and Medicine: An Historical and Contemporary Analysis of the Medical Sector in Great Britain.* London, Martin Robertson, 1978.

2. V. Navarro. The political economy of medical care: an explanation of the composition, nature, and functions of the present health sector of the United States. *Int J Health Serv* 1975; 5(1): 65–94.

3. M. K. Bowler, R. T. Kudrle, T. R. Marmor, et al. The political economy on national health insurance: policy analysis and political evaluation. *J Health Polit Policy Law* 1977; 2(1): 100–133.

4. E. H. Helt. Economic determinism: a model of the political economy of medical care. *Int J Health Serv* 1973; 3 (3): 475–485.

5. L. B. Russell, C. S. Burke. The political economy of federal health programs in the United States: an historical review. *Int J Health Serv* 1978; 8(1): 55–77.

6. A. C. Laurell. Three decades of neoliberalism in Mexico: the destruction of society. *Int J Health Serv* 2015; 45(2): 246–264.

7. J. Breilh. Community medicine under imperialism: a new medical police? *Int J Health Serv* 1979; 9(1): 5–24.

8. L. Doyal. *The Political Economy of Health.* London, Pluto Press, 1979.

9. B. I. Castleman. The export of hazardous factories to developing nations. *Int J Health Serv* 1979; 9(4): 569–606.

10. B. J. Berman, J. M. Lonsdale. Crises of accumulation, coercion and the colonial state: the development of the labor control system in Kenya, 1919–1929. *Can J Afr Stud* 1980; 14(1): 55–81.

11. World Health Organization. Closing the gap in a generation: health equity through action on the social determinants of health. Final Report of the Commission on Social Determinants of Health (CSDH). 2008. www.who.int/social_determinants/final_report/csdh_finalreport_2008.pdf (accessed November 19, 2021).

12. T. Marmor, C. Wendt. Conceptual frameworks for comparing healthcare politics and policy. *Health Policy* 2012; **107** (1): 11–20.

13. C. Borrell, A. Espelt, M. Rodríguez-Sanz, et al. Politics and health. *J Epidemiol Community Health* 2007; **61**(8): 658–659.

14. R. Evans. *Toward a Healthier Economics: Reflections on Ken Bassett's Problems.* New York, Wiley, 1998.

15. C. H. Tuohy. *Accidental Logics: The Dynamics of Change in the Health Care Arena in the United States, Britain, and Canada.* New York, Oxford University Press, 1999.

16. R. R. Alford. Health care politics: ideological and interest group barriers to reform. *AJN* 1976; **76**(1): 77.

17. J. M. Lewis. *Health Policy and Politics: Networks, Ideas and Power.* East Hawthorn, IP Communications, 2005.

18. V. Lin. *Evidence-Based Health Policy: Problems and Possibilities.* New York, Oxford University Press, 2003.

19. J. W. Kingdon. *Agendas, Alternatives, and Public Policies.* Boston, Little, Brown, 1984.

20. V. Tangcharoensathien, S. Wibulpholprasert, S. Nitayaramphong. Knowledge-based changes to health systems: the Thai experience in policy development. *Bull World Health Organ* 2004; **82**(10): 750–756.

21. R. G. Evans. Going for the gold: the redistributive agenda behind market-based health care reform. *J Health Polit Policy Law* 1997; **22**(2): 427–465.

22. D. B. Hipgrave, K. Hort. Dual practice by doctors working in South and East Asia: a review of its origins, scope and impact, and the options for regulation. *Health Policy Plan* 2014; **29**(6): 703–716.

23. A. Bonica, H. Rosenthal, D. J. Rothman. The political polarization of physicians in the United States: an analysis of campaign contributions to federal elections, 1991 through 2012. *JAMA Intern Med* 2014; **174** (8): 1308–1317.

24. J. Doggett. Political donations: a health sector perspective on the AEC donations data. 2021. www.croakey.org/political-donations-a-health-sector-perspective-on-the-aec-donations-data (accessed November 19, 2021).

25. J. Daley. Gridlock: removing barriers to policy reform. Grattan Institute. 2021. https://grattan.edu.au/wp-content/uploads/2021/07/Gridlock-Grattan-Report.pdf (accessed November 18, 2021).

26. P. Jones, F. Zuberi. A long way from there to here: human rights approaches to HIV/AIDS in a local setting. *HIV AIDS Policy Law Rev* 2005; **10**(1): 14–19.

27. A. L. Stangl, D. Singh, M. Windle, et al. A systematic review of selected human rights programs to improve HIV-related outcomes from 2003 to 2015: what do we know? *BMC Infect Dis* 2019; **19**(1): 209.

28. United Nations Human Rights Office of the High Commissioner. AIDS epidemic still being driven by human rights violations – UN experts warn. 2016. www.ohchr.org/EN/NewsEvents/Pages/DisplayNews.aspx?NewsID=20055&LangID=E (accessed November 19, 2021).

29. United Nations Population Fund. International conference on population and development programme of action. 2014. www.unfpa.org/publications/international-conference-population-and-development-programme-action?page=0%2C0%2C1 (accessed November 19, 2021).

30. United Nations. 25 years after population conference, women still face challenges to "well-being and human rights", says UN Chief. 2019. www.un.org/development/desa/en/news/population/25th-anniversary-of-the-international-conference-on-population-and-development.html (accessed November 17, 2021).

31. Y. Huang. China's position in negotiating the Framework Convention on Tobacco Control and the revised International Health Regulations. *Public Health* 2014; **128**(2): 161–166.

32. D. Gleeson, J. Lexchin, R. Labonté, et al. Analyzing the impact of trade and investment agreements on pharmaceutical policy: provisions, pathways and potential impacts. *Global Health* 2019; **15** (Suppl. 1): 78.

33. S. N. Kiwanuka, E. Rutebemberwa, C. Nalwadda, et al. Interventions to manage dual practice among health workers. *Cochrane Database Syst Rev* 2011; **2011**(7): CD008405.

34. K. Z. Socha, M. Bech. Physician dual practice: a review of literature. *Health Policy* 2011; **102**(1): 1–7.

35. Financial Professions Center. How a modern private hospital was created in Vietnam. 2021. www.professionsfinancieres.com/How-a-modern-private-hospital-was-created-in-Vietnam (accessed November 17, 2021).

36. L. A. Parker, G. A. Zaragoza, I. Hernández-Aguado. Promoting population health with public–private partnerships: where's the evidence? *BMC Public Health* 2019; **19**(1): 1438.

37. C. P. Yu, D. K. Whynes, T. H. Sach. Equity in health care financing: the case of Malaysia. *Int J Equity Health* 2008; **7**: 15.

38. Global Alliance for Vaccines and Immunizations. How our support works. 2021. www.gavi.org/programmes-impact/our-support#ntk (accessed November 18, 2021).

39. World Health Organization. Urgent health challenges for the next decade. 2020. www.who.int/news-room/photo-story/photo-story-detail/urgent-health-challenges-for-the-next-decade (accessed November 19, 2021).

40. P. J. Hotez, K. M. V. Narayan. Restoring vaccine diplomacy. *JAMA* 2021; **325**(23): 2337–2338.

41. Australian Government, Department of Foreign Affairs and Trade. Political economy analysis. 2016. www.dfat.gov.au/sites/default/files/political-economy-analysis-guidance-note.pdf (accessed November 11, 2021).

42. D. Hudson, A. Leftwich. From political economy to political analysis. 2014. www.dlprog.org/publications/research-papers/

from-political-economy-to-political-analysis (accessed November 18, 2021).

43. E. Browne. Gender in political economy analysis. 2014. www.gsdrc.org/docs/open/hdq1071.pdf (accessed November 15, 2021).

44. C. Althaus, P. Bridgman, G. Davis. *The Australian Policy Handbook: A Practical Guide to the Policy-Making Process*, 6th. ed. London, Routledge, 2020.

45. A. Green. *An Introduction to Health Planning for Developing Health Systems*. Cary, Oxford University Press, 2007.

46. A. Green. The challenge of local implementation in Uganda's new nutrition policy. 2020. www.devex.com/news/the-challenge-of-local-implementation-in-uganda-s-new-nutrition-policy-96648 (accessed November 17, 2021).

Chapter 37

Better Health Systems for Better Outcomes

How to Make It Happen!

Sameen Siddiqi, Awad Mataria, Katherine Rouleau, and Meesha Iqbal

37.1 Introduction

Most health professionals make use of their expertise in analyzing, researching, and advising on different aspects of health systems and their development, while only a few go on to the stage of building health systems. A thorough knowledge and understanding of the diverse elements of health systems, while necessary, is not sufficient to build a well-functioning health system that lends itself to improved performance and better health outcomes.

This book has attempted to equip its readers with knowledge about a broad range of conceptual and applied features of the health system, including its goals and objectives, its components and functions and their interconnectedness, the dimensions of demand and supply, the importance of sectoral and multisectoral approaches, and their impact on system design and performance. It has endeavored to demystify some of the complexities associated with health systems for health professionals of various backgrounds – whether practitioners, policymakers, public health academics, or students – working in or for low- and middle-income countries (L&MICs).

The purpose of this chapter is to distill and bring together key lessons presented earlier in this book, and to complement them with additional lessons needed for health systems to make a difference to the lives of the people they serve. It highlights the importance of health systems beyond traditional models and frameworks; leadership in health; the changing role of Ministries of Health in the twenty-first century; the complexities of health system reforms; integrating health security as an additional goal of the health system; measuring, monitoring, and managing health systems; and empowering communities. These are essential to *making it happen!* Each section concludes with key messages for policymakers, managers, health care providers, and professionals striving to strengthen health systems in their countries.

37.2 Health Systems: Beyond Building Blocks and Control Knobs

It is convenient and instructive to analyze health systems using the Building Blocks and/or the Control Knobs frameworks to identify challenges and gaps in health system performance. Health systems are complex, and analyzing their different functions and components has proven useful to identify the challenges that hinder the achievement of their goals and objectives. Devising policies and strategies to enhance health systems performance requires acting simultaneously on all functions and components, while accounting for socioeconomic, demographic, epidemiological, and political influences.

Health systems are organic. Their frontiers are ever-expanding, not necessarily in terms of the rigid boundaries defined, for instance, in a national health accounts analysis, but in terms of their implications for the multifaceted nature of health. The last few decades have seen an evolution in the thinking around health systems from a narrow biomedical perspective to a much broader and holistic concept of health. It stands to reason that *"Health is a state of complete physical, mental, and social well-being and not merely the absence of disease or infirmity"* [1], as stated by the constitution of the World Health Organization in 1948, which continues to be the most widely accepted definition of health today.

While the frontiers and boundaries of the health system can change, its values do not, being embedded in the principles of the primary health care (PHC) approach as defined in the Alma-Ata Declaration of 1978 [2] and reinforced by the more recent Astana Declaration of 2018 [3]. The values of equity and fairness, intersectoral coordination, and community participation have stood the test of time and are universal and self-sustaining. However, in health forums these are often put on the back burner and overtaken by politically expedient decisions. While health systems should be firmly rooted in the philosophy, values, and principles of PHC, the means for delivering good-quality services with financial protection can vary widely based on local circumstances. For instance, by establishing context-relevant models of care and executing them well, publicly financed primary care services can be provided equally well by private health care providers to achieve public health goals. The COVID-19 pandemic and its consequences have highlighted the need to reshape health systems to integrate health security as an additional goal and enhance resilience of its functions and components.

There is a lot of evidence pointing toward the interrelatedness of SDG 3 (ensure healthy lives and promote wellbeing for all at all ages) and other health-related SDGs [4, 5]. Health systems need to function beyond their traditional remit by adopting a multisectoral approach to achieving the targets of health and health-related SDGs. There are 33 health-related indicators across all the SDGs that impact health, including better education for girls, tackling child malnourishment, and ensuring access to safe water [6]. The health systems of the future will likely be organized so as to enable multisectoral governance, information systems that monitor health-relevant indicators across sectors, the implementation of a combined package of sectoral and intersectoral interventions, and the progressive integration of *Health in All Policies* (HiAP) [7].

Systems thinking, the analytic process to understand how things are connected to each other as part of a whole entity [8], is increasingly becoming the way of appraising and tackling health problems. Understanding health systems through systems thinking approaches and methods helps not only in recognizing the dynamics of disease transmission or variations in health services, but also helps in addressing the multisectoral nature of health, and in acquiring a better understanding of how intended and unintended consequences can impact health outcomes. Health system managers now and in the future need to be adept with the concepts and approaches of systems thinking for rational decision-making. In this regard, their understanding of implementation science will be necessary to accompany efforts to transform health systems by continuously devising context-relevant strategies and options.

Key Messages

- The frontiers of health systems are ever-expanding and the thinking around health systems is not confined to biomedical models, but embraces the holistic concept of health.
- The values and principles of PHC are universal and cannot be compromised in reforming health systems, yet the means for delivering needed services can vary based on local context and circumstances, calling for devising context-relevant models of care.
- Health systems now and in the future will increasingly adopt a multisectoral approach to achieve the health and health-related SDGs and targets well beyond 2030.
- Health system policymakers and managers in L&MICs, now and in the future, need to be adept with the concept and approaches of systems thinking and implementation science for rational decision-making.

37.3 Leadership for Health: Imperative for Well-Performing Health Systems

Good leadership can conjure optimal performance even in a challenging environment, while poor leadership can have disastrous consequences despite adequate resources and favorable circumstances. An effective leader has the ability to motivate their team to work toward the achievement of a common goal. They are a cardinal member of the team who has the vision and capability to make others want to engage in realizing that vision. It is no surprise that leadership and governance are one of the building blocks of the health system and are critical for ensuring well-performing health systems.

Health systems are complex, and without deliberate leadership can gravitate toward becoming inaccessible, inefficient, and unfair to the people. Health leaders should be able to successfully steer through such vicissitudes as the system goes through a reformative process. There is no dearth of literature on leadership for health and a deep exploration of this topic is beyond the scope of this chapter [9–12]; however, four attributes are considered as essential for successfully leading reforms of the health system.

First, the leader should have the vision to spearhead the development of a health system. Health reforms are medium to long term and require the leader to have a clear vision of where they would like the system to be over an extended time horizon. The vision should be underscored by the right set of values that promote equity, efficiency, and quality, but also greater participation. It is important for a leader to recognize that the vision and values for health should be well aligned with the overall vision and values of the state and its constitutional ethos, and at the same time be reinforced by a well-thought-through strategy and a roadmap for implementation. There are too many examples of the vision remaining unfulfilled and unimplemented. Indeed, there is more to leadership than just having a vision or upholding a set of values.

Second, there are many leadership styles, such as command and control or autocratic, democratic or participative, laissez-faire or delegative, and others [13]. While all leadership styles can produce results, those that promote trust, teambuilding, delegation, and a sense of achievement in the workforce are more likely to build sustainable health systems. Astute leaders often show flexibility in using different leadership styles to respond to various situations, and for getting the best out of the team and the circumstances.

Third, given the complexity of health systems, leaders should have a sound technical understanding of the issues, the sagacity to fathom the political underpinnings and implications, and the ability to recognize the interests of different stakeholder groups. A balanced approach that gives due importance to technical and political considerations and contemplates stakeholders' interests, especially those whose voices often go unheard, is likely to beget the best decision by the leader.

Fourth, too often leaders get trapped in lengthy processes or are preoccupied with self-aggrandizement and lack concern for results or outcomes for improving people's health. A committed leader should have an obsession for results and the desire to leave a legacy behind even if the opportunity presents itself for a limited duration. Building an equitable and resilient health system that extends coverage and financial protection to all, while protecting against emergencies, especially for the vulnerable and marginalized segments of the population, is a legacy that every health leader can aspire to leave.

While most consider leadership to be associated with authority or position, leadership in health is earned and not given. A community health worker who demonstrates a high level of responsibility and commitment to ensuring safe care and delivery for pregnant women in her jurisdiction is a better leader than a high-level policymaker who seems not to understand or care about the health of the population under his/her mandate. Sometimes, leaders with good intentions are looking for quick wins or "low-hanging fruit," largely because they would like to show results in the short run. Such leaders should be supported to achieve the short-term results within the context of a longer-term, evidence-informed strategy.

Finally, leadership, management, and governance are interwoven, and one is unlikely to function well without the others for improving performance of the health system. Leaders will be unable to translate their vision into actions on the ground unless they can create teams of competent managers and promote good governance. As frequently stated, a leader does the "right things," a manager does "things right" [14], and to add, good governance provides the "right environment" to do the right things.

Key Messages

- An inspirational leader has the ability to motivate their team to achieve a common goal.
- Leaders in health should:
  - have the vision and values for developing a health system;
  - promote trust, teambuilding, and delegation, and encourage team members;
  - understand technical issues and their political implications, and the interests of different stakeholders; and
  - seek to achieve measurable results and strive to leave a legacy behind.
- Leaders do the "right things," managers do "things right," and good governance provides the "right environment" to do the right things. The three are interwoven.

37.4 The Changing Role of Health Ministries in the Twenty-First Century and Post-COVID-19

As health systems and systems thinking have evolved, so has the role of Ministries of Health (MOHs), especially in L&MICs. While the stewardship and governance of the health system will remain central to the leadership role of the MOH, many of the traditional responsibilities of the MOH will give way to newer ones in the twenty-first century [15]. It will not be "business as usual" and the national MOHs and their state-level departments will need to undergo institutional reforms to keep pace with the ever-increasing demands for better health.

The MOH will increasingly move away from directly delivering health care, to adopting a more holistic approach to health. While this is not meant to undermine the importance of service delivery, there is enough evidence to demonstrate that the MOH should oversee, monitor, and regulate instead of delivering personal health services.

Concomitantly, there should be increased recognition of the importance of cost-effective population-level or nonpersonal interventions that fall within the realm of common public goods [16]. The MOH should increasingly turn attention to building its capacity in raising awareness about major public health problems among the population through advocacy, health promotion, and social marketing approaches. Informing the public about the risk of tobacco use, overcoming vaccine hesitancy against COVID-19, and the use of family planning services are some examples of essential population-level interventions. At the same time, the MOH will need to enhance their legislative and regulatory capacity in areas such as disease surveillance, monitoring water quality, or introducing taxation on unhealthy foods. These are best embodied in the essential public health functions (EPHF) and International Health Regulations (IHR) as the primary responsibility of the state for achieving public health goals nationally and globally (see Chapter 32). An approach that ensures enhanced oversight, advocacy, and regulatory capacity, and becoming increasingly responsive and accountable, requires a different skill set and competencies in the MOH.

The need for multisectoral engagement in health is well established [17–19]. Such an arrangement requires good leadership, commitment from all sectors, and efficient coordination. For instance, providing a built environment in terms of parks, walkways, and bike paths for better health would require advocacy with and coordination between the MOH and the local government. While the MOH would seem to be the natural institution to lead multisectoral engagement in health, in many L&MICs they lack the ability to do so. Hence, it requires a major cultural shift along with structural changes and newer capacities in MOH to discharge this responsibility in an effective manner.

One collaborative approach, called *Health in All Policies*, integrates and articulates health considerations into policymaking across sectors to improve the health of communities and its people [7]. It recognizes that health is created by a multitude of factors beyond health care that are often beyond the scope of traditional public health activities [7]. Five key elements of HiAP have emerged as vital to its success [20]: (1) promoting health, equity, and sustainability by incorporating these into specific policies, programs, and processes, and embedding them into government decision-making processes; (2) supporting multisectoral collaboration among partners to recognize the links between health and other policy arenas, breaking down silos and building new partnerships; (3) benefiting multiple partners by building upon the idea of "co-benefits" and "win–wins"; (4) engaging a variety of stakeholders, such as community members, policy experts, advocates, private sector representatives, and funders; and (5) creating permanent structural or procedural changes to enable agencies to better relate to each other and facilitate government decisions. Related to HiAP is the concept of whole-of-government and whole-of-society approaches to health [21], which denote public service agencies working across portfolio boundaries to achieve a shared goal and an integrated government and societal response to particular issues. Approaches can be formal and informal. They can focus on policy development, program management, and service delivery [22].

The need for building partnerships for improved population health with other government sectors, the for- and not-for-profit private sector, civil society, and academic institutions is well established and is already being implemented in many L&MICs. Three categories of partners deserve special mention.

- First, engagement with the private sector, which by definition is diverse and is critical for achieving public health goals such as UHC. The public sector needs to better understand the strengths and capabilities and the need to monitor and support the private sector for these partnerships to flourish (see Chapters 27 and 28).

- Second, the MOH has to regularly present their case to the Ministries of Finance and Planning to mobilize resources – although a tough ask as most MOHs lack the capacity to negotiate and put a strong case before the institutions that control the public purse. Learning the lingo of Ministries of Finance and Planning will be critical in making the case for health. The latter could be achieved by presenting the case for investing in health in terms of lives saved and burden of disease (in disability-adjusted life years [DALYs]) averted, cost-effectiveness and financial protection, and contribution to economic growth and development, which are much better understood by planners and financiers.

- Third, the MOH, especially in countries that rely on substantial external assistance, need the institutional capacity to negotiate and coordinate with development partners – bilateral and multilateral donors, UN agencies, and international NGOs – to minimize duplication and inefficiencies, and to maximize the effectiveness of development aid (see Chapter 35). For this to happen, the MOH require newer capacities and ways of working that demand demonstration of greater skills in leadership and coordination, communication and negotiation, monitoring and management, and building accountable and transparent public sector management.

Ministry of Health staff in most countries are a mix of public health professionals and clinicians (technocrats), career civil servants (bureaucrats), and policymakers (politicians). The balance of power and influence of each varies in different countries, and they often do not work in unison. One undesirable consequence, perhaps a legacy of the colonial era, is delayed decision-making and adherence to intricate rules and procedures, with little emphasis on results and outcomes. This requires a paradigm shift in terms of improving efficiency within the system, giving due attention to monitoring, and a renewed focus on results and outcomes.

> **Key Messages**
>
> - MOHs will continue to be the stewards of the health system and need to move away from delivering health services, as feasible, to adopting a holistic approach to health.
> - MOHs need to turn their attention to building oversight, advocacy, and regulatory capacity that require a different skill set and be increasingly accountable.
> - Leading multisectoral engagement in health requires a cultural shift along with structural and capacity changes in the MOH by adopting HiAP, a whole-of-government and whole-of-society approach to health.
> - Effective engagement with the private health sector will require MOHs to have newer capacities in leadership and coordination, communication and negotiation, trust and teambuilding, and monitoring and management.
> - MOHs require a paradigm change by shifting attention from processes to achieving outputs and attaining targets.

37.5 Unraveling the Complexities of Health System Reforms

Health system reforms (also termed health sector reforms, or HSR) are a sustained process of fundamental change in policies and institutional arrangements of the health sector, usually guided by the government [23, 24]. Many countries have undergone HSR programs over the last 30 years, designed and financed principally by the World Bank and bilateral donors. HSRs are fundamentally structural reforms such as decentralization of health services, regulation of private health care providers, restructuring of the MOHs, and financing and payment reforms. An important characteristic of HSR is the political nature of these reforms that requires a thorough understanding of the health system and the stakeholders involved. Successful HSR enhances efficiency, quality, equity, financing, and sustainability of health care. It helps in defining priorities, refining policies, and reforming institutions through which policies are implemented, thereby improving the performance of the health system and ultimately the health of the population [23].

The overarching HSR that most L&MICs are currently undergoing are reforms toward UHC. Despite UHC being an overarching target of SDG 3 and being a global commitment, there are substantial technical and political challenges in designing, monitoring, and implementing health strategies toward its realization at the level of the countries. HSR require sound institutional capacity in the MOH in areas such as health policy and system analysis, financing and costing of interventions, legislation and regulation, and contracts and grants management. These capacities are lacking in MOHs in many L&MICs. Some of these functions require being at arms-length and having a degree of independence from the decision-makers in order not to lose impartiality. Many a time when they have been too close, the responsible units in the MOH have become overly influenced by policymakers instead of providing evidence and advice to them.

Health system reforms are medium- to long-term structural reforms that often span across governments and elections. Not only do they require high-level and continued political commitment, often by successive governments, but a thorough understanding of the politics and the political economy of these reforms (see Chapter 36). These reforms can be blocked by stakeholders, who perceive them to be harmful to their interests. For instance, reforms that involve decentralization of authority and responsibility to local governments, outsourcing of health services to NGOs, or regulation of prices of medicines inevitably are resisted by groups that feel loss of power, authority, or resources. Hence, HSR should be properly "marketed" to the stakeholders, their benefits communicated to the public, and strategies identified to deal with the blockers.

Political commitment to HSR, especially UHC reforms, may be meaningless unless backed by financial commitment. While external financing by multilateral or bilateral donors may be essential in the short run for some L&MICs, in the long run the sustainability of these reforms comes into question unless there is progressive increase in reliance on domestic resources by increasing what is called the *fiscal space for health*. Domestic resources are made available both by allocating more money for health but also by minimizing wastage, abuse, and fraud in the system, thereby spending available resources more efficiently and judiciously.

Key Messages

- HSR is a sustained process of fundamental change in policies and institutional arrangements of the health system to improve performance and outcomes.
- HSR can be technically complex and political in nature, which requires a thorough understanding of their political economy.
- Reforms toward UHC are overarching HSR that require sound technical capacity along with political and financial commitment for appropriate design, monitoring, and implementation.
- HSR requires sound institutional capacity in the MOH, with a degree of independence to avoid being overly influenced by decision-makers.
- Fiscal space for HSR can be enhanced by allocating more domestic resources but also by spending available resources more efficiently and judiciously.

37.6 Resilient Health Systems and Health Security

The overarching goal of the health system, achieving UHC, is well recognized and has been addressed throughout this book. Also, as stated earlier, health systems are dynamic and it is difficult to fix their ever-expanding boundaries (see Chapter 1). One such instance has been the recurring theme of ensuring health security and establishing resilient health systems. The SARS epidemic in Southeast Asia (2002–2004) and the Ebola epidemic in West Africa (2014–2016) have been telltale signs, which with the ongoing pandemic of COVID-19 have further reinforced the claim to consider health security as an additional goal of the health system. Indeed, pandemics and other emergencies not only cost lives but pose some of the greatest risks to the global economy and global security.

It is inevitable in the future that UHC and health security are considered as complementary goals of the health system [25] (see Chapter 3). *Health security* encompasses all activities required to minimize the danger and impact of acute public health events that endanger the collective health of populations living across geographical regions and international boundaries [26]. Accordingly, health security entails preventing avoidable outbreaks, early threat detection, and responding rapidly and effectively.

Related to health security, *health system resilience* is the capacity of health actors, institutions, and populations to prepare for and effectively respond to crises; maintain core functions when a crisis hits; be informed by lessons learned during the crisis; and reorganize if conditions require [27]. Thus, health systems are resilient if they protect human life and produce good health outcomes for all during a crisis and in its aftermath. Building resilient health systems requires a shift in thinking toward [28]: (1) quality of life rather than diseases; (2) mainstreaming equity at all health system levels; (3) ensuring people-centeredness in all policies and actions; (4) integrating EPHF and common good for health as the first step in health system rebuilding; (5) strengthening intersectoral collaboration; (6) acting on and leveraging social determinants of health; all while (7) ensuring flexibility and continuous learning to facilitate correcting the course of action all along [25, 29].

Health security is a global public health issue that requires health systems to be resilient by investing in EPHF and by meeting the obligations of IHR (see Chapter 32) [30, 31]. *EPHF* have been defined as the indispensable set of actions, under the primary responsibility of the state, that are fundamental for achieving the goal of public health, which is to improve, promote, protect, and restore the health of the population through collective action. On the other hand, the purpose and scope of the *IHR* is to prevent, protect against, control, and provide a public health response to the international spread of disease in ways that are commensurate with and restricted to public health risks, and which avoid unnecessary interference with international traffic and trade [31, 32].

Building capacities in EPHF and IHR are clearly interdependent, the former responding primarily to strengthening in-country capacities while the latter meet the obligations of a binding instrument of international law. Assessing the existing status of the EPHF and IHR would be the first logical step toward building resilient health systems and enhancing health security. There is a plethora of tools available for assessing EPHF, while the Joint External Evaluation tool has been the most widely used for assessing IHR [33, 34].

A concept related to EPHF is the Common Goods for Health (CGH). These are population-based functions or interventions that require collective financing and governance and contribute to health and economic progress with a clear economic rationale based on market failures. These interventions (1) focus on public goods, which by definition are nonrival and nonexclusionary; or (2) have large social externalities [30]. The interventions that fall within the CGH include policy and coordination, taxes and subsidies, regulations and legislation, and information analysis and communication [16].

While contemporary thinking is much more developed in advancing health systems toward UHC, that for health security is catching up. Health systems of the present and the future will be looking at UHC and health security as the overarching goals. Assessment of the role and contribution of health systems toward enhancing health security, locally as well as globally, will be an integral component of health system performance assessment, and health system strengthening interventions will increasingly address both UHC and health security. Together UHC and health security when achieved will contribute to making the world fairer and safer.

Key Messages

- Pandemics and other health-related emergencies not only cost lives but pose huge risks to global economy and security. Health security and UHC are increasingly being considered as complementary goals of the health system.
- **Health security** encompasses all activities required to minimize the danger and impact of acute public health events that endanger the collective health of populations living across geographical regions and international boundaries.

- **Health system resilience** is the capacity of health actors, institutions, and populations to prepare for and effectively respond to crises, maintain core functions when a crisis hits, be informed by lessons learned during the crisis, and reorganize if the conditions require.
- Enhancing health security requires health systems to be resilient by investing in EPHF, CGH, and IHR.

37.7 Measuring, Monitoring, and Managing Health Systems: The Key to Effective Implementation

Better health systems for better outcomes demand sound measurement and regular monitoring strategies to enable decision-makers to track performance and continuously correct the course of action. The ability to monitor and evaluate health systems functions is of paramount importance to correctly implement targeted interventions and assess their desired impact. Measuring, monitoring, and evaluation are thus necessary components of managing health systems, and key for effective implementation. As Peter Drucker says, *"If you can't measure it, you can't manage it"* [35].

Evidence-based decision-making requires accurate and timely information that encompasses health status, health system inputs, processes, outputs, and outcomes, and health determinants. The purpose of health information systems (HIS) is to generate valid and reliable data that tracks health system performance and progress against identified priorities, evaluates impact of interventions, and ensures transparency and accountability. Each variable of the collected data comes at a cost, and it is thus necessary that countries select a core set of indicators, based on contextual priorities and resources.

The WHO Global List of 100 core health indicators based on four domains – health status, risk factors, service coverage, and health system – is a good reference point for countries to decide relevant indicators for national use [36]. It is imperative that once collected, data is converted into actionable information through proper analyses, tailored to the target audience, and disseminated in a timely fashion to inform decision-making. For instance, improving service provision requires data pertaining to populations' access to essential services, availability and distribution of health workers, and quality of care for informing decisions. Such data should be collected from the public and private sectors to develop contextually appropriate strategies.

Low- and middle-income countries should strengthen the national and subnational HIS by formulating a clear and comprehensive policy for beefing up health data systems in the country. It is important to develop a centralized health information infrastructure that integrates multiple independently operating HIS (see Chapters 8 and 22) to avoid fragmentation, duplication, or conflicting results. An independent, well-resourced health information agency should focus on building institutional capacity for collecting relevant data and processing it into useful information from multiple sources, including centralized HIS, demographic and health surveys, censuses, population surveillance, national health accounts, civil registration, and other sources of vital statistics. Use of new digital technologies and transition to an electronic health information system (EHIS) is inevitable in L&MICs as the available evidence confirms their effective role in improving health care with minimal financial resources [37]. However, the transition calls for caution: lack of administrative and policy support, inadequate technical capacity, and user resistance can hinder effective implementation [38].

Measuring and monitoring is critical for program implementation, and requires a holistic approach to strengthening HIS. Several areas in L&MICs will be key for reforming HIS in the future: (1) transforming "routine" health information systems to become "robust" sources of timely, valid, and reliable information that is readily available and used to inform decisions; (2) providing the necessary legal and regulatory framework to collect information on different aspects of the work of private providers, including disease surveillance; (3) strengthening the system for civil registration and vital statistics, including cause-of-death reporting at all levels of care, given its critical importance to governments in crafting policies, plans, and programs; (4) transitioning from siloed vertical to integrated HIS and progressively transitioning toward collecting information from other sectors aligned with health-related SDG goals, targets, and indicators; (5) building digital health infrastructure to transition from paper-based to electronic health records for ready access to "live" information; and (6) building institutional capacity and creating demand for implementation science and research among academics, managers, and policymakers for evidence-informed decisions (see Chapters 14 and 23).

Key Messages

- Evidence-based decision-making requires having accurate and timely information on health status, health system and services, and health determinants.
- The WHO Global List of 100 core health indicators is a good reference point for countries to select the relevant indicators for national and subnational use.
- Countries should aim for a centralized health information infrastructure that integrates multiple independently operating HIS to avoid fragmentation, duplication, or conflicting results.
- Use of digital technologies and transitioning to electronic HIS is inevitable for improved and timely access to information.
- Other priorities include upgrading routine HIS, providing a legal framework to seek information from the private health sector, strengthening civil registration and vital statistics, and building institutional capacity for implementation science.

37.8 Empowering and Giving Voice and Choice to the People: Last But Not Least

The necessary engagement of people in the prioritization, planning, and delivery of health-enabling actions and services, as individuals and communities, is at the core of the Alma-Ata Declaration [2] and the Declaration of Astana [3]. This is further evidenced in the inclusion of community engagement as one of the three components of PHC [39] and as one of the four strategic levers of the WHO PHC Operational Framework [40]. Beyond academic and political circles focused on health systems, the fact that people should be engaged as co-creators of their own health is so obvious that its mention can seem superfluous. Yet, moving beyond broad endorsement to the implementation of effective community engagement and, ultimately, to improved health outcomes requires explicit intent and purposeful action. This includes actions focused on mechanisms to "bring people into the process of engagement," on establishing conditions that cultivate effective engagement, including adequate and appropriate utilization of services, and on processes that demonstrate and monitor community engagement.

In addition, effective community engagement requires deliberate efforts to include those who are marginalized and excluded, as well as a shift from the mere provision of information to involvement in decision-making and relationship building at the institutional and individual levels. Cultivating a health workforce able to engage with the community at the macro, meso, and micro levels is essential to the full realization of PHC.

Participatory governance is a tested strategy for engaging people and has been identified as a key pathway to involve citizens in the public policy process (see Chapter 29). It is purported to enhance empowerment (intrinsic benefit) and improve accountability, increase government responsiveness, and even lead to better public services (extrinsic benefits) [41]. Within the health system, and beyond, participatory governance efforts implemented in L&MICs include public hearings, participatory budgeting, and planning and decision processes such as *assemblées sanitaires* (health assemblies) and others. While there are many examples of success, evidence about the extrinsic benefits of participatory governance is mixed and suggests that participation alone is necessary but not sufficient to result in health improvements. This is due in part to the multiple steps, diverse stakeholders, and long processes involved in moving from the prioritization of an issue to the outlining of a possible solution, the establishment of related legal frameworks, the implementation of a solution, and the generation of improved outcomes, regardless of the issue at hand. Any of these steps can be undermined by performative action devoid of true transformative potential or intent. At a minimum, then, effective participatory governance requires civil society actors to be able to engage and public officials willing to receive and include the perspective of civil society. This in turn requires a minimum level of social capital, security, and institutional capacity.

Being transparent and gaining the trust of communities are critical for people to remain engaged in shaping health services and to utilize those services appropriately, in addition to participatory governance. Trust between the public and the health system has been identified as a central determinant of health system resilience, as highlighted during the Ebola epidemic and more recently the COVID-19 pandemic [42]. A lack of transparency, consistency, and quality have been linked to a lack of trust and, in turn, to poor utilization of needed services. As in the case of participatory governance, while transparency and quality in the planning and delivery of health services is essential to cultivating trust, it is not always sufficient [42]. Furthermore, trust needs to be cultivated at the institutional and individual levels. In the former, it includes giving attention to systemic and structural sources of bias and discrimination and engaging the community in outlining solutions. This is particularly important as well as challenging for those most marginalized and excluded.

Being responsible and accountable for people's health is as important as engaging communities through participatory mechanisms and nurturing ongoing engagement through the cultivation of trust. To demonstrate effective engagement requires purposeful, rigorous, and consistent monitoring and evaluation. A number of recently developed PHC performance tools include indicators of community engagement to guide implementation and enable accountability. Examples of modes of community engagement to guide health system strengthening include mechanisms to engage communities in decision-making and the delivery of services, and health needs and assets assessment that include participatory analysis of health determinant and monitoring of health equity indicators [43].

Key Messages
• Health systems need to engage the community in planning and delivery to perform optimally and achieve the expected health outcomes.
• In addition to accurate and empowering information, effective engagement requires mechanisms to participate in decision-making and the development of trusting relationships.
• Various mechanisms of participatory governance have been used to engage communities.
• Deliberate efforts are required to include the voices and participation of those most marginalized, at risk, or left behind.
• Accountable health systems should be able to demonstrate how – and how well – they engage the communities they serve.

37.9 Conclusion

Books do not build health systems, people do! We hope that this book has helped you open the door for building health systems in places where you serve. Not everyone gets the opportunity to be a system builder, yet everyone can contribute to building health systems. For that to happen, it is essential to be a system thinker and to appropriately analyze, synthesize, interpret, and ultimately resolve the complexities of a health system. If this book has helped you acquire the necessary knowledge and skills to do so, it has served its purpose.

While the required knowledge and skills are essential, inculcating appropriate attitudes and behaviors is as important. Here are some closing thoughts as you embark on the journey to fix health systems in the real world. *Becoming a better listener* and paying attention to the views of those lower in the hierarchy may help you find the solution to the problem you are looking at. While evidence for informed decisions is essential, do not suffer from what is called *"paralysis by analysis"* – the inability to take decisions due to excessive rumination over a problem such that it defies choosing an option. *Implementation is the key.* Unless put into practice, policies and plans are only as good as the paper they are written on. Despite the risk of getting your hands dirty or fingers burned, implementation is the only way to achieve results. *Do not be afraid of failure*; at the same time, *do not throw caution to the wind* while making decisions. Be realistic in your expectations and be prepared to learn from your mistakes. Finally, a *problem-solving approach beyond problem identification is crucial to making health systems work in low- and middle-income countries!*

References

1. World Health Organization. Constitution. 2021. www.who.int/about/governance/constitution (accessed November 10, 2021).

2. World Health Organization. Declaration of Alma-Ata. 1978. https://cdn.who.int/media/docs/default-source/documents/almaata-declaration-en.pdf?sfvrsn=7b3c2167_2 (accessed December 13, 2021).

3. World Health Organization. Declaration of Astana. 2018. www.who.int/docs/default-source/primary-health/declaration/gcphc-declaration.pdf (accessed December 13, 2021).

4. W. Aftab, F. J. Siddiqui, H. Tasic, et al. Implementation of health and health-related sustainable development goals: progress, challenges and opportunities –

a systematic literature review. *BMJ Glob Health* 2020; **5**(8): e002273.

5. S. Siddiqi, W. Aftab, F. J. Siddiqui, et al. Global strategies and local implementation of health and health-related SDGs: lessons from consultation in countries across five regions. *BMJ Glob Health* 2020; **5**(9): e002859.

6. World Health Organization. SDG health and health-related targets. 2015. www .who.int/gho/publications/world_health_ statistics/2016/EN_WHS2016_Chapter6 .pdf (accessed November 10, 2021).

7. CDC. Health in All Policies. 2016. www .cdc.gov/policy/hiap/index.html (accessed November 10, 2021).

8. D. H. Peters. The application of systems thinking in health: why use systems thinking? *Health Res Policy Syst* 2014; **12**: 51.

9. C. A. Figueroa, R. Harrison, A. Chauhan, et al. Priorities and challenges for health leadership and workforce management globally: a rapid review. *BMC Health Serv Res* 2019; **19**(1): 239.

10. R. O. Ayeleke, A. Dunham, N. North, et al. The concept of leadership in the health care sector. 2018. www.intechopen.com/ chapters/60565 (accessed November 10, 2021).

11. AdventHealth University. 5 types of leadership styles in healthcare. 2020. https://online.ahu.edu/blog/leadership-styles-in-healthcare (accessed November 10, 2021).

12. G. R. Ledlow, J. H. Stephens. *Leadership for Health Professionals: Theory, Skills, and Applications.* Burlington, Jones & Bartlett Learning, 2017.

13. C. L. Giltinane. Leadership styles and theories. *Nurs Stand* 2013; **27**(41): 35–39.

14. P. F. Drucker. Quotable quotes. 2021. www .goodreads.com/quotes/18976-management-is-doing-things-right-leadership-is-doing-the-right (accessed November 10, 2021).

15. V. Sriram, K. Sheikh, A. Soucat, et al. Addressing governance challenges and capacities in ministries of health. 2020. https://hsgovcollab.org/system/files/2020-05/FINAL-WEB-3442-OMS-HSGF-WHO-WorkingPaper.pdf (accessed November 10, 2021).

16. A. Soucat. Financing common goods for health: fundamental for health, the foundation for UHC. *Health Syst Reform* 2019; **5**(4): 263–267.

17. C. Kanchanachitra, V. Tangcharoensathien, W. Patcharanarumol, et al. Multisectoral governance for health: challenges in implementing a total ban on chrysotile asbestos in Thailand. *BMJ Glob Health* 2018; **3**(Suppl. 4): e000383.

18. K. Rasanathan, S. Bennett, V. Atkins, et al. Governing multisectoral action for health in low- and middle-income countries. *PLoS Med* 2017; **14**(4): e1002285.

19. C. D. Willis, J. K. Greene, A. Abramowicz, et al. Strengthening the evidence and action on multi-sectoral partnerships in public health: an action research initiative. *Health Promot Chronic Dis Prev Can* 2016; **36**(6): 101–111.

20. Becker's Healthcare. 5 key elements of a "health in all policy" approach. 2013. www.beckershospitalreview.com/quality/ 5-key-elements-of-a-health-in-all-policies-approach.html (accessed November 10, 2021).

21. World Health Organization. Whole-of-government, whole-of-society, health in all policies, and multisectoral. 2016. www .who.int/global-coordination-mechanism/ dialogues/glossary-whole-of-govt-multisectoral.pdf (accessed November 10, 2021).

22. Australian Government. The whole of government challenge: chapter findings. 2020. https://legacy.apsc.gov.au/whole-government-challenge (accessed November 10, 2021).

23. World Health Organization. Health sector reform: issues and opportunities. 2000. https://apps.who.int/iris/bitstream/ handle/10665/127574/WP_HlthSecRefm_ Final%20Version.pdf;sequence=1 (accessed November 10, 2021).

24. P. Berman. Health sector reform: making health development sustainable. *Health Policy* 1995; **32**(1–3): 13–28.

25. World Health Organization. Building health systems resilience for universal health coverage and health security during the COVID-19 pandemic and beyond. WHO Position Paper. 2021. www .who.int/publications/i/item/WHO-UHL-PHC-SP-2021.01 (accessed January 24, 2021).

26. World Health Organization. Health security. 2022. www.who.int/health-topics/health-security/#tab=tab_1 (accessed January 24, 2022).

27. M. E. Kruk, M. Myers, S. T. Varpilah, et al. What is a resilient health system? Lessons from Ebola. *Lancet* 2015; **385**(9980): 1910–1912.

28. A. S. Masten. Ordinary magic: resilience processes in development. *Am Psychol* 2001; **56**: 227.

29. A. Mataria, R. Brennan, A. Rashidian, et al. "Health for All by All" during a pandemic: "protect everyone" and "keep the promise" of universal health coverage in the Eastern Mediterranean Region. *East Mediterr Health J* 2020; **26**(12): 1436–1439.

30. A. S. Yazbeck, A. Soucat. When both markets and governments fail health. *Health Syst Reform* 2019; **5**(4): 268–279.

31. World Health Organization. International Health Regulations (2005). 2008. www .who.int/publications/i/item/97892415804 10 (accessed January 24, 2022).

32. PAHO. Public health in the Americas: conceptual renewal, performance assessment, and bases for action. www3.paho.org/hq/index.php?option=com_content&view=article&id=4036:salud-publica-en-americas-nuevos-conceptos-analisis-desempeno-bases-para-accion&Itemid=2080&lang=en (accessed January 24, 2022).

33. World Health Organization. Assessment of essential public health functions in countries of the Eastern Mediterranean Region Assessment tool. 2017. https:// applications.emro.who.int/dsaf/EMROPub_ 2017_EN_19354.pdf?ua=1 (accessed January 24, 2022).

34. World Health Organization. Joint External Evaluation Tool, International Health Regulations (2005). 2016. https://apps .who.int/iris/bitstream/handle/10665/2043 68/9789241510172_eng.pdf (accessed January 24, 2022).

35. P. Drucker. If it cannot be measured, it cannot be managed. https://spec-india.medium.com/if-it-cannot-be-measured-it-cannot-be-managed-peter-drucker-7662da0a49dc#:~:text=Responses-,%E2%80%9CIf%20it%20cannot%20be%20measured%2C%20it%20cannot,be%20man aged%E2%80%9D%20%E2%80%94%20Peter%20Drucker.&text=Key%20Performance%20Indicators%20(KPI)%20have,isn't%20feasible%20at%20all (accessed January 21, 2022).

36. World Health Organization. 2018 Global reference list of 100 core health indicators (plus health-related SDGs). 2018. https:// apps.who.int/iris/handle/10665/259951 (accessed January 21, 2022).

37. F. Aminpour, F. Sadoughi, M. Ahamdi. Utilization of open source electronic health record around the world: a systematic review. *J Res Med Sci* 2014; **19**(1): 57–64.

38. J. M. Gesulga, A. Berjame, K. S. Moquiala, et al. Barriers to electronic health record system implementation and information systems resources: a structured review. *Procedia Computer Science* 2017; **124**: 544–551.

39. World Health Organization & United Nations Children's Fund (UNICEF). A vision for primary health care in the 21st century: towards universal health coverage and the Sustainable Development Goals. 2018. https://apps.who.int/iris/handle/106 65/328065 (accessed December 13, 2021).

40. World Health Organization. Operational framework for primary health care: transforming vision into action. 2020. www .who.int/publications/i/item/97892400178 32 (accessed December 13, 2021).

41. J. Speer. Participatory governance reform: a good strategy for increasing government responsiveness and improving public services? *World Dev* 2012; **40**(12): 2379–2398.

42. S. K. Kittelsen, V. C. Keating. Rational trust in resilient health systems. *Health Policy Plan* 2019; **34**(7): 553–557.

43. World Health Organization. *Voice, Agency, Empowerment: Handbook on Social Participation for Universal Health Coverage*. Geneva, WHO, 2021. www .uhcpartnership.net/wp-content/uploads/ 2021/08/9789240027794-eng.pdf (accessed March 10, 2022).

Index

Printed in the United States
by Baker & Taylor Publisher Services